CORPVS MEDICORVM GRAECORVM

EDIDERVNT

ACADEMIAE BEROLINENSIS HAVNIENSIS LIPSIENSIS

V 4, 1, 2

GALENI

DE PLACITIS HIPPOCRATIS ET PLATONIS

EDIDIT, IN LINGVAM ANGLICAM VERTIT, COMMENTATVS EST

PHILLIP DE LACY

LIBRI I–V

BEROLINI IN AEDIBVS ACADEMIAE SCIENTIARVM MCMLXXX

GALEN

ON THE DOCTRINES OF HIPPOCRATES AND PLATO

EDITION, TRANSLATION AND COMMENTARY

BY

PHILLIP DE LACY

FIRST PART: BOOKS I–V

SECOND EDITION

AKADEMIE-VERLAG · BERLIN 1981

Erschienen im Akademie-Verlag, DDR-1080 Berlin, Leipziger Straße 3—4

Lizenznummer: 202 · 100/244/80
Offsetdruck: VEB Druckerei „Thomas Müntzer", 5820 Bad Langensalza
Bestellnummer: 753 092 2 (2028/21/I) · LSV 0886
Printed in GDR
DDR 98,— M

VORWORT

Für die Textkonstituierung der vorliegenden Ausgabe der Galenschrift De placitis Hippocratis et Platonis wurden von ihrem Herausgeber Ph. DeLacy zum erstenmal auch der älteste griechische Textzeuge, der Hamilton. 270 aus dem 13. Jh., und die gesamte heute noch greifbare arabische Tradition dieses Werkes herangezogen. Sie stellt somit eine allen Anforderungen der modernen Textkritik genügende Edition dieses Textes dar. Ihr Wert gegenüber der letzten Ausgabe der Schrift (erschienen Leipzig 1874) wird noch dadurch erhöht, daß dem griechischen Text eine englische Übersetzung, die erste modernsprachige Übersetzung dieser Schrift überhaupt, und ein vor allem auf sachliche Probleme orientierter Kommentar beigegeben sind, die auch dem Nichtphilologen den Zugang zu diesem medizingeschichtlich wie philosophiehistorisch gleichermaßen bedeutsamen Werk ermöglichen.

Mit dem Erscheinen dieser Edition wird einem seit langem bestehenden Desiderat der internationalen Forschung entsprochen, da Galens Schrift Über die Lehrmeinungen des Hippokrates und des Platon einer der vielseitigsten Texte des Corpus Galenicum ist, der Interesse bei den Vertretern verschiedenster Fachrichtungen für sich beanspruchen darf. Ausgehend von den physiologischen Lehren des Arztes Hippokrates und des Philosophen Platon, die für Galen jeweils auf ihrem Gebiet die unübertroffenen Autoritäten darstellten, entwickelt der Pergamener in diesem Werk in kritischer Auseinandersetzung mit den Theorien seiner unmittelbareren Vorgänger sowohl in der Medizin wie in der Philosophie seine eigenen Lehren auf dem Felde der Physiologie. Die Hauptthemen bilden die Lehren vom Ursprung der Blutgefäße und Nerven, von den drei Seelenteilen und den mit ihnen verbundenen geistigen und physischen Prinzipien im menschlichen Körper sowie die Sinnesphysiologie, speziell die Lehre vom Sehen.

Entsprechend der skizzierten Anlage der Schrift finden wir in ihr einen nahezu lückenlosen Überblick über die Behandlung der genannten Themen in der Antike vom 5. Jh. v. u. Z. bis ins 2. Jh. u. Z. und eine Fülle von wörtlichen Zitaten aus sonst verlorenen Werken, vor allem stoischer Provenienz. Ihre besondere Bedeutung erlangt sie jedoch dadurch, daß sie wie kaum ein anderer medizinischer Text deutlich macht, wie eng Medizin und Philosophie im Altertum miteinander verbunden waren und wie außerordentlich fruchtbar sich diese Verbindung auf die Entwicklung medizinischer Theorien in der Antike ausgewirkt hat.

Die Redaktion
des Corpus Medicorum Graecorum
Jutta Kollesch

CONTENTS

ABBREVIATED REFERENCES

AJP = American Journal of Philology

Anon. Lond. = H. Diels, Anonymi Londinensis ex Aristotelis Iatricis Menoniis et aliis Medicis Eclogae. Supplementum Aristotelicum III, 1. Berlin, 1893 (The Greek text was reprinted, with English translation and notes, in W. H. S. Jones, The Medical Writings of Anonymus Londinensis, Cambridge, 1947.)

Bake, 1810 = J. Bake, Posidonii Rhodii Reliquiae Doctrinae. Leiden, 1810

Bardong, 1942 = K. Bardong, Beiträge zur Hippokrates- und Galenforschung, Nachrichten von der Akademie der Wissenschaften in Göttingen. Phil.-hist. Kl., 1942, pp. 577–640

Baumgarten, 1962 = H. Baumgarten, Galen Über die Stimme. Diss. Göttingen, 1962

CAH = Cambridge Ancient History

CMG = Corpus Medicorum Graecorum

Cobet, 1882 = C. G. Cobet, Ad Galenum, Mnemosyne N. S. 10 (1882), pp. 178–192

Daremberg, Thèse = C.-V. Daremberg, Exposition des connaissances de Galien sur l'anatomie, la physiologie et la pathologie du système nerveux. Paris, 1841

Diels, 1875 = H. Diels, Jenaer Literaturzeitung, 1875, no. 9, pp. 154–155 (Rev. of Müller's edition of PHP)

Diels, 1894 = H. Diels, GGA 1894, pp. 293–307 (Rev. of Kaibel, Stil und Text der Πολιτεία Ἀθηναίων)

Diels, 1905 = H. Diels, Die Handschriften der antiken Ärzte, I. Abh. Berlin, 1905, No. 3

Diels, 1907 = H. Diels, Erster Nachtrag zu den ... Katalogen. Abh. Berlin, 1907, No. 2

D.-K. = H. Diels and W. Kranz, Die Fragmente der Vorsokratiker. 6th edition. 3 vols. Berlin, 1951–1952

Domański, 1900 = B. Domański, Die Psychologie des Nemesius (Beiträge zur Geschichte der Philos. des Mittelalters III 1), Münster, 1900

Durling, 1961 = R. J. Durling, A Chronological Census of Renaissance Editions and Translations of Galen, Journal of the Warburg and Courtauld Institutes, 24 (1961), pp. 230–305

Edelstein, 1936 = L. Edelstein, The Philosophical System of Posidonius, AJP 57 (1936), pp. 286–325

Edelstein-Kidd = L. Edelstein and I. G. Kidd, Posidonius, Vol. I: The Fragments. Cambridge, 1972

Gal. Anat. = Galen, De anatomicis administrationibus (References to the Greek text of Books I to IX. 5 are identified by volume and page of Kühn's edition. For the rest, preserved only in Arabic, reference is made to the German translation of M. Simon [Vol. II of his edition, Leipzig, 1906]. The chapter divisions of Books IX to XV, introduced into the English translation of these books by W. L. H. Duckworth, M. C. Lyons, and B. Towers [Galen On Anatomical Procedures, the Later Books, Cambridge, 1962], have also been given.)

Gal. UP = Galen, De usu partium corporis humani (Passages are identified by volume and page of Kühn. Reference is made in some instances to the edition of G. Helmreich [2 vols., Leipzig, 1907–1909] and to the English translation

of Margaret T. May [Galen On the Usefulness of the Parts of the Body, 2 vols., Ithaca, New York, 1968].)
GGA = Göttingische Gelehrte Anzeigen
Haas, 1907 = A. E. Haas, Antike Lichttheorien, Archiv f. Geschichte d. Philosophie 20 (N. F. 13) (1907), pp. 345–386
Harris, 1973 = C. R. S. Harris, The Heart and the Vascular System in Ancient Greek Medicine from Alcmaeon to Galen. Oxford, 1973
Herbst, 1911 = W. Herbst, Galeni Pergameni de Atticissantium Studiis Testimonia. Diss. Leipzig, 1911
Hirzel, Unters. = R. Hirzel, Untersuchungen zu Ciceros philosophischen Schriften. 3 vols. Leipzig, 1877–1883
Ḥunain, Questions = Le livre des questions sur l'œil de Ḥonaïn ibn Isḥāq, ed. P. Sbath and M. Meyerhof, Mémoires présentés à l'Institut d'Égypte, Cairo, 1938, vol. XXXVI
Ḥunain, Ten Treatises = The book of the Ten Treatises on the Eye Ascribed to Hunain Ibn Is-hâq (809–877 A. D.), ed. M. Meyerhof, Cairo, 1928
Ilberg, RM 1889 = J. Ilberg, Über die Schriftstellerei des Klaudios Galenos I, RM 44 (1889), 207–239
Ilberg, BPW 1889 = J. Ilberg, BPW 9 (1889), cols. 1261–1264 (Rev. of Petersen, Diss.)
Ilberg, 1905 = J. Ilberg, Aus Galens Praxis, Neue Jahrbücher 15 (1905), pp. 276–312
Jaeger, Nemesios = W. Jaeger, Nemesios von Emesa. Berlin, 1914
Joly, 1970 = Hippocrate, De la nature de l'enfant, ed. R. Joly, in: Hippocrate, XI, Collection Budé, Paris, 1970, pp. 53–83
Joly, 1972 = Hippocrate, De l'aliment, ed. R. Joly, in: Hippocrate, VI, 2, Collection Budé, Paris, 1972, pp. 140–147
K. = Claudii Galeni Opera Omnia, ed. C. G. Kühn. 20 volumes. Leipzig, 1821–1833 (Reprinted, with a bibliographical supplement by K. Schubring [vol. XX, pp. V–LXII], Hildesheim, 1965. References are to volume and page.)
Kalbfleisch, 1892 = C. Kalbfleisch, In Galeni De Placitis Hippocratis et Platonis Libros Observationes Criticae. Diss. Berlin, 1892
L. = E. Littré, Œuvres complètes d'Hippocrate. 10 volumes. Paris, 1839–1861 (Reprinted Amsterdam, 1961–1962. References are to volume and page.)
LSJ = Liddell-Scott-Jones-McKenzie, A Greek-English Lexicon
Mugler, 1964 = C. Mugler, Dictionnaire historique de la terminologie optique des Grecs. Paris, 1964
Müller, 1871 = I. Müller, Quaestiones Criticae de Galeni Libris περὶ τῶν καθ' Ἱπποκράτην καὶ Πλάτωνα δογμάτων. Progr. Erlangen, 1871
Müller, 1874 = Claudii Galeni De Placitis Hippocratis et Platonis Libri Novem recensuit et explanavit Iwanus Mueller. Vol. I. Prolegomena critica, textum Graecum, adnotationem criticam versionemque Latinam continens. Leipzig, 1874
Müller, Beweis = I. Müller, Über Galens Werk vom wissenschaftlichen Beweis. Abh. Bayer. Akad. 1895, No. 2
Nauck = A. Nauck, Tragicorum Graecorum Fragmenta. 2nd edition, 1889 (Reprinted, with supplement by B. Snell, Hildesheim, 1964.)
Nock, 1959 = A. D. Nock, Posidonius, Journal of Roman Studies 49 (1959), pp. 1–16
Petersen, 1888 = J. Petersen, In Galeni De Placitis Hippocratis et Platonis Libros Quaestiones Criticae. Diss. Göttingen, 1888
PHP = Galen, De Placitis Hippocratis et Platonis
PIR = Prosopographia Imperii Romani
[Plut.], Hom. = Ps.-Plutarch, De vita et poesi Homeri, Plutarchi Moralia, ed. Bernardakis, vol. VII, pp. 329–462
Pohlenz, 1898 = M. Pohlenz, De Posidonii libris περὶ παθῶν, Jahrb. für class. Philol. Supplbd. 24 (1898), pp. 535–634
Pohlenz, 1906 = M. Pohlenz, Das dritte und vierte Buch der Tusculanen, Hermes 41 (1906), 321–355

Pohlenz, 1921 = M. Pohlenz, Poseidonios' Affektenlehre und Psychologie, Nachr. von der k. Gesellschaft der Wissenschaften zu Göttingen. Philol.-Hist. Kl. 1921, pp. 163–194

Pohlenz, 1926 = M. Pohlenz, GGA 1926, pp. 273–306 (Rev. of Reinhardt, Kosmos und Sympathie)

Pohlenz, Die Stoa = M. Pohlenz, Die Stoa. Geschichte einer geistigen Bewegung. 2 vols. Göttingen, 1948. Nachträge, 1955

RE = Pauly-Wissowa, Real-Encyclopädie der classischen Altertumswissenschaft

REG = Revue des Etudes Grecques

Reinhardt, 1921 = K. Reinhardt, Poseidonios. Munich, 1921

Reinhardt, 1953 = K. Reinhardt, Poseidonios. RE 22 (1953), cols. 558–826

Rhazes, al-Ḥāwī = Rhazes, *Kitābu l-Ḥāwī fi ṭ-ṭibb*, Vols. I–XX, ed. Hyderabad-Deccan, 1955–1967

RM = Rheinisches Museum für Philologie

Scr. min. = Galenus, Scripta Minora. 3 volumes, edited by I. Marquardt, I. Müller, and G. Helmreich. Leipzig, 1884–1893 (Reprinted Amsterdam, 1967.)

Siegel, 1968 = R. Siegel, Galen's System of Physiology and Medicine. Basel, 1968

Siegel, 1970 = R. Siegel, Galen on Sense Perception. Basel, 1970

Solmsen, 1961 = F. Solmsen, Greek Philosophy and the Discovery of the Nerves, Museum Helveticum 18 (1961), pp. 150–167, 169–197

Steckerl = F. Steckerl, The Fragments of Praxagoras of Cos and his School. Leiden, 1958

SVF = H. von Arnim, Stoicorum Veterum Fragmenta. 4 volumes. Leipzig, 1905–1924 (References are to volume and page, unless otherwise indicated.)

TAPA = Transactions and Proceedings of the American Philological Association

TGF = see Nauck

Verbeke, Pneuma = G. Verbeke, L'évolution de la doctrine du pneuma du stoicisme à S. Augustin. Paris and Louvain, 1945

Vogt, 1910 = S. Vogt, De Galeni in libellum κατ' ἰητρεῖον commentariis. Diss. Marburg, 1910

Walzer, 1962 = R. Walzer, Greek Into Arabic. Cambridge, Mass., 1962

Wellmann, 1885 = E. Wellmann, Codex Hamilton 329 (Galenos), RM 40 (1885), 30–37

INTRODUCTION

I. The sources for the text

A. Manuscripts, editions, emendations

1. Manuscript Hamilton 270

Hamilton 270 (401 in the catalogue of the Greek manuscripts in the
H Berlin Collection) (=H): see Die Handschriften-Verzeichnisse der Königlichen Bibliothek zu Berlin. Vol. XI: Verzeichnis der gr. Handschriften, II, ed. C. De Boor (Berlin, 1897), pp. 231f. Described by De Boor, who dates it in the 13th century. (Wellmann, 1885, p. 30, assigned it to the 15th, Petersen, 1888, pp. 11f., to the 14th–15th.) It was identified by De Boor as the manuscript formerly in the Convent of S. Michele, near Venice; see Diels, 1905, p. 74. Müller knew of its existence but failed to locate it; see his introduction, p. 15. It was discovered and first described by Wellmann.

The manuscript has suffered losses and other damage. 128 folios are extant, containing the text from 130.20 to *806.14*[1], with the exception of 234.18–238.20 (one lost folio), 258.27–266.10 (two lost folios), and *769.7–780.4* (two lost folios). The order of the folios has been disturbed; Wellmann reestablished the correct sequence as 14–21, 13, 1–4, 22, 11, 31–36, 12, 23–30, 5–10, 37–114, 121–122, 115–120, 123–128. After 30, one folio is lost; after 10, two folios are lost; and after 120, two folios are lost.

Ms. H was made up of ternions and quaternions, which were numbered. The first extant gathering, a quaternion (fol. 14–21), was originally the fifth. The sixth was a ternion (fol. 13, 1–4, 22); the seventh and eighth were quaternions (fol. 11, 31–36, 12; 23–30). The ninth was a quaternion whose first and last folios have been lost; the six remaining are fol. 5–10. The tenth lacks the first folio only; the seven that survive are fol. 37–43. The next eight quaternions (11–18) are complete and in order: fol. 44–107. The 19th gathering is also a complete quaternion (fol. 108–114, 121). The 20th was a quaternion containing fol. 122, 115–120, and a final folio now lost. The 21st began with a folio now lost, continued with 123–128, and concluded with a folio now lost. This gathering would then have ended approximately at the top of p. *811*, and the remainder of Book IX (pp. *811–827*) would have required four additional folios.[2]

[1] Numbers in italics refer to Books VI–IX in I. Müller's edition, which are to be published in CMG V 4.1.3.

[2] Fol. 127 contains 71 lines in Müller's text; fol. 128 contains 63 lines. From the end of fol. 128 to the end of Book IX there are 315 lines, equivalent to five folios of 63 lines each. The final folio, of course, may have been only partly filled.

The four lost gatherings at the beginning of the work could easily have contained the whole of Book I and the beginning of Book II. Indeed the portion of Book II now lost in H (pp. 102–130.20) is close to the average length of a quaternion.[1] Another quaternion (the third gathering) would easily contain the portion of Book I preserved by Ms. C (pp. 72.28–100.7). The two initial gatherings could have contained the rest of Book I; if both were quaternions, the first book must have been rather long, even longer than the ninth. On this hypothesis the entire work originally occupied 22 gatherings, of which the sixth was a ternion, the 22nd a binion or partial ternion or quaternion. One of the first four may also have been a ternion. The remainder were quaternions.[2]

The gatherings were numbered while H was still intact. By the time that M or its parent and the parent of Ald. were copied from it, it had lost Book I, but the remainder was still in order. Many folios had been damaged, however, and in the interval between the copying of the parent of Ald. and the copying of M or its parent some of the damaged letters had been retraced.[3] Subsequently the manuscript disintegrated. Several folios were lost, and the remainder ere reassembled in their present arrangement. Holes appeared in the two folios that had now become the first and the last (1 and 128)[4], and the folios of the eighth quaternion (23–30, containing pages 204.30 –234.18) lost an upper corner. The damage of this last period may be repaired from M and Ald., which derive from an earlier stage.

Ms. H is the source also of two sets of excerpts, one set preserved in Par. Suppl. Gr. 634 (Q) and Borbon. Gr. 229 III D 15 (N), the other in Par. 2283 (p). As neither set contains excerpts from Book I, we may assume that they postdate the loss of that book. See below, pp. 24–26; 29–30.

The manuscript from which H was copied contained variants, some of which appear in H as superscriptions by the first hand; see for example[5]:

1 Most of the preserved quaternions contain between 34 and 37 pages of Müller's text. The shortest contains 30 pages, the longest, 42.

2 Wellmann, 1885, p. 31, supposed that the first three quaternions would be too great for Book I; in his view, Book I would require no more than 16–20 folios, whereas 26 or 27 must be accounted for. He calculated the length of a book at 1,200 to 1,500 lines in Müller's text, and he calculated further that 1,500 lines would fill not more than 20 folios. My calculations are somewhat different. The first 1,164 lines of Book IX occupied 16.5 folios in H, or 70.5 lines per folio; the whole book (1,486 lines), therefore, would have required slightly over 21 folios. Furthermore, Wellmann failed to notice that one of the gatherings of Book II is a ternion; his estimate of folios to be accounted for must accordingly be reduced by two.

3 See below, p. 17.

4 See for example 156.31–32; 158.22; *803.13–14*; *804.16*.

5 For other examples see 150.30; 228.20; 254.33; 280.9; 284.18; 288.30; 350.5; *498.7*; *582.9*; *632.1*; *730.4*; *735.5*. For variants that go back to the common ancestor of H CL see below, pp. 33–34.

342.7 ἀνθέλκειν M (e corr.) R Ald.: ἀνθέλκων ML: ἀνθέλκ̃// H

342.8 στασιάζειν MR Ald.: στασιάζων L: στασιάζ̃// H

350.3 παρὰ MR Ald. L: $\overset{ἐ}{π}$αρὰ (i. e. περὶ or παρὰ) H

690.12 ταὐτὰ Ald.: ταῦτα MR: ταῦ̓τὰ (i. e. ταῦτα or ταὐτὰ) H

Sometimes the variants are side by side:

156.33 μὲν L: μόνον μὲν H MR: μόνον $H^{3?}$ Ald.

544.6 πρώτῳ Ald.: προτέρω πρώτω H MR

744.16 ἕλοιντο νίκην ὀλυμπιονίκην H MR Ald.: [ἕλοιντο νίκην] 'Ολυμπιονίκης Einarson

At 234.17 the variant is in the margin: δὲ H (in textu) Ald.: τε H in mg.: τε δὲ MR.

Several doublets in H can be inferred (where H is lost) from the readings of M and Ald., though here of course the variant could be the work of a corrector of H:

114.1 τροπικῶν C: τροπικῶν τριῶν MR Ald.

120.24 τὴν φάρυγγα C: τὴν τραχη (τραχῆ R) ἀρτηρίαν τὴν φάρυγγα M: τὴν τραχεῖαν ἀρτηρίαν τὸν φάρυγγα Ald.

264.14 ἐπειδάν Ald.: ἐπεὶ δὴ δάν M: ἐπειδὴ δ' ἄν R

264.15 νομίζῃ Kühn: νομίζοι M (super lin.) Ald.: νομίζειν M (in textu) R

774.4 δεῖ Cornarius: ἀεὶ δὴ MR Ald.

820.10 τι Cornarius: τοι τι MR Ald.: τοιοῦτον R[2]

The presence of double readings in the source of H points to editorial activity.[1] An editor's hand may be detected also in passages where the inherited text was thought to be faulty and an attempt was made at emendation:

250.21 διαλεχθέντα scripsi: διελέχθη H MR Ald.: διαλεχθῇ C

741.8 δύναται Cornarius: δύναται εἶναι H MR Ald.

At several points the scribe of H left blanks, presumably because he could not read the text before him. Two of these blanks were
H^s filled in by a different hand (H^s): 164.29 ὁμολογοῦμεν – 166.3 τρέφον, and 168.17 ἕτερα – 170.12 ἀρτηρίαν. In the former passage the supplement does not fill the space provided; in the latter, it runs over a bit. Thus it is evident that the supplements postdate the initial copying. The source of H^s in these passages is unknown. Its peculiarities include $\overset{ε}{π}$ for πε (not περι) and $\overset{''}{π}$ for περι (not παρα); for the latter see the critical notes to 170.6 and 8.

A short lacuna at 224.12 (6 letters) was filled by $H^{2?}$ with a ten-letter word (θεογονίαις). Other blanks have not been filled. At 166.10

[1] Cf. also 144.22 γενήσεται H^3 L: γε κινήσεται H Ald.: κινήσεται MR. The parent of H probably had γε superscribed as a correction over κι.

is a space for 150 letters, in which a later hand, probably H^{s}, has mistakenly written οὐ λείπ(ει). At 356.12 there is a lacuna of six or seven letters. At 128.29–30, where H is missing, both M and Ald. omit 21 words but leave a blank of only 5–7 letters; here M has written λείπει in the margin. Were it not for the lacuna, the omission would be explicable simply as a leap of the eye from one pair of words to an almost identical pair (see the critical note ad loc.).

Two passages were written by hands other than that of the principal scribe: folios 84^{v} and 85^{r} (*594.6* οὐχ ἕτερόν to *598.6* τριπλοῦν), and 125^{r} (*790.5* μηδὲ τὸ πτύαλον to *791.15* ὡς ἐν ὅλῳ). These hands are not the same, and both are different from H^{s}. De Boor, p. 231, supposed that these passages represent pages that were inadvertently passed over by the principal scribe and subsequently supplied; but as there is no evidence of crowding or expanding the lines to fill the spaces (each passage is an exact fit), it is more probable that at these points the principal scribe received temporary relief.

Ms. H makes extensive use of abbreviations, often omitting terminations or flexional endings.[1] Its source may have done the same. Some of the errors in H could have arisen from the misinterpretation of abbreviations, for example:

258.5 ὀρϑότατα Ald.: ὀρϑότητα H MR
718.14 δυομένου R^{2} Cornarius: δυομένον H MR Ald.
798.2 φιλοσόφοις R Ald.: φιλοσόφα H M

There are some intrusive words in H that may best be explained as derived from scholia in the parent manuscript: καϑόλου at 130.30, ἀληϑῶς at 302.35, and τὸ στοιχεῖον at *665.17*.

At 104.22 a gloss has dislodged the correct reading: μοχϑηρῶς C: ψευδῶς M Ald. (see Kalbfleisch, 1892, pp. 11–12).

Possibly the summary that appears in MR and C at the beginning of Book II was also present in H and its source; see below, p. 35.

H was carefully corrected by the first hand and again by a second hand (H^{2}). The second hand also added marginalia, as at 132.17: H^{2}

[1] Abbreviations in H were often misinterpreted by the copyists; for example, at *687.2–3* H reads πικρο$^{\tau\tau}$′, ὀξυ$^{\tau\tau}$′. In M and R this becomes πικροτάτης, ὀξύτητος, and in the Aldine, πικρότητος, ὀξύτατον. Cornarius restored the correct reading from Plato. Other examples include

300.8–9 συνωνυ$^{\mu}$′ H: συνωνυμίας Ald.: συνωνυμία M
692.1 ἱππο$^{\kappa\rho\tau'}$ H: ἱπποκράτην R: ἱπποκράτους M Ald.
717.8 χειμ^{ῶ} καὶ ϑ$^{ερ'}$ H: χειμῶνος καὶ ϑέρεος R Cornarius (χ. καὶ ϑέρους M): χειμῶνα καὶ ϑέρος Ald.
718.13 πάλ$^{\ddot{x}}$ (=πάλιν) H: πάχιον MR Ald. (the first leg of the apex was taken with the λ to form χ, the second leg was read as ον, and the two dots supplied the ι).

See also below, p. 22.

ὅτι ὁ ζήνων ἀρχηγ(έτης) ἐστὶ τῆς τῶν στωϊκῶν αἱρέσεως.[1] Corrections H³ not easily assignable to either H or H² have been designated H³. The corrections of H and H² are remarkably good; their source appears to be, for the most part, an authentic manuscript tradition rather than editorial ingenuity. The first hand probably corrected his own errors by reference back to his original; the source of H² and H³ is unknown. In rare instances the reading of H is preferred to the correction of the first hand:

244.39 ὁρμῶν H R Ald.: ὅρμον corr. H: ὅρμων MR (e corr.)
252.14 αὔτὸν H: αὐτὸν H (e corr.) MR Ald. C
736.11 ἀλλήλων H: ἀλλήλοις H (e corr.) Ald. (MR desunt)
793.16 λεγόμενα H: λελεγμένα H (e corr.) MR Ald.

The correction of H in this last instance appears to be an editorial attempt to make sense of a corrupt passage;[2] the others probably reflect ambiguities in the parent manuscript. H² is sometimes inferior to H; see 224.26; *507.11*, and

144.13 ἀπō προθέσεως H: θέσεως H² MR Ald.: προθέσεως L
286.18 ἐπιφέρει H MR Ald.: ἐπιφέρῃ H²
496.11 ἀγυμνασίας H Ald. L: ἀγυμναστίας H² MR

Such errors suggest that H² misread his source. Elsewhere he appears to have emended to the sense, e. g. 138.35 ἥπερ H² p: εἴπερ H MR Ald. L.

There is no clear evidence that any of the correctors of H attempted to remove errors in the quotations from Homer, Hippocrates or Plato by consulting manuscripts of those authors. An ambiguous case is *698.15* αἰδοίων καὶ ἵδρωα (ἴδρωα Ald.) H² Ald.: καὶ αἰδοίων ἱδρώσεις H: καὶ αἰδοίων ἵδρωα MR. H² might have got his correction from a text of Hippocrates or from Galen's commentary on the Aphorisms; but it is also possible that the variants were in the ms. of PHP that was available to him. Another ambiguous case is the correction of ἅμα to ἅμμα in the quotations of Timaeus 70 b 1. At 174.11 the correction is made by H², at *575.9* by H; at *569.1* the error remains uncorrected.

The corrections of H, H² and H³ were made before M and the parent of the Aldine were copied, but one or the other copy sometimes adopted the original reading of H rather than the correction. Thus M has the older reading at

164.8 ὅθεν H³ Ald. L: ὅταν H MR
270.25 ἔτι H (e corr.) Ald.: ἔστι H MR

[1] The same note appears in R; one would infer that it was also in M, but it cannot be seen on the photostat of M available to me. H³ also added marginalia.

[2] The correction of H was more successful at 146.2: ἠρωτημένον H (e corr.) MR Ald.: ἐρωτημένον H: ἐρωτώμενον L. At 196.31 the reading in H κεκοσμεῖσθαι points to a lost variant κοσμεῖσθαι.

685.16 πομφόλυγες H (e corr.) Ald.: -γγ- H MR (H made the correction currente calamo)
803.1 αὐτῆς H (e corr.) Ald.: αὐτοῖς H MR

The Aldine has the older reading at 244.39 (quoted above, p. 16); 186.20 (below, p. 34), and

288.9 ὀρεκτῶν MR: ὀρεκτικῶν H Ald.: ὀρεκῶν (sic) $H^{3?}$
662.5 διηνέχθη H (e corr.) MR: διηνέχθην H Ald.

The majority of these readings testify to the editorial superiority of the Aldine over M. On occasion, however, both M and Ald. retain an inferior reading of H; see 138.35 (above, p. 16), 144.22 (p. 14, n. 1), and

220.17 καὶ διανοεῖσθαι H^2: καρδίαν νοεῖσθαι H: καὶ καρδίαν νοεῖσθαι MR Ald.
714.5 φησὶ e corr. H: φημὶ H MR Ald.
726.6 διαιωρούμενον e corr. H (ω super lin.): διαιρούμενον H MR Ald.

They retain the inferior reading of H^2 at 224.26: δὴ ῥὰ H: δ' ἦρα H^2 MR Ald.

Examples of errors introduced by the retracer (H^r; see above, p. 13) and adopted by M include: H^r

674.14 οὕτως H Ald.: ὄντως H^r MR
734.8 φύσιν H Ald.: φησὶν H^r MR

The presence of these readings in M and their absence in Ald. suggest that the parent of Ald. was copied from H before the retracing was done; see Petersen, 1888, p. 14. There are retracings also at *718.1–6*.

Where H is damaged, the Aldine sometimes preserves words that M omits, and sometimes M has the more complete text. For example, at 348.25 the words from οὔτ' ἐμνήσθη to ἀντειπεῖν are barely legible in H; the Aldine has them, but M shows a lacuna of 15 letters followed by πεῖν. In the next line, both M and Ald. leave a blank for the words μακρῶν, μᾶλλον, but M has the following δέ, whereas the Aldine does not. At 350.28, M has a lacuna of 30 letters in place of the words διακαιομένων ἐπιθυμούντων τε πόματος. In H the word ἐπιθυμούντων is completely gone, but the rest can be made out (ἐπιθυμούντων is attested by L, which has the passage undamaged). The Aldine contains a lacuna and two misreadings: συγκαιομένων + lacuna of 14 letters + περὶ πόματος. At *726.15* H is again damaged; one can make out ὑπολαβ. ⁚ . . The Aldine got it right: ὑπολαβεῖν, but M erred: ὑπολάβοι, which R altered to ὑπολάβοιτο. Cf. also

108.17 τῷ ζητουμένῳ Ald. C: lac. 10 litt. M (H deest)
134.18 οὐδὲν H Ald. L: οὐ χρὴ M: οὐ χρῆ R (the letters δεν are indistinct in H).

Some crude interlineations in H at 178.20 may be subsequent to the copying of M.

H is the source of MR Ald. QN FP p.

2. Manuscript Marcianus 284

M Marcianus 284 (= M): see A. M. Zanetti and A. Bongiovanni, Graeca D. Marci Bibliotheca codicum manuscriptorum per titulos digesta, p. 136. A fifteenth century manuscript that once belonged to Bessarion. See Müller's discussion of it in Quaest. Crit., 1871, pp. 5–7, and on pp. 70–72 of his edition. Müller collated it.

M contains on folios 12–83 Books II through IX of PHP. Its descent from H was established by Wellmann, 1885, p. 34, and further confirmed by Petersen, 1888, p. 13. At one point the scribe of M turned two pages at once, thus omitting folios 117ᵛ and 118ʳ of H (*753.1–757.15*). Wellmann was probably right when he said that H is "die unmittelbare Vorlage von M", as some of the errors in M are best explained on the assumption that the scribe was actually looking at H. For example, at *713.13* H has a correction: the first hand wrote ἐξομόργ then corrected γ to ξ and added the ending -εως. The scribe of M first wrote ἐξομόσεως (the letter ξ superimposed on γ in H gives the illusion of a sigma, with curlicues below and above); then he noticed that he had skipped the rho and added it as a superscription above the omicron. The Aldine here is with the correction of H: ἐξομόρξεως; R, as usual, follows M: ἐξομόρσεως.

M's departures from H sometimes agree with the Aldine or with L. The former will be discussed below, pp. 22–23, the latter are probably mere coincidence:

152.33 λυπῶν H Ald.: λοιπῶν MR L
154.8 λοιπὸν H Ald. L (e corr.): λοιπῶν MR L
172.15 ζητήσομεν H Ald.: ζητήσωμεν MR L
176.4 αὐτὸν τῶν H Ald.: αὐτῶν τῶν MR L

In general, M is useful only for those passages where H is no longer extant (see above, p. 12) or has suffered damage subsequent to the copying of M (see above, p. 13). Most of the departures of M from H are the result of carelessness; on rare occasions M has the better reading, for example at 278.35: δ' ἐτυγχάνομεν M: δὲ τυγχάνομεν H R Ald. The manuscript contains corrections by the first hand M² and at least one subsequent hand (M²). For examples of corrections of M see below, p. 19 (*689.13*; *715.2*), and for M², pp. 19 (246.13–14) and 21 (118.17), and the critical notes to 120.31–33.

Müller reports (1871, pp. 5–6; 1874, p. 71) that M contains marginalia in red as well as in black. The marginalia in red are barely visible in the photostats available to me; but it is worth noting that the majority of those identified by Müller as red are present also in R, and in H where H is extant. Examples are

134.5 οὐχ ὑπὸ τοῦ ἐγκεφάλου φησὶν ὁ γαληνὸς ἐκπέμπεσθαι· ἀλλ' ὑπὸ τῆς ἐν τῶ ἐγκεφάλω κατ' αὐτὸν οὔσης αἰσθητικῆς καὶ λογικῆς ψυχῆς H^3 in mg. M in mg. R in mg.
182.26 ὅρα ὅτι ὕστερος πλουτάρχου γαληνός $H^{2?}$ in mg. M in mg. R in mg.
224.21 οὐθ' ἑνὸς ὄντος τοιούτου H^2 in mg. M in mg. R in mg. (In this passage Müller states that the red hand in M is multo recentior; but the pattern is the same.)

M is the source of R and of the excerpts preserved in F and P.

3. Manuscript Mosquensis 467

Mosquensis 467 (= R) was formerly in the Bibliotheca Sanctissimae Synodi and is now in the Historical Museum in Moscow. It was copied in Venice by Ambrosius Leo of Nola in 1518, and was at some time the property of Maximus, Bishop of Cythera. It is described by Archimandrite Vladimir, Sistematičeskoe opisanie rukopisej Moskovskoj Sinodal'noj (Patriaršej) Biblioteki, Vol. I: Rukopisi grečeskija (Moscow, 1894), p. 705. R

Ms. R was listed by Diels, 1905, p. 74, but was not known to Müller. Like M, it contains (1^r–96^r) Books II through IX. It exhibits many of M's errors; for example, omissions at 250.19–20 (καταβάντα – εἰρηκέναι), *491.4* (κἂν – χρησόμεθα), *693.12–13* (τοῦτο – χειμῶνι), and *708.12–13* (πᾶν – θερμότητα). Omissions in R at *654.14–16* (αἰδεσθῆναι – μόνος) and at *737.13–15* (ὁ 'Αδείμαντος – ἔφην) correspond exactly to lines in M. A correction at *703.8–11* by the first hand of R establishes without question that R is a copy of M: after πυρετῶν in *703.11*, M jumped back to πυρετῶν in line *8* and continued with ἄμεινον γὰρ ἦν, repeating the entire passage. The scribe of R wrote πυρετῶν ἄμεινον γὰρ, then noticed the error, expunged ἄμεινον γὰρ, and continued with οὐδ' ἐγγὺς. Similarly, at 108.21, M has
προκειμ
τῶ προβλήματι (the scribe first omitted προκειμένῳ, then wrote it above the line). R wrote τῶ προκειμένω βλήματι. R has marginalia from M also; see above.

Ms. R usually follows corrections in M, as at 246.13–14: προστάττει M: προστάττη H M^2 R: πράττη Ald. *689.13*: διωρίσθαι Müller ex Hippocr.: διορεῖσθαι H M: διηρῆσθαι M (e corr.) R; διηρεῖσθαι Ald. But at *715.2*, R is with M: ἐνίας H M (e corr.) Ald.: ἐνία MR.[1]

[1] Where R does not follow the corrections in M, it is possible that they were not yet made when R was copied. An example is 184.6 τοιοῦτον H M^2 Ald. L: τοιοῦ MR.

When the first hand of R differs from M, it is often the result of editorial activity; R tried to correct some of the many errors in M, or at least what he took to be errors; cf. *505.5* and

234.9–10 ταὗτά τοι H Ald.: ταῦτα τά τοι M: ταύτῃ τοι R
266.12 κεκινῆσθαι Bas.: κεκινεῖσθαι H M Ald.: γε κινεῖσθαι R
290.14 διὰ τὸν R Ald.: διτὸν H M
300.6 φησὶ R Ald.: φύσει H M
494.12 λέγοιντ' R Ald.: λέγοιτ' H M: λέγοντ' L
660.9 πραγματείαν R Ald.: πραγμάτων M: πραγ$^{\mu\tau'}$ H
691.8 ἔχοντι R Cornarius: ἔχοντος H M Ald.
708.2 χυμῶν R Ald.: ψυχῶν H: ψυμῶν H (e corr.) M

It will be noted that these readings of R sometimes coincide with readings of the Aldine.[1] Another example of such agreement is *693.6* ἀλλοιουμένους H M: ἀλλοιωμένους R Ald.: ἠλλοιωμένους Müller.

The scribe of R may also have drawn on a manuscript source, perhaps H itself; but the evidence is inconclusive. He was resourceful enough to have hit on the right reading independently. See for example

643.8 ὁρατῶν H R Ald.: om. M: αἰσθήσεων p
690.10 ἀνθρώπω H R: ἀνθρώπου M Ald.

R and L share an easy error at 144.20: they omit τῶν after πάντων.

R^2 A second hand (R^2) introduced a large number of readings, some probably taken from manuscript or other sources, some clearly of his own devising. Examples of the latter are

106.22 ψιλὴν Ald. C: ὑψιλὴν MR, del. R^2 (H deest)
110.17 αὐτῶν MR Ald. C: γρ αὐτοὶ R^2 (H deest)
120.20 ἐκφύσησιν MR Ald. C: ἔκφυσιν R^2 (H deest). R^2 perversely introduces this change wherever the word occurs.
130.10 ἐκφανὴς M C: ἐμφανὴς Ald.: ἐκ φωνῆς R: ἡ φωνὴ R^2 (H deest)
134.4 ἐκ R^2 Bas.: ἀπὸ H MR Ald. L
238.28, 29 παρουσίας H MR Ald.: παρόντος R^2
314.24 εἴρηται H MR L: εἴρεται R^2
679.4 γῆς H Ald. Q: τῆς MR: τῆς γῆς τε καὶ R^2
684.9 αὐτῶν H MR Ald.: αὐτῷ R^2
699.13 παχυτάτοισι H Ald.: παντάτοισι MR: παντάπασι R^2

See also the critical notes to 264.1; 292.14; 296.14.

R^2 sometimes agrees with the Aldine; see the critical notes to 122.29; *716.12*, and

[1] For other passages where M is with H, and R Ald. have the correct reading, see *684.3–4*; *686.13*. See further below, p. 23 n. 1.

106.6 παρενσημαίνουσα C: ἀπῆρεν σημαίνουσα MR (-μαίν- ex -μεν- corr. R): παρεμφαίνουσα R^2 Ald. (H deest)
262.6 ῥῆσις R^2 Ald.: χρῆσις MR (H deest)
684.15 Ἱπποκράτους R^2 Ald.: ἱπποκράτην MR: ἱππο$^{κτ'}$ H
697.10 ἧρος Ald.: ἥρως H M: ἥρος R: $_{ϑ}$ἥρος R^2
704.7 εἴωϑα R^2 Ald.: εἴωϑεν MR: εἴῶ H

or with Cornarius (e. g. at 316.27; *508.13*) or with some other manuscript:

110.16 ἀποδείξεως C: ἴσως ἀποδείξεως R^2: δείξεως MR Ald. (H deest)
110.17 ὧν R^2 Ald. C: τῶν MR (H deest)
118.17 ϑέσιν R^2 Ald. C: ϑέσι γαρ M: ϑέσει γαρ M^2: ϑέσιν γὰρ R
152.9 μοι H MR^2 Ald. L: om. R
643.8 εὐλαβήϑῃ R^2 p Ald.: εὐλαβήϑην H MR

R^2 may have consulted a text of Plato at

679.3 τεττάρων γὰρ H R^2 Ald.: τεσσάρων γὰρ Q: lac. 6 litt. M, lac. 8 litt. R
706.10 ἀναιμωϑέντος H Ald.: ἀναιμοϑέντος MR: ἀνεμοϑέντος R^2: ἀνεμωϑέντος Cornarius ex Platone

R^2 also introduced marginal comments, as at 130.2: τοῦ ζήνωνος λόγος περὶ φωνῆς.

4. The Aldine edition

The Editio Princeps is the Aldina (Venice, 1525) (= Ald.). PHP is in Vol. I, edited by Asulanus. The edition is described and evaluated by Müller, 1874, pp. 14–38. **Ald.**

The Aldine, like M and R, contains PHP II through IX and is a primary source for those passages where H is lost. Müller had seen that M and Ald. had a common source, which we now know to be H. But whereas M is derived directly from H, Ald. gives evidence of one or more intervening steps. For example, at 248.16 the Aldine has admitted into the text the words ὡραῖον τι, which are not in H or MR. Wellmann, 1885 (p. 36) identified the insertion as a misplaced marginal comment; but there is no such comment in H or MR. It must therefore have been written by a reader in the margin of a manuscript intermediate between H and the Aldine.

The Aldine is not from M, and M is not from the parent of Ald. They differ in their interpretation of ambiguous or damaged passages in H, and in their choice between double readings in H.[1] In general, the parent of the Aldine was more judicious than M.

[1] For examples see above, p. 14, p. 15 n. 1, and p. 16. Sometimes they differ also in their efforts to emend:

It is necessary, however, to posit some kind of contact between M and the Aldine (or its parent). Pohlenz, 1898, p. 550, note 5, called attention to several passages in which M and Ald. agree in a reading that differs from the reading of H.[1] Many more passages can be cited to illustrate the same phenomenon; they are too numerous to be coincidental. Consider the following examples:

246.13 ἐκεῖνο H: ἐκεῖνος MR Ald.
276.19 ἔτι H: ὅτι MR Ald.
298.38 ἀλλήλας H: ἀλλήλοις MR Ald.
348.1 δ' οὖν H L: δ' αὖ MR Ald.
621.17 ἔμπτωσιν H: ἔκπτωσιν MR Ald.
684.5 τὸ H: καὶ τὸ MR Ald.
697.7 ἂν H: δὲ M Ald.: δ' R
711.4 ὃ H: ἐπὶ MR Ald.
780.11 ἀδιήθητον H: ἀήθητον MR Ald.
799.1 κατὰ τύχην H: κατὰ τὴν τύχην MR Ald.
802.6 τῆς εἰς H: εἰς om. M Ald.: τῆς εἰς om. R
803.3 ὅλην H: ὅσα MR Ald.

In all of these passages the reading of H is unobjectionable; M and Ald. share a corruption.

Very rarely a reading of M Ald. is superior to that of H:

665.4 τούτων MR Ald.: τούτου H ut vid.

M and the Aldine also agree sometimes in their misinterpretations of abbreviations in H. For examples see *718.13* (quoted above, p. 15 note 1), and

226.17 ἀθηναι^{ς}' (= ἀθηναίης) H: ἀθηναίη MR Ald.
228.32 ὅπς (= ὅπως) H: ὅπερ MR Ald.
266.29 με$^{γλ'}$ (= μεγάλα) H: μεγάλων MR Ald.
298.10 νοσω^{δ}' (= νοσώδους) H: νοσώδου MR Ald.

In at least one instance a mistaken reading of MR appears in the Aldine alongside the correct reading. This points to the Aldine (or its parent) as the borrower:

798.2 δ' οὔτ' H: δ' ἄν τ' MR: δ' οὔτε δ' ἄν τ' Ald.

Other doublets in the Aldine could have had a similar origin:

780.10 πάντα HR: πάντ^{α}ες M: πάντα ἐς Ald.

292.24 ἐπιθυμητικήν H: ἐπιθυμητικοῦ MR: ἐπιθυμητικόν R[2]: ἐπιθυμικόν Ald.
652.7 ἐδείκνυον Ald.: ἐνδεικνύων MR: ἐνδεικνύον H

[1] Of the seven passages mentioned by Pohlenz only three (240.18–19; 248.2; 282.7) actually illustrate his point. In the other four (242.30; 268.16–17; 338.10; 352.14) he was misled by inadequate information about the readings of H, M, and the Aldine.

812.11 αὐτοὺς MR: ἂν τοὺς αὐτοὺς Ald. (H deest)
815.6 τίμαιον MR: τιμαῖον τι μᾶλλον Ald. (H deest)

The similarities of M Ald. on the one hand, and of R Ald. on the other[1], do not admit of a single explanation; there was probably more than one set of borrowings. R often differs from both, as at *690.10* (see above, p. 20); but R is between M and Ald. at

709.6 ἀ(π)ολλυμένου H: ἀλλυομένου M: ἀλλοιομένου R: ἀλλοιουμένου R^2 Ald.

Quite apart from the readings that it shares with M or R, the Aldine gives evidence of extensive editorial activity. Quotations from Homer and Plato were checked against the text of these authors and corrections were introduced. Corrections of this kind, however, were sporadic.[2] I have not identified the sources used by the Aldine editor for Homer and Plato; they could well have been the Aldine editions of those authors (the Aldine Plato appeared in 1513[3], the Aldine Homer in 1504). I have detected no examples of such corrections in the quotations from Hippocrates (the Aldine Hippocrates did not appear until 1526).

The Aldine shares an error with L at *508.1*: εὐτροφίαν H M: εὐτροπίαν R: ἀτροφίαν Ald. L.

The Aldine also has a large number of successful emendations; see for example the critical notes to 244.16; 246.12, 24, 36; 248.19; 258.5, 14; 290.15; 306.19, 23; 322.10; 326.18; 328.4, 24; 334.6. Not all new readings, of course, were successful, for example

657.16 ἀπεδείχθη H MR: ἀποδείξεων ἐδείχθη Ald.
661.4 μετὰ H MR: κατὰ Ald.
690.3 ψαύοντι H MR: ψαυούσῃ Ald.

In passages where H is lost and the text depends on M Ald. (with or without CL), editorial modifications in the Aldine are more difficult to detect. When the Aldine has a good reading and M a poor one, either Ald. corrected, or M corrupted, the reading of H:

264.12 περί τινων Ald.: περίτιμον MR (H deest)

[1] The Aldine is in unique agreement with R or R^2 most often in the correction of errors (cf. above, pp. 20 and 21); but R Ald. agree in error at *693.6* (above, p. 20), and R^2 Ald. at 106.6 (above, p. 21).

[2] Examples may be found in the critical notes; for Homer see the notes to pages 236; 278; *663* etc.; and for Plato, notes to pages 310; 312; *683*; *751*; *774*; *775* etc. At 344.23–24 the Aldine editor may have used his Plato text for supplying the words αὐτοῦ τοῦ διψῶντος and ἄγοντος ὥσπερ, which are present in L but damaged in H (MR leave lacunas). Cf. also *812.9* πέρι Diehl: περὶ MR: εἰπόντων περὶ Ald. with ms. Y of Plato. The text of Hesiod is corrected at 224.25.

[3] See Petersen, 1888, p. 14.

264.19 μέγιγα Ald. (voluit μέγιστα): μέγιστοι MR (H deest)
264.20 ἐμπαθῶς Ald.: ἐμπαθῶν MR: ἐκ παθῶν R²

But here again the Aldine is sometimes the corruptor:

106.31 γῶ MR: ἐγὼ Ald.: γε C
236.19 καθ' ἕν γε Müller (καθ' ἓν F): καθήγε MR: καθ' ἕτερον Ald.

A copy of the Aldine, now at Jena, was annotated by Cornarius. Mewaldt (CMG V 9.1, pp. XXI–XXIII) notes that Cornarius bought a copy of the Aldine in 1532. His corrections were presumably entered between that date and 1550, when he published a translation of PHP. He had some knowledge of the Basileensis (1538); at *526.5* he credits the reading καὶ λεπτότερον to Bas., and at 106.5 he rejects the reading ἐπιστημονικόν, which is otherwise known only from the margin of the Basileensis. At 116.6 Cornarius and Bas. (in mg.) propose ἐπίστασθαι in place of καταστήσασθαι (R² here wrote ἐπι over κατα, thus hinting at a possible link with Bas. or Cornarius). On the whole, however, there is very little connection between Cornarius and the Basileensis.

Cornarius made a systematic check of quotations from Homer, Plato, and Hippocrates against the texts of those writers. I have not discovered what sources he used. His corrections of Hippocrates may have come in part from other works of Galen; see for example

695.4 αὐτοῦ H: αὐτέου Hippocrates: αὐτῷ Cornarius and Galen (CMG V 9.1, p. 44.28)

Cornarius also introduced many conjectures of his own. Sometimes he is in agreement with R (cf. *691.8*) or R² (316.27), with F (*714.14, 15*) or Q (*675.4*), or with Ricci (358.6, 22); but there is no clear evidence that he actually used any of them.

5. The manuscripts of the excerpts

Three sets of excerpts from PHP have survived. One set is found in mss. Q and N, which were unknown to Müller.

Q Paris. Suppl. Gr. 634 (=Q). Described by H. Omont, Inventaire sommaire des manuscrits grecs de la Bibliothèque Nationale, Vol. III, p. 287, and dated by Omont in the 14th century. See also G. Helmreich, Handschriftliche Studien zu Galen (Progr. Ansbach, 1910), pp. 5, 15, 16–18. On folios 19–26 Q contains, along with other material, the following passages from Book VIII of PHP:

663.2 ὀνομάζεται to *664.7* οὐσίαν
664.9 ἕκαστον to *664.12* προσαγορεύομεν
670.10 τὰ μὲν τοῦ to *670.13* ὕδατος
671.4 τὸ μὲν τῆς to *671.7* τριγώνων

671.9 εἶτα φησὶ to *671.10* τεσσάρων
673.17 καὶ μὴν καὶ to *675.6* γεννᾶται
679.3 τεσσάρων to *680.6* αἷμα
681.11 ἄχρι to *683.2* αὐτό

Borbonicus Graecus 299 III D 15 (=N). Described by S. Cyrillus, Codices Graeci MSS Regiae Bibliothecae Borbonicae descripti atque illustrati. Vol. II (Naples, 1832), pp. 388–389. Listed by Diels, 1907, p. 31. Dated in the 14th century. Ms. N contains (folios 174–184) the same excerpts as Q. N

Excerptors in general feel less obligation than other copyists to reproduce exactly the text before them; and if we grant to QN a reasonable degree of freedom in this regard, there is no reason to suppose that they had any source other than H (or a relative of H). Their departures from H include the following:

663.15 δὲ τὸ H MR Ald.: δὲ αὐτῆς τὸ QN
663.16–664.1 τούτων πάλιν H MR Ald.: πάλιν τούτων QN
664.10–11 μηκέτι χωρῇ H MR Ald.: μηκέτ' ἐγχωρῇ QN
671.6 post ὀκτάεδρον add. τοῦ ἀέρος QN
671.7 post εἰκοσάεδρον add. τοῦ ὕδατος QN
671.9 καὶ φησί H MR Ald.: εἶτα φησὶ QN
671.10 δυοῖν γενέσθαι H MR Ald.: ἐξ γινόμενον QN
674.7 ὁπόσα H MR Ald.: ὅσα QN
674.13 μὲν om. QN
679.5 καὶ μέντοι καὶ H MR Ald.: καὶ QN
679.8–9 ξηρόν . . . ψυχρόν H MR Ald.: ψυχρόν . . . ξηρόν QN
679.13 ἡ ξανθὴ καὶ μέλαινα χολή H MR Ald.: ξανθὴ χολὴ καὶ μέλαινα QN
681.15 ἐπ' ἀμφοῖν om. QN
682.13 καὶ om. QN

See also the critical notes to *674.1*; *675.3–5*; *679.3, 7*; *680.4*.

Mss. QN have no evident ties with M or the parent of the Aldine. When H differs from M or Ald., they are normally with H; and their agreements with M or Ald. against H are mostly trivial:

670.11 κυβοειδῆ Q F Ald.: κυμοειδῆ H MR
671.4 τεττάρων H MR: τεσσάρων QN Ald.
674.3 πλεόνων H Ald.: πλειόνων QN MR
674.13 ὡς ὕλη H (ut vid.) Ald.: ὕλη QN: ἐν ὅλῃ H^r MR
τὸ συγκείμενον H QN Ald.: προκείμενον H^r: προκείμενα MR
674.14 οὕτως H (ut vid.) QN Ald.: ὄντως H^r MR
675.4 ἔχοντι QN Cornarius: ἔχοντες MR Ald.: ἐχο$\overset{\tau}{\upsilon}$ H
679.7 ἀπὸ H (e corr.) QN Ald.: ἅπαν H: ἃ παρὰ MR

Ms. N is more remote than Q from H, and it is not unlikely that N derives from Q. Q stands between H and N at *674.3*: φάσκοντες H MR

Ald.: φάσκοῦ Q: φάσκοντα N. Cf. also *664.1*: αὖθις H MR Ald.: αὖ θις Q: αὖ N. Sometimes N abbreviates: *675.5–6* χολὴ ξανθὴ καὶ μέλαινα γεννῶνται H MR Ald.: χ. ξ. καὶ μ. γεννᾶται Q: διτταὶ χολαὶ N. A few of N's readings may be regarded as attempts to emend:

664.5 ἐλαχίστην H Q MR Ald.: ἐλάχιστόν N
679.13 μὲν H Q MR Ald.: μὲν γὰρ N
682.7 φθορᾶς H Q MR Ald.: φθορὰν N
682.17 τῶν ἄλλων H (e corr.) Q MR Ald.: τῶν ἀλλήλων H: ἀλλήλων N

A second hand in N has added some explanatory material:

664.7 ἀριστοτέλους N^2 (annot. marginal. ad οὐσίαν)
664.11 δέξασθαι super lin. N^2 (super τομὴν)
670.11 κύβος ἐστὶ σχῆμα στερεὸν ὑπὸ ἓξ ἴσων τετραγώνων καὶ ἰσοπλεύρων περιεχόμενον N^2 in mg.
671.6 ἴσων καὶ ἰσοπλεύρων super lin. N^2 (post ἓξ)
καὶ ἴσων (post ἰσοπλεύρων) add. N^2
671.7 τὸ δὲ δωδεκάεδρον ὑπὸ δώδεκα πενταγώνων ἴσων καὶ ἰσοπλεύρων καὶ ἰσογωνίων περιεχόμενον N^2 in mg.
ἴσων καὶ ἰσοπλεύρων super lin. N^2 (post τριγώνων)

A second set of excerpts is preserved in mss. F and P.

F Laur. 74,12 (= F). Described by Bandini, Catalogus Codicum Manuscriptorum Bibliothecae Mediceae Laurentianae, Vol. III (Florence, 1770; reprinted Leipzig, 1961), cols. 100–101. Bandini dates it in the 15th century. It was known to Müller, who used a collation made by J. Deutschke; see Müller, 1874, pp. 74–75.

On folios 1–20 ms. F contains 50 excerpts from Books II to IX of PHP. These excerpts often depart from the exact wording of the text. They sometimes give way to summary or paraphrase and are occasionally interrupted by editorial comment. Each excerpt is accompanied by a marginal heading.

Detailed information about the extent of the excerpts may be found in Müller, 1871, pp. 13–14 (under his discussion of P). I shall give only page and line of the new text.

1. 154.33 to 156.15
2. 160.34 to 162.6
3. 166.11–15
4. 170.6–24 (omitting most of 170.7–8, 10–17)
5. 170.33 to 172.10
6. 174.5–21 (omitting 174.7–10)
7. 176.19–28
8. 198.23–38
9. 212.33 to 214.3
10. 236.16–21

11. 284.33 to 286.4
12. 288.30 to 290.5
13. 302.17–23
14. 308.26–34
15. 310.7 to 312.21 (omitting 310.22–312.10)
16. 312.29–36
17. 324.2–9
18. 324.18–23
19. 324.26–28; 326.20–24[1]
20. 336.16 to 340.6 (omitting 338.1–2, 3–7, 16–22, 23–340.12)
21. *501.7* to *502.4* (followed by Theodorus' scholium)
22. *566.9* to *568.13* (omitting *567.5–14*; *568.2–11*)
23. *569.9* to *570.5*
24. *571.5* to *577.3* (omitting *571.13–574.4*; *574.12–575.2*; *575.9–576.3*)
25. *588.8* to *589.9*
26. *590.10* to *591.1*
27. *591.11* to *592.1*
28. *594.15* to *595.5*
29. *602.16* to *603.9*
30. *626.17* to *632.2* (omitting *627.8–10*; *627.15–628.7*; *628.11–629.3*; *630.3–632.1*)
31. *637.13* to *639.4*
32. *643.14* to *644.7*
33. *666.12* to *669.2* (omitting *667.1–6*; *667.12–668.6*; *668.9–669.1*)
34. *669.9* to *674.7* (omitting *670.15–671.2*; *672.8–10*; *673.3–16*)
35. *685.14* to *688.10* (omitting *686.15–687.11*; *688.5–10*)
36. *702.14* to *708.2* (preceded by a scholium, and omitting *703.5–12*; *704.2–707.10*)
37. *708.8–11* (paraphrase)
38. *711.10* to *728.7* (omitting *711.13–712.9*; *712.9–714.9*; *715.3–717.9*; *718.3–12*; *718.12–719.2*; *719.3–12*; *719.15–721.3*; *721.9–722.1*; *722.6–724.1*; *724.5–726.14*; *727.4–728.3*)
39. *730.4–10*
40. *736.6* to *738.7* (omitting *736.10–12*; *737.1–4*; *737.5–738.6*)
41. *739.2* to *740.9* (omitting *739.9–740.8*)
42. *740.9* to *743.1* (omitting *741.1–742.7*)
43. *765.5* to *776.7* (omitting *766.7–8*; *768.1–11*; *769.2–770.9*; *771.3–7*; *771.13–775.9*)
44. *791.5* to *792.3*
45. *793.5* to *794.1*
46. *794.11–15*
47. *810.14* to *811.9*
48. *811.13* to *813.9* (omitting *812.10–813.2*)

[1] Müller's 19th excerpt might better be considered two distinct excerpts, the second with the heading, Ποσειδωνίου τοῦτο.

49. *814.7–13*

50. *815.3–10* (omitting *815.6–9*; excerpt 50 precedes 49 in F).

P Paris. Gr. 2277 (=P). Described by Omont, Inventaire sommaire des Manuscrits Grecs de la Bibliothèque Nationale, Vol. II, pp. 228–229. Omont dates it in the 15th–16th centuries. It was known to Müller, who collated it in 1870, shortly before the outbreak of the war between France and Germany. See Müller, 1871, p. 12; 1874, pp. 75–76.

Ms. P contains (folios 111^{r}–134^{r}) the same excerpts, scholia and marginalia as F. It is clearly a copy of F; many of its errors are readily explained as misreadings of F's rather careless writing. An example is *717.13* οὖν H M (R deest) Ald. F (ante corr.): ὀπ̄π P (the line of deletion drawn by F made the loops of υν look like a double π).

Petersen, 1888, p. 10, pointed out that the excerpts in F and P derive from M. They have no special relation with R, which also derives from M but postdates F. F introduces new readings rather freely, and sometimes with happy results; see the critical notes to 286.1; 290.4; 310.15, 18; 336.21; 338.11; *670.4*. F also agrees at times with H, Q, Ald. and others against M; for examples see the critical note to 310.16 and

162.2 περαίνοιτ' H FP Ald. L: περαίνειτ' MR
162.6 τινος ἀπροαιρέτου H FP Ald. L: τινας προαιρέτου MR: τινος προαιρέτου R^2
166.11 ἐπιλανθανόμενος H MR Ald.: ἐπιλαθόμενος FP p (L deest)
198.36 οὓς H FP Ald.: ὡς MR
212.36 σπλάγχνῳ R^2 FP Ald.: σπλάγχνον MR: σπλάγχν̄ H
310.22 ψυχῆς H MR: ψυχὴν FP Ald. Plato
670.1 δὲ H FP Ald.: om. MR
671.8 σχήματα H (e corr.) MR Ald.: σώματα H FP
688.10 ὀξείας τε H MR: ὀξύς τε καὶ FP: ὀξὺς καὶ Ald.
724.4 καὶ οὐχ H (e corr.) FP Ald.: οὐχ H MR

A correction by F^2 is the preferred reading at 166.13 φήσαντι F^2P (super lin.): φήσαν̄ H M: φήσαντα R: φήσαντος FP (in textu) Ald.: φήσασι Wachsmuth.

F has two scholia attributed to Theodorus. The first (to *502.1–4*) is as follows:

Θεόδωρος
ἐπιδεδεῖχθαι μὲν τοῦτο ἐν τοῖς ἔμπροσθεν λέγει· οὐδαμοῦ δὲ ἀποδειχθὲν φαίνεται πρόσθεν, πλὴν ὅσον διαφόρους ταῦτ' εἶναι δυνάμεις δέδεικται· τοῦτο δὲ καὶ Ἀριστοτέλην ὁμολογεῖν καὶ αὐτός φησιν. εἶτα καὶ ἀναβαλόμενος τὴν περὶ τούτου ἀπόδειξιν εἰς τὸ ἕκτον βιβλίον τουτί, πῶς ἐπιδεδεῖχθαι ταὐτὸ ἐν τοῖς ἔμπροσθεν λέγει; οὐ μὴν ἀλλ' οὐδὲ ἐν τοῖς ὕστερον λόγοις φαίνεται ἀποδεικνὺς τοῦτο. ἄλλως δὲ πρὸς Ἀρίστωνα καὶ Χρύσιππον τὸν λόγον ποιούμενος ἐξεῖναί φησιν ἀκούειν τὸ τῆς οὐσίας ὄνομα καὶ ὡς ὕπαρξίν τε καὶ τελειότητα βελτίστην τῆς ἑκάστου φύσεως

[γε] σημαῖνον: ἀλλὰ τοῦτο κατασκευαστικὸν μὲν ἂν εἴη τοῦ οἰκείου λόγου, οὐχὶ δὲ καὶ τοῦ ἐναντίου ἀνασκευαστικόν, εἴπερ ὡς μὲν πλείους ἂν εἶεν οὐσίαι ὡς δὲ μία. ὡς μὲν γὰρ ὕπαρξις, πλείους· ὡς δὲ τὸ ὑποκείμενον ἢ τὸ συνεκτικόν, μία.

8–10] *cf.* PHP 588.13–14 Müller

9 τε *sscr.* F 10 γε *delevi*

The text of the second scholium (at *688.10*) is as follows:

Θεόδωρος
τὰ Πλάτωνος ταῦτα οὐδὲ Γαληνὸς ἐπαινεῖ, ὡς μὴ συμφωνοῦντα τοῖς Ἱπποκράτους λόγοις. «τὸ μὲν οὖν ἐκ πυρὸς ὑπερβολῆς μάλιστα νοσῆσαν σῶμα συνεχῆ καύματα καὶ πυρετοὺς ἀπεργάζεται, τὸ δὲ ἐξ ἀέρος ἀμφημερινούς, τριταίους δὲ ἐξ ὕδατος διὰ τὸ νωθέστερον ἀέρος καὶ πυρὸς αὐτὸ εἶναι, τὸ δὲ γῆς τέταρτον ὂν νωθέστατον τούτων ἐν τετραπλασίαις περιόδοις χρόνου καθαιρόμενον τεταρταίους πυρετοὺς ποιῆσαν ἀπαλλάττεται μόλις.» δῆλον γὰρ ὅτι «ἐπὶ μὲν τῶν ἀμφημερινῶν ὁ φλεγματώδης πλεονάζει χυμὸς ὑγρὸς καὶ ψυχρὸς ὤν, ἐπὶ δὲ τῶν τριταίων ὁ τῆς ξανθῆς χολῆς ἄκρως θερμὸς καὶ ξηρός, ὥστ' ἐπὶ τούτου μὲν ἐχρῆν εἰρῆσθαι πλεονάζειν τὸ τοῦ πυρὸς στοιχεῖον· ἐπ' ἀμφημερινοῦ δὲ ⟨τὸ⟩ τοῦ ὕδατος.» ἄτοπον δ' οἴεται Γαληνὸς κἀκεῖνο τοῦ Πλάτωνος, τὸ ἐκ συντήξεως ἁπαλῆς σαρκὸς γενέσθαι ποτὲ φλέγμα· καὶ ὀρθῶς γε. «ἡ γὰρ τοῦ φλέγματος γένεσις ἐκ τροφῆς φύσει ψυχροτέρας ἐνδεῶς ὑπὸ τῆς ἐμφύτου θερμασίας κατεργασθείσης ἀποτελεῖται· τηκομένη δὲ σὰρξ ὅμοιόν τι ποιεῖ σύντηγμα τὴν μὲν χρόαν τῇ ὠχρᾷ χολῇ ἐπὶ τὸ λευκότερον ῥέπον,» τὴν δὲ σύστασιν «παχύτερον» καὶ τὴν ὀσμὴν «δυσωδέστερον, καί τινα γλισχρότητα πολλάκις» καὶ «λιπαρότητα» ἔχον.

12 τὸ *add.* F²P 16 μὲν *inser.* F 18 *ante* καὶ^III^ *add. et del.* ἔχον F

A third set of excerpts is contained in p.

Paris. Gr. 2283 (= p). Described by Omont, Inventaire sommaire, Vol. II, p. 229. Omont dates it in the 16th century. Müller examined it and found it of little use; see Müller, 1871, pp. 14–15; 1874, pp. 76–77. p

On folios 108^r^ to 113^v^, ms. p has excerpts from PHP II–IX. Most of the excerpts are short, and they often distort the text. Some are paraphrases or summaries. Infrequently p introduces some slight improvement.

Folios 108^r^ to 109^v^ contain quotations or paraphrases of some forty passages from PHP II, the longest of which runs from 110.23 τὰ μὲν ἐπιστημονικὰ to 112.2 τὰ σοφιστικά. Other excerpts of more than minimal length include 128.4 ὅτι ἡ καρδία πηγὴ to 128.8 ἐπιδείξει and 138.34 σολοικίζειν to 140.3 ἀδιανόητά γε. There is a Latin gloss on fol. 108^v^: τυποῦν· formare.

Folios 109^{v} to 110^{v} contain about twenty passages from Book III, the longest being a fairly continuous transcription of 230.14 ὥσπερ γὰρ to 230.27 κοιλιῶν. Book IV is quickly passed over, with no heading and only nine very short excerpts (fol. 110^{v}). Book V supplies 16 excerpts (fols. 110^{v} to 111^{r}), one of moderate length: from 308.17 τὸ δὲ κάλλος to 308.25 κανόνα. Book VI provides ten excerpts, of which the longest is from *496.16* θυμὸς to *497.4* πάθη. From Book VII (fols. 111^{v} to 113^{r}) the excerpts are more extensive: sixteen passages, including *609.2* ἡ κατὰ ποιότητα to *609.9* κατὰ χώραν; *643.3* πολύ τι ἄμεινον to *644.9* γίνεσθαι; *644.13* ἀλλοιοῦται to *645.12* κινήσεως. Folio 113^{r} contains four excerpts from Book VIII; and finally, on folio $113^{r,v}$, are thirteen passages from Book IX, the longest of which are *796.8* ἀνάγεται to *797.1* ἄρχεσθαι, *801.2* διαγινώσκειν to *801.10* παρακολουθοῦντας, and *806.11* οὐδὲ ἁπλῶς to *807.5* δεξιά.

Ms. p, like QN and FP, belongs to the group H MR Ald., but its precise affiliation is obscure. It is sometimes with M or R or both, sometimes with H, rarely with the Aldine:

110.25 ὅσοις Ald. C: ὅσα MR p (H deest)
116.1 μὴ μόνον Ald. C: μὲν μόνον MR (R^{2} deperd. in mg.): οὐ μόνον p
126.22 οὖν τοῦτο Müller: τοῦτο MR p Ald.: οὖν C
126.24 συντόνως M p Ald. C: συντόμως R
126.25 ὑπὸ MR p Ald.: ἀπὸ C
128.7 οὐχ MR p C: om. Ald.
138.35 ἧπερ H^{2} p: εἴπερ H MR Ald. L
150.35 μήτι L: μήτοι MR Ald.: μήτι^{οι} H p
150.35–36 δὴ ταῖς ἀρτηρίαις H Ald. L: διὰ ταῖς ἀρτηρίαις MR: διὰ τὰς ἀρτηρίας p
166.11 ἐπιλανθανόμενος H MR Ald.: ἐπιλαθόμενος FP p
168.17 ἀπὸ τῶν H^{s} Ald.: om. MR p
198.19 ἀποσχέσθαι H p Ald.: ἀποδέχεσθαι MR
230.25 φήσει H: φύσει MR p Ald.
643.8 ὁρατῶν H R Ald.: om. M: αἰσθήσεων p
εὐλαβήθη R^{2} p Ald.: εὐλαβήθην H MR

Ms. p has the accepted reading at 200.17 and *496.17*.

[Par. 2278.] Ackermann's Historia Literaria Claudii Galeni, as printed in Vol. I of Kühn's edition of Galen, mentions on p. XCII three manuscripts of PHP: Paris. 2278 "cui tamen liber I. deest", Marc. 284 (= M), and Cantab. (= C). Diels, 1905, p. 74, lists Par. 2278, but in brackets and with a query. The only Paris manuscripts of PHP known to me are the three collections of excerpts, 2277 (P), 2283 (p), and Suppl. Gr. 634 (Q). It seems probable that Ackermann's manuscript is to be identified with 2277 or 2283, both of which have excerpts from Books II–IX but not from I.

6. Manuscripts Cantabrigiensis Caius College 47/24 and Laurentianus 74,22

No. 47/24 in the Library of Gonville and Caius College, Cambridge (= C). Described by Montague Rhodes James, A Descriptive Cata- C logue of the Manuscripts in the Library of Gonville and Caius College, Vol. I (Cambridge, 1907), pp. 39–40. See also Müller, 1871, pp. 9–12; 1874, pp. 42–45, 73–74. James dates the manuscript in the 15th century. It was acquired by Caius in Paris (in 1543, by Müller's calculations) and brought by him to Cambridge. Müller used a collation made for him by M. Schanz.

The manuscript is a miscellany, the third item of which comprises nine folios of PHP: a quaternion (folios 1–8) that carries the letter beta (= 2) on 1ʳ and the number XXV on 8ᵛ and contains pp. 72.28 to 132.15 ἀπέδειξαν, and a single folio (9) that contains a part of PHP IV, from 248.22 ⟨ὄνομα καὶ κ⟩ατὰ to 256.19 ἀγ⟨αθὸν εἶναι⟩ κα⟨θάπερ⟩. C alone preserves the surviving portion of PHP I (pp. 72.28–100.7), which was first edited, with Latin translation, by Caius, Cl. Galeni Pergameni nobilissimi medici libri aliquot (Basileae, 1544). There is a copy of this book at Cambridge with corrections that are thought to be in Caius' own hand.[1] Also probably in Caius' hand is a marginal note on fol. 1ʳ: Ms hunc Jo. Caius edidit Basil. 1544 et latinum fecit in 4to. This note is written in a slate-colored ink much the same in appearance as that used for a number of corrections and retracings in the text, e. g. the οὐ of οὐδὲ at 76.4 and the θ of θρόμβον at 78.4. At 92.1 it was probably Caius who consulted a text of Aristotle and wrote the marginal comment, οὐ περὶ ζώων ἱστορίας οὐδὲ περὶ γεννήσεως ἀλλὰ περὶ ζώων μορίων.

No. 74,22 in the Laurentian Library (=L). Described by A. M. L Bandini, Catalogus Codicum Manuscriptorum Bibliothecae Mediceae Laurentianae, Vol. III (Florence, 1770; reprinted Leipzig, 1961), cols. 124–125. See also Müller, 1871, pp. 7–9; 1874, p. 72. Müller used a collation made for him by H. Kruse.[2]

Ms. L contains fragmentary portions of several of Galen's works. From PHP it has two quaternions, one (folios 15–21) containing PHP 132.15 χρύσιππόν to 190.7 ἔτι δὲ θ.ρ. . ., but lacking 168.15 τῷ μορίῳ to 170.29 μὲν γὰρ. This missing portion of the text corresponds to the sixth folio of the quaternion, which is blank and lacks a folio number (it is between numbered folios 19 and 20).[3] The other quater-

[1] Readings from this copy may be found at 78.11, 21, 30; 88.35. I am grateful to Richard Durling for informing me of the existence of this copy and securing photographs of it.

[2] In a few passages (e. g. 184.29), where L is badly damaged, I have accepted from Müller's app. crit. readings of L that are illegible to me. These readings presumably come from Kruse's collation.

[3] As the length of the missing text is much less than the amount normally contained

nion (folios 22–29) contains PHP 306.17 μὴ τοίνυν to *508.5* γι⟨γνόμε-νον⟩. The earlier quaternion has the letter gamma (=3) at the beginning (15^{r}) and the number XXVI at the end (21^{v}). The other has the number XXVIIII at the end (29^{v}); there is no Greek number visible on 22^{r}, the lower margin of which is damaged.

The folios of the two quaternions in L were at one time marked consecutively with the letters of the Latin alphabet, the first having the letters A to H (the blank folio is marked F), the second I to Q (there is no J). Someone, recognizing that the quaternions are not consecutive, inserted eight blank folios between 21 (H) and 22 (I). There is similar interleaving between the fragmentary texts contained in the earlier portions of the manuscript. After the interleavings the folios were numbered consecutively. In an earlier numbering the folios of PHP (including all the blanks) extend from 22 to 45; these numbers, however, have been deleted, and a second series (lower right hand margin of the rectos) gives to these folios the numbers 24–47.

Müller recognized C and L as two parts of the same manuscript.[1] The second quaternion, preserved in C, is a perfect match with the third quaternion preserved by L. Each of the extant quaternions contains between 68 and 75 pages of Müller's text; and the gap between the end of the third and the beginning of the sixth is about 150 pages. At the midpoint of the gap (p. 248.22) begins the isolated folio (9) preserved in C; one may conclude, therefore, that it was originally the first folio of the fifth quaternion.

Müller pointed out that the whole of PHP would have required ten quaternions in the original CL. If the first quaternion contained about 70 Müller pages, Book I must have been rather long (70+31 pages). The evidence of H points to the same conclusion (see above, p. 13).

The date of the disintegration of CL is not known. The separation of C from L, however, may be reasonably placed in the interval between the publication of the Aldine (1525) and the acquisition of C by Caius; for both C and L have marginal notes, apparently by the same hand, giving the location of the fragments in the Aldine. These notes are on folios 4^{v} and 9^{r} of C, and 15^{r} and 22^{r} of L.

Ms. L (or a twin of L) was apparently known to Alexander Justinianus, whose notes on the text of PHP appear as marginalia in the Juntine Latin edition. At 348.30 he cites αὐτῶν as a manuscript variant; this is the reading of L but not of H MR Ald. (which read αἰτιῶν).

Ms. CL is not a copy of H. It is generally inferior to H, but sometimes it preserves the better reading. See for example the critical notes to 122.18–19 (M Ald.); 134.14; 140.4, 21; 146.30; 150.10;

on a folio of L (about nine of Müller's pages), we must suppose that the scribe of L was copying from a defective original and deliberately left the folio blank. See the observations of Kruse as reported by Müller, 1871, p. 8.

[1] See Müller, 1871, pp. 10–11; 1874, pp. 73–74; Petersen, 1888, pp. 6–7.

180.21; 250.12, 19; 308.4; 312.13; 336.21; 340.8; 342.25; 348.4; 356.20; *499.16*. It is consistently better than H in its retention of certain poetic forms, such as κραδίη (158.24; 178.8, and passim), and στήθεσσι (176.2; 178.21, and passim). It also has a better Plato text at 354.33 and possibly at 338.1.

The errors of CL are in part mechanical, in part the result of unsuccessful editorial revision. The mechanical errors are of the usual varieties; perhaps it is enough to mention only a few that rest on a misreading of the letter π (see Bast, Commentatio Palaeographica [Leipzig, 1811], who however does not mention the confusions found here):

136.1 ἀποκεκρυμμένον H: αὐτῷ κεκρυμμένον L
144.7 ὅπως H: οὕτως L
150.35 οὐδ' ἐπὶ H: οὐδέν τι L

Examples of unsuccessful emendation in CL include the addition of ὡς at 104.20 and of ὅτι at 120.4, and the substitution of αὐτόματοι for αὐτοὶ at 112.25. At 108.21 an editor may have been trying to correct a mechanical error (λήμματα . . . προβλήματι); see also 126.2 (ἀπόλλοιτο) and 146.2 (quoted above, p. 16 note 2).

Some of the errors in CL point to double readings in its source. See for example 84.26 and

122.14 ἐν ταῖς Wilamowitz: ἐπὶ ταῖς M Ald.: ἐν ταῖς ἐπὶ C
136.11 πρὸ τῆς φάρυγγος H: . . . της τοῦ φάρυγγος L

The noun φάρυγξ regularly has the feminine article in H, the masculine in L. The present passage indicates that the archetype had the feminine, and the masculine in L is an editorial change. The editor overlooked the passage at 120.24, where C retains the feminine: τὴν φάρυγγα (see above, p. 14).

144.19 ἀπέραντον H: ἀπεράντω· ψευδῆ L
254.18 εἴποι H: εἴποι (ε ssscr.) C

At one point (84.38) a marginal note has found its way into the text of C.

The common archetype of CL and H was probably minuscule, though the evidence is slight, and both manuscripts have uncial corruptions. There is a misreading of minuscules, in my opinion, at 110.26: κυήσεως scripsi: μυήσεως M Ald. C (H deest). But C has an uncial corruption at 114.10 δεηθεὶς M Ald.: δεήσειε C (H deest), and L at 162.33 κοιλίη H Ald.: κοιλία M: κοινῇ L. H preserves an uncial corruption as a doublet at 284.18 παύεται sscr. H: γίνεται H in textu (ΠΑΥΕΤΑΙ : ΓΙΝΕΤΑΙ). Perhaps the uncial corruptions that survive in C were also preserved as variants in the minuscule archetype.

That the archetype had double readings is indicated further by such passages as 106.6 παρενσημαίνουσα C: ἀπῆρεν σημαίνουσα M:

παρεμφαίνουσα Ald. (H deest). At 106.26, where this Chrysippean passage is repeated, M Ald. C have παρεμφαίνουσα. This latter reading may originally have been a gloss on the rare word παρενσημαίνουσα. Consider also the following:

106.11 λεγομένην M (in textu) Ald.: λέγομεν M (in mg.) C (H deest)
110.5 δή Diels: ἤ M: δὲ Ald.: δὲ ἤ C. δή was corrupted to δέ, and a superscribed ή was interpreted as a separate word.
116.20 ἐστιν ἐν αὐτῇ, τοῦτ' ἔστιν scripsi: ἐστιν ἐν αὐτῇ M Ald.: τοῦτ' ἐστὶν C. One or the other of the two phrases appeared as a superscription in the archetype. The copyists took it to be an alternative rather than a supplement.
126.22 οὖν τοῦτο Müller: τοῦτο M Ald.: οὖν C
130.1 εἴση Ald.: εἰσι M: εἴσι^{η} C
186.20 ἀμαλῆσι Müller ex Homero: ὁμαλῆσι L: ἁπαλῆσι H (e corr.) M: ἁπαλοῖσι H Ald.
338.2 οἵαις Charterius ex Platone: αἷς H: οἷα L. The archetype had the dative singular corrected by a superscription to the dative plural. Something similar may have happened at 112.22.
350.19 παρελθεῖν Müller: π́ροελθεῖν H: προέλθεῖν L. The redundant accent is a vestige of the abbreviation for παρα. H has a similar doublet at 192.6.

An interesting example of corruption in the archetype is the Chrysippean definition of ὄρεξις, quoted four times, at 238.36–37, 250.9 and 11–12, and 342.30. It seems probable that Chrysippus wrote ἐπί τινος ὅσον χρὴ ἥδοντος. These words appear in H as ἐπί τι ὅσον χρὴ ἧδον (238.36–37), or ἐπί τι ὅσον χρὴ ἧδον αὐτῶ (250.9, 11–12), or ἐπί τι ὅσον χρὴ ἥδοντος (342.30). They appear in CL as ἐπί τι ὡς ὧν χρὴ ἥδη ὄντος αὐτῶ (250.9, 11–12), or ἐπί τι ὅσον χρὴ ἥδη ὄντος αὐτῶν (342.30). CL is lacking at 238.36–37. A possible explanation of the variants is that τινος was corrupted to τι before ὅσον. ἥδοντος was then changed to ἧδον, in order to agree with τι, but the original reading was preserved in a superscribed οντος. Similarly, the lost second syllable of τινος, if superscribed, could have generated ὡς in CL; but the following ὧν remains unexplained. The word αὐτῶ(ν) added at the end of the phrase might have originated as an interpretation of the superscribed οντος, or it may have first arisen at 250.9 as a doublet for οὕτω, which follows immediately. The presence of the intrusive αὐτῶ(ν) in both H and CL indicates that it was already in the archetype.

The archetype of H CL was damaged at 164.29–166.4, and again at 166. 10. Both H and L left blank spaces, though H was able to read more than L (or L's parent). A supplementary hand (H^{s}) supplied the missing words in the first lacuna, whether by a more careful reading of the archetype or from some other source is impossible to say (see above, p. 14).

There is no clear evidence of cross correction between H and the parent of CL, and most of the similarities between CL and the descendants of H are probably coincidental; see above, p. 18, and 160.7 αὐτῷ H: αὐτὸ MR Ald. L. Even the summary of the contents of Book II that is preserved in MR and C might have been in the archetype.[1] It is strange, however, that there are no such summaries for the other books.

Ms. CL contains corrections by the first and by later hands. C has also a few Latin glosses. Some of the corrections in C may have been made by Caius; see above, p. 31. Examples of corrections in CL may be found in the critical notes to pages 74, 78, 80, 104, 112, 134, 136, 160, 250, 336, 338, 340, 356 etc. The corrections at 338.1 and 354.33 might have resulted from consultation of a text of Plato, that at 92.4 may have been taken from Aristotle.

The textual tradition may be illustrated by the following stemma:

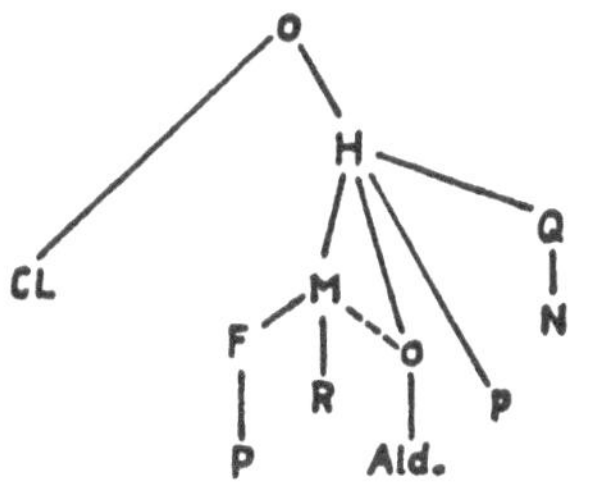

7. Editions after the Aldine

Since the Aldine (1525) the Greek text of PHP has been printed in the following editions:

1. Galeni Pergameni . . . opera omnia. 5 vols. Edited by Camerarius, Fuchs, and Gemusaeus. Basel, 1538. Vol. I contains PHP II–IX on pages 253–342. The text is based on the Aldine; see Müller, 1874, pp. 38–42. Emendations that first appear in the Basileensis are identified in the critical notes of the present edition by the symbol "Bas.". There are a few variant readings printed in the margin of Bas.; some are not found elsewhere, others appear in R² or Cornarius. In at least

[1] The text of the summary is as follows: κεφάλαια τῶν ἐν τῷ δευτέρῳ βιβλίῳ· ὅτι τῶν ἠρωτημένων λόγων ὑπὸ τοῦ (τοῦ om. MR) χρυσίππου περὶ τοῦ τῆς (τοῦ τῆς om. MR) ψυχῆς ἡγεμονικοῦ, τινῶν (τινὰ MR) μὲν οὐκ ἀληθές (ἀληθῆ MR) τι τῶν λημμάτων ἐστί, τινῶν δὲ οὐκ οἰκεῖον (οὐκ om. C: οὐ κοινῶνα MR?: οὐκ οἰκοῖα R²): ὅτι τὰ (τὰ om. MR) τοῦ (τοῦ in textu om. C) ζητουμένου πράγματος οἰκεῖα πρὸς ἀπόδειξιν λήμματα κατὰ ψιλὴν καὶ μόνην τὴν οὐσίαν τοῦ προκειμένου σκέμματος γίγνεται: ὅτι τῶν οὐκ οἰκείων λημμάτων τρεῖς εἰσι διαφοραί, καὶ ὅτι σαφοῦς (σαφοῦσιν MR?: σαφῆς R²) ἕνεκα διδασκαλίας ὠνόμασται τὰ μὲν γυμναστικά τε καὶ διαλεκτικά, τὰ δὲ πιθανά τε καὶ ῥητορικά· τὰ δὲ σοφιστικά, ὡς γίνεσθαι (γίγνεσθαι C) τὰς πάσας διαφορὰς τῶν λημμάτων τέσσαρας· ἀποδεικτικήν· γυμναστικήν· ῥητορικήν· σοφιστικήν (ante σοφιστικήν add. καὶ MR).

one instance Cornarius borrows from Bas.: at *526.5* his note reads, "καὶ λεπτότερόν Bas.". See above, p. 24, and the notes to *513.1–2*; *526.13*; *529.16*; *591.3*. In still other passages the marginal reading in Bas. restores the text of H MR, for example, *549.13*: ἡ μήτρα H MR Bas. (in mg.) Cornarius: ἡμετέρας Ald. Bas. (in textu). Of the readings peculiar to Bas. (in mg.) an example is *512.1* φάναι H MR Ald. Bas. (in textu): εἶναι Bas. in mg.

2. Caius' edition and translation of the remains of Book I; see above, p. 31.

3. Operum Hippocratis Coi et Galeni Pergameni ... Renatus Charterius edidit. Paris, 1679. 13 vols. PHP is in Vol. V, pp. 78–274. Charterius combined the remains of Book I with Books II–IX. He also provided a Latin translation of the whole, adapting the translation of Book I from Caius, and using Guinterius Andernacus for the rest.[1] He divided each book into chapters, following the division of the Juntine Latin Galen. Charterius took the Greek text of Book I from Caius, and the rest from the Basileensis. He corrected a large number of errors, many of them in quotations from Plato and the Greek poets. See for example the critical notes to 186.21; 226.6, 16–20; 236.7, 8; 272.8; 278.15; 282. 20, 22; 350.2, 6, 7. The defects of Charterius' edition were set forth at great length by Müller, 1874, pp. 45–60.

4. Claudii Galeni Opera Omnia. Ed. C. G. Kühn. 20 vols. Leipzig, 1821–1833. PHP I–IX is in Vol. V, pp. 181–805. Kühn, following Charterius, gave the Greek text and a Latin translation. He corrected a substantial number of errors that had escaped his predecessors. Yet he did not succeed in producing a dependable edition; see Müller, 1874, pp. 60–69.

5. Claudii Galeni De Placitis Hippocratis et Platonis libri novem. Ed. I. Müller. Vol. I. Leipzig, 1874. Vol. I contains a long introduction, the Greek text with critical notes, and a Latin translation. The projected second volume was never published. In establishing his text Müller used manuscripts M C L F P p. He also consulted the printed editions, the marginalia of Cornarius, and all other sources available to him. Thus his text is significantly better than anything earlier. Unfortunately it was soon rendered obsolete by the discovery of the Hamilton manuscript (see above, p. 12) and by other advances in the study of Galen. Prior to the appearance of his edition Müller published Quaestiones Criticae de Galeni libris Περὶ τῶν καθ' Ἱπποκράτην καὶ Πλάτωνα δογμάτων, Erlangen, 1871, 1872.

8. Emendations made by modern authors

In addition to the editors of printed editions, a number of others have contributed to the improvement of the text.

[1] Andernach's translation of PHP II–IX was first published at Paris, 1534. For further information on 16th century Latin translations see Durling, 1961.

1. Cornarius entered emendations in a copy of the Aldine now at Jena. See above, p. 24.

2. The Latin Galen edited by A. Ricci and V. Trincavelli (Venice, 1541–1545) contains in Sect. 1, Pt. 2, pp. 929–1242, Andernach's translation of PHP II–IX, with variant Greek readings printed in the margins. I am indebted to Richard Durling for information about these readings, which he assigns to Ricci. Some of them are based on Andernach's Latin; see for example the critical note to 194.23. Others are found in Cornarius (e. g. 304.20; 358.6, 22), and still others are clearly original (e. g. 172.21; 202.21; *709.14*).

3. The fourth edition of the Juntine Latin Galen (Venice, 1565) contains a revised version of Feliciano's translation of PHP[1], with the variant readings of Alexander Justinianus in the margin. At least one of these readings appears to be taken from manuscript L (see above, p. 32). Others were anticipated by Ricci and Cornarius. But in several places Al. Just. is himself credited with a successful emendation; cf. 280.4; 296.23; 340.18; *547.13*.

4. Through the courtesy of the editorial office of CMG a transcript was provided of marginal annotations entered by H. Schöne in his copy of Müller's edition. All readings ascribed to Schöne are from this source, with the exception of three (at 136.29; 162.34; 264.7) which he published in Sitzungsberichte Berlin, 1924, p. 106.

5. Readings credited to Benedict Einarson were transmitted by him to the editor in the form of comments on the typescript of this edition.

6. Readings assigned to Rusch are from F. A. Rusch, Galen, De Placitis Hippocratis et Platonis, Book VIII. Dissertation, Northwestern University, Evanston, Illinois, 1968.

7. Readings assigned to Jouanna have been taken from Jacques Jouanna, Hippocrate, La Nature de l'homme. CMG I 1.3, Berlin, 1975.

Readings have been cited also from the following publications:

Alexanderson: B. Alexanderson, Bemerkungen zu Galens Comm. nat. hom., Comm. acut., De temperamentis und De placitis, Eranos LXVIII (1970), pp. 61–75

Aly: W. Aly, Hesiods Theogonie. Heidelberg, 1913

von Arnim, SVF[2]

Bake, 1810

Baumgarten, 1962

Bergk: Th. Bergk, Die Geburt der Athene, I, Fleckeisens Jahrbücher 6 (1860), pp. 289–319. Readings are assigned to Bergk also at PHP 276.30 and 288.2 on the authority of Müller, 1874.

Boissonade: A reading at 226.21 is assigned to Boissonade on the authority of Jacoby.

Bywater: I. Bywater, ATAKTA, Journ. of Philol. 10 (1882), p. 71

[1] This translation was first published at Basel, 1535; see Durling, 1961, p. 258.

[2] For bibliographical details see the list of Abbreviated references, above, pp. 9–11.

Castiglioni: L. Castiglioni, Decisa Forficibus VI, Rendiconti Ist. Lomb. 82 (1949), pp. 119–128
Charitonides: Ch. Charitonides, ΚΡΙΤΙΚΑ, ΠΛΑΤΩΝ 3 (1951), p. 88
Cobet: C. G. Cobet, Variae Lectiones, Leiden, 1873, p. 294; also Cobet, 1882
Diehl: E. Diehl, Proclus Diadochus in Plat. Tim. Comm. 3 vols., Leipzig, 1903–1906. Reprinted Amsterdam, 1965
Diels: Diels, 1875; also, readings assigned to Diels by Kalbfleisch, 1892.
Dombartus: A reading at *732.6* is assigned to Dombartus on the authority of Müller, 1874.
Edelstein, 1936
Edelstein-Kidd
Gomperz: A reading at *779.8* is assigned to Th. Gomperz on the authority of H. Kühlewein, Hippocratis Opera, I. Leipzig, 1895.
Greenhill: W. Greenhill, Emendationen zum Texte des Galen, Henschel's Janus 1 (1846), pp. 625–638
Helmreich: G. Helmreich, Neue Philol. Rundschau, 1890, pp. 35–37 (review of Petersen's dissertation)
Herbst, 1911
Hermann: G. Hermann, Allgemeine Schulzeitung 10 (1833), col. 923; also Opuscula, Vol. VI (Leipzig, 1835)
Hirzel, Unters.
Ilberg, BPW 1889
Jacoby: F. Jacoby, Hesiodi Carmina I: Theogonia. Berlin, 1930
Jaeger, Nemesios
Kalbfleisch, 1892
Kontos: K. Kontos, ΚΡΙΤΙΚΑ ΚΑΙ ΓΡΑΜΜΑΤΙΚΑ, ΑΘΗΝΑΙΟΝ 7 (1878), p. 111
Marquardt: J. Marquardt, Philol. Anzeiger, 1875, pp. 87–91 (review of Müller's edition of PHP); also Galenus, Scr. min., Vol. I, Praefatio
Meineke: A. Meineke, Fragmenta Comicorum Graecorum, I: Historia Critica Comicorum Graecorum (Berlin, 1839), p. XII
Mewaldt: J. Mewaldt, Galenos über echte und unechte Hippocratica, Hermes 44 (1909), p. 111
Müller, Beweis
Musgrave: S. Musgrave, Euripidis Tragoediae et Epistolae ... accedunt Fragmenta. Vol. II (Leipzig, 1779), p. 478
Nauck, TGF
Petersen, 1888
Pohlenz, 1898, 1921, and Die Stoa
Porson: R. Porson, Adversaria. Leipzig, 1814
Powell: J. Powell, Collectanea Alexandrina. Oxford, 1925
Recens. anon.: Reviewer of Müller, 1874 in Literarisches Centralblatt, 1875, cols. 49–51 (identified as Hultsch by Marquardt, Scr. min., Vol. I, p. XLV)
Reinhardt, 1921, 1953

Renehan: R. Renehan, Lectiones Galenicae, RM 108 (1965), pp. 61–70
Ruhnken: A reading at 226.20 is assigned to Ruhnken on the authority of Müller. The remainder are from D. Ruhnken, Epistola critica in Homeridarum Hymnos et Hesiodum ad virum clarissimum Ludov. Casp. Valckenarium (Leipzig, 1827), pp. 154–155.
Scaliger: A reading at 332.27 is assigned to Scaliger on the authority of Wachsmuth, who cites it from Stephanus, Poes. philos., p. 217.
Schöne: see above, p. 37
Solmsen, 1961
Troost: K. Troost, Zenonis Citiensis de rebus physicis doctrinae fundamentum. Berlin, 1891
Usener: H. Usener, Epicurea. Leipzig, 1887
Valckenaer: Euripidis Hippolytus . . . adnotatibus instruxit L. C. Valckenaer (Leiden, 1768), p. 198
Wachsmuth: C. Wachsmuth, Commentatio I de Zenone Citiensi et Cleanthe Assio. Progr. Göttingen, 1874
Wifstrand: A. Wifstrand, Eikota 6. Lund, 1957
Wilamowitz: Readings assigned to Wilamowitz are from Petersen, 1888, except the reading at 280.31, which is from Pohlenz, 1898, p. 550, and the readings at 332.27–28, which are from Hermes 54 (1919), p. 68.
Wyttenbach: Readings assigned to Wyttenbach are taken from Bake, 1810, pp. 260–286.

B. Indirect tradition

1. References to the title

The title in H and CL always has the form περὶ τῶν Ἱπποκράτους καὶ Πλάτωνος δογμάτων. This form is found also in other works of Galen that make specific reference to PHP. I have noted the following passages:

Ars med. 37 (I 409 K.)
Anat. vii. 8 (II 615 K.)
UP i. 16; iv. 13; vi. 11, 18; vii. 17; viii. 4, 6, 11; xv. 5; xvi. 3 (III 45; 310; 462; 501; 589; 625; 642; 667; IV 239; 277 K.).[1]
De respir. usu 5 (IV 510 K.)
De foet. form. 5 (IV 679 K.)
An in art. nat. sang. cont. 8 (IV 732 K.)

[1] At Gal., UP iv. 13; xv. 5; xvi. 3 (III 310; IV 239, 277 K.) τε is added before καί. At ix. 4 (III 699 K.) the phrase is ὁπότ' ἐξηγούμεθα τά θ' Ἱπποκράτους καὶ Πλάτωνος δόγματα. At i. 16 Helmreich reports (Vol. I, p. 33.3 of his edition) that ms. C (Par. 985) gives the title in the form περὶ τῶν καθ' Ἱπποκράτην καὶ Πλάτωνα δογμάτων (see below).

De san. tuend. i. 8. 12 (CMG V 4.2, p. 19)
De sympt. caus. i. 2 (VII 91 K.)
De plenit. 3 (VII 523 K.); cf. 10 (VII 563 K.): τῆς (sc. πραγματείας) τῶν Ἱπποκράτους καὶ Πλάτωνος δογμάτων
De marcore 5 (VII 683 K.)
De loc. aff. i. 1; iii. 5; iii. 9 (VIII 19; 159; 174 K.)
De praesagit. ex puls. iv. 12 (IX 425 K.)
Meth. med. i. 2; ix. 10; xii. 5 (X 14; 635; 840; 842 K.)
De simpl. med. temp. et fac. v. 9 (XI 731 K.)
In Hipp. Prorrhet. comm. i. 4 (CMG V 9.2, p. 17)
In Hipp. Progn. comm. i. 23 (CMG V 9.2, p. 236)
In Hipp. Epid. VI comm. iii. 18; v. 5 (CMG V 10.2.2, pp. 153; 271; 274)
De libr. prop. 1, 2, 13 (Scr. min., Vol. II, pp. 96, 100, 122 Müller = XIX 15, 20, 46 K.)

At the beginning of Books II through VI, the Aldine gives the title in the form, περὶ τῶν καθ' Ἱπποκράτην καὶ Πλάτωνα δογμάτων. This same form is also found once in ms. M (at the beginning of Book II), once in F (introducing the first excerpt), and twice in Q (attached to the excerpts that begin at *664.9* and *673.17*). It appears also as a variant in Gal., UP i. 16 (see above, p. 39 n. 1).

Nemesius, De nat. hom. 7 (p. 180 Matth.), refers to PHP in the following way: Γαληνὸς δὲ συμφώνως Πλάτωνι περὶ τῆς ὄψεως ἐν τῷ ἑβδόμῳ τῆς Συμφωνίας λέγει ....

There are also several references to PHP in Galenic works preserved only in Arabic or Latin versions. These references are consistent with the form found in H and CL. They are as follows:

In Hipp. Epid. II comm. iv (CMG V 10.1, p. 317.8–9)
In Hipp. Epid. III comm. i. 40 (CMG V 10.2.1, p. 58.22)
In Hipp. Epid. VI comm. viii (CMG V 10.2.2, p. 506.6–7)
De moribus, p. 26.6 Kraus (cf. Walzer, 1962, p. 144 n. 5)
Compend. Tim., pp. 55; 88 Kraus-Walzer
De propr. plac. (ms. Paris. Lat. 6865, fol. 172^v, col. 1, and 173^v, col. 1) [1]

2. Other testimonia

a) Galen

Galen does not quote verbatim from PHP in any of his other works, so far as I know. He refers to it frequently, however. To those passages mentioned above, in which the title is given, should perhaps be added Gal., De foet. form. 6 (IV 699, 701, 702 K.). Other passages that

[1] I am indebted to B. Einarson for information about this Latin version of Gal., De propr. plac. Einarson collated from photographs three Latin mss. that contain the work: Paris. 6865, Biturigensis 299, and Malatestianus S. V: 4.

mention the central thesis of PHP but do not refer to the work specifically may be found listed in the note to PHP *490.1–491.1*.

b) Oribasius

Oribasius (IV A. D.) quotes or alludes to the following passages:

PHP	Coll. med. rel.
126.28–31	XXIV. 3.6–8 (CMG VI 2.1, p. 12.8–17)
	lib. inc.
558.3–8	8.25 (CMG VI 2.2, p. 87.18–21)
560.3–6	8.28 (CMG VI 2.2, p. 88.6–8)
561.2–5	8.25 (CMG VI 2.2, p. 87.21–23)
562.5–11	8.25 (CMG VI 2.2, p. 87.23–28)
562.15–563.3	8.26 (CMG VI 2.2, p. 87.28–31)
564.8–11	8.27 (CMG VI 2.2, p. 87.31–34)
565.2–5	8.27 (CMG VI 2.2, pp. 87.34–88.1)
565.10–566.1	8.28 (CMG VI 2.2, p. 88.1–6)
596.9–597.12	59.4 (CMG VI 2.2, p. 160.18–35)
604.13–605.3	59.3 (CMG VI 2.2, pp. 159.32–160.4)
605.3–8	59.4 (CMG VI 2.2, p. 160.6–10)
605.15–606.1	59.4 (CMG VI 2.2, p. 160.10–12)
679.13–680.6	1.5–6 (CMG VI 2.2, pp. 75.21–76.5)

c) Nemesius of Emesa

Nemesius of Emesa (IV A. D.) borrowed from several of Galen's works, including PHP. See Pohlenz, 1898, pp. 597–608; Domański, 1900; Jaeger, Nemesios. In De nat. hom. 7 (pp. 180.5–181.9 Matth.) Nemesius cites by number the seventh book of PHP (see above, p. 40) and gives an abridgement of pages *615.15–617.2*. Other passages of PHP that are either borrowed or closely paraphrased by Nemesius are the following:

PHP	De nat. hom. (ed. Matthaei)
491.12–14	ch. 16 (p. 216.12–15)
492.3–6	16 (pp. 216.15–217.1)
492.8–9	16 (p. 217.4–5)
493.1–5	16 (p. 217.7–11)
494.2–3	16 (p. 217.11–12)
494.11–13	16 (pp. 217.14–218.1)
495.6–7	16 (p. 218.1–2)
623.4–7	7 (p. 181.10–13)
623.11	7 (p. 183.1–2)
625.1	7 (p. 182.11)
626.2–6	6 (pp. 174.3–175.1)
626.10–13	11 (p. 199.2–5)
626.17–627.1	6 (p. 175.6–8)
635.5–6	6 (pp. 175.16–176.1)
643.6–8	7 (p. 179.14–16)

d) Renaissance forgeries

The Renaissance forgeries, [Gal.], In Hipp. De alim. comm. iv (XV 224–417 K.)[1] and [Gal.], In Hipp. Epid. II comm. v (XVII A 303–479 K.)[2] contain excerpts from PHP:

PHP	In Hipp. De alim. comm.
82.20–21	XV 388.16–389.2 K.
164.2–6	XV 387.8–13 K.
164.2–7	XV 243.7–14 K.
258.13–14	XV 303.13–15 K.
543.12–14	XV 270.10–12, 361.6–7 K.
559.11–14	XV 244.10–12 K.
605.3–7	XV 263.13–16 K.
676.6–677.8	XV 252.5–253.2 K.
809.15–810.7	XV 308.8–16 K.
817.13–818.2	XV 278.9–279.1 K.
	In Hipp. Epid. II comm.
158.10–15	XVII A 314.17–315.6 K.[3]

The forger or forgers probably used printed texts, Caius for PHP I and perhaps Bas. for the rest.[4] A reading from [Gal.], In Hipp. De alim. comm. is quoted in the critical note to *809.15*. The commentary on Epid. II, according to Wenkebach, shows the influence of Foesius.

e) The Arabic translation

The Arab translator Ḥunain ibn Isḥāq (809–873 A. D.) in his missive to ʿAlī ibn Yaḥyā gives the following record of PHP and its Syriac and Arabic translations[5]: "His book On the doctrines of Hippocrates and Plato. He wrote this book in ten[6] sections. He pursues in it the aim of showing that Plato in most of the things he says agrees with Hippocrates because he took them over from him, and that

[1] See H. Diels, Sitzungsb. Berlin, 1914, pp. 128–129.

[2] See E. Wenkebach, Pseudogalenische Kommentare zu den Epidemien des Hippokrates, Abh. Berlin 1917, philos.-hist. Kl., No. 1, pp. 23–52.

[3] The parallel was noted by Müller, Beweis, p. 56 note 73.

[4] At PHP *676.8*, [Gal.], In Hipp. De alim. comm. has καὶ γὰρ συντίθεται with Bas., and at *677.6* it has καὶ γλῶττα with Ald. Bas. At *543.13*, where αὐτοῖς (the reading of H) was corrected by Cornarius to ὃ τοῖς, De alim. comm. has ὃ τοῖς at XV 361.6 K., but ὃ αὐτοῖς at XV 270.10.

[5] Über die syrischen und arabischen Galen-Übersetzungen, ed. G. Bergsträßer, Abh. f. d. Kunde d. Morgenlandes XVII. 2, Leipzig, 1925, no. 46. Another recension of Ḥunain's missive as described by Bergsträßer (Neue Materialien zu Ḥunain ibn Isḥāq's Galen-Bibliographie, Abh. f. d. Kunde d. Morgenlandes XIX. 2, Leipzig, 1932) has only insignificant textual variants. For further bibliography on Ḥunain see G. Strohmaier, Ḥunayn b. Isḥāḳ al-ʿIbādī, The Encyclopaedia of Islam, new ed., III, pp. 578–581; M. Ullmann, Die Medizin im Islam, Leiden, Köln, 1970, pp. 115–119.

[6] For this assertion, which contradicts Galen's own statement, see below, p. 44.

Aristotle was wrong where he disagreed with both of them. He explains in it all that is necessary in regard to the faculty of the leading soul, which is the source of thinking, imagination, and memory, and in regard to the three principles from which the faculties governing the body originate, and other matters from various disciplines. Ayyūb[1] had translated this book into Syriac, nobody else had translated it before. A number of Greek manuscripts were in my possession. Other matters prevented me from dealing with them. Then I translated it into Syriac and I added a treatise to it which I wrote in order to excuse Galen for what he had said in the seventh section of this book.[2] Ḥubaiš[3] translated it into Arabic for Muḥammad ibn Mūsā."

These translations have not survived, so far as is known. Excerpts, however, are contained in the following works, and no doubt in others as well. Some quotations are taken not from the translation itself, but from "summaries" (*ǧawāmi'*) made by Ḥunain and not mentioned in his letter to 'Alī ibn Yaḥyā.

1. Ḥunain's "Ten treatises on the eye" contain borrowings from PHP VII between pp. *608.7* and *642.6*.[4] They are recorded in the testimonia. Some of the same material is also found in Ḥunain's "Questions on the eye".[5]

2. The huge collection of excerpts made by Rhazes (born 865 A. D.) in his *Kitābu l-ḥāwī* (Liber continens) contains a number of more or less literal quotations from PHP[6]:

PHP	al-Ḥāwī
72.3–76.4	vol. XIII, p. 43.1–12[7]
122.29–124.5	vol. III, p. 180.6–9
148.24–26	vol. XII, pp. 217.12–218.2

1 Ayyūb ibn al-Abraš ar-Ruhāwī (died after 832 A. D.), see Ullmann, op. cit., pp. 101–102.

2 Cf. Ibn abī Uṣaibi'a, *'Uyūnu l-anbā'*, ed. A. Müller, Vol. I, Cairo, 1882, p. 198.30. A passage of this treatise is preserved in Ibn al-Muṭrān, *Bustānu l-aṭibbā'*, Ms. Bethesda/Maryland A8, fol. 58v11–59r12, Ms. Tunis (Zaitūna-Aḥmadiyya) 5400, fol. 24r24–24v13; partly translated by F. Rosenthal, Das Fortleben der Antike im Islam, Zurich, Stuttgart, 1965, pp. 45–46.

3 See Ullmann, op. cit., p. 119.

4 Ed. M. Meyerhof, Cairo, 1928, cf. pp. XLI and 20–39 (Arabic pp. 89–111) – another reference given by Meyerhof pp. XLII and 53 is erroneous. This work of Ḥunain is the source of Constantinus Africanus, De oculis and of its twin, the so-called Galeni Liber De oculis a Demetrio translatus. See P. Pansier, Constantini monachi Montiscassini Liber de oculis (Collectio Ophthalmologica Veterum Auctorum, fasc. VII), Paris, 1909–1933; and J. Hirschberg, Über das älteste arabische Lehrbuch der Augenheilkunde, Sitzungsb. Berlin, 1903, No. 49, pp. 1080–1094.

5 Le livre des questions sur l'œil de Ḥonaīn ibn Isḥāq, ed. P. Sbath and M. Meyerhof (Mémoires présentés à l'Institut d'Égypte, Vol. XXXVI), Cairo, 1938.

6 Ed. Hyderabad-Deccan, 1955 sqq. (at our disposal Vols. I–XX); references are due to Ullmann, op. cit., p. 40, and F. Sezgin, Geschichte des arabischen Schrifttums, Vol. III, Leiden, 1970, p. 106.

7 The mutilated Greek text begins in the very middle of this excerpt. A more complete version of this passage is found in Ibn al-Muṭrān, see below, p. 45.

PHP	al-Ḥāwī
526.4–7	vol. XII, p. 224.5–10
611.11–13 (cf. *612.12*)	vol. II, p. 219.5–7
693.7–10; *696.13–15*	vol. I, p. 84.14–15
755.4–10	vol. XIII, p. 178.2–6
756.3–9	vol. XIII, p. 178.7–10
758.11–16	vol. XIII, p. 235.3–7 (cf. p. 178.11–15)
758.16–759.3	vol. XIII, pp. 178.16–179.2
759.16–761.1	vol. XIII, p. 235.7–9 (cf. p. 179.3–7)
777.1–778.15	vol. IV, pp. 218.17–219.7
778.1–15	vol. IV, pp. 182.14–183.2
785.3–787.4	vol. XIII, pp. 235.17–236.5 (cf. p. 179.9–16)

Rhazes also quotes a passage from "the tenth book of the opinions of Hippocrates and Plato" (Vol. I, p. 17.2–4): "He said: All physicians when treating a spasm on both sides or a shivering in the whole body or a disorder or a laxness in the whole body from the lower part of the face (?) are aiming (?) by their cure at the back of the head." The Arabic text is surely corrupt and the Latin version of little help.

3. The philosopher al-Fārābī (died 950 A. D.) refers in his "Rhetoric" to an argument made by Galen in "the last chapter of PHP". The curious passage may be quoted in full[1]: "Sometimes the orator seeks to give preeminence to himself and to depreciate his adversaries with regard to something which has nothing to do with the theme of his speech, and he praises himself and depreciates his adversaries with regard to other things outside the theme about which they are arguing, as Galen did when he boasted by mentioning the preeminence of his father and his country, and when he depreciated his adversaries by mentioning the faults of their fathers and their countries. For in the book De methodo medendi, where he contradicts Thessalus the physician, he speaks of the meanness of his father's profession[2], and as he did in the last chapter of his book On the opinions of Hippocrates and Plato, where he attacks Mendapius (?)[3], who had argued against some of his statements in his book. For he depreciates him in that he hailed from villages distant from the great cities, and he praises himself in that he lived in the big city of Rome which is, as many poets had said, 'the little world'." These polemics are not found in the ninth book or elsewhere in PHP. One might assume that the expression "the last chapter" means that tenth book mentioned by Ḥunain and Rhazes. Galen here is said to defend himself against an adversary who attacked some of his statements made previously in PHP. This hints at the

[1] *Kitābu l-ḫiṭāba*, ed. J. Langhade, Mélanges de l'Université Saint-Joseph (Beirut), XLIII (1967), pp. 127.11–129.2 (reference due to Ullmann, loc. cit.); the same text in: J. Langhade and M. Grignaschi, Deux ouvrages inédits sur la rhétorique, Beirut, 1971, pp. 71 and 73.

[2] The statement is correct, cf. X 10.5 Kühn.

[3] Or Mendaberius (?), the two mss. read MNDBRYS and MNDBWYS.

possibility that Galen added this tenth book later in life and after De libris propriis where he explicitly indicates the number of books in PHP to be nine.[1] One must further assume that this tenth book, like the beginning of Book I, has been lost in the Greek textual tradition.[2]

4. 'Alī ibn Riḍwān (died 1068) in his "Useful book on how to teach the medical art" gives a further testimonium[3]: "There came into my possession his tract On the theories of Hippocrates and Plato, which I investigated. There I found him stating that only two types of man can understand what he says. The first are those who have been trained in geometry and have thus acquired for themselves a capacity for proof which prevents them from accepting erroneous statements. The second type are those with training in logic, who know its rules, so that none of their objects escapes them." The reference here could be to PHP VIII, *652.16–657.11*, where Galen chides his opponents for their lack of training in logic and their inability to follow a geometrical proof. The need for prior training in logic is a commonplace in Galen; see for example PHP II, 102.28–104.2; 112.8–12; 140.21–23; VII, *588.1–3*; IX, *742.12–13*; *817.7–8*.

5. Some quotations from PHP and from Ḥunain's summaries are found in Ibn al-Muṭrān's (died 1191 A. D.) unsystematic anthology of medical authors called "The garden of physicians and the meadow of the educated". One passage dealing with anatomical research on the heart precedes in Ibn al-Muṭrān the story of the slave of Maryllus just at the beginning of the preserved Greek text.[4] Though no explicit reference is given it seems to have been taken from the lost portion of Book I too.[5] The version of the story is more complete here than that given by Rhazes, though Ibn al-Muṭrān states that he quotes it after Ḥunain's summaries, not after the work itself.[6] Other testimonies corresponding to the Greek text are:

PHP	Ibn al-Muṭrān Ms. Bethesda	Ms. Tunis
80.4–9	fol. 9ʳ3–10	fol. 5ʳ15–21
619.9–15	fol. 6ʳ11–13	fol. [illegible]ᵛ20–22
620.9–621.2	fol. 12ᵛ5–13ʳ2	fol. 7ʳ5–15
625.16–626.1	fol. 13ʳ9–10	fol. 7ʳ20–22

6. Moses Maimonides (1139–1204 A. D.), the great Jewish philosopher and court physician to 'Alī son of sultan Saladin, quotes some passages from PHP in his Medical Aphorisms.[7] The Hebrew trans-

[1] Script. min., Vol. II, p. 122.18.

[2] [Similarly now M. Ullmann, Orient. Literaturzeitung LXXII (1977), cols. 194–195.]

[3] Engl. translation by M. C. Lyons, The *Kitāb al-Nāfi'* of 'Alī ibn Riḍwān, The Islamic Quarterly vi (1961), p. 67 (reference due to Ullmann, Die Medizin).

[4] See below, p. 72.

[5] See below among the fragments of Book I, p. 70.

[6] See above, p. 43.

[7] See Ullmann, op. cit., p. 167.

lation made by Nathan ha-Meati in Rome ca. 1280[1] has been checked with the Arabic text as extant in the Ms. Gotha 1937:

PHP	Hebrew text, ed. Muntner	Ms. Gotha
78.34–80.11	xxiv. 55[2]	fol. 237^{v}1–12
94.11–13, 16–17, 19–21	i. 10	fol. 12^{v}3–10
94.21–27	i. 11	fol. 12^{v}10–16
94.32–96.2	i. 12	fol. 12^{v}16–13^{r}4[3]
126.23–25	xxv. 71	fol. 271^{r}4–10
186.1–3	xxiv. 56	fol. 237^{v}12–16
579.6–16	xxiv. 57	fol. 237^{v}16–238^{r}9

f) The Latin translations

Several sixteenth century Latin translations were made from the Greek. All are subsequent to the first printed Greek texts. They are sometimes useful in interpreting obscure passages. Mention has already been made of Caius (above, p. 31), Andernach (p. 36), and Feliciano (p. 37). To these should be added Cornarius (below, p. 59), and Rasarius (see Durling, 1961, pp. 285–286).

II. Composition of PHP

A. Date of composition

Galen wrote the first six books of PHP during his first stay in Rome (A. D. 162–166). He wrote the last three books during his second stay, in the interval between his return to Rome (169) and the Emperor's return from the German campaign (176). In De libr. prop. 1–2 Galen informs us that the first six books were written at the urging of Boethus, a Peripatetic and a consular, who took them (along with the first book of UP) to Syria Palestina, where he was to be governor (ἄρξων), and where he died. Completion of the work was delayed by the death of Boethus and by other obstacles that Galen encountered after his return from Rome to Pergamum in 166.

[1] Ed. by S. Muntner, Moshe ben Maimon, (Medical) aphorisms of Moses, Jerusalem, 1959; cf. M. Steinschneider, Die hebräischen Übersetzungen des Mittelalters, Berlin, 1893, p. 766.

[2] References to chapters and paragraphs according to Muntner's edition.

[3] The three paragraphs following i. 12 (i. 13, 14, and 15) are also designated as having the same source as i. 12. In fact, however, they are from De motu musculorum, I, and are therefore omitted here.

When he was recalled to Rome in 169, he persuaded Marcus Aurelius to allow him to remain in the city, while Marcus was engaged in the war against the Germans. The war proved to be longer than anticipated, and in the interval Galen found time to complete PHP and UP and to write a number of other works. Thus A. D. 176, the date of the Emperor's return, is the latest possible date for the completion of PHP.[1]

The internal evidence is not wholly in accord with these dates. Books I–VI contain references to works of Galen that were probably written after 166, and Books VII–IX to works written after 176. The following works are cited in PHP I–VI (listed in the order in which they are first mentioned):

De usu part.	PHP 88.8
De anat. administr.	88.8–9
De motu musc.	94.18
De nerv. diss.	98.33
De demonstr.	102.27
De recta nom. rat.	104.20–21
De voce	122.4
De thorac. pulmon. motu	124.21
De caus. respir.	124.27
De respir. usu	128.14
De Hipp. anat.	*516.3–4*
De nat. fac.	*546.5–6*
De semine	*559.4*
De usu puls.	*564.15*

There is also reference to a projected treatise on the genuine works of Hippocrates (*517.10–11*), and possibly also to a work on cartilages (122.7–9), to the lost De coloribus (*565.9*), and to certain projected Hippocratic and Platonic commentaries (*577.9–10*).[2]

Of the works on the list, Books II–XVII of UP, along with De motu musc., De respir. usu, De nat. fac., De usu puls., and possibly De semine were written after 166; see Ilberg, RM 1889, pp. 217–218; Bardong, 1942, pp. 633–634. One must suppose, therefore, either that Galen had begun them before 166, or that he inserted references to them at some later date. The simplest explanation, offered by Il-

[1] The basic work on the chronology of Galen's writings was done by J. Ilberg. For PHP see especially RM 1889, pp. 217–218, 228–229. In a later article (Ilberg, 1905) he corrected his earlier dating of the first stay in Rome. Discussions of chronology may be found also in Vogt, 1910, pp. 1–8; Bardong, 1942; and J. Mewaldt, "Galenos" (2), RE 7 (1912), cols. 578–581. See also the useful entry "(Aelius) Galenus" in PIR IV^2 (1952), pp. 4–6, and, for Boethus, "Flavius Boethus", PIR III^2 (1943), p. 140. W. Weber in CAH XI^2 (1954), p. 362, dates Marcus' return to Rome in November, 176.

[2] The reference here may be to Galen's commentary on the Timaeus; see the note to *565.9*.

berg, is that at the time when he undertook the completion of PHP he made some additions to the books already written.

Books VII–IX contain references to the following additional works:

De virt. diff.	PHP *596.5–6*; cf. *662.8–13*
De instr. odor.	*626.15*
De part. homoeom. diff.	*684.11–13*
De elem. sec. Hipp.	*692.1*
De crisib.	*704.5*
De febr. diff.	*704.5–6*
In Hipp. Aph. comm.	*711.5–6*
Adv. Lycum	*711.6–7*
In Hipp. De off. med. comm.	*733.6–7*
In Hipp. De acut. victu comm.	*777.12–13*
De anim. speciebus	*825.11*

There is also a reference (*686.5–6*) to a projected work on the medical passages in Plato's Timaeus.

Of the items on this second list, Bardong (p. 630) would assign three (De crisib., De febr. diff., In Hipp. Aph. comm.) to the end of the period within which PHP was completed, and three (Adv. Lycum, In Hipp. De off. med. comm., In Hipp. De acut. vict. comm.) to the period after 176. It seems probable, therefore, that Galen revised the last three books of PHP at some time subsequent to the period in which he says they were written.[1] The extent of the revision is impossible to determine.

B. The plan of PHP

Although Galen's initial statement of his purpose in writing PHP has been lost, it is evident that he intended to show not only that Plato and Hippocrates agreed in their views of the powers that control the activities of animals, but also that their views were correct, and that their proofs were "scientific". This much is accomplished in Books I–VI. Whether the subjects discussed in Books VII–IX (sense-perception, elements, and methods of inquiry) were included in the initial plan is not clear, but it seems probable that Galen did not intend to limit himself to the discussion of the three powers.

[1] See Vogt, 1910, p. 8; and with reference to Gal., Adv. Lycum, E. Kind, "Lykos", RE 13 (1927), cols. 2413–2415. G. Strohmaier, Über die Verschiedenheit der homoiomeren Körperteile, in arab. Übers. hrsg., übers. u. erl., CMG Suppl. Or. III, Berlin, 1970, p. 34, gives reason to believe that the reference to De part. hom. diff. may also be a later insertion.

Thus the first two testimonies to the lost portion of Book I indicate that his plan was to include all points of agreement between Hippocrates and Plato.

The work is in large part polemical. Galen defends the position of Hippocrates and Plato against all who reject it. He begins in Book I his discussion of the rational part of the soul, and he tells us early in Book II (102.8–104.2) that his plan was to divide the refutation of mistaken views into two parts, first, the refutation of those who base their arguments on false premises (for example, that the heart is the source of the nerves), and second, the refutation of those whose reasoning is faulty. This division forms the plan of the first two books (cf. *651.7–16*). Presumably Galen intended then to proceed in Book III to the discussion of the other two parts of the soul (cf. 156.15–19).

At the beginning of Book III, however, Galen announces a change of plan. The first two books had evidently been circulated, and an "eminent sophist" had accused Galen of not answering all the arguments used by Chrysippus to prove that the rational part of the soul is in the heart. Galen decided, therefore, at the urging of his friends, to continue the refutation of Stoicism in the third book (cf. 168.26–170.2; 204.34–206.2; 214.30–33; 232.24–29; *581.8–582.5*), and to postpone to Book IV the discussion of the virtues, which was to have been included in Book III (168.23–24).[1] He selected as a target for his criticism Chrysippus' work On the Soul. Before he had completed the third book he decided to extend the criticism of Stoicism into Book IV, with an attack on Chrysippus' theory of the affections and on his treatment of conflicts between the affections and reason (214.27–30; cf. *583.15–584.4*; *653.6–654.8*). His chief target in the fourth book is Chrysippus' work On the Affections.

As it turned out, the discussion of the affections was not confined to a single book (cf. 290.20–27). The expansion resulted, in part at least, from a decision to strengthen his case by pointing out that even the Stoic Posidonius rejected the Chrysippean theory of the affections in favor of the Platonic view (cf. *584.4–7*). Posidonius' name first appears at 248.3, about one-fourth of the way through Book IV, and his disagreements with Chrysippus occupy a prominent place in the latter half of the book (cf. 264.17–270.9; 280.18–290.27). He continues to be a central figure in the first two-thirds of Book V, until finally, at 336.15, the refutation of Chrysippus is concluded.

It must have seemed to Galen that the long digression on Stoicism provided an adequate account of both the rational and the spirited parts of the soul. At any rate, after concluding the digression he does not go on to discuss the spirited part but rather rounds out

1 Whether this proposed discussion of the virtues was itself a modification of the plan announced at 156.15–19 is not clear. No doubt Galen planned to adopt Plato's scheme in Republic IV, where the four principal virtues are defined in terms of the three parts of the soul. See 156.9–11; 354.21–25, and finally *588.1–596.3*, where the virtues are actually discussed in Platonic terms.

Book V with a presentation of the arguments that Plato used in Republic IV to differentiate the three parts of the soul. At the very end of the book (358.20–22) he announces that in the next book he will prove that the three parts occupy different positions in the body.

At the beginning of Book VI the argument is again interrupted long enough for Galen to clear up some ambiguities. After first restating his overall purpose, he goes on to explain in what sense one may speak of the activities (ἐνέργειαι) and the affections (πάθη) of the parts of the soul (*491.8–499.10*). Then he raises the question whether the three parts should be called parts (μέρη) or forms (εἴδη), and on the authority of Plato he states that they are both parts and forms (*499.11–506.3*). After these preliminaries he turns to the proof that each of the parts has its own place in the body, the rational in the head, the spirited in the heart, and the desiderative in the liver. Dismissing the first two items as already proved, he spends the remainder of the book (*506.6–580.6*) on the liver and veins. At the end he takes a parting shot at Chrysippus (*577.15–580.6*).

Books VII, VIII, and IX exhibit the same looseness of structure as the earlier books. Book VII begins with a backward look at the long digression on Stoicism (*581.1–588.1*), then turns to the discussion of the virtues that had been promised in Book III (168.23–24). This discussion (*588.1–596.9*) is cut short, however, with a promise of a separate work on the virtues (*596.4–6*). The rest of VII is about the brain, the nerves, and the sense organs, including a long passage on vision.

The eighth book, like the seventh, begins with a recapitulation (*649.1–662.13*). Galen summarizes the content of Books I–VI and puts the blame for their length on his adversaries. He does not include Book VII in the summary, apart from a very brief reference to the discussion of the virtues (*662.6–13*).[1] The remainder of VIII presents an account of the four elements. This topic has no direct connection with the psychological doctrines presented in the earlier books; rather, it is introduced as another instance of agreement between Hippocrates and Plato (cf. *662.14–663.1*). In the course of the discussion Galen quotes extensively from both sources.

The ninth book deals with yet another point of similarity between Hippocrates and Plato: their views on the correct method of "distinguishing between similars" (*729.5–6*). At the end of the book (*813.13–827.5*) Galen indicates how this method is relevant to the inquiry about the three parts of the soul. Thus he brings the entire work to an appropriate conclusion.

[1] The separate work on the virtues, promised in VII, has now been written. There must have been an interval, though perhaps not a very long one, between the writing of VII and VIII.

C. Morphology, syntax, style

Galen's aim was to conform to the best standards of Attic Greek.[1] Departures from these standards are not infrequent, however, and the editor is often faced with the question whether or not to remove an irregularity by emendation. Since no comprehensive study of Galen's language and style has yet been made, and since in other respects Galen's works give indications of hasty writing, it is the practice in this edition to be rather tolerant of irregularities, especially when they cannot be readily accounted for on palaeographical grounds.

Ionic forms:

Ionic forms sometimes appear in Galen's text, usually in proximity to quotations from Hippocrates. In general they have been retained, since it is possible that they were intended as deliberate echoes of Hippocratic language. Examples may be found at 164.3; *697.6*, *7*; *779.10*; *782.5*, *9*; *783.15*. At *817.1* (ἰητρικήν) there is no nearby quotation to account for the form. A curious reversal is found at *717.9–10*: the Hippocratic passage has a non-Ionic phrase (εἰς ἑαυτόν), whereas Galen in his comment uses the Ionic ἐς ἑωυτόν. Descendants of H have restored normal usage.

Other variations in spelling and morphology:

Variations between γίνομαι and γίγνομαι, ἐς and εἰς, and the like, have been allowed to stand, though usually one or the other form is dominant. Thus γίγνομαι is far more frequent than γίνομαι. μικρός is found after both vowels and consonants, σμικρός only after vowels, with the exception of σμικρύνοντι at *514.1*. τέτταρες outnumbers τέσσαρες three to one. The accusative case of the proper nouns Ἀριστοτέλης and Ἱπποκράτης presents a special problem, as these names are usually abbreviated. In those passages where they are written in full, ms. CL prefers the accusative in -η (82.2 is an exception), H the accusative in -ην.[2] When H and CL differ in a matter of this kind, the reading of H has been adopted, unless otherwise noted.

The forms μηθέν and οὐθέν occur only in quotations from Chrysippus. See for example 224.21; 274.37; 284.13. There is one instance (340.14) of the comparative ὀλιγώτερον, and one (*556.10*) of οἴδασι. The form παρεβίασεν is allowed to stand at 170.1; see LSJ s. v. παρα-

[1] See especially G. Herbst, 1911.

[2] H writes ἀριστοτέλην at *508.13* and ἱπποκράτην at *665.16*. In each case the following word begins with a consonant. CL has ἀριστοτέλη at 90.27 and 92.23, ἱπποκράτη at 96.7 and 148.33, but ἱπποκράτην at 82.2. H has the dative ἱπποκράτη at *665.17* and *666.13*, but ἱπποκράτει at *685.4*; *745.2*; *765.2*, *6*.

βιάζομαι. The dual ἔστον has been admitted as an emendation at 292.14; compare Gal., Meth. med. iii. 3 (X 178.9 K.) and De nat. fac. iii. 15 (Scr. min., Vol. III, p. 253.16). Perhaps it is a platonism (see PHP *631.1* and *8*).

Unaugmented pluperfects are not uncommon[1], for example at 112.26; 144.10; 232.21; *662.1*. At 268.2 the form βέβλητο is used by Posidonius in a paraphrase of the Iliad.

The unassimilated form πάνκαλον appears to be the correct reading at *781.11* (H has πᾶν καλόν), and παλινκοτέῃ is found at *787.3*. Both are in quotations from Hippocrates.

The spelling ἔννατος at *501.5* and *504.2* has been tacitly corrected.

Some syntactical items:

ἄν is found with the future indicative after ὥστε at 78.13–14. In spite of Marquardt's defense, the reading has not been allowed to stand; see the note ad loc.

ἀπάρχομαι governs an infinitive at 204.24.

δείκνυμι is followed by an infinitive in the sense of "show that" at *520.1*; *597.13–14*, and of "show how" at *765.13*; see Kühner-Gerth II 2, p. 71. ἐπιδείκνυμι is followed bv an infinitive at 170.31–32; *764.1–2*; *821.6–7*, and by emendation at *587.11–13*.

Sometimes neuter plural subjects take plural verbs, e. g. at *729.6–7*; *766.3*, *6*; *808.13*. This construction is found also in quotations from Hippocrates; cf. *694.8* and Gal., In Hipp. De off. med. comm. ii. 23 (XVIII B 777 K.).

An infinitive takes the place of a finite verb at *668.2–4* (συγχεῖσθαι after ὡς in oratio obliqua). Chrysippus especially seems to have favored the infinitive; cf. 104.30; 170.12, 15; 172.26; 174.5; 200.29.

There are some questionable instances of neuter participles used as accusative absolutes: 74.17 γενόμενον, 150.30 ἀποδεδειγμένον, *528.7* θεωρούμενον, *556.2* κωλῦον, *681.13* γιγνόμενον, and *783.10* δυνάμενον. The first two and the last two have been removed by emendation.

There is a lack of parallelism in the syntactical units connected by μέν and δέ at *529.11–15*, where a participial phrase is correlated with a finite verb.

Hapax legomena:

656.1 ἀντιτεχνίτης
106.6 παρενσημαίνουσα (Chrysippus; not in LSJ).

Hiatus:

It is well established that Galen accepted the avoidance of hiatus as a principle of style. H. Diels, 1875, p. 155, first pointed out that

[1] See G. Helmreich, Acta Sem. Erlang. 2 (1881), p. 304.

this principle applies to PHP, and J. Petersen, 1888, pp. 37–52, examined in some detail the violations, real or apparent, that one finds in PHP. He drew up a list of conditions under which hiatus appears to be tolerated, and in a number of places he attempted to eliminate improper hiatus by altering the text.[1] But the boundary that divides proper from improper hiatus is not at all distinct, and the assumption that all instances of improper hiatus result from textual corruption puts an impossible burden on the editor.[2] Perhaps it is more prudent to assume that in the main Galen avoided hiatus, employing for that purpose the familiar devices of later Greek prose, but that he was not so enslaved to the principle that he felt constrained to follow it on every occasion.

Galen's conscious use of devices for avoiding hiatus may be seen in the following examples, which could be multiplied many times over. When a vowel precedes, he uses λέλεκται rather than εἴρηται (cf. *637.14*; *770.10*), and πᾶς rather than ἅπας (cf. *510.13*; *550.10*).[3] When a vowel follows, he uses μέχρι περ and ἄχρι περ rather than μέχρι and ἄχρι (cf. *551.3*; *560.13*), and ἀποδεικνύειν rather than ἀποδεικνύναι (cf. 104.1; 198.33).

Under certain circumstances, however, hiatus is tolerated. The least ambiguous of these are the following:

1. In quotations from other authors, and in close paraphrases of such quotations.
2. In technical and formulaic language. Examples may be found at 80.22; *530.11*; *555.10*; *661.2*.
3. In certain set phrases, such as εὖ ἔχει, εὖ οἶδα, εἰ οὕτως ἔτυχε, εἴη ἄν, τί or τι ἄν, τί or τι ἄλλο.
4. Where elision or aphaeresis is possible, for example after ἄρα, ἔτι and οὐκέτι, verb forms ending in -μεθα, participles ending in -τα, nouns ending in -μα; and before ἐχρῆν (*528.11*).
5. After καί, μή, and the article, and before and after ἤ.
6. In a pause. See Petersen, 1888, p. 46; Marquardt, Scr. min., Vol. I, pp. L–LI.

In a number of other situations hiatus is found in the manuscripts, but infrequently, as though avoidance were preferred but not required:

7. After εἰ, ὅτι and διότι, περί, πρό, τί and τι.
8. Before ὡς and ὥσπερ, perhaps made tolerable by the slight pause that often precedes these words. As one would expect, καθάπερ is often used in place of ὥσπερ after vowels, rarely after consonants.

[1] On Galen's avoidance of hiatus see also Marquardt, Scr. min., Vol. I, pp. XLVII–LV; C. Kalbfleisch, Galeni Institutio Logica, pp. VII–VIII.

[2] An example of the kind of rewriting that would be required if hiatus were to be eliminated is offered by Einarson in the critical note to *519.9–11*.

[3] The forms of ἅπας are by far the more frequent when a consonant precedes. See Kalbfleisch, Inst. Log., pp. VII–VIII, and Diels, 1894, pp. 297–305.

9. After words ending in the diphthongs -αι, -ει, and -οι. Examples include nouns (e. g. *509.1*; *519.9*; *797.8*), adjectives and participles in -αι and -οι (e. g. *519.10*; *816.4*); the pronouns μοι and σοι (*787.11*; *733.12*); the adverb ἐκεῖ (138.31) and the conjunction καίτοι (84.2); and verb forms in -αι and -ει (e. g. 96.2; *665.5, 11*; *819.1*). In some instances hiatus of this kind is softened by a pause, but there is a substantial residue that yields to no easy explanation.[1] At *497.7* hiatus after ἐπεὶ has been removed by emendation; but at 90.8 the emendation ⟨ἐκφύεσθαι⟩ ἐκ introduces hiatus.

10. After -η (including δή) and -ῃ. See for example 90.14–15; 108.1; 110.5; 138.30; 170.6; 248.18; 256.18; *506.7*; *523.12–13*; *531.15*; *720.13*; *723.1*; *797.9*; *819.1*. Hiatus follows ᾗ at *758.6* and *7* in semi-technical language. At *652.7* and *656.15* there is hiatus after ταύτῃ in an argument. Hiatus has been removed by emendation after ἤδη at *581.8*.

11. After -ου. See 168.29; 214.17; 276.29; 306.10; *519.14*; *536.3*; *715.7*; *777.15–16*; *819.11*. Hiatus follows τούτου at *689.9*; it has been removed by emendation after πρώτου at *534.15* and after τούτου at *535.8*.

12. After -ω and -ῳ. See 92.25; 104.3; 108.26; 254.23; 280.15; 318.28; 348.7; *800.8*. It follows ᾧ at *554.12*. It has been removed by emendation after πω at 220.3 and after ᾧ at *546.9* and *616.6*.

13. After relative and personal pronouns. Petersen (p. 52) lists relative pronouns among the words after which hiatus is permitted, but the instances are few: once after ὅ (218.34), twice after ἅ (102.20; 284.24), twice after ᾗ (see paragraph 10, above), and twice after ᾧ (see paragraph 12, above). Marquardt, Scr. min. I, p. LI, lists personal pronouns also; but here the instances are even less numerous: once each after μοι and σοι (see paragraph 9, above) and once after σε (*554.17*).

14. After numerals. See Marquardt, Scr. min. I, p. LV. Again the examples are few: once after μιᾷ (*660.14*), three times after δύο (190.11, 21; 318.20), once after εἴκοσι (*663.7*), and once after τέτταρα in the phrase δὶς δύο τέτταρα εἶναι (*655.13*).

15. After forms of οὗτος. See Marquardt, Scr. min. I, p. LI. Hiatus after ταύτῃ was mentioned above in paragraph 10, after τούτου in paragraph 11. Hiatus after αὗται at *753.14* has been removed from this category by the emendation of αὗται to αὐταί. Hiatus after τοῦτο and ταῦτα falls under paragraph 4, above. There is no instance of hiatus after τούτῳ or οὗτοι.

16. After αὐτό. Petersen, p. 43, lists four examples: 152.7; 186.3; *603.8*; *612.2*. At *526.6* αὐτό before ἐστι is deleted by emendation.

[1] It is perhaps worth noting that hiatus before οὐ (οὐκ, οὐχ), οὐδέ, οὐδείς, and οὔτε often involves these diphthongs; see 248.1; 272.15; 280.30; 306.8; 324.29; 342.22; *509.1*; *518.1*; *551.12*; *734.14*; *765.3*; *805.1*. The same is true of hiatus before οὖν; cf. *491.2*; *616.9*; *651.1*. Hiatus before οὖν has been removed by emendation at *519.13*.

17. Before the article. All instances fall under some one of the headings already mentioned, except αὖ αἱ (306.12).

18. Before ἐστί. Hiatus before ἐστί, although fairly common, is not indiscriminate. In some twenty instances the preceding vowel is -ᾰ (e. g. 274.5 ἄγνοιά; 330.24 αὐτά; *559.10* τινά; *586.11* πρᾶγμά; *744.12* οἷά; *805.14* πάντα). In five cases the preceding word is ἄλλο (78.18; 260.14; 274.18; 284.27; *521.11*), and in three it is τοῦτο (218.32; *589.4*; *674.12*). Another half dozen instances occur in technical passages (definitions or syllogisms): 134.12; 142.28; 144.3; 250.11; *493.2*; *496.3* (at *656.9* the hiatus is removed by emendation). Of the remainder, one falls under paragraph 10 (ψυχή ἐστι, 306.5), one under paragraph 11 (προκειμένου ἐστί, *595.12*), one under paragraph 14 (εἴκοσί ἐστι, *663.7*), one under paragraph 16 (*526.6*), and one under paragraph 7 (εἰ ἔστιν, *798.12*).

19. Before εἶναι. See Marquardt, Scr. min. I, p. LV. All examples fall under one or another of the headings already mentioned.

20. Before ὑπάρχειν and ἔχειν. See Marquardt, Scr. min. I, p. LV. All instances fall under one or another of the headings already mentioned.

21. Before οὐ, οὐκ, οὐχ, οὐδέ, οὐδείς, οὔτε. Here hiatus is fairly common, especially after diphthongs. For diphthongs in -ι see above, note to paragraph 9. Other examples include διδομένου οὐκ (*536.3*); κόρυζα οὐδέ (140.10); ἑτέρωθι οὐ (82.37).

22. Before ἄν. See Marquardt, Scr. min. I, p. LV. All instances fall under one or another of the headings already mentioned.

23. Miscellaneous. Not otherwise accounted for are ἀμετρία αἶσχος (304.8), μηδετέρα οὖσα (*554.14*) and ἀπεφήνατο ἄγειν (*643.5*).

It is evident that the above list of the kinds of hiatus encountered in the manuscripts of PHP does not rest on any precisely formulated principle of classification, and the considerations relevant to the study of hiatus in Galen are far from clear. In the absence of firm guidelines, hiatus has generally been allowed to stand, except where some further consideration made emendation desirable.

D. Quotations from other authors

1. Hippocrates

At the time of writing PHP Galen had completed at least two works on Hippocrates, De elementis ex Hippocratis sententia, and De Hippocratis anatomia, and had perhaps begun the commentary on the Aphorisms (see above, p. 48). But PHP antedates the major commentaries, and in it Galen quotes from the Hippocratic corpus with less discrimination than in his later works. At *577.5–6*, for example, he assigns to Hippocrates a passage from De acut. morb. victu which in his commentary on that work (CMG V 9.1, pp. 305–306) he rejects as spurious. He also quotes passages from Epid. II as by Hippocrates (*571.13–574.4*; *576.12–13*), although in his commentary on Epid. II he holds that Thessalus compiled this work from Hippocrates' notes (cf. CMG V 10.1, pp. 155, 310; XVIII A 529 K.). He raises the question of authenticity in PHP only with reference to De natura hominis (cf. *516.13–16*; *665.17–666.4*), and even there he is not entirely consistent. Thus at *710.6* he uses De nat. hom. 12 as evidence for Hippocrates' view, even though this chapter belongs to that part of the work that he had rejected as spurious (see note to *516.13–14*).

In the text of the quotations editorial change has been kept at a minimum. Non-Ionic forms have been accepted, for example ὀνόματα (*689.14*), γίγνονται (*694.8*), εἰς (*695.2*).[1] The title of De natura hominis appears both as περὶ φύσεως ἀνθρώπου and as περὶ φύσιος ἀνθρώπου; cf. *666.1, 4, 6* (see CMG V 9.1, p. IX n. 3). The abbreviated quotation at *732.14–733.5* has not been expanded, as Galen himself might be responsible for the omissions. The departures of Galen's text from the manuscripts of Hippocrates have not been recorded.

2. Plato

The quotations from Plato in PHP show no consistent alignment with any of the other witnesses to the Platonic text. PHP appears to preserve a few ancient variants, for example the addition of δή before διψῇ in Rep. 439 a 9 (PHP, p. 344.21); and at 348.5 the evidence of mss. H and L points (as Einarson saw) to the reading σημαίνει γε rather than σημαίνει γάρ (Rep. 440 a 7). Editors of Plato should note that Burnet and Diès were mistaken in citing Galen as authority for the reading διαφθορᾶς διαφοράν in Sophist 228 a 8; the passage is quoted twice in PHP (302.19; 310.26), and in each case the text is corrupt.

Several Platonic passages are quoted more than once in PHP, and no doubt in most instances the differences are due to textual corruption. Thus ἅμμα (Tim. 70 b 1) alternates with ἅμα at 174.11; *569.1*, and *575.9* (see above, p. 16). When there is a possibility that the variation may go back to Galen himself, it has been allowed to stand, e. g. κάεσθαι (Tim. 85 b 6) at *705.14*, but καίεσθαι at *688.5*; and νῦν δή (Rep. 437 c 1) at *498.12*, but νῦν at 338.31. A comparison of PHP 338.25–340.6 (where Galen quotes Plato, Rep. 437 b 1 – d 1) with *498.4–499.4* (where he quotes the same passage a second time) will illustrate the problems that would be encountered if one attempted to reconstruct Plato's text from the evidence of PHP alone.

[1] Galen himself admitted Attic forms in Hippocratic texts; see Gal., In Hipp. De fract. comm. i. 1 (XVIII B 322 K.).

3. Chrysippus

PHP is a major source of verbatim quotations from Chrysippus. The textual problems raised by these quotations are especially difficult, for several reasons. First, Galen may have had a poor text of Chrysippus. In view of his hostility to Stoicism, it seems unlikely that he made as careful a study of Stoic texts as he did of the texts of Hippocrates and Plato. Second, too few Chrysippean texts have survived to provide an adequate basis for the study of his language and style. The fragments preserved in PHP are themselves among the most useful for this purpose, and little help can be got from other sources. Third, Chrysippus' Greek is difficult. Galen complains of his solecisms and his lack of clarity (cf. PHP 138.34–140.1; 192.25–194.10), and even the students of the Stoic Epictetus compared reading Chrysippus to reading Latin (Arrian, Epict. Diss. i. 17.16). It is not always possible, therefore, to draw the line between Chrysippus' Greek and textual corruption. An example may be found at 104.29–31. Finally, when Galen quotes the same Chrysippean passage more than once, the text is often found to vary. In the definition of appetition (ὄρεξις) the differences are apparently the result of textual corruption (see above, p. 34). In another passage, quoted three times (152.23–27; 170.23–27; 220.5–9), the variations may result from Galen's carelessness, and the same may be true, in part at least, of the passage quoted at 152.29–33 and 172.20–24. Other examples may be found at 222.3–6 (repeated at 234.31–236.1); 222.10–13 (repeated at 236.5–8), and 284.10–13 (repeated at 288.19–24).

A special feature of the material that Galen takes from Chrysippus is that it includes scores of verses from the Greek poets, from Homer to Menander. Some of these lines are not otherwise preserved (e. g. the hexameters at 180.14–15; 182.31; 236.3), others depart from the standard text of the poets (e. g. the lines from the Iliad quoted at 178.13–14 and 286.15–16). The passages quoted from Hesiod on the birth of Athena include nineteen lines (PHP 226.4–22) not known from any other source. They have been the subject of much controversy, the resolution of which pertains more to Hesiodic than to Galenic scholarship. In general, it is evident that the information provided by PHP about the poetic texts available to Chrysippus has only limited value because of the many textual uncertainties.

4. Posidonius

The quotations from Posidonius in PHP have had an important place in scholarly controversies about that philosopher's modifications of Stoic doctrine. The publications of Pohlenz and Reinhardt contain rather full discussions of them, and of the two, Pohlenz is in general the more helpful. The study of Posidonius' philosophy has been greatly facilitated by the publication of the fragments, edited by I. Kidd from the papers of L. Edelstein.

III. Editorial conventions

A. Critical notes

The critical notes have been made as brief as possible. All readings from the testes potiores (H, CL, and M Ald. where H is lost) have been recorded, with the following exceptions:

1. Some of the damaged and illegible letters in H are not reported, when the restoration is certain. Damaged passages in CL are sometimes not reported when the space and traces of writing are consistent with the reading of H.

2. Many of the abbreviations in H and CL are not reported, if the correct expansion is evident. It is not mentioned, for example, that at *492.7* L has the correct reading (ἑκατέρου), whereas H has an abbreviation (ἑκα$^{\tau\rho'}$) that was misinterpreted by both M (ἑκάτερον) and Ald. (ἑκατέρων).

3. Many minor errors in accents and breathings are not reported, e. g. φᾶτο (286.34), ἡρόφιλος (*651.3*), κᾶν (for κἄν, *665.15*).

4. Word divisions such as μὴ δὲ μίαν (*641.1*) and παρὰ χρῆμα (*549.11*) are not reported.

5. Trivial miswritings by H are sometimes ignored, for example *657.3* βλία H: βιβλία corr. H (βι super lin.).

6. In the variation between elided and unelided vowels (τοῦτο, τοῦτ'; δὲ, δ', and so forth), between the presence and absence of -ν (including τοσοῦτο, τοσοῦτον), between γιγν- and γιν-, -σσ- and -ττ-, κἀκ and καὶ ἐκ, and other matters of this kind, the differences between H and CL are sometimes not reported. In such cases the reading of H (or M, where H is lost) is adopted.

Readings from sources other than the testes potiores are quoted only when they are accepted or are otherwise of special interest. No attempt has been made to signalize the errors in Müller's apparatus, and many of his unsuccessful conjectures have been passed over in silence. Similarly, no mention is made of his successful emendations that have been confirmed (and supplanted) by the readings of H.

B. Division into books, chapters, sections

The division into books is clearly Galen's own, as he refers to them in the text by number; see for example *651.8, 11*; *653.12–13*; *657.7*. The books were first divided into chapters by the publishers of Latin translations.[1] The earliest division known to me is that of Cornarius (Lyons, 1550). A different division was made in the Juntine edition of 1565 and was adopted, with modifications (e. g. at 258. 23–25), by Charterius, who introduced it into the Greek text as well. Kühn followed Charterius. Müller omitted chapter numbers but retained paragraph divisions that correspond in general to the chapters in Kühn.[2] The numbered chapters in the present edition are taken from Kühn.

The division of chapters into sections is new with the present edition.

First and foremost let me express my gratitude to the Zentralinstitut für Alte Geschichte und Archäologie of the Akademie der Wissenschaften der DDR for undertaking the publication of this edition in the Corpus Medicorum Graecorum. Work on the preparation of the edition was supported at various stages by Northwestern University, Cornell University, the University of Pennsylvania, and the National Institutes of Health. The assistance received from these sources is gratefully acknowledged.

To the officers of the National Medical Library, the Library of Gonville and Caius College, the Bibliothèque Nationale, the Biblioteca Nazionale at Naples, the Laurentiana, the Marciana, the Staatsbibliothek in Berlin, and the Historical Museum in Moscow, thanks are due for providing copies of manuscripts and for granting permission to use them.

It is not possible to list by name all the many friends and colleagues who have helped with specific problems. My greatest debt is to Professor B. Einarson, who followed the work through all its stages. Einarson's emendations of the Greek text are recorded in the critical apparatus; his many other contributions must remain unnoted.

Special thanks go to Dr. G. Strohmaier of the Akademie der Wissenschaften der DDR. Dr. Strohmaier provided the section on Arabic materials in the Introduction and the translations from Arabic texts in the edition and commentary.

[1] A bibliography of Renaissance Latin translations of PHP may be found in Durling, 1961.

[2] There are exceptions; for example, Müller introduced a new paragraph at 146.28, where there is no chapter break in Kühn.

Finally, it is a special pleasure to acknowledge the patient and unfailing assistance of Dr. J. Kollesch and her colleagues in the editorial office of the Corpus Medicorum Graecorum.

Philadelphia, January 15, 1977 Phillip De Lacy

ΓΑΛΗΝΟΥ

ΠΕΡΙ ΤΩΝ ΙΠΠΟΚΡΑΤΟΥΣ ΚΑΙ ΠΛΑΤΩΝΟΣ ΔΟΓΜΑΤΩΝ

ΒΙΒΛΙΑ Α′–Ε′

GALEN

ON THE DOCTRINES OF HIPPOCRATES AND PLATO

BOOKS I–V

CONSPECTVS SIGLORVM ET COMPENDIORVM

H	= Hamilton 270
H^2, H^3, H^s, H^r	= eiusdem codicis correctores (cf. supra, pp. 14–17)
C	= Cantabrigiensis Caius coll. 47/24
L	= Laurentianus 74,22
M	= Marcianus 284
R	= Mosquensis 467
Q	= Parisinus Suppl. Gr. 634
N	= Borbonicus Gr. 229 III D 15
F	= Laurentianus 74,12
P	= Parisinus Gr. 2277
p	= Parisinus Gr. 2283
Ald.	= editio Aldina, Venetiis, a. 1525
Bas.	= editio Basileensis, a. 1538
Caius	= editio Cai, Basileae, a. 1544
Chart.	= editio Charterii, Lutetiae Parisiorum, a. 1679.
Kühn	= editio Kühnii, Lipsiae, a. 1823
Müller	= editio Mülleri, Lipsiae, a. 1874
Corn.	= Cornarius in Aldinae exemplari suo nunc bibliothecae universitatis Ienensis proprio
Al. Just.	= Alexandri Justiniani lectiones vel emendationes in quarta editione Juntina

ΓΑΛΗΝΟΥ

ΠΕΡΙ ΤΩΝ ΙΠΠΟΚΡΑΤΟΥΣ ΚΑΙ ΠΛΑΤΩΝΟΣ ΔΟΓΜΑΤΩΝ

ΒΙΒΛΙΟΝ ΠΡΩΤΟΝ

Testimonia et fragmenta ad primi libri initium pertinentia

I. Hippocratis et Platonis comparatio

ἀλλὰ γὰρ οὐ πρόκειταί μοι κατὰ τήνδε τὴν πραγματείαν οὔτε ἀθροίζειν ἁπάσας τῶν ἀνδρῶν τὰς ῥήσεις οὔτ' ἐξηγεῖσθαι, μέλλοντί γε δι' ἑτέρων ὑπομνημάτων ἰδίᾳ ποιεῖσθαι τὰς ἐξηγήσεις, ὅπερ δὲ ἐναρχόμενος εἶπον, ἐπισκέψασθαί τε καὶ κρῖναι τὰ δόγματα μόνον εἴτε κατὰ πάντα ἀλλήλοις ὁμολογοῦσιν εἴτε καὶ μή.

Ἐπειδὴ περὶ πάντων ὧν ἀμφότεροι λέγουσιν ὁ Ἱ π π ο κ ρ ά τ η ς καὶ ὁ Π λ ά τ ω ν ἐπισκέψασθαι προὔκειτο, λέλεκται δ' ἤδη περὶ τῶν μεγίστην δύναμιν ἐχόντων εἰς ἰατρικήν τε καὶ φιλοσοφίαν, καιρὸς ἂν εἴη τραπέσθαι πρὸς τἄλλα.

II. De facultatibus nos regentibus

Προὔκειτο μὲν ἐξ ἀρχῆς ἐπισκέψασθαι περὶ τῶν διοικουσῶν ἡμᾶς δυνάμεων, εἴτ' ἐκ τῆς καρδίας μόνης ὁρμῶνται σύμπασαι, καθάπερ Ἀ ρ ι σ τ ο τ έ λ η ς τε καὶ Θ ε ό φ ρ α σ τ ο ς ὑπελάμβανον, εἴτε τρεῖς ἀρχὰς αὐτῶν τίθεσθαι βέλτιον, ὡς Ἱ π π ο κ ρ ά τ η ς τε καὶ Π λ ά τ ω ν ἐδόξαζον. ἐπεὶ δὲ Χ ρ ύ σ ι π π ο ς οὐ περὶ τῶν ἀρχῶν μόνον ἠμφισβήτησε πρὸς τοὺς παλαιούς, ἀλλὰ καὶ περὶ τῶν δυνάμεων αὐτῶν οὔτε τὴν θυμοειδῆ συγχωρήσας ὑπάρχειν οὔτε τὴν ἐπιθυμητικήν, ἔδοξε χρῆναι τὴν τούτου πρότερον δόξαν ἐπισκεψαμένους οὕτως ἐπανέρχεσθαι πάλιν ἐπὶ τὸ προκείμενον ἐξ ἀρχῆς, ὡς ἐγκέφαλός τε καὶ καρδία καὶ ἧπαρ ἀρχαὶ τῶν διοικουσῶν ἡμᾶς δυνάμεών εἰσιν.

Ὅτι μὲν ἀναγκαῖόν ἐστιν οὐ φιλοσόφοις μόνον ἀλλὰ καὶ ἰατροῖς, ὅσοι γε μὴ ἀλογίστως ἅπτονται τῆς τέχνης, ἐσκέφθαι περὶ τῶν διοικουσῶν ἡμᾶς δυνάμεων ὁπόσαι τέ εἰσι κατὰ γένος ὁποία τέ τις ἑκάστη κατ' εἶδος ἐν τίνι τε μάλιστα τοῦ ζῴου μορίῳ καθίδρυται, διὰ τοῦ πρώτου δέδεικται λόγου.

Περὶ τῶν Ἱ π π ο κ ρ ά τ ο υ ς καὶ Π λ ά τ ω ν ο ς δογμάτων ἐπισκέψασθαι προθέμενοι πρῶτον μὲν ἐδιδάξαμεν ἀναγκαιότατον ὑπάρχειν ἰατρικῇ

6–10] PHP 577.7–12 Müller 11–14] PHP 729.1–4 Müller 16–25] PHP 490.1–491.1 Müller 26–30] ***infra,*** **p. 168.4–8 31–66.2] PHP 649.1–4 Müller**

1–3 γαληνοῦ περὶ τῶν ἱπποκράτους καὶ πλάτωνος δογμάτων βιβλίον πρῶτον ἀκέφαλον ***in mg. add.*** **C³?**

GALEN

ON THE DOCTRINES OF HIPPOCRATES AND PLATO

BOOK I

Testimonies and fragments of the beginning of Book I

I. The comparison of Hippocrates and Plato

But it is not my purpose in this treatise either to assemble all the passages from these men or to interpret them, since I intend to present my interpretations separately in other treatises. My present purpose, as I stated at the outset, is to examine and judge their views only in respect to the question whether or not they agree with each other on every point.

Since it was my purpose to look into all points of agreement between Hippocrates and Plato, and I have already spoken of the matters of major importance for medicine and philosophy, it is now time to turn to those that remain.

II. Inquiry into the powers that govern us

It was my purpose at the beginning to inquire about the powers that govern us, whether they all have the heart as their only source, as Aristotle and Theophrastus supposed, or whether it is better to posit three sources for them, as Hippocrates and Plato believed. But since Chrysippus disputed with the ancients not only about the sources but also about the powers themselves and did not admit the existence of either the spirited or the desiderative (power), I decided that I must first examine his view and then return to my original plan, which was to show that the brain, the heart, and the liver are the sources of the powers that govern us.

In the first book I pointed out that it is necessary not only for philosophers, but also for all physicians who approach the art rationally, to have inquired about the powers that govern us, how many they are in kind, what is the specific nature of each, and in what part of the animal each power mainly resides.

When we undertook to examine the teachings of Hippocrates and Plato, we first showed that it is most necessary for medicine τε καὶ φιλοσοφίᾳ, εἴτε πλείους εἰσὶ δυνάμεις αἱ διοικοῦσαι τὸν ἄνθρωπον εἴτε μία, βεβαίως ἐξευρεῖν.

Περὶ τῶν Ἱπποκράτους καὶ Πλάτωνος δογμάτων ἐπισκέψασθαι προθέμενος ἀπὸ τοῦ πρώτου κατὰ τὴν δύναμιν ὑπηρξάμην, ᾧ καὶ τἄλλα σχεδὸν ἅπαντα τὰ κατὰ μέρος ἀκολουθεῖν ἔδειξα, τοῦτο δέ ἐστι τὰ περὶ τῶν διοικουσῶν ἡμᾶς δυνάμεων ὁπόσαι τέ εἰσι τὸν ἀριθμὸν ὁποία τέ τις ἑκάστη καὶ τόπον ὅντιν' ἐν τῷ ζῴῳ κατείληφεν.

οὐδὲν γὰρ οὕτως ἐναργές ἐστιν ὡς τὸ δυνάμεις τινὰς ἐν ταῖς ἡμετέραις εἶναι ψυχαῖς ἐφιεμένας φύσει, τὴν μὲν ἡδονῆς τὴν δὲ κράτους καὶ νίκης, ἃς ἐναργῶς ὁρᾶσθαί φησι κἀν τοῖς ἄλλοις ζῴοις ὁ Ποσειδώνιος, ὥσπερ καὶ ἡμεῖς ἐπεδείξαμεν εὐθὺς ἐν ἀρχῇ τοῦ πρώτου γράμματος.

III. De demonstratione

... παρεκάλουν τε διὰ τοῦ πρώτου τῶνδε τῶν ὑπομνημάτων ἐν ἐκείνῃ (sc. τῇ ἀποδεικτικῇ μεθόδῳ) γυμνάσασθαι πρότερον, ὅστις ὁτιοῦν ἀποδεικνύειν ἐπιχειρεῖ.

ἀλλ' ἀπό γε τῶν προαιρετικῶν ἀρξάμενοι καθ' ἃς καὶ τὸ καλούμενον ἰδίως ἡγεμονικόν ἐστι τῆς ψυχῆς, ἕνα λόγον ἐδείκνυμεν ἠρωτῆσθαι μόνον ἐπιστημονικῶς ἀπ' αὐτοῦ τοῦ ζητουμένου τῆς οὐσίας ἔχοντα τὰς προτάσεις, ὄντα τοιοῦτον· «ὅπου τῶν νεύρων ἡ ἀρχή, ἐνταῦθα καὶ τὸ τῆς ψυχῆς ἡγεμονικόν.» αὕτη μὲν ἡ τοῦ λόγου κυριωτάτη πρότασις ὡμολογημένη πᾶσιν ἰατροῖς τε καὶ φιλοσόφοις· ἡ δ' οἷον πρόσληψις αὐτῆς ἀληθὴς μὲν «ἡ ἀρχὴ τῶν νεύρων ἐν τῷ ἐγκεφάλῳ», ψευδὴς δὲ «ἡ ἀρχὴ τῶν νεύρων ἐν καρδίᾳ», γράφειν μὲν ταύτην τὴν πρότασιν ἢ καὶ λέγειν τοῖς ἀπείροις ἀνατομῆς δυναμένου τινός, οὐ μὴν δεῖξαί γε δυναμένου.

IV. De animae principiis

οὐ γὰρ τὴν κατὰ δύναμιν ἀρχὴν ἐνδείκνυται τοῦτο συγχωρηθὲν ὑπὲρ ἧς νῦν ζητοῦμεν, ἀλλὰ τὴν κατὰ γένεσιν. – εἴρηται δέ μοι καὶ διώρισται σαφῶς ὑπὲρ τῆς διαφορᾶς τῶν ἀρχῶν ἐν τῷ πρόσθεν λόγῳ.

ἆρ' οὖν ὅτι κατὰ τὴν πρώτην διάπλασιν ἐκ καρδίας ἡ γένεσις αὐτῶν ἐστι, διὰ τοῦτ' ἀρχὴν ἕξουσι τὴν καρδίαν αἱ φλέβες; ἀλλ' οὔτε περὶ τῆς τοιαύτης ἀρχῆς ἡ ζήτησις ἦν, ὡς ἐν τῷ πρώτῳ γράμματι κατ' ἀρχὰς εὐθέως διώρισται.

ἐφεξῆς δ' ἐπὶ τὴν ζήτησιν αὐτῶν τραπόμενοι κατὰ τὸν ἀποδεικτικὸν νόμον ἔννοιαν ὁμολογουμένην ἔφαμεν εἶναι τοῦ τῆς ψυχῆς ἡγεμονικοῦ τὸ κατάρχον αἰσθήσεώς τε καὶ κινήσεως τῆς κατὰ προαίρεσιν.

3–7] *infra*, p. 102.4–8 8–11] *infra*, p. 288.14–18 14–16] *infra*, p. 102.28–104.2 17–25] PHP 650.4–15 Müller 27–29] *infra*, p. 160.31–34 30–33] PHP 544.3–7 Müller 34–36] PHP 649.5–8 Müller and philosophy to discover with certainty whether the powers that govern man are one or more than one.

Having proposed to investigate the teachings of Hippocrates and Plato, I began with the doctrine that is first in importance, from which I showed that very nearly all particular details follow; this is their teaching about the powers that govern us, their number, the nature of each, and the place that each occupies in the body.

Nothing is so evident as that there are certain powers in our souls, one of which naturally pursues pleasure, the other mastery and victory. These powers, Posidonius says, are clearly seen also in the lower animals; and we too made this same point at the very beginning of the first book.

III. The apodeictic method

... and throughout the first book of this treatise I exhorted everyone who undertakes any demonstration first to train himself in that (sc. scientific) method.

Beginning our inquiry with the voluntary movements which are the province of that part of the soul that is specifically designated as governing, we showed that only one argument was formulated scientifically, having its premises from the essence of the very thing being investigated. It is the following: "Where the beginning of the nerves is, there is also the governing part of the soul." This, the primary premise of the argument, has been agreed to by all physicians and philosophers. Its added premise, as it were, "The beginning of the nerves is in the brain" is true; but "The beginning of the nerves is in the heart" is false. You can write this latter premise, you can even say it to persons unfamiliar with anatomy; but you cannot prove it.

IV. The first principles of the soul

For this (premise), if granted, does not point to the beginning that pertains to power, which is what we are now looking for, but that which pertains to origin. – In the preceding book I discussed and clearly distinguished the different kinds of beginnings.

Could he say that the veins have the heart as their source because at their first formation their origin is from the heart? But the inquiry, as initially defined at the beginning of the first book, was not concerned with this kind of source.

Then, turning to the investigation of these powers by the law of scientific proof, we said that it is a generally acknowledged concept that the source of perception and voluntary movement belongs to the governing part of the soul.

V. De anatomia nervorum

μακροτέρων οὖν λόγων ἐδεήθημεν εὐθὺς ἐν τῷ πρώτῳ βιβλίῳ διὰ τοὺς ἃ μηδ' ὅλως εἶδον ὡς ἀκριβῶς ἰδόντας ἐπιχειρήσαντας γράφειν, ἠναγκάσθημέν τε καὶ νεύρων καὶ ἀρτηριῶν ἀνατομὴν ἐπὶ κεφαλαίων ἐν αὐτῷ διελθεῖν.

οὐκ ὀκνήσομεν δὲ κἀνταῦθα τὴν ἀνατομὴν ἑρμηνεῦσαι τῶν ἀρτηριῶν, ὥσπερ ἔμπροσθεν τῶν νεύρων.

ἀλλ' εἰ καὶ νεῦρά τις εἶναι συγχωρήσειεν αὐτὰ καὶ μὴ νευρώδη σώματα, τό γε τὴν καρδίαν ὑπάρχειν νεύρων ἀρχὴν οὐκ ἐξ ἀνάγκης ἕπεται μὴ δυναμένων ἡμῶν ἐπιδεῖξαι μηδὲν νεῦρον εἰς μηδὲν μόριον τοῦ σώματος ἀπ' αὐτῆς φερόμενον, ὡς ἔμπροσθεν ἐδείξαμεν ἀπ' ἐγκεφάλου τε καὶ νωτιαίου.

φαίνεται γάρ, ὡς ἔμπροσθεν ἐδήλωσα, τὰ μὲν ἐξ ἐγκεφάλου τῶν νεύρων ἄντικρυς ἐκπεφυκότα, τὰ δὲ ἐκ τοῦ νωτιαίου μυελοῦ, νωτιαῖος δὲ αὐτὸς ἐξ ἐγκεφάλου.

... ὡς ἔμπροσθεν ἐδήλωσα τὴν τῶν νεύρων εἰς ἅπαντα τοῦ ζῴου τὰ μόρια νομήν ...

... ἀλλ' ὡς ἔμπροσθεν εἴρηται σμικρὸν (sc. νεῦρον) ἀπ' ἐγκεφάλου κατιὸν εἰς αὐτὴν (sc. τὴν καρδίαν) ἐμφύεται.

ὅτι μὲν γὰρ ἀρχὴ νεύρων ἁπάντων ἐγκέφαλός τε καὶ νωτιαῖος καὶ ὡς αὐτοῦ τοῦ νωτιαίου πάλιν ἐγκέφαλος, ἀρτηριῶν δ' ἁπασῶν καρδία, φλεβῶν δ' ἧπαρ, καὶ ὡς τὰ μὲν νεῦρα παρ' ἐγκεφάλου τὴν ψυχικὴν δύναμιν, αἱ δ' ἀρτηρίαι παρὰ καρδίας τὴν σφυγμικήν, αἱ φλέβες δ' ἐξ ἥπατος τὴν φυτικὴν λαμβάνουσιν, ἐν τοῖς Περὶ τῶν Ἱπποκράτους καὶ Πλάτωνος δογμάτων ἀποδέδεικται.

VI. Stoicorum refutatio

ἄντικρυς μὲν ψευδῆ τὰ τοιαῦτα, περὶ ὧν ἐν τῷ πρώτῳ βιβλίῳ διῆλθον ἐπὶ πλέον, ὅταν ἤτοι μηδὲν τῶν ἀλόγων ζῴων ἐπιθυμεῖν τις ἢ θυμοῦσθαι φάσκῃ, καθάπερ οἱ ἀπὸ τῆς Στοᾶς, ἢ πάλιν ἐκ καρδίας πεφυκέναι τὰ νεῦρα.

ἠξίουν τε μηδὲν οὕτω φυλάττεσθαι κατὰ τὸν λόγον ὡς τὸ τοῖς ἐναργῶς φαινομένοις ἐναντία τίθεσθαι, καθάπερ οἵ τε μηδὲν ἄλογον ζῷον ἐπιθυμεῖν ἢ θυμοῦσθαι φάσκοντες οἵ τε τὴν ἀρχὴν τῶν νεύρων ὑπάρχειν ἐν τῇ καρδίᾳ. ἀποτετόλμηται γὰρ ἅπαντα τὰ τοιαῦτα πρὸς ἀνθρώπων ἀνατρέψαι φιλονεικούντων ὅσα καλῶς εἴρηται τοῖς παλαιοῖς, ὑπὲρ τοῦ

2–5] PHP 651.7–11 Müller 6–7] *infra*, p. 82.18–19 8–12] *infra*, p. 96.24–28 13–15] *infra*, p. 80.30–32 16–17] *infra*, p. 86.8–9 18–19] *infra*, p. 96.13–14 20–25] Gal. UP i. 16: I, pp. 32.23–33.4 Helmr. = III 45.9–15 K. 27–30] *infra*, p. 102.22–25 31–70.2] *infra*, p. 102.8–15

V. The anatomy of the nerves

So we needed an extended discussion already in the first book because of those (men) who tried to write of things they did not see at all, as if they saw them with precision; and we were compelled to give in that book a summary of the anatomy of nerves and arteries.

But we shall not hesitate here again to explain the anatomy of the arteries, as we did earlier of the nerves.

But even if one should admit that they are nerves, not nerve-like structures, it does not follow of necessity that the heart is the source of nerves, since we cannot point to any nerve passing from it to any part of the body in the way that we earlier pointed out their passage from brain and spine.

For it is obvious, as I demonstrated earlier, that some nerves grow out directly from the brain, others from the spinal cord, and the spinal cord itself from the brain.

. . . as I had earlier explained the distribution of nerves to all parts of the body . . .

. . . but a small one (sc. nerve), as we said before, descends from the brain and grows into it (sc. the heart).

In the treatise On the Doctrines of Hippocrates and Plato it was demonstrated that the source of all nerves is the brain and spinal cord and that the source of the spinal cord itself is again the brain, the source of all arteries is the heart, of all veins the liver, and that the nerves receive psychic power from the brain, the arteries the power of pulsation from the heart, and the veins the power of growth from the liver.

VI. Refutation of Stoic errors

Patently false are premises such as those discussed at some length in the first book, when one says, as the Stoics do, that no irrational animal feels desire or anger, or again, that the nerves grow from the heart.

And in this discussion I thought proper to avoid nothing so carefully as making assertions contrary to what is clearly observed, as those men do who assert that no irrational animal feels desire or anger, and also those (who say) that the source of the nerves is in the heart. All such notions have been boldly advanced by men who were ambitious to overthrow all the excellent teachings of the ancients, in νεωτέραν αἷρεσιν ἰδίαν συστήσασθαι. τὰ μὲν οὖν τοιαῦτα τῶν ψευσμάτων ἐν τῷ πρώτῳ βιβλίῳ διήλεγξα.

ὁ δὲ Χρύσιππος ἅμα τοῖς ἄλλοις Στωϊκοῖς ἐπὶ μὲν τῶν ἀλόγων ζῴων ὁμόσε χωρεῖ πρὸς τὸ δόγμα μηδ' ἐπιθυμεῖν φάσκων· καί μοι περὶ τῆς ἀναισχυντίας τοῦ λόγου πρόσθεν εἴρηται.

οὐδὲν γάρ, ὡς οἴεται, τῶν ἀλόγων ζῴων οὔτε τὸ θυμοειδὲς οὔτε τὸ ἐπιθυμητικὸν οὔτε τὸ λογιστικὸν ἔχει ἀλλ' ὡς εἴρηταί μοι καὶ κατὰ τὸ πρῶτον γράμμα, παρὰ πᾶσαν τὴν ἐνάργειαν ἀφαιροῦνται τῶν εἰρημένων ἁπάντων αὐτὰ σχεδὸν ἅπαντες οἱ Στωϊκοί.

ἐπεδείξαμεν οὖν ἤδη καὶ διὰ τοῦ πρώτου βιβλίου περὶ τῆς πρὸς ἑαυτὸν ἐναντιολογίας τοῦ Χρυσίππου.

VII. De corde nudando

Εἴρηται δέ μοι καὶ πρόσθεν ὡς οὐ χρὴ συντιτράναι τοῦ θώρακος οὐδετέραν κοιλότητα γυμνοῦντας τὴν καρδίαν. εἰ γὰρ δὴ τούτου τύχοι τις, οὐ μόνον ἢ θλίβειν ἢ θλᾶν ἤ τι τοιοῦτον ἕτερον ἐργάζεσθαι βουληθεὶς δυνήσεται κατορθοῦν, ἀλλὰ καὶ βουληθεὶς ἀθρόως ὅλην ἐξελεῖν οὐκ ἀτυχήσει τῆς χειρουργίας.

ἐὰν οὖν ἅμα τε τοῦτο ποιήσῃς καὶ τέμῃς ὄρθιον, ὡς εἴρηται, τὸν δεξιὸν θώρακα, τῆς δεξιᾶς κοιλίας τῆς καρδίας ἐναργῶς ὄψει τὸν σφυγμόν.

إشارة إن أحببت أن تشقّ عن قلب حيوان تستثبت حال نبض القلب والعروق الضوارب الناشئة منه عيانا فينبغى أن تفعل ذلك فى بيت هواءه حارّ فإنّه إن لقى القلب الهواء البارد أتلف الحيوان بسرعة ولم يبق النبض على مجرى طبيعته لكن يحدث اختلاف وتشوّش كثير فينبغى أن يكون ذلك الفعل فى حمّام أو بيت شبيه به

3–5] *infra*, p. 214.22–24 6–9] *infra*, p. 190.31–35 10–11] *infra*, p. 200.13–15 13–17] *infra*, p. 126.18–22 18–19] PHP 554.15–17 Müller 20–23] Ibn al-Muṭrān (*cf. supra*, p. 45): cod. Bethesda (=B), fol. 6r14–6v1 cod. Tunis (=T), fol. 3v22–4r1

21 *post* بيت *add.* يكون T 22 *ante* البارد *add.* الحار T 23 يشبه T

order to found a newer school of their own. In the first book I thoroughly refuted fabrications of this kind.

But in the case of the irrational animals Chrysippus and the other Stoics boldly attack this view, claiming that the animals do not even experience desire; I mentioned earlier the shamelessness of this statement.

He holds that none of the irrational animals has the spirited or desiderative or rational part; as I said also in the first book, every Stoic, so far as I know, contrary to all clear evidence deprives them of all these (parts).

Already in the first book we showed how Chrysippus contradicted himself.

VII. Exposing the heart

I also said earlier that when exposing the heart one must not at the same time pierce either of the two chest cavities. If a person should succeed in this, not only will he be able successfully to press or crush the heart or do anything else of the sort if he so wishes, but even if he wishes to remove the whole (heart) all at once he will not fail in his surgery.

If you do this and at the same time make an incision straight up the right side of the thorax as I described, you will clearly see the pulsation of the right ventricle of the heart.

If you want to lay the heart of an animal bare to ascertain distinctly the condition of the pulsation of the heart and of the arteries coming from it, you must do this in a house in which the air is warm. For if the heart is affected by cold air, the animal soon contracts an injury and the pulse does not remain in its natural course, but becomes disordered and greatly disturbed. It is necessary that this procedure takes place in a bath or a similar building.

Libri primi quod exstat

137 M. 5. . . . τὸ πάμ-

Rhazes

المقالة الأولى من آراء أبقراط وأفلاطن

كان غلام فى صدره ‹ناصور› قد بلغ إلى العظم الذى فى وسط قصه وكشفنا عن عظم القصّ جميع ما يحيط به

فوجدناه قد أصابه فساد

فاضطررنا إلى قطعه

وكان الموضع الفاسد منه الموضع الذى عليه مستقرّ غلاف القلب

فلمّا رأينا ذلك توقّفنا توقّفا شديدا فى انتزاع العظم الفاسد

وكانت عنايتنا باستبقاء الغشاء المغشّى له من داخل وحفظه على سلامته

† بكلّ † ما اتّصل من

Ibn al-Muṭrān

حكاية من الكتاب المذكور

واتّفق لنا أنّ عليلا كان فى صدره ناصور قد كان بلغ إلى العظم الذى فى وسط قصّه فلمّا التمسنا مداواته كشفنا عن عظم القصّ جميع ما يحيط به من الأجسام فوجدنا القصّ قد أصابه فساد الجوهر فاضطرّنا ذلك إلى قطعه وكان الموضع الفاسد من القصّ هو الذى عليه مستقرّ غلاف القلب وهو الموضع الذى من عادتنا أن نفتحه فى التشريح الذى نريد فيه الكشف عن القلب فلمّا رأينا ذلك توقّفنا توقّفا شديدا فى انتزاع العظم الذى كان قد فسد وكانت عنايتنا إنّما هى باستبقاء الغشاء المغشّى له من داخل وحفظه على سلامته غير أنّا لم نجد هذا الغشاء سليما لا آفة به أصلا كان ما هو منه

3–74.23] Rhazes, al-Ḥāwī (*cf. supra*, p. 43) vol. XIII, p. 43.1–12

3–76.10] Ibn al-Muṭrān (*cf. supra*, p. 45) cod. Bethesda, fol. 6v2–7r3 cod. Tunis, fol. 4r1–15

3–76.13] *cf.* Gal. Anat. vii. 12–13: II 631–633 K.

28–130.20 Τοιοῦτος *om.* H 28–100.7 *om.* M *Ald.*

5 ناصور *addidi* 28 *fort.* فكل *scribendum est*

5 [عليلا *fort.* غلاما, *cf. Rhaz.* 6 ناصورا BT: *correxi* قد *om.* T 17 أن نفتحه *om.* T 18 نريد *om.* T 19 فيه *om.* B *ante* القلب *add.* غلاف T 20 فوقفنا T 23 وقد كانت T 25 *ante* على *add.* عليه T 27 *post* آفة *add.* T كان, *ut vid.*

The extant part of Book I	*Rhazes*	*Ibn al-Muṭrān*
	The first book of "The Doctrines of Hippocrates and Plato":	Story from the book mentioned:
	A young boy had a fistula in his chest which had penetrated to the bone in the middle of his sternum.	It happened to us that a patient had a fistula in his chest which had penetrated to the bone in the middle of his sternum. When we undertook treating
	We removed from the bone of the sternum all that surrounds it and we found it already affected by the corruption.	him we removed all the surrounding bodies from the bone of the sternum. We found that the sternum was already affected by the corruption of the substance.
	So we were compelled to cut it out. The corrupted place in it was the place at which the pericardium is attached.	This compelled us to cut it out. The corrupted place in the sternum was the place at which the pericardium is attached. This is the place that we usually open in dissection when our aim is to lay the heart bare.
	Seeing this, we were very hesitant about extracting the corrupted bone, our purpose being only to preserve the membrane that covers the bone on the inside and to keep it intact. . . .	Seeing this, we were very hesitant about extracting the bone that was corrupted, our purpose being only to preserve the membrane that covers the bone on the inside and to keep it intact. But we did not find this membrane sound and unaffected by any damage.
5. . . . at all. But	The parts of this	The parts

Libri primi quod exstat	*Rhazes*	*Ibn al-Muṭrān*
V 181 K. παν. | ἀλλὰ κἀκείνου τὸ συνεχὲς τῷ στέρνῳ διασεσήπει, καὶ ἦν οὕτω σαφῶς θεάσασθαι τὴν καρδίαν ὡς κἀν ταῖς τῶν ζῴων ἀνατομαῖς, ἐπειδὰν ἑκόντες αὐτὴν γυμνώσωμεν.	هذا الغشاء بالقصّ كان قد عفن أيضا قال وكنّا ننظر إلى القلب نظرا بيّنا مثل ما نراه إذا كشفنا عنه بالتعمّد فى التشريح	متّصل بالقصّ قد عفن فكنّا ننظر إلى القلب نظرا بيّنا كمثل ما نراه إذا كشفنا غنه بالتعمّد فى عمل التشريح
2 τὸ μὲν οὖν παιδάριον ἐσώθη σαρκωθέντων τε τῶν περὶ τὸ στέρνον καὶ συμφύντων ἀλλήλοις καὶ ⟨εἰς⟩ τοιοῦτον ἐπίθεμα γενομένων τῆς καρδίας οἷόν περ ἡ ἔμπροσθεν ἦν κορυφὴ τοῦ χιτῶνος.	قال فسلم ذلك الغلام ونبت اللحم فى ذلك الموضع الذى ‹قطع له› من القصّ حتّى امتلأ واتّصل بعضه ببعض وصار يقوم من ستر القلب وتغطيته بمثل ما كان يقوم به قبل ذلك رأس غلاف القلب	وسلم ذلك الغلام ونبت اللحم فى ذلك الموضع الذى قطع له من القصّ حتّى امتلأ واتّصل بعضه ببعض وصار يقوم من ستر القلب وتغطيته بمثل ما كان يقوم به من قبل ذلك رأس غلاف القلب
3 καὶ οὐ χρὴ θαυμάζειν εἰ γυμνωθείσης 182 τῆς καρδίας | ἐσώθη τὸ παιδάριον. οὐδὲν γὰρ περιττότερον ἢ	قال وليس هذا بأعجب من الجراحات التى ينثقب بها الصدر	قال وليس ينبغى لك أن تتعجّب من أن يكون القلب قد تعرّى وانكشف والغلام أفلت فإنّه لم يحدث هناك من العلّة

9–11] *cf.* PHP 554.11 Müller

3 κἀκείν^x C: *corr. Caius* 4 τὸ] τ. C: *suppl. Caius* 5 διεσεσήπει *Chart.* 8 κἂν C: *corr. Caius* 10 αὐτὴν γυμνώσωμεν *scripsi*: αὐ. . γυμνώ...εν C: ἀναγυμνώ. . .εν C²: ἀναγυμνῶμεν *Caius* 16 εἰς *addidi* 16–17 τοιοῦτ. . . . .θεμα C: *suppl.* C²: τοιούτου ἐπιθέματος *Müller*: τοιούτων ἐπιθεμάτων *recens. anon.* 17 γενόμενον C: *corr. Caius* 19 ἔμπροσθεν] ἔμ. . . . . C: *suppl.* C² 22 γυμνωθείσης] ει *ex* η *corr.* C

13 قطع له *addidi sec. Ibn al-Muṭrān et vers. Lat. Rhazis* (. . . in quo facta fuit incisio de torace) 18 رأس غلاف] بغلاف *editio*: *correxi sec. Ibn al-Muṭrān et vers. Lat. Rhazis* (. . . caput cellule cordis)

3 متّصلا BT: *correxi* 25 الحلّة, *ut vid.*, B

	The extant part of Book I	*Rhazes*	*Ibn al-Muṭrān*
	also the part (of the pericardium) that touches the sternum had mortified, and the heart could be seen as clearly as in the dissection of animals, when we deliberately lay it bare.	tunic that were connected with the sternum were also rotten. He said: We saw the heart clearly as we see it when we deliberately lay it bare in a dissection.	which are connected with the sternum were rotten, so that we saw the heart as clearly as we see it when we deliberately lay it bare during a dissection.
2	Now the young boy survived, as the parts around the sternum took on flesh and grew together and formed a covering over the heart similar to the apex of the tunic that had covered it before.	He said: This young boy recovered and flesh grew at that place where the sternum had been excised, so that it was filled and its parts became connected with each other. It now served as a protection and cover for the heart, as did the apex of the pericardium before.	This young boy recovered. The flesh grew at that place where the sternum had been excised, so that it was filled and its parts became connected with each other. It now served as a protection and cover for the heart, as did the apex of the pericardium before.
3	And there is no cause for surprise that the young boy recovered after the exposure of his heart. His condition was no more extreme	He said: This is not more astonishing than the wounds whereby the chest is pierced.	He said: You must not be surprised that the heart was bare and exposed and the young boy survived. For no more dam-

Libri primi quod exstat

διάθεσις εἶχε τῶν
ὁσημέραι γινομένων
εἰς τὸν θώρακα συν-
4 τρήσεων. οὐ μὴν οὐδὲ
ὁ περικάρδιος ἴδιον
ἐξαίρετον ἐπιφέρει
τινὰ κίνδυνον, ὥσ-
περ που καὶ Ἡρό-
5 φιλος εἴρηκε καὶ ἄλλοι πολλοὶ τῶν ἰατρῶν. οὔτε οὖν τὸ παιδάριον
138 ἐκεῖνο παρ' / ὅλην τὴν θεραπείαν ἐβέβλαπτο τὴν ἐνέργειαν οὔθ' ὁπόταν
ζῷον ὁμοίως ἀνατέμνωμεν.
6 Τίνος οὖν ἕνεκα ταῦτ' εἴρηταί μοι; τοῦ τὴν καρδίαν αἵματος εἶναι με-
στὴν τηνικαῦτα κατ' ἀμφοτέρας τὰς κοιλίας. τῷ τοῦτο δῆλον; εἰ τρώσαις
7 αὐτήν, εὐθὺς ἐκχεῖται τὸ αἷμα. ἐχρῆν δέ γε κατὰ τὸν Χρύσιππον ἢ τὸ
πνεῦμα πρότερον ἐκκενούμενον φαίνεσθαι κἄπειθ' οὕτως ἕπεσθαι τὸ
αἷμα, ἢ μηδὲ ὅλως ἕπεσθαι, καθάπερ οὐδὲ ἐπὶ τῶν κατὰ τὸν ἐγκέφαλον
ἕπεται κοιλιῶν, ἀλλ' ἐπειδὰν ἐκκόψαντες τὸ κρανίον ἀφέλωμεν τὴν
παχεῖαν μήνιγγα καὶ γυμνώσαντες ἅπαντα τὸν ἐγκέφαλον ἐπιχειρῶμεν
τιτρώσκειν ἥντινοῦν αὐτοῦ κοιλίαν, οὔτε ἐν τῷ παραχρῆμα φαίνεται
8 κατ' αὐτὰς αἷμα περιεχόμενον οὔθ' ὕστερον ἑπόμενον. οὕτως δὲ κἀπὶ
183 τοῦ τεθνεῶτος ἤδη ζῴου κατὰ μὲν | τὴν ἀριστερὰν κοιλίαν τῆς καρδίας
οὐκ ἔσθ' ὅπως οὐκ ἂν εὕροις αἵματος θρόμβους, ἐν δὲ ταῖς κατὰ τὸν
ἐγκέφαλον οὐχ εὑρήσεις, πλὴν εἰ θλασθέντος αὐτοῦ σὺν τῷ κρανίῳ τῶν
139 9 ἐν αὐτῷ / τινες ἀρτηριῶν ἢ φλεβῶν διασπασθεῖεν. οὕτω δὲ κἀπὶ τῶν
τιτρωσκομένων κατὰ τὴν ἔκφυσιν τοῦ νωτιαίου βο[λ]ῶν εὑρίσκεταί ποτε
10 διαδιδόμενον εἴς τινα τῶν προσθίων κοιλιῶν αἷμα. καὶ οὐδὲν οὐδ'
ἐνταῦθα θαυμαστὸν αὐτῆς τῆς ὀπισθίου κοιλίας τιτρωσκομένης καὶ
πολλῶν καὶ μεγάλων αὐτῇ συντιτρωσκομένων ἀγγείων ἀφικνεῖσθαί
11 ποτε καὶ μέχρι τῶν προσθίων τὸ αἷμα. δύναιτο δὲ ἂν ἐνίοτε καὶ βρόχῳ
πνιγέντος τοῦ ζῴου διὰ τὴν ὑπερβάλλουσαν βίαν ῥαγῆναί τι τῶν
κατὰ τὸν ἐγκέφαλον ἀγγείων, οἷα δὴ πολλάκις ὁρᾶται γιγνόμενα καὶ

Ibn al-Muṭrān

شيء أكثر ممّا يكون في كل يوم من الجراحات التي تثقب الصدر ومع هذا فليس يأتي من قبل غلاف القلب خاصّة شيء من الإشراف على التلف كما يأتي من قبل باقي أجزائه

11–13] *cf.* Gal. Anat. vii. 12: II 631.9–13 K. In Hipp. De off. med. comm. i. 1: XVIII B 643.14 K. 15–19] SVF II, p. 246 25] *cf.* Gal. Anat. ix. 1: II 709.5–6 K. 26–27] *cf. infra*, p. 126.28–29; PHP 607.1–2 Müller Gal. Anat. ix: II, p. 13 Simon

4 الخراجات T: *sine punct.* B 7–8 شيء
من] شحم B 8 التلف]
التكلف B 9 كيما B

12 οὔθ' ὁπόταν] οὔθ. :̣ό C: *suppl. Einarson*: οὔτε ἄν τι *Caius* 22 αὐτὰς] αὐτὴν *Müller* περιεχόμενον] προχεόμενον *recens. anon.* 24 ὅπου C: *corr. recens. anon.* 27 βολῶν C: *corr. Caius*

The extant part of Book I	*Ibn al-Muṭrān*
than the perforations of the chest that occur every day. Nor does the pericardium bring any exceptional danger of its own, as indeed Herophilus and many other physicians have remarked. So that	age occurred than is caused by those wounds which happen 4 every day and pierce the chest. So from the pericardium taken by itself nothing fatal results, as it does from the other parts of the heart. 5

young boy had suffered no impairment of function through the whole course of treatment, nor does an animal when we lay it open in the same way.

What was my purpose in speaking of this? To show that at that 6
moment both ventricles of the heart are filled with blood. What is the evidence for this? If you pierce the heart, blood immediately flows out. But on Chrysippus' view, either the pneuma should be 7
observed escaping first, and then blood should follow, or no blood should follow at all, no more than it does in the ventricles of the brain; for when we have cut open the cranium and removed the dura mater and laid bare the whole brain, and then set about piercing any of its ventricles, blood is neither observed to be enclosed in them at the moment of piercing nor to follow later. It is the same with an animal 8
already dead. You cannot avoid finding clots of blood in the left ventricle of the heart, but you will not find them in the ventricles of the brain, unless the brain was crushed along with the cranium and some of the arteries or veins in it were torn open. And similarly when cattle 9
are wounded at the point where the spinal cord grows out from the brain, blood is sometimes found spreading to one of the anterior ventricles. Here too there is no cause for surprise that when the 10
posterior ventricle has itself been wounded and many large vessels along with it, blood should at times reach as far as the anterior ventricles. Even when an animal is strangled with a noose, one of the ves- 11
sels in the brain could on occasion burst from the excessive force, the sort of thing that we often observe happening in any other part,

καθ' ὁτιοῦν ἄλλο μέρος ὑπὸ πλήθους αἵματος ἢ χύσεως ἀναρραγέν-
τος ἀγγείου· εἰ δὲ ἐν ὕδατι πνιγείη τὸ ζῷον, οὐκ ἂν ὁμοίως ἀγγεῖον
12 ῥαγείη. κατὰ μέντοι τοὺς ἄλλους ἅπαντας θανάτους τῶν ζῴων οὐκ ἂν
εὕροις ἐν ἐγκεφάλου κοιλίᾳ περιεχόμενον θρόμβον, ὥσπερ ἐν τῇ καρδίᾳ
διαπαντός.
184 13 Ἀλλὰ τὰ μὲν | ἐπὶ τῶν τεθνεώτων ἐκ περιουσίας εἰρῆσθαί μοι δοκῶ.
ἐπάνειμι δὲ αὖθις ἐπὶ ⟨τὰ⟩ ζῶντα ζῷα καὶ δείκνυμί σοι γυμνωθείσης τῆς
140 καρδίας οὐ / μόνον εἰ σμίλην καθείης εἰς τὴν ἀριστερὰν κοιλίαν, αἷμα
προχεόμενον εὐθέως, ἀλλὰ κἂν γραφεῖον ἢ βελόνην ἤ τι τοιοῦτον ἕτερον.
14 καίτοι γε εἴπερ ἀναγκαῖον ἦν, ἐχρῆν ἐκκενωθῆναι τὸ πνεῦμα πρότερον,
ἵνα ἀκολουθήσῃ τὸ αἷμα· τὸ γὰρ στεγνὸν τῆς ὀπῆς ἂν εἰς χρόνου μῆκος
15 οὐ σμικρὰ συνετέλεσεν. ἀλλ' οὐχ ὧδ' ἔχει τἀληθές· ἕπεται γὰρ αὐτίκα
μάλα τῷ τρώσαντι τὸ αἷμα, ὥστε οὐκ ἄν, οὐδὲ εἰ πάνυ σφόδρα ταχύνοις
ἐν τῇ χειρουργίᾳ, δυνηθείης ποτὲ ἀναίμακτον ἐξαρπάσαι τὸ τρῶσαν.
ᾧ δῆλον ὡς πλήρης ἐστὶν αἵματος ἡ ἀριστερὰ κοιλία.
6. Τὸ γὰρ ὑπὸ τῶν περὶ τὸν Ἐρασίστρατον λεγόμενον, ὡς πρὶν μὲν
τοῦ γυμνωθῆναι πνεῦμα μόνον ἐν αὐτῇ περιείχετο, γυμνωθείσης δὲ παρεμ-
πίπτει τὸ αἷμα, οὐδὲν ἄλλ' ἐστὶν ἢ ἀνθρώπων λόγος ἀναισχύντων πρὸς
2 τὸν ἔλεγχον. ἀλλὰ καὶ τοῦτ' αὐτῶν ἐλέγξαι τὸ ἀναισχύντημα ῥᾷστόν
185 *141* ἐστιν. εἰ γὰρ δὴ παρὰ φύσιν εἰς τὴν πνευματικὴν | κοιλίαν τῆς / καρδίας
ἐκπέπτωκε τὸ αἷμα, πάντ' ἐχρῆν, οἶμαι, συγκεχύσθαι τὰ κατὰ φύσιν
αὐτῆς ἔργα καὶ μήτε τὰς ἀρτηρίας ἔθ' ὁμοίως σφύζειν ἵν' ἐκ τοῦ παρ'
αὐτῆς ἐπληροῦ⟨ν⟩το πνεύματος, ἀπολωλέναι τε παμπόλλας ἐνεργείας,
3 ὡς ἂν τῆς πηγῆς αὐτῶν οὐκέτι οὔσης. — Ἐρασίστρατος μὲν γὰρ
ζωτικοῦ πνεύματος, Χρύσιππος δὲ τοῦ ψυχικοῦ πνεύματος πλήρη
4 φησὶν εἶναι τὴν κοιλίαν ταύτην. — ἀλλ' οὐδὲν ὅλως τὸ ζῷον καταλαμβάνει
σύμπτωμα. καὶ τοῦτ' ἔνεστι τῷ βουλομένῳ μαθεῖν παρ' ἡμῶν, ὥσπερ
ἀμέλει πολλάκις ἐδείξαμεν οὐκ ὀλίγοις τῶν ἀπιστούντων εὐθὺς ἀντιπα-
ραβάλλοντες αὐτοῖς ἐφ' ἑτέρου ζῴου, πολλάκις δὲ καὶ καθ' ἓν ὁτιοῦν
⟨καὶ⟩ ταὐτόν, ὁπόσα τε καὶ ὁποῖα καταλαμβάνει τὸ σύμπ[τ]αν σῶμα
5 παθήματα κοιλίας ἐγκεφάλου τρωθείσης. καίτοι τί λέγω τρωθείσης; εἰ
γὰρ καὶ πρὶν τρῶσαι θλίψεις ἡντινοῦν αὐτῶν ἀκίνητόν τε καὶ ἀναίσθητον,
6 ἄπνουν τε καὶ ἄφωνον εὐθὺς ἔσται τὸ ζῷον. οὕτω δὲ κἀπὶ τῶν ἀνθρώ-
186 πων αὐτῶν ἀνατιτραμένων φαίνεται συμ|πῖπτον. ἐν γὰρ τῷ τὰ κατεα-
142 γότα / τῶν ὀστῶν ἐκκόπτειν ὑποβάλλειν ἀναγκαζομένων ἡμῶν ἀσφαλείας

24–26] SVF II, p. 246 34–80.3] *cf.* Maimonid. Aph. xxiv. 55

7 τὰ *add. Schöne* 9 κἂν] καὶ *Müller* 11 στεγνὸν] στένον *(sic) Caius in mg.* 13 ταχύνης C: *corr. Müller* 14 δυνήσῃ C *(def. Marquardt, Scr. min. I, pp. XLV–XLVI)*: *corr. recens. anon.*: δυνήσαιο *Müller* 18 ἀλλ' C: *corr. Caius* 21 ἐμπε-πτώκει *Müller* (ἐμπεπτ *iam Caius in mg.*) 22 ἵν'] .ν' C: *suppl. Einarson*: ὡς ὅτ' *Caius* ἐκ *del. Müller* 23 ἐπληροῦτο C: *suppl. Caius* 24 οὔσης] ῥεούσης *(?) Schöne* Ἐρασίστρατος — 26 ταύτην *post* πνεύματος *(lin. 23) collocandum censet Schöne* 26 φασὶν C: *corr. Müller* 28 *post* πολλάκις *add.* μὲν *Müller* 30 καὶ[I] *add. Caius in mg.* σύμπταν *(ex* συμπτώματος *corr.)* C: *corr. Caius* 32 καὶ[I] *sscr.* C θλίψεις *e* σθλίψεις *radendo corr.* C 34 ἀνατιτραμένων] τρ *e corr.* C κα-τεαγότα] ε *e corr.* C

when a vessel is made to burst by a large quantity of blood or by its
flow. But if the animal were suffocated in water, the vessel would
not have burst in the same way. Indeed in all other deaths of animals 12
you do not find a blood clot enclosed in a ventricle of the brain, as you
do without exception in the heart.

But I have made these remarks about dead animals, I believe, 13
superfluously. I return now to the living and demonstrate to you
that when the heart is exposed, if you insert a lancet into the left
ventricle – and not only a lancet, but even a writing reed or needle
or any other such instrument – hemorrhage follows immediately. Yet 14
the pneuma would have had to be emptied out first, if that were
necessary, so that the blood could follow; for the constriction of the
opening would have contributed no little amount to the length of
time. But the truth is quite otherwise; blood follows instantaneously 15
on the piercing, so that even if you performed the operation with
very great speed you could never pull the instrument away unstained
by blood. This makes it clear that the left ventricle is full of blood.

6. For the statement of Erasistratus and his school, that
before being laid bare it contained only pneuma, and that blood slips
in after it has been laid bare, is nothing but the talk of men who are
shameless in the face of refutation. But this piece of shamelessness on 2
their part is also very easy to refute. If the blood had escaped unnatu-
rally into the pneumatic ventricle of the heart, then, in my opinion,
all the natural functions of this ventricle would have been disturbed,
the arteries would no longer be pulsating in order to be filled from its
pneuma, and very many activities would have been destroyed, as their
source would no longer exist. – Erasistratus says that this ventricle 3
is full of vital pneuma, Chrysippus of psychic pneuma. – But the 4
animal shows no symptoms whatever. Anyone who wishes may learn
this from me by the procedure I have often used to demonstrate pre-
cisely this point to no few doubters: I immediately show them by
way of contrast in another animal, or often in one and the same animal,
whatever it be, the number and nature of the disorders that lay hold
of the whole body when a ventricle of the brain is wounded. But why 5
do I say wounded? If even before inflicting a wound you apply pres-
sure on any one of the ventricles the animal will immediately lose
motion and sensation, breath and voice. And the same results are 6
seen in the case of human beings themselves who have undergone
trepanning. When we excise the broken fragments of bone we are

ἕνεκα τοὺς καλουμένους μηνιγγοφύλακας, εἰ βραχεῖ βιαιότερον ἐπιθλίψει
τις αὐτοῖς τὸν ἐγκέφαλον, ἀναίσθητός τε καὶ ἀκίνητος ἁπασῶν τῶν καθ'
ὁρμὴν κινήσεων ὁ ἄνθρωπος ἀποτελεῖται, οὐ μὴν τήν γε καρδίαν
7 γυμνωθεῖσαν θλιβόντων. ἀλλ' ἔγωγε οἶδα καὶ πυράγρᾳ ποτὲ χαλκέως
ἐπιτρέψας τινὶ περιλαβεῖν αὐτήν, ἐπειδὴ καὶ τῶν δακτύλων ἐξεπήδα
βιαίως παλλομένη· ἀλλ' οὐδὲν οὐδὲ τότε τὸ ζῷον ἔπασχεν οὔτε εἰς
αἴσθησιν οὔτε εἰς κίνησιν τὴν καθ' ὁρμήν, ἀλλ' ἐκεκράγει τε μεγάλα
8 καὶ ἀκωλύτως ἀνέπνει καὶ πάντα ἐκίνει σφοδρῶς τὰ κῶλα. μόνη γὰρ ἡ
τῶν ἀρτηριῶν βλάπτεται κίνησις οὕτω διαληφθείσης τῆς καρδίας, ἄλλο
δὲ οὐδὲν πάσχει τὸ ζῷον, ἀλλ' ἄχρι περ ἂν ζῇ καὶ κινεῖ πάντα τὰ μέλη
9 καὶ ἀναπνεῖ. ἐγκεφάλου δὲ οὕτω θλιφθέντος ἔμπαλιν ἅπαντα συμπίπτει·
σφύζουσι μὲν αἱ ἀρτηρίαι κατὰ φύσιν ἅμα τῇ καρδίᾳ, κινεῖται δὲ οὐδὲν
10 μέλος οὐδὲ ἀναπνεῖ τὸ ζῷον οὐδὲ ἐκφωνεῖ. ἤδη μὲν οὖν ἐκ τῶνδε
143 187 καὶ ἄλλο τι / μεῖζον | ἐκφαίνεται, τὸ μήτε τὴν καρδίαν ἐγκεφάλου τι
προσδεῖσθαι πρὸς τὴν οἰκείαν κίνησιν μήτε τὸν ἐγκέφαλον τῆς καρδίας.
11 οὐ μὴν τούτου γε ἕνεκεν ἐμνημόνευσα τῶν ἐκ τῆς ἀνατομῆς φαινομένων,
ἀλλ' ὅπως ἐπιδείξαιμι τὸ ψυχικὸν πνεῦμα κατὰ τὰς τοῦ ἐγκεφάλου
12 κοιλίας περιεχόμενον. ἔνθα νῦν καὶ μάλιστα μεμψαίμην ⟨ἂν⟩ τὸν Χρύσιπ-
πον, ὅτι βουλόμενος εἰλικρινές τι καὶ καθαρὸν εἶναι πνεῦμα τὸ κατὰ τὴν
ἀρχὴν τῆς ψυχῆς, οὐ προσηκόντως ἐν τῇ καρδίᾳ καθίδρυσεν αὐτό.
13 Καίτοι Χρύσιππον μὲν ἄν τις ἀποδέξαιτο μετρίως ἀποφηνάμενον
ὡς μήθ' ὅτι τῶν νεύρων ἀρχὴ ἡ καρδία τὴν γνῶσιν αὐτῷ χαρίζεται
μήτ' ἄλλο μηδὲν τῶν κατὰ τὸ πρόβλημα τοῦτο ζητουμένων· ὁμολογεῖ
14 γὰρ ἀπείρως ἔχειν τῶν ἀνατομῶν· Ἀριστοτέλει δέ γε καὶ Πραξαγόρᾳ
παρὰ τὸ φαινόμενον ἀποφαινομένοις ἀρχὴν τῶν νεύρων εἶναι τὴν καρ-
15 δίαν ἐγκαλέσειεν ἄν τις δικαίως. ὅτι μὲν γὰρ ἄλλα πολλὰ τῶν κατὰ τὰς
144 ἀνατομὰς ἀκριβῶς ἑωράκασιν, ἐξ ὧν ὑπελεί/ποντο συνταγμάτων ἔνεστι
188 καταμαθεῖν· | ὅτι δὲ ἤτοι παντάπασιν αὐτοὶ τυφλώττοντες ἢ τυφλοῖς
διαλεγόμενοι περὶ τῆς τῶν νεύρων ἀρχῆς ἔγραψαν, οὐ λόγοις χρὴ
16 μακροῖς κατασκευάζειν, ἀλλ' ἐπὶ τὴν αἴσθησιν ἰέναι. φαίνεται γάρ, ὡς
ἔμπροσθεν ἐδήλωσα, τὰ μὲν ἐξ ἐγκεφάλου τῶν νεύρων ἄντικρυς ἐκπε-
φυκότα, τὰ δὲ ἐκ τοῦ νωτιαίου μυελοῦ, νωτιαῖος δὲ αὐτὸς ἐξ ἐγκεφάλου.
17 βέλτιον οὖν ἦν οὐθ' ἁπλῶς ἀρχὴν τῶν νεύρων ἀποφήνασθαι τὴν καρδίαν,
ὅπερ Ἀριστοτέλης ἐποίησεν, οὔτε ἐκ πανουργίας τινὸς ἐπιβεβουλευ-

4–11] *cf.* Maimonid. Aph. xxiv. 55 4–9] Ibn al-Muṭrān, cod. Beth. A8, fol. 9r3–10 *et* cod. Tun. 5400, fol. 5r15–21 (*v. supra*, p. 43 adn. 2) 4–6] *cf.* Gal. Anat. vii. 14: II 635–636 K. 7–8] *cf. infra*, p.126.23–25 8–13] *cf. infra*, pp. 126.11–17; 210.20–26 8–11] *cf.* Gal. De loc. aff. v. 2: VIII 304 K. 14–15] *cf. infra*, pp. 128.3; 150.3–6 Gal. Anat. vii. 8: II 614 K. 18–24] SVF II, p. 246 21–82.25] Prax. fr. 11 Steckerl 24–26] *cf.* Arist. Hist. animal. iii. 5: 515 a 27–28 30–32] libri primi test., *v. supra*, p. 68.13–15

5 ἐπιτρίψας C: *corr. Caius* καὶ *del. Müller* 6 ἐπέσχεν C: *corr.* C2 8 σαφῶς C: σφοδρῶς *sscr.* C2 9 διαληφθείσης] θλιφθείσης *Al. Just.* 10 κινεῖ] ει *in* η *corr.* C μέλη] ελ *ex* ερ, *ut vid.*, *corr.* C 11 ἀναπνεῖ] ει *in* η *corr.* C 12 σφύζουσι] σι *e corr.* C 14 *ante* ἐγκεφάλου *add.* τοῦ *Müller* 14–15 τι προσδεῖσθαι] τινὸς δεῖσθαι C: *corr. Müller (cf. infra, p. 150.4)* 18 ἂν *add. Kühn* 22 ὡς *del. Müller* χαρίζεσθαι C: *corr. Einarson*: ἰσχυρίζεσθαι *(?) Schöne*

compelled for safety to insert underneath the instruments called
protectors of the dura mater, and if you press the brain with them a
little too heavily, the patient is rendered incapable of sensation and
of all voluntary movements; but this does not happen when pressure
is applied to the exposed heart. This I know: I once allowed someone 7
to hold a heart with a smith's tongs, since it jumped out of his fingers
because of the violent palpitation; but even then the animal suffered
no impairment of sensation or voluntary movement. It uttered a loud
scream, breathed without hindrance, and kept all its limbs in violent
motion. For when the heart is thus separated off, only the movement 8
of the arteries is impaired, and the animal is not otherwise affected;
as long as it survives it moves all its limbs and breathes. But when 9
pressure is applied to the brain in the manner described, all the symp-
toms are just the reverse: the arteries pulsate naturally along with
the heart, but no limb moves and the animal does not breathe or cry
out. Once these facts have been established, another more important 10
fact comes to light as a consequence, that the heart does not need the
brain at all for the exercise of its proper movement, nor the brain the
heart. But that was not my object in mentioning the evidence of ana- 11
tomy; it was rather to point out that the psychic pneuma is contained
in the ventricles of the brain. Here I would be especially critical of 12
Chrysippus: he intended that what occupies the place of authority
in the soul be unmixed and pure pneuma, but he stationed it in the
heart, where it does not belong.

You might nevertheless put up with Chrysippus, who modestly 13
declared that his heart did not vouchsafe to him either the knowledge
that it is the source of the nerves, or any other answer to the questions
that arise in connection with this problem; for he admits that he is
ignorant of anatomy. But when Aristotle and Praxagoras affirm, 14
contrary to anatomical observation, that the heart is the source of
the nerves, they deserve to be censured. One can learn from the trea- 15
tises they left that they observed with precision many other ana-
tomical matters; but when they wrote about the source of the nerves,
either they were completely blind themselves or they were addressing
a blind audience. No long arguments are needed to prove this; the
evidence of the senses is enough. For it is obvious, as I demonstrated 16
earlier, that some nerves grow out directly from the brain, others
from the spinal cord, and the spinal cord itself from the brain. It 17
would have been better, then, neither to state simply, as Aristotle
did, that the heart is the source of the nerves, nor to do so from a delib-

18 μένης, ὡς ὁ Πραξαγόρας. οὗτος γὰρ ὁ ἀνὴρ ἐπειδὴ μηδὲν ἑώρα νεῦρον
ἐκφυόμενον τῆς καρδίας, ἐφιλοτιμεῖτο δὲ πρὸς Ἱπποκράτην καὶ πάντως
ἐβούλετο τὸν ἐγκέφαλον ἀφελέσθαι τῆς τῶν νεύρων ἀρχῆς, οὐ σμικρὸν
ἀπετόλμησε ψεύσασθαι τὰς ἀρτηρίας φάμενος ἐν τῷ προϊέναι καὶ κατα-
σχίζεσθαι στενὰς γιγνομένας εἰς νεῦρα μεταβάλλειν· τοῦ γὰρ δὴ σώματος
αὐτῶν ὑπάρχοντος νευρώδους μὲν ἀλλὰ κοίλου, ⟨καὶ⟩ κατὰ τὴν ἐπὶ
145 πλέον ἐν τῷ ζῴῳ σχίσιν οὕτως γιγνομένων μικρῶν τῶν κοιλοτήτων / ὡς
189 ἐπιπίπτειν | ἀλλήλοις τοὺς χιτῶνας, ὁπόταν τοῦτο πρῶτον γένηται,
19 νεῦρον ἤδη φαίνεσθαι τὸ ἀγγεῖον. Ἐρασίστρατος μὲν οὖν οὐδὲ ἀντι-
λο[λο]γίας ἠξίωσε τὸν λόγον ὡς ἀναισχύντως ἀποτετολμημένον.

7. Ἐγὼ δὲ ἐπειδήπερ ἅπαξ κατέστην εἰς τὸ περὶ πάντων διασκέψα-
σθαι, βραχέα τῷ Πραξαγόρᾳ διαλεχθῆναι βούλομαι καὶ μάλισθ' ὅτι καὶ
Χρύσιππος ἐμνημόνευσε τἀνδρὸς ἀντιθεὶς τοῖς ἀπὸ τῆς κεφαλῆς ἄρχε-
2 σθαι τὰ νεῦρα νομίζουσιν. ὅτι γὰρ οὕτως ἐχρῆν ἔχειν τὸ φαινόμενον ἐκ
τῶν ἀνατομῶν ὡς ὁ Πραξαγόρας εἴρηκεν, εἰ μελ⟨λ⟩ήσει τις εὐλόγως
ἀρχὴν τῶν νεύρων ὑπολήψεσθαι τὴν καρδίαν, οὐδὲ ἡμεῖς ἀμφισβητοῦ-
3 μεν. ὅτι δὲ οὐχ οὕτως ἔχει, μυριάκις μὲν ἤδη τοῖς βουληθεῖσι γνῶναι
τἀληθὲς ἐπὶ τῶν ζῴων ἐδείξαμεν, οὐκ ὀκνήσομεν δὲ κἀνταῦθα τὴν
ἀνατομὴν ἑρμηνεῦσαι τῶν ἀρτηριῶν, ὥσπερ ἔμπροσθεν τῶν νεύρων.
4 ἐκφύεται μὲν γὰρ ἐκ τῆς ἀριστερᾶς κοιλίας τῆς καρδίας ἀρτηρία μεγίστη,
5 καθάπερ τι πρέμνον ἁπασῶν τῶν κατὰ τὸ ζῷον ἀρτηριῶν. ἀποβλα-
146 190 στάνει δὲ ἀπ' αὐτῆς / πρῶτον μὲν ἡ | τὴν καρδίαν περιστ[ρ]έφουσα· καὶ
6 δὴ καὶ ὀνομάζουσιν οὕτως αὐτὴν οἷς μέλει τῶν ἀνατομῶν. ἀλλ' οὐκ ἂν
εἴποις, ὦ γενναιότατε Πραξαγόρα, μειουμένην ἐν τῷ κατασχίζεσθαι
7 τὴν ἀρτηρίαν ταύτην εἰς νεῦρα τελευτᾶν. ἐφεξῆς δὲ τῆσδε δίχα σχι-
σθείσης τῆς μεγάλης ἀρτηρίας ἡ μὲν μείζων μοῖρα κατακαμφθεῖσα πρὸς
τὴν ῥάχιν ἐπὶ μέσων στηρίζεται τῶν σπονδύλων· ἡ δ' ἑτέρᾳ μετέωρος
8 εὐθὺ τῶν σφαγῶν ἀναφέρεται. πρώτας οὖν ἐπίσκεψαί μοι τὰς εἰς τὸν
θώρακα φερομένας ἀπ' αὐτῶν καὶ τόλμησον εἰπεῖν τινα μεταβάλλειν εἰς
νεῦρον. εἰσὶ μὲν γὰρ β' καὶ κ' τὸν ἀριθμόν, ἐν ἑκάστῳ μεσοπλευρίῳ μία,
9 συναποφύεται δὲ αὐταῖς ἀπὸ τοῦ νωτιαίου νεῦρα. καὶ φαίνεταί γε καθ'
ὅλον τὸν θώρακα καὶ συναποτεινόμενά τε καὶ συγκατασχιζόμενα ταυτὶ
τὰ δύο γένη τῶν ἀγγείων εἴς τε τὸν ὑπεζωκότα τὰς πλευρὰς χιτῶνα
καὶ τοὺς μεσοπλευρίους μῦς τρίτου τινὸς αὐτοῖς συναποφυομένου τε καὶ
10 συναποτεινομένου καὶ συγκατασχιζομένου φλεβώδους ἀγγείου. ἀλλ'
147 οὐδὲν τό γε νῦν εἶναι δέομαι / διεξέρχεσθαι περὶ φλεβῶν· ἀναμένει γὰρ
191 οὖν κἀκείνας | ἑτέρωθι οὐ σμικρὸς λόγος· ἐπὶ δὲ τὰς ἀρτηρίας αὖθις
11 ἐπάνειμι. καὶ καταλίπωμεν ἤδη τὰς κατὰ τὸν θώρακα μηδὲ αὐτοῦ τοῦ

11–14] SVF II, p. 246 18–19] libri primi test., *v. supra*, p. 68.6–7 25–28] *cf.* Gal. UP xvi. 10: IV 313–314 K. De ven. art. diss. 9: II 817–820 K. 37–84.28] Prax. fr. 11 Steckerl

6 καὶ *add. Müller* 7 ὡς *ex* ὧν *corr.* C 8 ὁπόταν] οπ *e corr.* C 9 ἀντιλολογίας C: *corr. Caius* 13 "*fortasse* ἀντιτιθεὶς *legendum*" *Müller* 15 μελήσει C: *suppl. Caius* 22 περιστρέφουσα C: *corr. Kühn* 25 τελευτᾶν] ευτ *ex* εστ, *ut vid., corr.* C 28 ἀναφέρεται] εται *e corr.* C πρώτας *ex* πρῶ[τ] *corr.* C 30 *post* μεσοπλευρίῳ *add.* μυΐ *Müller* 32 καὶ[I] *om. Caius* 33 τὰς] ας *e corr.* C

erate perverseness, as Praxagoras did. This man, since he did 18
not see any nerve growing out from the heart yet was ambitious to
compete with Hippocrates and wished at all costs to eliminate
the brain as source of the nerves, ventured on no inconsiderable
fiction: he said that as the arteries advance and divide they become
constricted and change into nerves; for since their body is nerve-
like but hollow, and the hollows get so small with the progressive
divisions in the animal that the tunics (of the artery) come together,
as soon as this happens, the vessel then appears as a nerve. Erasi- 19
stratus did not even think this account worthy of refutation, holding
it to be a piece of brazen effrontery.

7. But since I have this once become engaged in examining all
views, I wish to argue briefly with Praxagoras, especially because
Chrysippus too mentioned the man, opposing him to those who
hold that the nerves take their beginning from the head. Now we too 2
concede that the evidence of anatomy would have to be as Praxa-
goras stated it, if anyone is to suppose with good reason that the
heart is the source of the nerves. But the facts are otherwise, as we 3
have already demonstrated with animals on countless occasions to
those who wished to learn the truth. But we shall not hesitate here
again to explain the anatomy of the arteries, as we did earlier of the
nerves. The largest artery grows out from the left ventricle of the 4
heart, as it were the trunk of all the arteries in the animal. First to 5
branch off from it is the artery that encircles the heart like a crown,
and indeed people who are concerned with anatomy call it the coronary
artery. But you would not say, most noble Praxagoras, that this 6
artery, reduced in size by being split, turns at last into nerves. Next, 7
when the large artery divides, the larger portion turns down toward
the spine and attaches itself to the mid-line of the vertebrae; the other
rises up straight to the throat. Now first (I ask you) look at the ar- 8
teries that go from these to the thorax and say if you dare that some
one of them changes into a nerve. They are twenty-two in number,
one in each intercostal space, and paired with them in their distri-
bution are nerves from the spinal cord. Throughout the thorax these 9
two kinds of vessels are seen to be paired in their extensions and divi-
sions, and at the membrane that undergirds the ribs and intercostal
muscles a third venous vessel separates off with them and accompanies
them in their extensions and divisions. For the present there is no 10
need for me to go into detail about veins, for they too will be discussed
fully at another time. I return, then, to the arteries. And let us now 11
leave the arteries of the thorax, as even Praxagoras himself did

Πραξαγόρου τολμήσαντος ἐν θώρακι φάναι μηδεμίαν ἀρτηρίαν εἰς
12 νεῦρον μεταβάλλειν. — καίτοι εἴπερ ἐν θώρακι μὲν φαίνεται νεῦρα πάμπολ-
λα, μεταβάλλει δὲ οὐδὲ μία κατ' αὐτὸν εἰς νεῦρον ἀρτηρία, δῆλον ὡς οὐκ
13 ἔστιν ἐκ τῶν ἀρτηριῶν ἡ γένεσις τοῖς νεύροις. — ἀλλὰ γὰρ ἐπὶ τὰς
ἔξω τοῦ θώρακος ἴωμεν, ὧν πρώτη μέν ἐστι συζυγία τῶν ἐπὶ τὰς
ὠμοπλάτας ἀναφερομένων, ἀφ' ὧν οὐκ ὀλίγη μοῖρα καὶ πρὸς τὸν
νωτιαῖον εἴσω καταδύεται καὶ τοῖς ἐν τραχήλῳ μυσὶ διασπείρεται,
δευτέρα δὲ τῶν εἰς τὰς χεῖρας φερομένων ἀρτηριῶν, ἅς μοι καὶ μάλισθ' ὡς
14 ἀπονευρουμένας ὁ Πραξαγόρας αἰνίττεσθαι δοκεῖ. καίτοι φανερώτερόν
γε τῶν κατὰ τὸν θώρακα καὶ ταύτας ἰδεῖν ἔστιν, ὅσῳπερ καὶ μείζους
15 εἰσίν, εἰς ὅλα τὰ κῶλα κατασχιζομένας ἄχρι τῶν δακτύλων. ἀλλ' οὐδὲ
τούτων οὐδεμία φαίνεται νεῦρον γιγνομένη. καὶ γὰρ αἱ κατὰ τοὺς καρποὺς
148 τῶν χειρῶν, ὧν ἔθος ἡμῖν ἐστιν ἅπτεσθαι / πυρετῶν διαγνώσεως
192 ἕνεκα, | καὶ μεταξὺ τῶν δακτύλων λιχανοῦ τε καὶ μεγάλου μικραὶ μὲν
ὑπάρχουσι παντάπασιν, ἀλλ' οὔτε εἰς νεῦρον ἤδη μεταβεβλήκασιν
ἐναργῶς τε φαίνονται σφύζουσαι καὶ πρὸ τῆς ἀνατομῆς.

16 Ἀλλ' ἐν ταύταις μὲν ἴσως οὐ χρὴ πικρῶς διελέγχειν τὸν Πραξαγό-
ραν ἀλλά τι καὶ συγγνώμης νέμειν, εἰ μικρὰς ἀρτηρίας οὐκ ἐθεάσατο. —
17 καίτοι γε ὅταν εἰς νεῦρα μεταβάλλειν αὐτὰς φάσκῃ τὰς μικροτέρας, οὐκ
ἀμβλυωπίαν ὑποτιμᾶται δήπουθεν, ἀλλ' ὀξὺ βλέπειν ἐπαγγέλλεται. —
18 τῶν δὲ κατὰ τὰς μασχάλας ἀρτηριῶν, ἔστι δὲ καθ' ἑκατέραν χεῖρα μία,
μεγάλων τε οὐσῶν ἅμα καὶ τέτταρα ζεύγη νεύρων μεγάλων ἀμφ'
αὐτὰς ἐχουσῶν ἀναμνῆσαι βούλομαι τοὺς τὰ τοῦ Πραξαγόρου
19 πρεσβεύοντας. οὐδέπω μὲν γὰρ οὐδὲ ὑπήρξατο σχίζεσθαι κατὰ ταῦτα
τὰ μόρια τῶν ἀρτηριῶν οὐδετέρα, μεγάλα δέ ἐστιν οὕτως ἤδη τὰ νεῦρα
20 ὥστ' εἰ καὶ τυφλὸς εἴη τις, οὐκ ἂν λάθοιεν αὐτοῦ τὴν ἁφήν. πόθεν οὖν
149 ἐγεννήθη ταῦτα / καὶ τίνων ἀρτηριῶν ἀπεβλάστησε, δίκαιος λέγειν ὁ
21 Πραξαγόρας ἐστί. καίτοι τί προκαλοῦμαι λέγειν ἐκεῖνον ἐνὸν ἡμᾶς
193 εἰπεῖν | ἤδη τἀληθές, ὡς ἡ μὲν πρώτη συζυγία τῶν εἰρημένων τεττάρων
νεύρων ἀπὸ τοῦ νωτιαίου μυελοῦ σαφῶς ἀποβλαστάνει, καθ' ἃ συμβέ-
βληκεν ὁ τέταρτος τοῦ τραχήλου σπόνδυλος τῷ πέμπτῳ, ἡ δευτέρα δὲ
ἐφεξῆς αὐτῇ μεταξὺ τοῦ πέμπτου τε καὶ ἕκτου καὶ δὴ καὶ ἡ τρίτη μὲν ἵνα
συμβέβληκεν ὁ ἕκτος τῷ ἑβδόμῳ, ἡ τετάρτη δὲ ἐπ' αὐτῇ, τὸ δὲ τελευταῖον
ζεῦγος τῶν νεύρων ἐκ τῆς μεταξὺ χώρας ἐκφύεται τοῦ θ' ὑστάτου τῶν
τοῦ τραχήλου σπονδύλων καὶ τοῦ πρώτου τῶν ἐν τῷ θώρακι καὶ τοῦτ'
22 ἔστι τὸ εἰς ἄκρας ἰὸν τὰς χεῖρας. οὕτως γὰρ οἱ ἀνατομικώτατοι τῶν πρὸ
ἡμῶν ἔγραψαν, ὧν κἀν τοῖς πρώτοις λόγοις κἀν τοῖς νῦν ἐνεστῶσι
φυλάττω τὴν διδασκαλίαν [πληθυντικῶς], εἴ τί που παρεῖδον ἢ οὐκ
ἀκριβῶς ἐξειργάσαντο, παραλιπών· ἐν ἑτέρᾳ γάρ μοι πραγματείᾳ περὶ

24–25] *cf.* Gal. Anat. xiii. 9: II, p. 159 Simon

2 *post* καίτοι *addiderit* γ' *Einarson (cf. supra, p. 54)* 8 φερομένων] φερ *e corr.* C μοι *ex* μὴ *corr.* C 10 καὶ[I] *del. Müller* 12 αἱ] εἰ *Müller* 14 *post* καὶ[I] *add.* αἱ *Kühn* 18 νεμεῖν C: *corr. Kühn* 21 δὲ καθ' *ex* δὲ καὶ καθ' *corr.* C: δὲ ἀρτηρία καθ' *Müller* 23 αὐτὰς C: *corr. Kühn* 26 λάθη *in textu*, λαθεῖν *sscr.* C: λάθειεν *Caius*: *corr. Kühn* 28 καίτοι *ex* καί τι *corr.* C 30 καθὰ C: *corr. Schöne* 38 πληθυντικῶς *seclusi ut glossema ad verbum* παρεῖδον

not venture to say that in the thorax any artery changes to a nerve. –
Yet if very many nerves are observed in the thorax, and not one of the 12
arteries in it changes to a nerve, obviously the nerves do not come from
the arteries. – But let us proceed to the arteries outside the thorax, 13
the first of which is the pair rising to the scapulae, from which no
small part also penetrates deep into the spinal cord and spreads out
to the muscles in the neck. Second is the pair of arteries that pass to
the arms; these especially, it seems to me, are in Praxagoras' cryptic
remarks changed to nerves. But as these arteries are more easily ob- 14
served than those in the thorax, to the extent that they are also larger,
it is even more evident that they too divide and spread to all parts
(of the arms), as far as the fingers. But it is apparent that none of 15
these becomes a nerve either. The arteries in the wrist, which it is
our habit to touch in order to diagnose a fever, and those between
the index finger and thumb are very small; but they have not yet
changed to nerves, and even before dissection it is clear that they
pulsate.

Perhaps in the case of these arteries we should not expose Praxa- 16
goras mercilessly, but rather grant him some measure of pardon for
failing to see small arteries. – Yet when he says that it is precisely 17
the smaller arteries that change into nerves, he is not pleading dull-
ness of vision at all, but is claiming that his eyesight is acute. – But I 18
wish to remind Praxagoras' adherents of the arteries in the axillae,
one for each arm, which are large and have four pairs of large nerves
around them. Neither artery has yet even begun to divide at this 19
point, and the nerves are already so large that even if a person were
blind he could not fail to detect them by touch. Where did they come 20
from? What arteries did they grow out from? It is only right that
Praxagoras should tell us. Yet why do I challenge him to speak, 21
when I can myself give the correct account without further delay?
The truth is that the first pair of the four nerves just mentioned clearly
branches off from the spinal cord at the point where the fourth cervical
vertebra adjoins the fifth; the second pair, next after it, (branches
off) between the fifth and sixth vertebrae; the third pair where the
sixth adjoins the seventh; and the fourth after that. The final pair
of nerves grows out from the region between the last cervical vertebra
and the first thoracic; this is the pair that goes to the hands. This 22
is the account given by the best authorities on anatomy prior to our
time; I have held to their teaching, both in my earlier accounts and
in the present ones, passing over anything that they overlooked or
failed to work out in detail; for I shall speak of such matters in another

150 23 τῶν τοιούτων εἰρήσεται. οὔκουν ἀρτηρίας / χρὴ ζητεῖν ἐξ ὧν νεῦρα τῷ
λόγῳ γεννήσαντες ἢ τοὺς δακτύλους κινήσομεν ἢ τι τῶν κατὰ τὰς
24 χεῖρας ἕτερον. ἔχομεν γὰρ ἤδη τὰ νεῦρα καὶ πλείω καὶ μείζω τῶν ἀρτη-
194 ριῶν οὐκ ἐκ τῆς ἐκείνων τραγικῆς μεταμορφώσεως, | ἀλλ' ἐκ τοῦ νωτιαίου
μυελοῦ γεγενημένα.

25 Τὰ μὲν δὴ τοῦ Πραξαγόρου ψεύσματα πεφώραται σαφῶς ἤδη
καὶ οὐδὲν ἔτι Πραξαγόρου γ' ἕνεκεν ἐπὶ τὰς ἀρτηρίας ἰέναι χρὴ τῷ
26 λόγῳ. ἀλλ' ἐπειδήπερ ὑπεσχόμην, ὡς ἔμπροσθεν ἐδήλωσα τὴν τῶν
νεύρων εἰς ἅπαντα τοῦ ζῴου τὰ μόρια νομήν, οὕτω καὶ νῦν ἐκδιδάξαι
27 τῶν ἀρτηριῶν, ἐπὶ τὰς ὑπολοίπους αὖθις αὐτῶν τρέψομαι. καὶ πρώτας
μὲν τὰς ἐπὶ τοὺς μασθοὺς φερομένας προσθήσω τῷ λόγῳ, δευτέρας δὲ
τὰς ἄνω τοῦ θώρακος καὶ τρίτας τὰς κάτω καὶ τετάρτας ὅσαι τοῖς
σκέλεσι διανέμονται.

28 Αἱ μὲν δὴ τῶν μασθῶν ἀρτηρίαι τῆς ἐπὶ τὰς σφαγὰς ἀναφερομένης
ἀποφύονται, ἐπιβαίνουσαι δὲ τῷ στέρνῳ καλουμένῳ μικρὸν ὑποκάτω
τῆς τῶν κλειδῶν πρὸς αὐτὸ διαρθρώσεως ὑποφέρονται διαπαντὸς
αὐτῷ καὶ τελευτῶσαι διεκπίπτουσιν ἐκτὸς τοῦ θώρακος ὑπὸ τοῦ στήθους.
151 29 οὐ μὴν ἐνταῦθά γε ὅλαι / κατασχίζονται· φαίνεται γάρ τις αὐτῶν μοῖρα
δι' ἐπιγαστρίου κατιοῦσα κἀνταῦθ' εἰς πλείω σχιζομένη ταῖς ἀπὸ τῶν
30 βουβώνων ἀνιούσαις εἰς ταὐτὸν ἥκουσα. λελέξεται δὲ ὑπὲρ ἐκείνων
ὀλίγον ὕστερον, ἐπειδὰν ἡ τοῦ λόγου τάξις ὑποβάλλῃ. |

195 Νυνὶ δὲ ἐπὶ τὰς ἄνω κλειδῶν ἰέναι καιρὸς ἀρχὴν τῷ λόγῳ τήνδε θεμέ-
31 νους. ἐπειδὰν πρῶτον ἐκ τοῦ θώρακος ἀνασχοῦσα καὶ τὰς κλεῖς ὑπερβᾶσα
32 κατὰ μέσην γένηται τὴν σφαγὴν ἡ ὄρθιος ἀρτηρία, δίχα σχίζεται. τοὐν-
τεῦθεν δὲ τὸ γεννηθὲν ζεῦγος ἀρτηριῶν μεγάλων οὐκ ὀρθῶς μὲν ὀνομά-
ζονται καρωτίδες, ἀλλ' ἤδη κρατεῖ τοὔνομα διὰ τὴν πολλὴν ἄγνοιαν
33 ἁπάντων τῶν μεθ' Ἱπποκράτην φιλοσόφων τε καὶ ἰατρῶν. ἀλλ' ὅτι
μὲν οὗτοί τε κακῶς ὑπειλήφασι πάθημα τῶν εἰρημένων ἀρτηριῶν εἶναι
τὸν κάρον οὔθ' Ἱπποκράτης οὕτως ἐγίγνωσκεν, ἐν τῷ δευτέρῳ τῶνδε
152 τῶν ὑπομνημάτων / ἀναγκαῖόν ἐστί μοι διελθεῖν· ἐν δὲ τῷ παρόντι λόγῳ
τοῦ γε ὀνόματος οὐ φθονήσω ταῖς ἀρτηρίαις, ἀλλ' ὀνομαζέσθωσαν ἔτι
34 καὶ νῦν καρωτίδες. ὅστις δὲ ὁ τρόπος αὐταῖς ἐστι θέσεώς τε ἅμα καὶ
σχίσεως ἁπάσης τε τῆς εἰς τὰ τῶν κλειδῶν ἄνω μόρια διανομῆς, ἐγὼ
35 διηγήσομαι. φέρονται μὲν ἔτι καὶ νῦν ὄρθιαι, καθάπερ ἐξ ἀρχῆς ὥρμησαν,
196 36 τὸ δ' οἷον πρέμνον αὐτῶν εὐθὺ τῆς κεφαλῆς. ἀποβλαστήματα δὲ | κατὰ
τὸν τράχηλον ἀποπέμπουσι μικρὰ τοῖς ταύτῃ μυσίν. ἐπειδὰν δὲ πλησίον
37 ἤδη γένωνται τῆς γένυος, ἑκατέρα δίχα σχίζεται. καὶ οὕτως ἤδη τέτταρες
αἱ πᾶσαι γεννηθεῖσαι δύο μὲν εἰς γλῶττάν τε καὶ σύμπαν τὸ πρόσωπον

1–3] Prax. fr. 11 Steckerl 6–8] Prax. fr. 11 Steckerl 8–9] libri primi test., *v. supra*, p. 68.16–17 20–21] *v. infra*, p. 88.33–35 34–88.2] *cf.* Gal. UP xvi. 12: IV 332–334 K.

2 τοῖς δακτύλοις C: *corr. Caius* 10 τρέψωμεν C: τρέψωμαι *aut* τρέψομαι *Schöne* 11 τοὺς μασθοὺς *e* τοῦ μασθοῦ *corr.* C 19 πλείω] πλείους *Müller* 22 τῷ λόγῳ] τοῦ λόγου *Müller* 24–25 τοὐντεῦθεν δὲ τὸ] "*fortasse* τὸ ἐντεῦθεν δὲ" *Müller* 28 τε] γε *Müller* 29 οὔθ'] οὐδὲ *Müller* 30 ἐστί] ἔσται *Schöne* 31 γε] τε C: *corr. Kühn* 32 ὅστις δὲ] ὅς τισι C: *corr. Caius* 35 ἀποβλαστήματα *ex* ἀποβλάστημα *corr.* C

treatise. There is therefore no need to hunt for arteries from which we 23
first generate nerves theoretically and then move our fingers or any
other part of the arm. For we already have nerves that are larger 24
and more numerous than the arteries, produced not from a theatrical
transformation of arteries, but from the spinal cord.

The falsifications of Praxagoras have now been clearly exposed; 25
and there is no need, on his account, to pursue further the discussion
of the arteries. But since I promised that as I had earlier explained 26
the distribution of nerves to all parts of the body, so now I would
give a full account of the arteries too, I shall turn to those that remain.
I shall enlarge my discussion to include first, the arteries that go to 27
the breasts; second, those above the thorax; third, those below (it);
and fourth, those that are distributed to the legs.

The arteries of the breasts take their start from the artery that 28
rises to the throat. They reach the sternum, as it is called, a little
below its articulation with the clavicles, and they proceed under it
all the way, emerging finally outside the thorax at the base of the
chest. Yet they are not wholly dispersed there. A portion is seen de- 29
scending through the epigastrium, where it separates into several
(branches) and meets the arteries ascending from the groin. We shall 30
speak of those arteries a little later, when the order of the discussion
brings us to them.

It is now time to go to the arteries above the clavicles. We begin
our account as follows: as soon as the straight artery, ascending from 31
the thorax and rising above the clavicles, reaches the midpoint of
the throat, it divides into two branches. The pair of large arteries 32
produced by that division are incorrectly called carotid, but the name
has by now prevailed because of the great ignorance of all philosophers
and physicians since Hippocrates. In the second book of this treatise 33
I shall be compelled to explain in detail that they were wrong in
assuming stupor to be an affection of these arteries, and that Hippo-
crates did not share their view. But in the present account I shall
not begrudge the name to the arteries; let them even now be called
carotid. I shall now describe their position, their division, and the 34
whole of their distribution to the parts above the clavicles. They 35
continue to go straight on, as they did from the start, their "trunk"
as it were going directly to the head. At the neck they send off small 36
branches to the muscles there. But when they are already close to
the chin, each splits in two. Thus four arteries in all have now been 37
produced. Two of them branch out to the tongue and the whole of

ὅσον τε τὸ τῆς κεφαλῆς ἐκτὸς τοῦ κρανίου κατασχίζονται· δύο δὲ λοιπὸν
38 διεξερχόμεναι τὸ κρανίον εἰς τὸν ἐγκέφαλον ἔρχονται. καὶ δεῖ καὶ τῶνδε
μεμνῆσθαι τῶν ἀρτηριῶν· οὐ σμικρὸς γὰρ οὐδὲ αὐτὰς ἐκδέχεται
λόγος, ὅτι μηδὲ ἁπλῶς μηδὲ ὡς ἔτυχεν ἐπὶ τὸν ἐγκέφαλον ἀνίασιν, ἀλλ'
153 ὑπὸ τῇ παχείᾳ μή/νιγγι τὸ θαυμαστὸν ἐκεῖνο πλέγμα τὸ τῷ δικτύῳ
39 παραπλήσιον ἐργάζονται. νυνὶ δὲ ⟨οὔτε⟩ τούτων τῶν ἀρτηριῶν οὔτε
ἄλλης οὐδεμιᾶς ἀνάγκη λέγειν ἅπασαν τὴν ἐκ τῆς ἀνατομῆς γιγνωσκο-
μένην ἰδέαν· τῇ τε γὰρ Περὶ χρείας μορίων πραγματείᾳ καὶ τῇ Τῶν
40 ἀνατομικῶν ἐγχειρήσεων ἡ τοιαύτη διέξοδός ἐστιν οἰκειοτέρα. κατὰ δὲ τὸ
παρόν, ὅσον ὑπογράψαι χρήσιμον ὡς ἐκ τῆς ἀριστερᾶς κοιλίας τῆς καρ-
δίας αἱ ἀρτηρίαι πᾶσαι πεφύκασι, τὴν ἀνατομὴν αὐτῶν διέξειμι.
197 41 Ἡ μείζων μοῖρα τῆς μεγίστης ἀρτηρίας | ἐστήρικται μὲν ἐπὶ μέσης
τῆς ῥάχεως οὐ κατὰ τὸν νῶτον μόνον, ἀλλὰ καὶ τὴν ὀσφῦν ἅπασαν.
42 ἀποφύσεις δὲ πρώτας μέν, ὡς ἔμπροσθεν εἴπομεν, εἰς ὅλον ἀποστέλλει
τὸν θώρακα κἄπειτ', ἐπειδὰν ἤδη διεκπίπτῃ τὸ διάφραγμα, καὶ τούτῳ
43 ζεῦγος ἕτερον. ἐφεξῆς δὲ πρώτη τῶν κάτω τοῦ θώρακος ἀρτηρία διττὴ
μετ' αὐτὰς εὐθέως τὰς φρένας ἀποβλαστάνουσα τῆς ἐπὶ τὴν ῥάχιν
φέρεται πρὸς τῷ σπληνὶ καὶ γαστρὶ καὶ ἥπατι καὶ τοῖς ἐντέροις ἅπασι
154 44 καὶ παντὶ τῷ μεσαραίῳ διασπειρομένη. ἑξῆς δὲ κατὰ / συζυγίαν ἤδη
δύο μὲν εἰς τοὺς νεφροὺς μείζονες πολλῷ τῆς προειρημένης, ἄλλαι δὲ
δύο κατ' ἐπιγάστριόν τε καὶ τὰς ψόας, καθ' ἕκαστον σπόνδυλον ἓν
ζεῦγος ἄχρι τοῦ πλατέος ὀστοῦ, καὶ μέν γε καὶ εἰς τὰς μήτρας τε καὶ
45 ὄρχεις ἐντεῦθεν κατέρχονται καί τις ἄζυγὴς εἰς μεσεντέριον. ἀλλὰ καὶ εἰς
αὐτὸν εἴσω τὸν νωτιαῖον ἀπὸ τῆς μεγάλης ἀρτηρίας καθ' ὅλην τὴν
ῥάχιν ἐκφύονταί τινες ἀρτηρίαι μικραί, δύο καθ' ἕκαστον σπόνδυλον.
46 ἐπειδὰν δὲ κατὰ τὸ ἱερὸν ὀστοῦν γένηται, σχίζεται τοὐντεῦθεν ἤδη
198 μεγάλα μέρη. καὶ κατέρχεταί τις | εἰς ἑκάτερον σκέλος, ἐν τῇ παρόδῳ
τοῖς καθ' ἱερὸν ὀστοῦν ἀποβλαστήματα πέμψασα κύστει τε καὶ τῆς
μήτρας τοῖς κάτω καὶ ξυνελόντι φάναι τοῖς γεννητικοῖς ἅπασι μορίοις·
οὐδὲν γὰρ ἔτι δέομαι λέγειν οὐδ' ἐνταῦθα τὸν τρόπον τῆς διανομῆς.
47 ἀπὸ τούτων τῶν ἀρτηριῶν τῶν ἐπὶ τὰ σκέλη φερομένων, ἐπειδὰν πλησίον
ἥκωσι βουβώνων, ἀποφύεται μία καθ' ἑκατέραν ἄνω τοῦ σώματος ἰοῦσα
155 48 δι' ἐπιγαστρίου. / κατασχιζόμεναι δὲ ἐνταῦθα ταῖς ἀπὸ τῶν μαστῶν
καταφερομέναις εἰς ταὐτὸν ἥκουσιν, ὡς ἑνοῦσθαι τὰ⟨ς⟩ τέτταρα⟨ς⟩
τά⟨σ⟩δε. περὶ τούτων τῶν ἀρτηριῶν εἴρηταί μοι καὶ πρόσθεν, ἡνίκα
τὰς κατὰ τὸν θώρακα διῄειν τῷ λόγῳ.

12] *cf. supra*, p. 82.25–27 14] *cf. supra*, p. 82.28–31 35–36] *v. supra*, p. 86.14–20

1 λοιπὸν] λοιπαὶ *Müller* 4 μηδὲ ... μηδὲ] μήθ' ... μήθ' *Müller* 5 τῷ *deleverit Schöne (cf. infra, p. 92.14)* 6 ἐργάζεται C: *corr. Kühn* οὔτε[I] *add. Caius* 7 γιγνωσκομένην *ex* γιγνομένην *corr.* C[2] 14 πρώτας] πρῶτον *Müller* 16 πρώτῃ *Caius* 26 *post* ἤδη *add.* εἰς *Caius (cf. Petersen, 1888, p. 38; Helmreich, Neue Philol. Rundschau [1890], p. 36)* 27 *post* τις *add.* μοῖρα *Müller* 32 ἑκάτε-ρον *Caius (cf. infra, p. 90.1)* 34–35 τὰ τέτταρα τάδε C: *corr. Müller* 35 εἰρητό C: *corr. Caius in mg.*

the face and as much of the head as lies outside the cranium; the
other two pass through the cranium and reach the brain. These ar- 38
teries too must be kept in mind, for no small discussion follows on
them, as their ascent to the brain is not simple or random, but beneath
the dura mater they produce that remarkable interweaving that
resembles the fishnet. But at the moment there is no need to de- 39
scribe, for these arteries or any other, the entire form revealed by
dissection. Such a detailed account is more appropriate to my treatises
On the Use of the Parts, and On Anatomical Procedures. For the 40
present I shall explain the anatomy of them only so far as is useful
for showing that all the arteries grow from the left ventricle of the
heart.

The larger branch of the largest artery is firmly attached to the 41
middle of the spinal column not only along the back but also along
the whole of the lumbar region. But as I said before, it sends its first 42
branches to the whole thorax and then, just as it emerges from the
diaphragm, it sends a second pair also to that organ. Next, the first 43
of the arteries below the thorax, branching off just below the dia-
phragm from the artery that goes to the spine, proceeds on a double
course: in addition to the spleen, stomach, and liver, it is distributed
also to all the intestines and the whole mesentery. Next, two arteries, 44
now going in pairs, much larger than the one just mentioned, go to
the kidneys; others separate off by twos in the region of the epi-
gastrium and the muscles of the iliac region, a pair at each vertebra
as far as the sacrum, and from this same region arteries go to uterus
and testes, and an unpaired artery goes to the mesentery. And in 45
addition, the whole length of the spine, certain small arteries, two at
each vertebra, grow out from the large artery and pass inside the spinal
column itself. But when it reaches the sacrum it splits from there on 46
into large parts. And a branch goes down to each leg, sending off-
shoots, as it passes by, to the region of the sacrum, to the bladder,
to the lower parts of the uterus, and, in a word, to all the organs of
generation; for here again I need not now describe the manner in
which they are distributed. From these arteries that go to the legs, 47
as they approach the groin, arteries grow out, one from each, and go
up the body through the epigastrium. There they divide and go to 48
meet the arteries descending from the breasts, so that the four are
united. I mentioned those others earlier, when I was recounting the
arteries of the thorax.

49 Λοιπαὶ δὲ τῶν σκελῶν αἱ ἀρτηρίαι δύο, μία καθ' ἑκάτερον ἐνεχθεῖσα
βουβῶνα τοῖς ἐντὸς τοῦ μηροῦ παρατάττεται μέρεσιν ἄχρι τοῦ γόνα-
50 τος. ἀπὸ τούτων ἑκατέρας εἰς τοὺς καθ' ἑκάτερον τῶν μηρῶν μῦς αἱ
ἀρτηρίαι κατασχίζονται, τὸ δὲ ὑπόλοιπον αὐτῶν διὰ τῆς ἰγνύος ἐνεχθὲν
51 εἴς τε τὰ περὶ τὴν κνήμην ἅπαντα καὶ τὸν πόδα νενέμηται. καὶ οὐδὲν οὐδὲ
199 ἐνταῦθα δέομαι διέρχεσθαι τὸν τρόπον τῆς νομῆς, | ἀλλ' ἀρκεῖ βραχεῖ
λόγῳ δεδηλωκέναι τὰς ἐν τῷ ζῴῳ πάσας ἀρτηρίας ἀπὸ μιᾶς ἐκείνης πε-
φυκυίας, ἣν ⟨ἐκφύεσθαι⟩ ἐκ τῆς ἀριστερᾶς κοιλίας τῆς καρδίας, οἷον ἐκ
γῆς τι[νὸς] πρέμνον ἐλέγομεν.
52 Ἔστι δὲ καὶ ἑτέρα τις ἀρτηρία τῆς αὐτῆς κοιλίας ἐκφυομένη, φλε-
βώδης τὸν χιτῶνα. κατασχίζεται δὲ εἰς ὅλον αὕτη τὸν πνεύμονα τοῖς
156 ζῴοις ἅπασιν / οἷς πνεύμων ἐστίν· οἷς δὲ οὐκ ἔστιν, εἰς ἕτερόν τι μόριον
53 ἀνάλογον ὑπάρχον πνεύμονι, καθάπερ τοῖς ἰχθύσιν εἰς τὰ βράγχια. ταύτην
τὴν ἀρτηρίαν εἰκάσειεν ἄν τις τῷ τοῦ πρέμνου κάτωθεν ἐν αὐτῇ τῇ γῇ
ἐμπεριεχομένῳ μέρει τοῦ φυτοῦ· καὶ δὴ καὶ κατασχίζεσθαι ταύτην μὲν ὡς
ἂν εἰς ῥίζας τινὰς τὰς κατὰ τὸν πνεύμονα πεφυκυίας ἀρτηρίας, τὴν μεγάλην
δὲ τὴν εἰς ὅλον τὸ σῶμα νενεμημένην οἷόν περ κλάδους ἀπομερίζειν ἑαυτῆς
54 ἁπάσας τὰς κατὰ τὸ ζῷον ἀρτηρίας ὀλίγον ἔμπροσθεν εἶπον. οὕτως
γὰρ οἶμαι καὶ τὸν Ἱπποκράτην προσεικάσαντα ῥίζωσιν ἀρτηριῶν
ἀποφαίνεσθαι τὴν καρδίαν, ὥσπερ ἀμέλει τῶν φλεβῶν τὸ ἧπαρ. εἰρήσεται
200 δέ μοι | περὶ τῆς εἰκόνος ἐπὶ πλέον ἐν τοῖς ἑξῆς, ἐπειδὰν ὑπὲρ ἥπατός τε
55 καὶ φλεβῶν ὁ λόγος περαίνηται. νυνὶ δὲ ἀρκεῖ τὰ λεγόμενα πρὸς ἔνδειξιν
τοῦ καὶ τὰς ἀρτηρίας ἁπάσας ἀπὸ τῆς καρδίας ἐκπεφυκέναι καὶ μηδεμίαν
αὐτῶν εἰς νεῦρον μεταβάλλειν, ἀλλ' ἀρχὴν ἁπάντων τῶν νεύρων ὑπάρ-
χειν τὸν ἐγκέφαλον. /
157 8. Καταλιπόντες οὖν ἤδη τὸν Πραξαγόραν ἀναίσχυντα σοφιζό-
μενον αὖθις ἐπὶ τὸν Ἀριστοτέλη μεταβῶμεν, ἐπειδὴ καὶ αὐτὸς ἐκ τῆς
καρδίας φύεσθαί φησι τὰ νεῦρα. συγκεχυμένως δὲ εἴρηται καὶ ἀδιορίστως
2 δὶς πρὸς αὐτοῦ περὶ τῆς τῶν νεύρων ἀρχῆς. ἐχρῆν γὰρ οἶμαι τὸν ἀπὸ
καρδίας αὐτὰ φύεσθαι φάσκοντα δεῖξαι πῶς εἰς ἕκαστον τοῦ ζῴου μόριον
ἀπ' αὐτῆς ἔρχεται [τὸ] νεῦρον, ὥσπερ ἡμεῖς ὀλίγον ἔμπροσθεν ἐπεδεί-
ξαμεν ἀρτηρίαν, οὐ τὸ ἁπλῶς γε τοῦτο εἰπεῖν μόνον αὔταρκες ὑπολα-

8–9] *v. supra*, p. 82.20–21 18–20] Hipp. De alim. 31: CMG I 1, p. 82.13 = p. 144.15 Joly *cf. infra*, PHP 520.2–4; 570.17 Müller 20–22] *cf. infra*, PHP 509.14–512.13; 519.13–520.14; 521.15–522.6 Müller 26–28] Prax. fr. 11 Steckerl 27] *cf. supra*, p. 80.24

1 τῶν σκελῶν αἱ] αἱ τῶν σκελῶν *Müller* 2 παρατάττεται] τ^{I} *et* ται *e corr.* C: παρατέταται *Caius* μέρεσιν] μέρεσ *e corr.* C 3 αἱ *del. Müller* 6 διανομῆς *Marquardt* 8 ἐκφύεσθαι *addidi (cf. supra, p. 82.20)* 9 τινὸς C: *corr. Müller (cf. supra, p. 82.21 et infra, PHP 514.11; 518.12; 531.10 Müller)* λεγόμενον C: *correxi* (ἐλέγομεν φύεσθαι *Caius*) 10 ἐκφυομένη] η *ex* ης, *ut vid., corr.* C 11 αὐτή C: *corr. Kühn* 12 εἰς *add. supra lin.* C^{2} 13 βρογχία C: *corr. Einarson* 18 *ante* ὀλίγον *add.* ἃς C^{2} *in mg.* 21 περὶ *add. supra lin.* C^{2} 22 περαίνεται C: *corr. Caius* 26 Καταλιπόντες] ο *ex* ω *corr.* C 27 Ἀριστοτέλην *Müller (cf. supra, p. 51)* 29 αὐτὸν C: *corr. Caius* 31 τὸ *del. Petersen (cf. infra, p. 98.4)* ὕστερον C: ἔμπροσθεν *sscr.* C^{2} 32 *ante* ἀρτηρίαν *add.* τὴν *Müller* οὐ τὸ] ὡς C: ὡς τὸ C^{2}: *corr. Caius*

There remain the two arteries of the legs; one passes along each 49
groin and lies close to the inner parts of the thigh as far as the knee.
From each of these are divided off the arteries to the muscles in each 50
thigh; what remains passes through the back of the knee and spreads
out to the whole region of the shin and the foot. Here too I need not 51
trace the manner of distribution; it is enough to have shown in a brief account that all the arteries in the animal arise from that one artery which, as we pointed out, grows out from the left ventricle of the heart like a tree trunk from the earth.

There is, besides, another artery growing out from the same 52
ventricle, whose covering is like that of a vein. It spreads to the whole of the lungs in all animals that have lungs; in those that do not, it goes to some other part analogous to the lungs; in fish, for example
to the gills. You might compare this artery to the lower part of a tree 53
trunk enclosed in the earth itself. Indeed, as I said just now, it is divided into the arteries of the lungs as into roots of a sort, while the large artery that spreads to the whole body sends off from itself, like
branches, all the arteries in the animal. This was the comparison, I be- 54
lieve, that Hippocrates made when he said that the heart is the *rhizōsis* of the arteries, precisely as the liver (is the *rhizōsis*) of the veins. I shall speak later at greater length of the comparison, when an
account is given of the liver and veins. The present remarks are enough 55
to indicate not only that all arteries grow out from the heart but also that none of them changes into a nerve; rather, the source of all the nerves is the brain.

8. Let us now leave Praxagoras propounding his shameless sophistries and return to Aristotle, since he too says that the nerves come from the heart. He spoke twice of the origin of the nerves in
a confused and imprecise way. For the man who says that they come 2
from the heart should, in my opinion, have pointed out the route by which a nerve passes from the heart to each part of the body, just as we pointed out the route of the arteries just now; he should not have supposed that the simple assertion is by itself sufficient.

3 βεῖν. ὅθεν ⟨ὅπερ⟩ ἐν τῷ τρίτῳ Περὶ τῶν ἐν τοῖς ζῴοις ἔγραψεν οὐδαμῶς
ἦν πρέπον Ἀριστοτέλει. παραγράψω δὲ τὴν ῥῆσιν αὐτήν· «ἔχει
201 δὲ καὶ νεύρων πλῆθος ἡ καρδία, καὶ τοῦτο εὐλόγως· ἀπὸ | ταύτης
γὰρ αἱ κινήσεις, περαίνονται δὲ διὰ τοῦ θ' ἕλκειν καὶ ἀνιέναι· δεῖ
158 4 οὖν / τοιαύτης ὑπηρεσίας τε καὶ ἰσχύος.» ὅτι μὲν γὰρ «δεῖ τοιαύτης
ὑπηρεσίας τε καὶ ἰσχύος» ἐκείνῳ τῷ μέλει τοῦ σώματος ὃ τὴν ἀρχὴν τῆς
ψυχῆς ἐν ἑαυτῷ περιέχει, πρόδηλον ἅπαντι· τὸ μέντοι τὴν καρδίαν τοῦτ'
εἶναι τὸ μέλος οὐ μόνον οὐκ ἀπέδειξεν ὁ Ἀριστοτέλης ἀλλ' οὐδὲ πι-
θανῶς ἐπεχείρησεν, εἰ μὴ ἄρα τὸ νεύρων ἔχειν πλῆθος αὐτὴν ἱκανὸν
5 εἶναι γνώρισμα νομίζει τοῦ νεύρων ὑπάρχειν ἀρχήν. ἀλλ' οὕτω γε καὶ
τὰς χεῖρας καὶ τοὺς πόδας ἀρχὰς ὑποληψόμεθα νεύρων. ἂν γὰρ ἱκανὸν
εἶναι νομίσωμεν ἔνθ' ⟨ἂν⟩ ᾖ νεῦρα πολλά, τοῦτ' ἀρχὴν τίθεσθαι νεύρων,
6 οὐδὲν ἡμᾶς κωλύσει καὶ ταῦτα τὰ μόρια νεύρων ἀρχὰς ὑπολαβεῖν. οὕτω
δὲ καὶ τὸ τῷ δικτύῳ παραπλήσιον πλέγμα τὸ ὑπὸ τῇ παχείᾳ μήνιγγι τῶν
ἀρτηριῶν ἀρχὴν ἐροῦμεν, οὐ τὴν καρδίαν· ἀναρίθμητον γάρ τι πλῆθος
ἀρτηριῶν ἐστι κατ' ἐκεῖνο τὸ πλέγμα.
7 Ταυτὶ μὲν οὖν ἐκ περιουσίας εἰρήσθω μοι πρὸς τὸ μηδ' εἰ πολλὰ
202 159 κατὰ τὴν | καρδίαν ἐφαίνετο νεῦρα, πάντως ἄν τιν' / ἐκ τούτων τίθεσθαι
8 δικαίως ἀρχὴν ἁπάντων τῶν κατὰ τὸ σῶμα τοῦ ζῴου νεύρων. ἐπεὶ
δ' οὐδ' ἔχει νεῦρα πολλά, μεῖζον ἂν ἔτι γίγνοιτο τῷ Ἀριστοτέλει τὸ
ἄτοπον. εἰσὶ μὲν γάρ τινες ἐν αὐτῇ νευρώδεις διαφύσεις, οὐ μὴν ἤδη γέ
9 πω καὶ νεῦρα. δειχθείη δὲ ἂν οὐ διὰ μακρῶν τοῦτο κατ' αὐτὸν τὸν
Ἀριστοτέλη. οὗτος γοῦν ἐστιν ὁ διδάξας ἡμᾶς εἰς τὴν ἐνέργειάν τε
καὶ χρείαν ἀποβλέπειν ἑκάστου τῶν ὀργάνων, οὐκ εἰς τὴν κατασκευήν,
10 ἐπειδὰν ὅ τί ποτέ ἐστιν αὐτῷ τὸ εἶναι σκοπώμεθα. τὸ γοῦν ὀφθαλμῷ
εἶναι τί ποτέ ἐστιν ἐρωτηθέντες, ἀποκριναίμεθ' ⟨ἂν⟩ «ὀργάνῳ ὀπτικῷ».
οὐ γὰρ δὴ τό γ' ἐκ τοσούτων τε καὶ τοιούτων ὑγρῶν χιτώνων τε καὶ
ὑμένων καὶ μυῶν ὡδί πως συγκειμένων κατεσκευάσθαι τὴν οὐσίαν αὐτὴν
εἶναι βούλεται τῶν ὀφθαλμῶν ὁ Ἀριστοτέλης, ὀρθότατα γινώσκων, ὡς
11 καὶ πρὸς ἡμῶν ἐν ἑτέροις ἐπιδέδεικται. νυνὶ δὲ οὐδὲ οἶμαι δεῖσθαι εἴς γε
160 τὰ / παρόντα τῆς παρ' ἡμῶν ἀποδείξεως αὐτοῦ τοῦ Ἀριστοτέλους
12 δοξάζοντος οὕτως. εἰ μὲν γὰρ πρὸς ἄλλον τινὰ τὸν λόγον ἐποιούμην,
203 ἐπειρώμην ἂν ἐπιδεικνύειν ὡς ταῖς | ἐνεργείαις τε καὶ χρείαις ἕκαστον τῶν
13 μορίων, οὐ τῇ τοῦ σώματος ἰδέᾳ κρίνεται. ἐπειδὴ δὲ πρὸς Ἀριστοτέλη

2–5] Arist. De part. animal. iii. 4: 666 b 14–16 *cf.* iii. 3: 665 a 10–13 De motu animal. 10: 703 a 14–24 13–14] *cf. supra*, p. 88.4–6

1 ὅπερ *addidi*, ὡς *addiderit Einarson*, ὃ *add. Caius* τῶν ἐν τοῖς ζῴοις] τῶν ἐν τοῖς ζῴοις μορίων *Caius*: ζῴων μορίων *Müller* 4 δὲ] καὶ C: *del.* C²: *corr. Caius ex Arist.* θ' *del.* C²: *om. Arist.* 9 τὸ] τῶν C: *corr.* C² 10 καὶ *inser.* C 12 ἂν *add. Müller* 15 οὐ τὴν καρδίαν *del. Müller* 18 ἐφαίνετο] αι *e corr.* C 21 διαφύσεις *coni. Caius (cf. infra, p. 96.19)*: διαστάσεις C 23 Ἀριστοτέλην *Müller* 25 αὐτὸ C: *correxi* τὸ^II] τῶ C: *corr. Diels* 26 εἶναι] ἵνα ᾖ C: *corr. Diels* ἂν *add. Müller* 28 καὶ μυῶν ὡδί πως *add. supra lin.* C² συγκείμενον C: *corr.* C² κατεσκευάσθαι *in* κατασκευάσθαι *mut.* C 29 ὀρθότατα] ὀρθὰ ταῦτα C: ὀρθώτατα C²: *corr. Kühn* 30 πρὸ C: *corr.* C² οὐδὲ] οὐκ *Müller* 34 ἰδέᾳ] ε *e corr.* C ἀριστο^τλ' C: *suppl. Caius*: Ἀριστοτέλην *Müller*

Thus Aristotle's remarks in the third book of his treatise On the 3
(Parts) of Animals were quite unworthy of him. I shall transcribe
the actual passage: "The heart also has a large number of nerves,
and reasonably so, for movements begin from it and are carried out
by pulling and slacking; therefore it needs service and strength of
this sort." Now it is clear to all that the member of the body which 4
encloses the soul's source "needs service and strength of this sort".
But not only did Aristotle fail to demonstrate that the heart is
this member; his argument is not even plausible, unless he actually
supposes that the presence of a large number of nerves in the heart
is sufficient token that (the heart) is source of the nerves. But by that 5
reasoning we shall accept even the hands and the feet as sources of
nerves. For if we consider it sufficient to postulate that whatever
place has a large number of nerves is a source of them, nothing will
prevent us from accepting these parts too as sources of nerves. And 6
by that reasoning we shall also say that the net-like web that lies
under the dura mater, and not the heart, is the source of the arteries;
for there is a countless multitude of arteries in that web.

Let this then be an argument from abundance, that even if a large 7
number of nerves were to be seen in the heart, it would be quite wrong
to make it, on that account, the source of all the nerves in the animal's
body. But since the heart does not even have a large number of nerves, 8
Aristotle's position becomes even more absurd. There are in it
certain nerve-like strands, but we cannot go so far as to call them
nerves. And this could be demonstrated at no great length on Ari- 9
stotle's own principles. Thus it was he who taught us to look to the
action and use of every organ, not to its structure, when we investigate
its 'being'. If asked, "What is 'being' for the eye?", we would answer, 10
"It is that it be an organ of sight". Certainly Aristotle does not intend
that the formation of the eye from moist bodies and tunics and
membranes and muscles, so many in number, of such and such kinds,
and arranged in such and such a way, is the very 'essence' of the eye;
and in this his judgment is entirely correct, as I have pointed out in
other works. But for our present purpose no proof, I think, is required 11
of me, as Aristotle himself accepts this view. If I were answering 12
someone else, I would attempt to point out that each part is distin-
guished by its actions and uses, not by its bodily form. But since I am 13

διαλέγομαι τὸν αὐτὸν οὕτως γινώσκοντα πολὺ πρότερον ἡμῶν, ἀναμνῆ-
σαι χρὴ μόνον ὧν αὐτὸς ἔν τε τῷ δευτέρῳ Περὶ ψυχῆς κἀν τῷ Περὶ μο-
ρίων ἀπεφήνατο, τὸ ταὐτὸν καὶ τὸ ἕτερον ὄργανον ἐκ τῶν ἐνεργειῶν καὶ
14 χρειῶν, οὐκ ἐκ τῆς τοῦ σώματος ἰδέας κρίνεσθαι βουλόμενος. εἰ μὲν γὰρ
ὀπτικὸν εἴη τὸ ὄργανον, ὀφθαλμός ἐστι, κἂν ἑτέρως ἔχῃ κατεσκευα-
σμένον ἀνθρώποις τε καὶ καρκίνοις· εἰ δὲ βαδιστικόν, σκέλος, ἄν τ' ἐλέ-
15 φαντος ἄν τ' αἰγὸς ἄν τε οἰὸς ἄν τε ἀνθρώπου τύχῃ. εἰ δὲ ταῦθ' οὕτως
ἔχει, κρινέσθω σοι τὸ νεῦρον, Ἀριστότελες φίλτατε, μὴ τῇ τοῦ σώ-
ματος ἰδέᾳ, καθάπερ τοῖς πολλοῖς καὶ ἀγυμνάστοις περὶ λόγον, ἀλλ'
ἐνεργείᾳ τε καὶ χρείᾳ. /
161 9. Τρία γάρ ἐστιν ὄργανα παραπλήσια μὲν ἀλλήλοις τὴν μορφὴν
τοῦ σώματος, οὐκ ὀλίγον δὲ ἐνεργείαις τε καὶ χρείαις διαλ⟨λ⟩άττοντα·
204 προσαγορεύεται δὲ αὐτῶν | τὸ μὲν νεῦρον, τὸ δὲ σύνδεσμος, τὸ δὲ τένων.
2 τὸ μὲν δὴ νεῦρον ἐξ ἐγκεφάλου πάντως ἢ νωτιαίου πέφυκεν αἴσθησιν
ἢ κίνησιν ἢ τὸ συναμφότερον οἷς ἂν ἐμφύηται παράγον· ὁ σύνδεσμος δὲ
ἀναίσθητος μέν ἐστιν, ἡ χρεία δὲ αὐτοῦ κατὰ τοὔνομα. λοιπὸς δὲ τένων
πέρας ἐστὶ νευρῶδες μυὸς ἐκ συνδέσμου καὶ νεύρου γεννώμενος, ὡς ἔν
τε τοῖς Περὶ μυῶν κινήσεως ἡμῖν ἐπιδέδεικται κἀν ταῖς ἀνατομικαῖς
3 ἐγχειρήσεσι. νεῦρον μὲν δὴ πᾶν ἀκριβῶς ἐστι στρογγύλον, οἱ τένοντες
δὲ οὐχ ἅπαντες, ἔτι δὲ μᾶλλον οἱ σύνδεσμοι· πλατύνονται γὰρ οἱ πλείους
4 αὐτῶν εἰς ὑμένος ἰδέαν. ἀλλ' ὑμὴν μὲν ἅπας ἀκριβῶς ἐστι λεπτὸς καὶ
5 μαλακός, σύνδεσμος δὲ καὶ σκληρὸς καὶ παχὺς τοὐπίπαν. ἔνιοι μὲν αὐτῶν
νευροχονδρώδεις ὀνομάζονταί τε καί εἰσιν· οὔτε δὲ ὑμὴν οὔτε νεῦρον
162 οὔτε τένων εἰς τοσαύ/την ποθ' ἥκει σκληρότητα, ἀλλὰ τῶν μὲν νεύρων
ἔνια καὶ πάνυ μαλακὰ τὴν φύσιν ἐστίν, εἰς αἴσθησιν ἐπιτήδεια μόνην,
205 ἔνια δὲ εἰ καὶ σκληρότερα τούτων ὑπάρχει κατὰ | τὴν τοῦ σώματος
6 οὐσίαν, ἀλλὰ παμπόλλῳ γε ἀπολείπεται συνδέσμου σκληρότητος. οὕτω
δὲ καὶ οἱ ὑμένες εἰ καὶ διαφέρουσιν ἀλλήλων κατὰ σκληρότητα, συνδέσμων
7 ἀπολείπονται πάμπολυ. οἱ τένοντες δὲ σύγκεινται μὲν ἔκ τε τῶν συνδέσμων
καὶ τῶν νεύρων τῶν σκληροτέρων, ἐν τῷ μέσῳ δὲ εἰκότως ἀμφοῖν εἰσι,
τοσούτῳ νεύρου σκληρότεροι τὴν οὐσίαν ὑπάρχοντες ὅσῳ συνδέσμου
8 μαλακώτεροι. ἅπαντα δὲ ταῦτά ἐστι τὰ τρία γένη λευκὰ καὶ ἄναιμα

4–6] *cf.* Gal. UP viii. 4: III 627–630 K. Meth. med. i. 5: X 43 K. 11–96.2] *cf.* Gal. Anat. i. 3: II 233 K. xiv. 2: II, pp. 169–170 Simon De motu musc. i. 1, 2: IV 368–369; 374–376 K. UP i. 17; xii. 3: III 47; IV 9 K. De ossibus ad tir., prooem.: II 739 K. De bon. mal. sucis 4: CMG V 4.2, pp. 402–403 Meth. med. vi. 4: X 408–409 K. De part. homoeom. diff. 2: CMG Suppl. Or. III, p. 55 [Gal.] Def. med. 86: XIX 366 K. 11–13, 16–17, 19–21] *cf.* Maimonid. Aph. i. 10 15–16] *cf.* Gal. Anat. i. 10: II 267–268 K. 16–17] *cf.* *infra*, lin. 29–30; p. 98. 24–25 Nemes. De nat. hom. 4, 27: pp. 148, 251 Matth. 21–27] *cf.* Maimonid. Aph. i. 11 22–23] *cf.* Gal. Anat. vii. 10: II 619 K. UP vi. 19: III 502 K. 24–27] *cf.* *infra*, PHP 619.10–15 Müller 32–96.2] *cf.* Maimonid. Aph. i. 12

2 ὧν *ex* ὡς *corr.* C Περὶ^{II}] πρώτῳ περὶ ζῴων *Müller* 3 τὸ^{I} *om. Müller* 7 τύχοι C: *corr. Kühn* 12 διαλάττοντα C: *corr. Caius* 15 ἐμφύηται] ἐμ *ex* ἐκ *corr.* C^2 16 *ante* τένων *add.* ὁ *Müller* 17 νευρώδους C: *corr. Caius* 22 καὶ^{I} *inser.* C 26 τὴν *add.* C^2 32 μαλακώτεροι] κώ *ex* κό *corr.* C

answering Aristotle, who himself recognized this fact long before
our time, I need only mention what he said in the second book of his
work On the Soul and in his work On the Parts (of Animals), his inten-
tion being to distinguish identity and difference in organs by their
actions and uses, not their bodily form. If the organ is the instrument 14
of sight, it is an eye, even though it is differently constructed in men
and in crabs; if it is the instrument for walking, it is a leg, whether it
happens to belong to an elephant or a goat or a sheep or a man. But if 15
that is so, dear Aristotle, then you must differentiate a nerve not by
its bodily form as the majority, who are untrained in reasoning, do but
by its action and use.

9. There are three structures similar to each other in bodily form
but quite different in action and use. One is called 'nerve', another
'ligament', and the third, 'tendon'. A nerve in every case grows from 2
the brain or spinal cord and conveys sensation or motion or both to
the parts to which it is attached. A ligament is without sensation; its
use is expressed by its name. Finally, a tendon is the nerve-like termi-
nation of a muscle, the product of ligament and nerve, as we pointed
out in On the Movement of the Muscles and Anatomical Procedures.
Now every nerve is exactly round, but not all tendons, and even less 3
the ligaments; for most of them are flattened in the form of a mem-
brane. But every membrane is quite thin and soft, whereas a ligament 4
is for the most part both hard and thick. Some ligaments are neuro- 5
cartilaginous and are so named; but no membrane or nerve or tendon
ever reaches such a degree of hardness. Some nerves are by nature very
soft, suitable only for sensation; others, though harder than these in
their physical substance, yet fall far short of the hardness of a tendon.
It is the same also with membranes: even though they differ from one 6
another in hardness, they fall far short of ligaments. Tendons are 7
formed of ligaments and the harder nerves, and they lie, reasonably
enough, in the middle; they are as much harder than a nerve in their
substance as they are softer than a ligament. All these three classes 8

καὶ ἀκοίλια καὶ εἰς ἶνας εὐθείας λυόμενα πλὴν τῶν πάνυ σκληρῶν
9 συνδέσμων· οὐ γὰρ οἷόν τε τούτους ἀναλῦσαι εἰς ἶνας. εἰ γοῦν οὕτως
ὀνομάζειν ἐθέλεις ὡς Ἱπποκράτης ὠνόμαζε, τὸ μὲν αἴσθησίν τε καὶ
κίνησιν παρέχον ἤτοι νεῦρον ἢ τόνον – ἄμφω γὰρ αὐτὸ προσαγορεύει –,
163 τὸ δὲ ἀναίσθητον σύνδεσμον, εἰς ὃν δὲ / ὁ μῦς τελευτᾷ, τένοντα, δείξω
10 σοι σαφῶς οὐκ ἔχουσαν πλῆθος νεύρων τὴν καρδίαν· εἰ δὲ καὶ συγχεῖν
βούλοιο τὰς προσηγορίας ὡς οἱ πλεῖστοι τῶν μεθ' Ἱπποκράτη, κάλει
μὲν ἅπαντα νεῦρα, διαφορὰς δὲ ἐν αὐτοῖς λέγε τριττάς, αἰσθητικὰ μὲν
206 καὶ προαιρετικὰ | τὰ ἐξ ἐγκεφάλου καὶ νωτιαίου πεφυκότα, συνδετικὰ
δὲ τὰ ἀναίσθητα καὶ τρίτα ἔτι πρὸς τούτοις τὰ ἐκ τῶν μυῶν ἀπονευ-
ρουμένων φυόμενα.

10. Καὶ οὕτως δὲ δείξομεν οὐκ ἔχουσαν ἀξιόλογα τὸ μέγεθος ἢ τὸ
πλῆθος αἰσθητικά τε καὶ προαιρετικὰ νεῦρα τὴν καρδίαν ἐναργῶς, ἀλλ'
ὡς ἔμπροσθεν εἴρηται σμικρὸν ἀπ' ἐγκεφάλου κατιὸν εἰς αὐτὴν ἐμφύεται.
2 τί ποτε οὖν ἐστι τὸ πρὸς Ἀριστοτέλους εἰρημένον «ἔχει δὲ καὶ νεύρων
πλῆθος ἡ καρδία»; οὔτε γὰρ φιλοψευδὴς ὁ ἀνὴρ οὔτε παντάπασιν
ἄπειρος τῆς ἀνατομῆς, ἵνα καὶ τοῦτόν τις ὥσπερ τοὺς περὶ τὸν Χρύ-
3 σιππον ἑτέροις ἐψευσμένοις ἠκολουθηκέναι νομίσειεν. ἐμοὶ μὲν δοκεῖ τὰς
ὑπὸ Ἡροφίλου νευρώδεις διαφύσεις ὠνομασμένας αὐτὸς οὐ νευρώδεις
164 4 ἀλλ' ἄντικρυς εἰρηκέναι νεῦρα. πέρατα δ' / ἐστὶ ταῦτα τῶν ἐπὶ τοῖς
στόμασι τῆς καρδίας ὑμένων, ὑπὲρ ὧν Ἐρασίστρατος μὲν ἀκριβῶς
5 ἔγραψεν Ἡρόφιλος δὲ ἀμελῶς. συμφύονται δὲ καὶ συνδοῦνται δι' αὐτῶν
πρὸς τὴν καρδίαν οἱ ὑμένες οὗτοι καὶ ἡ χρεία γε κατὰ τοὺς συνδέσμους |
207 6 αὐτοῖς, οὐ κατὰ τὰ νεῦρα. ἀλλ' εἰ καὶ νεῦρά τις εἶναι συγχωρήσειεν
αὐτὰ καὶ μὴ νευρώδη σώματα, τό γε τὴν καρδίαν ὑπάρχειν νεύρων
ἀρχὴν οὐκ ἐξ ἀνάγκης ἕπεται μὴ δυναμένων ἡμῶν ἐπιδεῖξαι μηδὲν νεῦρον
εἰς μηδὲν μόριον τοῦ σώματος ἀπ' αὐτῆς φερόμενον, ὡς ἔμπροσθεν ἐδείξαμεν
7 ἀπ' ἐγκεφάλου τε καὶ νωτιαίου. δοκεῖ δή μοι δύο μὲν ἐνταῦθα ὑποθέμενος
ὀρθῶς ὁ Ἀριστοτέλης, ἓν μὲν ὡς ἰσχύος δεῖ τινος οὐκ ἀγεννοῦς εἰς
τὰς κατὰ προαίρεσιν ἐνεργείας, ἕτερον δὲ ὡς οὐδεμιᾶς τοιαύτης ἰσχύος

3–4] *cf.* Hipp. De artic. 11: IV 108 L. Gal. Anat. xiv. 2: II, p. 169 Simon De motu musc. i. 1: IV 369 K. In Hipp. De artic. comm. i. 46, 52: XVIII A 380–381; 387 K. Ruf. Onom. 211: p. 163 Daremberg-Ruelle 5] *cf.* Gal. In Hipp. De artic. comm. ii. 3: XVIII A 428 K. In Hipp. De fract. comm. iii. 54: XVIII B 620 K. Compend. Tim. 22: p. 89 Kraus-Walzer 7–11] *cf.* Gal. In Hipp. Epid. VI comm. i. 2: CMG V 10.2.2, p. 9 9–10] *cf.* Gal. De loc. aff. iii. 8: VIII 168–169 K. In Hipp. Epid. VI comm. iv. 7: CMG V 10.2.2, p. 197 10–11] *cf.* Gal. UP i. 16; x. 8: III 46; 797 K. De motu musc. i. 1: IV 368 K. De bon. mal. sucis 4: CMG V 4.2, p. 403 De loc. aff. ii. 8: VIII 99 K. Meth. med. vi. 4: X 411 K. (*cf.* Herbst, 1911, pp. 122–123) 14] libri primi test., *v. supra*, p. 68.18–19 *cf.* Gal. Anat. vii. 8: II 613 K. De nerv. dissect. 10: II 844 K. 16–18] SVF II, p. 246 24–28] libri primi test., *v. supra*, p. 68.8–12

1 ἶνας *ex* οἶνας *(?) corr.* C 2 οὐ *ex* εἰ *corr.* C ἶνας] ας *e corr.* C 3 ἐθέλοις *Müller* 5 ὃν] ὃ *Müller* 7 Ἱπποκράτην *Müller* 15 ἔχει] χε *e corr.* C 16 ὁ *add.* C² 17 ἵνα] ὥστε ἂν *Müller* τοῦτον *ex* τούτων *corr.* C 18 ἑταίροις *(ex -ους corr.)* C: *corr. Kühn* ἠκολουθηκέναι] ἠ *e corr.* C 19 Ἡροφίλου] ο[I] *ex* ρ, *ut vid.*, *corr.* C αὐτὰς C: *corr. Herbst*: ταύτας *Schöne*

are white, bloodless and solid, and all are separable into straight fibres except the very hard ligaments; for they cannot be divided into
fibres. Thus if you are willing to give them the names that Hippo- 9
crates gave them, calling the one that provides sensation and motion either 'nerve' or 'tone' – he uses both names –, the one that lacks sensation 'ligament', and the one in which the muscle terminates 'tendon', I shall demonstrate clearly to you that the heart does not
have a large number of nerves; but if you want to confuse the names, 10
as most men have done since Hippocrates' time, call them all 'nerves' but say that there is a three-fold distinction among them, those from the brain and spinal cord being sensory and volitional, those without sensation being ligamentous, and third, in addition to these, are those that grow from the muscles as they turn into 'nerves'.

10. Even then we shall show that the heart clearly does not have 'sensory and volitional' nerves of any consequence in size or number, but a small one, as we said before, descends from the brain and grows
into it. Just what, then, did Aristotle mean, that "the heart also has 2
a large number of nerves"? He was not a man to delight in falsehood, nor was he totally unacquainted with dissection, that he might be thought, like Chrysippus, to have followed the mistakes of others.
My opinion is that what Herophilus called 'nerve-like strands' 3
Aristotle termed not 'nerve-like' but simply 'nerves'. These are the 4
terminations of the membranes at the openings of the heart, of which Erasistratus gave a precise account, Herophilus a careless one.
These membranes are attached and tied to the heart by the strands, 5
whose use is that of ligaments, not of nerves. But even if one should 6
admit that they are nerves, not nerve-like structures, it does not follow of necessity that the heart is the source of nerves, since we cannot point to any nerve passing from it to any part of the body in the way that we earlier pointed out their passage from brain and spine.
In my opinion Aristotle here used two correct premises, the first, 7
that some considerable strength is needed for voluntary actions, and the second, that the brain does not possess any such strength. But

ἐγκεφάλῳ μέτεστιν, ἐπ' αὐτοῖς δὲ τρίτον ἐξ αἰσθήσεως προσλαβὼν τὸ
πλῆθος τῶν ἐν τῇ καρδίᾳ νευρωδῶν συνδέσμων, οὐκέθ' ὑπομεῖναι περὶ
165 τὴν κατὰ μέρος ἀνατομὴν ἀσχοληθῆναι καὶ ζητῆσαι πῶς εἰς / ἕκαστον
τοῦ σώματος μόριον ἐκ καρδίας ἀφικνεῖται νεῦρον, ἀλλ' ὡς ἄντικρυς ἑπό-
8 μενον ἐν οἷς εἶπον ἀποφήνασθαι. πολλὰ γὰρ δὴ τοιαῦτα καὶ παρὰ τοῖς
ἰατροῖς ἔστιν εὑρεῖν ἀνατομικὰ θεωρήματα μοχθηρῶς γεγραμμένα, μὴ
208 βουληθέντων αὐτῶν ἀναμεῖναι τὸ φαι|νόμενον ἐκ τῆς ἀνατομῆς, ἀλλ'
9 ἐξ ἀκολουθίας μέν τινος ἐλπισάντων ὡς ἑωρακότων. οὕτω δή μοι καὶ
ὁ Ἀριστοτέλης ἐσφάλθαι φαίνεται δύο μὲν ἀληθῆ θέμενος λήμματα,
10 τὸ δὲ τρίτον ἐγγὺς ἀληθείας πιθανόν. ἀληθῆ μὲν οὖν εἶναί φημι τό τε
δεῖν ἰσχύος τινὸς τοῖς κινήσουσιν ὀργάνοις τὰ τοῦ ζῴου μέλη καὶ τὸ
μηδὲν ἀπ' ἐγκεφάλου φαίνεσθαι τοιοῦτον, πιθανὸν δέ, οὐκ ἀληθές,
ὡς ἐν τῇ καρδίᾳ πλῆθος εἴη νεύρων.
11 Ἀλλ' ἡμεῖς γε δεῖξαι δυνάμεθα τὸ καλῶς μὲν ὑπ' αὐτοῦ τῷ λόγῳ
γνωσθὲν ὄργανον ὑφ' οὗ χρὴ κινεῖσθαι τὰ τοῦ ζῴου μέλη, διότι δ' ἠμέλησε
ζητῆσαι κατὰ τὰς ἀνατομὰς αὐτό, διὰ τοῦτ' ἐκφυγόν τε τὴν διὰ τῶν
166 12 αἰσθήσεων εὕρεσιν / ἄγνωστόν τε μεῖναν τἀνδρί. τῶν μὲν γὰρ νεύρων
οὐδέν ἐστι τοιοῦτον, οἱ δὲ ὀνομαζόμενοι μύες ὑποδεχόμενοι ταῦτα κι-
13 νοῦσι τὰ μέλη. καὶ δόξειεν ἂν οἷον μοχλοῦ τινος ἔχειν δύναμιν ὁ μῦς ὡς
πρὸς τὸ νεῦρον. ὥσπερ γὰρ ὅσα ταῖς χερσὶν οὐχ οἷοί τ' ἐσμὲν κινῆσαι
βάρη, διὰ τῶν μοχλῶν αὐτὰ κινοῦμεν, οὕτω καὶ τὰ τοῦ σώματος μέλη
209 14 τοῖς νεύροις ἀδυνατοῦντες κινεῖν τοὺς μῦς | προσεκτησάμεθα. λυόμενον
γὰρ εἰς ἶνας ἐν ἑκάστῳ μυῒ τὸ νεῦρον ἀναμίγνυταί τε καὶ διαπλέκεται ταῖς
ἐκ τῶν συνδέσμων ἰσίν, εἶτα ἐξ ἀμφοῖν ἕν τι νευρῶδες σῶμα γεννηθὲν
ἐκφύεται τοῦ σώματος ⟨τοῦ⟩ μυὸς ὁ προσαγορευόμενος τένων· — οὕτως
γὰρ οὐχ Ἱπποκράτης μόνον ἀλλὰ καὶ Ὅμηρος αὐτὸν ὀνομάζουσιν· —
ὅστις τένων ὀργάνων ἐκφυόμενος ἀνάλογον ἕξει τῷ τοῦ μοχλοῦ πέρατι
15 τῷ ψαύοντι τῶν βαρῶν. οὐδ' ἔστιν οὐδὲν εὑρεῖν ἐν τῷ σώματι μέλος
167 ὃ κατὰ μὲν τὴν ἡμετέραν κινεῖται προαίρεσιν, οὐ προτέτακται / δὲ αὐτοῦ
16 τις μῦς ἀπ' ἐγκεφάλου δεχόμενος νεῦρον. ὅστις δὲ καὶ περὶ τοῦδε πεισθῆναι
ἐθέλει βεβαίως, τούτῳ γέγραπται πρὸς ἡμῶν ὑπομνήματα δύο, κατὰ μόνας
ἑκάτερον, ἓν μὲν ἅπαντας τοὺς μῦς ὁποία τ' ἐστὶν ἐνέργεια καθ' ἕκαστον
ἀκριβῶς διδάσκον, ἕτερον δὲ τὴν τῶν νεύρων εἰς αὐτοὺς νομὴν διηγού-
17 μενον. οὐ μὴν ἀλλὰ καὶ ἐν Ταῖς ἀνατομικαῖς ἐγχειρήσεσι καὶ τοῖς Περὶ
χρείας μορίων ὑπομνήμασιν ἐπὶ πλέον ὑπὲρ ἁπάντων τούτων διέξιμεν.

5] *cf. supra*, p. 92.2–5 24–25] *cf. supra*, pp. 94.16–17; 96.5 26] *e. g.* Hom. Od. iii. 449 Il. v. 307 32–33] Gal. De motu musc.: IV 367–464 K. *cf. etiam* De musc. dissect.: XVIII B 926–1026 K. 33] Gal. De nerv. dissect.: II 831–856 K.

1 ἐξ αἰσθήσεως *inser.* C 5 ἐν *del. Müller* 5–6 *per verba* τοιαῦτα — εὑρεῖν *linea producta est, quasi delendi causa, in* C 8 μὲν *del. Müller* 11 μέλη] μένη C: *corr.* C[2] 14 τὸ *del. Müller* αὐτῶ C: *corr. Caius* 15 μέλη] μένη C: *corr. Caius* 16 ἐκφυγόν τε] ἐκφεύγοντος C: *corr. Al. Just.* 19 μέλη] μένη C: *corr. Caius* δείξειεν C: *corr. Caius* 24 εἴτε C: *corr. Caius* γεννη C: *corr. Caius* 25 τοῦ[II] *add. Kühn* μῦς C: *corr. Caius* 27 ὀργάνων] αν *e corr.* C 31 ἐθέλοι C: *corr. Müller* 33 διδάσκον] ον *ex* ων *corr.* C

when he adds to these as a third, taken from sense-perception, the
large number of nerve-like ligaments in the heart, he no longer had the
patience to concern himself with the particulars of anatomy and to
inquire how a nerve proceeds from the heart to each part of the body;
he asserts it as if it were directly entailed in the passage that I cited.
Indeed in the works of physicians, too, one may find many such 8
anatomical speculations, incorrectly stated, because they were not
willing to await the evidence of dissection but anticipated it by some
inference, as if they had seen it. So I think that Aristotle was also 9
misled when he posited two true premises and a third plausibly close
to the truth. I call true the statements that the organs which are to 10
move the animal's limbs need a certain strength and that no such
organ is observed (coming) from the brain; I call plausible, but not
true, the statement that there are many nerves in the heart.

But we can point to the organ required to move the animal's 11
limbs, an organ which he rightly recognized in theory but which,
since he did not take the pains to search for it by dissection, eluded
discovery by observation and remained unknown to him. For none of 12
the nerves is that kind of organ; the limbs are moved by the muscles,
as they are called, which receive the nerves. And the muscles in rela- 13
tion to the nerves would seem to have the power of a kind of lever, as
it were. For just as we use levers to move weights that we cannot move
with our hands, so we have muscles in addition to nerves, since we
cannot move the limbs of the body with the nerves. The nerve in each 14
muscle separates into fibres and mixes and intertwines with the
fibres from the ligaments, and then a single nerve-like structure, the
product of their union, grows out from the body of the muscle, the so-
called tendon. – It is given this name not only by Hippocrates but
also by Homer. – This tendon, growing out from the organs of the
body, will be analogous to the end of a lever in contact with heavy
weights. You cannot find in the body any limb moved by our volition 15
which does not have placed before it some muscle that receives a
nerve from the brain. As an aid to the person who wishes to be firmly 16
convinced of this I have written two separate treatises, one instructing
him in all the muscles and explaining in detail the activity of each,
the other describing how the nerves are distributed to them. And in- 17
deed I shall give a rather full account of all these matters both in my
Anatomical Procedures and in my work On the Use of the Parts.

18 Ὥστ' οὐδενὸς ἔτι προσδεῖν ἡμῖν ἔοικεν ⟨ὁ λόγος⟩, ἀλλ' ὁμολο-
210 γούμενος | ἑαυτῷ τε καὶ τοῖς ἐναργῶς φαινομένοις ὑπάρχει⟨ν⟩ πᾶσιν ἀρχὴν
19 τῶν νεύρων ἐγκέφαλον τιθέμενος. οὕτω δὲ καὶ τῶν ἀρτηριῶν ἐπεδείξαμεν
ἀρχὴν ὑπάρχουσαν τὴν καρδίαν· ὅτι δὲ καὶ τῶν φλεβῶν ἀρχὴ τὸ ἧπάρ
20 ἐστιν ἐν τοῖς ἐφεξῆς ἀποδειχθήσεται. ἐνταῦθ' οὖν ἤδη καταπαύσας τὸ
πρῶτον βιβλίον ἐπὶ τὰ συνεχῆ τοῖς ἀποδεδειγμένοις ἐν αὐτῷ κατὰ τὸ
δεύτερον τρέψομαι. /|

4–5] *v. infra*, **PHP lib. VI**

1 ὁ λόγος *post* ἔοικεν *add. Einarson, post* τιθέμενος *(lin. 3) Müller* ὁμολογουμένως C: *corr. Einarson* 2 ὑπάρχει C: *suppl. Schöne* 6 ἑαυτῶ C: *corr. Caius*

Thus it seems to me that the account needs nothing more; it is 18
consistent with itself and with all that is clearly observed when it
postulates that the brain is the source of the nerves. And similarly we 19
have shown that the heart is the source of the arteries. Later we shall
also prove that the liver is the source of the veins. I therefore now 20
bring the first book to a close and turn in the second to the matters
that come next after those here demonstrated.

ΓΑΛΗΝΟΥ

ΠΕΡΙ ΤΩΝ ΙΠΠΟΚΡΑΤΟΥΣ ΚΑΙ ΠΛΑΤΩΝΟΣ ΔΟΓΜΑΤΩΝ

ΒΙΒΛΙΟΝ ΔΕΥΤΕΡΟΝ

168 211 1. Περὶ τῶν Ἱπποκράτους καὶ Πλάτωνος δογμάτων ἐπισκέ-
ψασθαι προθέμενος ἀπὸ τοῦ πρώτου κατὰ τὴν δύναμιν ὑπηρξάμην,
ᾧ καὶ τἄλλα σχεδὸν ἅπαντα τὰ κατὰ μέρος ἀκολουθεῖν ἔδειξα, τοῦτο δέ
ἐστι τὰ περὶ τῶν διοικουσῶν ἡμᾶς δυνάμεων ὁπόσαι τέ εἰσι τὸν ἀριθμὸν
ὁποία τέ τις ἑκάστη καὶ τόπον ὅντιν' ἐν τῷ ζῴῳ κατείληφεν· ἠξίουν τε
212 μηδὲν οὕτω φυλάττεσθαι κατὰ τὸν λόγον | ὡς τὸ τοῖς ἐναργῶς φαι-
νομένοις ἐναντία τίθεσθαι, καθάπερ οἵ τε μηδὲν ἄλογον ζῷον ἐπιθυμεῖν
169 ἢ θυμοῦσθαι φάσκοντες οἵ τε τὴν / ἀρχὴν τῶν νεύρων ὑπάρχειν ἐν τῇ
2 καρδίᾳ. ἀποτετόλμηται γὰρ ἅπαντα τὰ τοιαῦτα πρὸς ἀνθρώπων ἀνα-
τρέψαι φιλονεικούντων ὅσα καλῶς εἴρηται τοῖς παλαιοῖς, ὑπὲρ τοῦ νεω-
τέραν αἵρεσιν ἰδίαν συστήσασθαι. τὰ μὲν οὖν τοιαῦτα τῶν ψευσμάτων
ἐν τῷ πρώτῳ βιβλίῳ διήλεγξα· νυνὶ δὲ ἐπὶ θάτερον εἶδος λόγων ὧν ποι-
οῦνται ἔγνωκα μεταβὰς ἐπιδεῖξαι σαφῶς, καθόσον οἷός τ' εἰμί, πῇ ποτε
σφάλλονται.

2. Διελέσθαι δὲ ἴσως ἄμεινον ἕνεκα σαφηνείας εὐθὺς ἐν ἀρχῇ τοῦδε
τοῦ γράμματος, ἥτις ἐστὶν ἡ διαφορὰ τῶν λόγων οἷς χρῶνται πάντες οἱ
2 κακῶς ὁτιοῦν μεταχειριζόμενοι πρόβλημα. φημὶ δὴ τῶν λημμάτων ἃ ἕνεκα
τοῦ συμπεράσματος λαμβάνουσιν, [ὡς] τὰ μὲν ἄντικρυς εἶναι ψευδῆ, τὰ
3 δὲ οὐκ οἰκεῖα τοῦ προκειμένου σκέμματος· ἄντικρυς μὲν ψευδῆ τὰ τοιαῦτα,
περὶ ὧν ἐν τῷ πρώτῳ βιβλίῳ διῆλθον ἐπὶ πλέον, ὅταν ἤτοι μηδὲν τῶν
213 ***170*** ἀλόγων ζῴων ἐπι|θυμεῖν τις ἢ θυμοῦσθαι φάσκῃ, / καθάπερ οἱ ἀπὸ τῆς
Στοᾶς, ἢ πάλιν ἐκ καρδίας πεφυκέναι τὰ νεῦρα· τὰ δὲ οὐκ οἰκεῖα τῶν
λημμάτων ὁπόσα τὴν φύσιν ἐστίν, εἴρηται μὲν ἐπὶ πλεῖστον ἐν τοῖς
Περὶ ἀποδείξεως ὑπομνήμασιν, ἐν οἷς ἅπασαν ἐδήλωσα τὴν ἀποδεικτικὴν
μέθοδον ὁποία τίς ἐστιν παρεκάλουν τε διὰ τοῦ πρώτου τῶνδε τῶν

4–8] libri primi test., *v. supra*, p. 66.3–7 8–15] libri primi test., *v. supra*, pp. 68.31–70.2 9–10] *cf. supra*, p. 100.2 10–11] *cf. infra*, lin. 23–25 11–12] Prax. et Arist., *cf. supra*, pp. 80.24–26; 90.26–28 22–25] libri primi test., *v. supra*, p. 68.27–30 25–104.8] *cf.* Prantl, Gesch. d. Logik I 569 n. 27–104.2] *cf.* Prantl, Gesch. d. Logik I 562 n. 28–104.2] libri primi test., *v. supra*, p. 66.14–16

1–3 Γαληνοῦ περὶ τῶν καθ' ἱπποκράτην καὶ πλάτωνα δογμάτων. ἀρχὴ τοῦ δευτέρου βιβλίου M: Γαληνοῦ περὶ τῶν καθ' ἱπποκράτην καὶ πλάτωνα δογμάτων. βιβλίον δεύτερον *Ald.*: *om.* C 6 τὰ *om.* C 11 θυμοῦσθαι] θυμοῦντες C: *corr.* C[3] 12 ἀποτετολμῆσθαι C 16 οἷον C 20 δὴ] δὲ C 21 λαμβάνουσιν *om.* C ὡς *om. Ald.* 22 τῷ προκειμένῳ σκέμματι *Müller* 23 ὧν] τῶν M 24 φάσκει *Ald.*: φάσκουσι M 25 πάλιν] πάντ' C 26 λημμάτων] προβλημάτων C 27 ἅπασιν *Ald.* ἐδήλωσαν *Ald.*: ἐδηλ^ω C

GALEN

ON THE DOCTRINES OF HIPPOCRATES AND PLATO

BOOK II

1. Having proposed to investigate the teachings of Hippocrates
and Plato, I began with the doctrine that is first in importance, from
which I showed that very nearly all particular details follow; this is
their teaching about the powers that govern us, their number, the
nature of each, and the place that each occupies in the body. And in
this discussion I thought proper to avoid nothing so carefully as
making assertions contrary to what is clearly observed, as those men
do who assert that no irrational animal feels desire or anger, and also
those (who say) that the source of the nerves is in the heart. All such 2
notions have been boldly advanced by men who were ambitious to
overthrow all the excellent teachings of the ancients, in order to found
a newer school of their own. In the first book I thoroughly refuted
fabrications of this kind; I have decided now to pass on to the other
kind of argument that they use and to show as clearly as I can where
their error lies.

2. Perhaps for the sake of clarity it is better right at the start of
this book to distinguish the different arguments that all men use when
they argue badly about any problem whatever. With reference to the 2
premises that they posit in order to draw a conclusion, I say that some
are patently false, others are not appropriate to the question before
them. Patently false are premises such as those discussed at some 3
length in the first book, when one says, as the Stoics do, that no
irrational animal feels desire or anger, or again, that the nerves grow
from the heart; inappropriate premises were enumerated according to
their nature at great length in my treatise On Demonstration, where
I explained what scientific method is in its entirety; and throughout

ὑπομνημάτων ἐν ἐκείνῃ γυμνάσασθαι πρότερον, ὅστις ὁτιοῦν ἀποδεικνύειν ἐπιχειρεῖ.

4 Γεγράφθαι δὲ λέγω ὑπὲρ αὐτῆς ἄριστα τοῖς παλαιοῖς φιλοσόφοις τοῖς περὶ Θεόφραστόν τε καὶ Ἀριστοτέλην κατὰ τὰ Τῶν δευτέρων ἀναλυτικῶν βιβλία καὶ διὰ τοῦτο πρὸς ἐκείνους μὲν οὐδὲ μακρὸν ἔσεσθαι
5 τὸν λόγον ἐλπίζω περὶ τῶν τριῶν ἀρχῶν τοῦ ζῴου· τὰ γὰρ ἰδιωτικά τε καὶ ῥητορικὰ λήμματα αἰδοῦνται παραλαμβάνειν εἰς ἀποδείξεις ἐπιστημονικάς, ὧν πέπλησται τὰ Χρυσίππου βιβλία ποτὲ μὲν ἰδιώτας ἐπικαλούμενα μάρτυρας ὧν ὑποτίθεται λημμάτων, ἔστι δὲ ὅτε ποιητὰς ἢ τὴν βελτίστην ἐτυμολογίαν ἤ τι ἄλλο τοιοῦτον, ἃ περαίνει μὲν οὐδέν,
171 ἀναλίσκει / δὲ καὶ κατατρίβει μάτην ἡμῶν τὸν χρόνον αὐτὸ τοῦτο μόνον
214 ἐν|δεικνυμένων αὐτοῖς, ὡς οὐκ ἔστιν ἐπιστημονικὰ τὰ τοῦ συμπεράσματος λήμματα, μετὰ ταῦτα δὲ καὶ συγκαταβαινόντων τε καὶ συμπαλαιόντων αὐτοῖς ὑπὲρ τοῦ δεῖξαι καὶ τοὺς ἰδιώτας καὶ τοὺς ποιητὰς οὐδὲν ἧττον
6 ἡμῖν ἢ ἐκείνοις μαρτυροῦντας, ἀλλ' ἔστιν ὅτε καὶ μᾶλλον. οὕτω δὲ καὶ τὴν ἐτυμολογίαν, ἐπειδὰν ἄγωμεν μακροτέραν σχολήν, ἐπιδείκνυμεν αὐτοῖς
7 οὐδὲν μᾶλλον ἐκείνοις ἤπερ ἡμῖν μαρτυροῦσαν. ἀλλ' ὅτι μὲν ἀλαζών ἐστι μάρτυς ἡ ἐτυμολογία πολλάκις μὲν ὁμοίως μαρτυροῦσα τοῖς τἀναντία λέγουσι τῶν ἀληθῶν, οὐκ ὀλιγάκις δὲ τοῖς ψευδομένοις μᾶλλον ἤπερ τοῖς ἀληθεύουσιν, ἐν ἑτέρᾳ πραγματείᾳ δέδεικταί μοι, τῇ Περὶ ὀνομάτων ὀρθότητος, ἔνθα καὶ περὶ τῆς ἐγὼ φωνῆς ἐπέδειξα τὸν Χρύσιππον
8 ἐτυμολογοῦντα μοχθηρῶς. τί ἂν οὖν ἔτι δεοίμην ὑπὲρ τῶν αὐτῶν ἐνταῦθα διεξιέναι; Χρυσίππῳ μὲν γὰρ καὶ τοῦτο φίλον, οὐ δὶς ἢ τρίς,
172 ἀλλὰ καὶ τετράκις, ἐνίοτε καὶ πεντάκις ὑπὲρ / τῶν αὐτῶν ἐν διαφερούσαις πραγματείαις διέρχεσθαι· φυλάξαιτο δὲ ἄν τις αὐτὸ τῶν χρόνου φειδομένων.

215 9 Ἃ δ' οὖν ὑπὲρ τῆς ἐγὼ φωνῆς ἔγραψεν ἐν τῷ πρώτῳ | Περὶ ψυχῆς ὁ Χρύσιππος ὑπὲρ ἡγεμονικοῦ διαλεγόμενος, ἤδη παραγράψω γνω-
10 ρίσματος ἕνεκα λημμάτων οὐκ οἰκείων τῷ προκειμένῳ σκέμματι. «Οὕτως δὲ καὶ τὸ ἐγὼ λέγομεν, κατὰ τοῦτο δεικνύντες ἑαυτοὺς ἐν ᾧ φαίνεσθαι διάνοιαν εἶναι, τῆς δείξεως φυσικῶς καὶ οἰκείως ἐνταῦθα φερομένης· καὶ ἄνευ δὲ τῆς κατὰ τὴν χεῖρα τοιαύτης δείξεως νεύοντες εἰς αὐτοὺς τὸ ἐγὼ

6–15] SVF II, p. 237 8–15] *cf. infra*, pp. 196.12–16; 220.32–33; 232.17–20; PHP 578.4–6 Müller 11] *cf. infra*, p. 232.16; PHP 578.12–13 Müller Müller, Beweis, p. 22 n. 24 15–21] *cf.* Prantl, Gesch. d. Logik I 567 n. 20–26] *cf.* SVF II, p. 237 23–24] *cf. infra*, p. 194.1–2 27–106.6] SVF II, p. 245

2 ἐπιχειροῖ *Müller* 3 δ' ἔλεγον *Petersen* 4 τοῖς *om.* M ἀριστο (τλ' supra lin.) C κατὰ τὰ] κατὰ M *Ald.*: τὰ C: *corr. Müller* 5 ἀναλυτικῶν] -ῶν *ex* -ῶ *corr.* M 8 ἐπικαλούμενον C 9 ὑποτίθενται C 11 δὲ *om.* M 12 ἐνδεικνυομένων M *Ald.*: ἐνδεικνυμένων *ex* -νομένων *corr.* R: ἐνδεικνύμενον C 15 ἢ ἐκείνοις] ἐκείνοις C: ἐκείνων *Einarson* 17 οὐδὲν — ἤπερ *del.* C² *ante* ἐκείνοις *add.* ἢ C 20 *ante* ἐν *add.* ὡς C τῇ Περὶ] τῆς περὶ *Ald.*: τῆς περὶ τῶν C 22 μοχθηρῶς] ψευδῶς M *Ald.* τί ἂν] τί μὲν *Ald.*: τί C 29 λημμάτων — σκέμματι *om. in textu* M *Ald.*, *in mg. add.* M 30 δὲ *add. supra lin.* M² αὐτοὺς *Ald.* ἐν ᾧ φαίνεσθαι] ἐν τῷ ἀποφαίνεσθαι τὴν M *Ald.*: ἐν ᾧ ἀποφαίνομαι τὴν *Petersen*: ἐν τῷ ἑαυτῶν ἀποφαίνεσθαι τὴν *Einarson*: ἐν τῷ λέγειν, εἰς τὸ ἐκεῖ ἀποφαίνεσθαι τὴν *v. Arnim*: ἐν τῷ λέγειν 'ἐμοὶ τοῦτο προσήκει, τοῦτο ἐγώ σοι λέγω' εἰς τὸ ἀποφαίνεσθαι ἐνταῦθα τὴν *Müller* 31 *ante* οἰκείως *add.* οὐκ C 32 αὐτοὺς M *Ald.* C: *corr. Kühn*

the first book of this treatise I exhorted everyone who undertakes any
demonstration first to train himself in that method.

I say that the best accounts of scientific demonstration were 4
written by the old philosophers, Theophrastus and Aristotle in
their Second Analytics. For this reason I anticipate that my reply to
them on the three ruling parts of animals will not be long; for they 5
would be ashamed to employ for scientific demonstrations the inexpert
and rhetorical premises with which the volumes of Chrysippus are
filled. Chrysippus sometimes calls on non-experts as witnesses to
the premises that he postulates; sometimes he calls on poets, or ety-
mology, that fine friend, or something else of the sort, things that prove
nothing but spend and waste our time to no purpose, as we make this
one point clear to them, that the premises of the syllogism are not
scientific, and then descend into the arena and wrestle with them in
order to demonstrate that the non-experts and the poets testify for us
no less, and sometimes even more, than for them. And similarly, when 6
we enjoy greater leisure, we shall prove to them that etymology
testifies no more for them than for us. Indeed I have shown in another 7
work, On the Correctness of Names, that etymology is an impostor,
often testifying equally for those who speak the reverse of the truth,
and not infrequently giving greater support to speakers of falsehoods
than of truths. In that work I showed further that Chrysippus gave
a faulty etymology of the word *egō* (I). Why then should I again 8
expound at length the same matters here? Chrysippus relishes this as
well: he discusses the same matters in different treatises not two or
three times, but also four and on occasion even five times; but anyone
who is sparing of his time would avoid it.

Accordingly, without further delay, I shall quote, as an illustra- 9
tion of premises inappropriate to the inquiry at hand, Chrysippus'
remarks on the word *cgō* (I) in his first book On the Soul, where he is
discussing the governing part of the soul: "We also say *egō* (I) in this 10
way, pointing to ourselves at that place in which thought appears to
be, the gesture being carried there naturally and appropriately; and
apart from such a gesture of the hand, we nod toward ourselves as

λέγομεν, εὐθὺς καὶ τῆς ἐγὼ φωνῆς τοιαύτης οὔσης καὶ κατὰ τὴν ἑξῆς
11 ὑπογεγραμμένην δεῖξιν συνεκφερομένης. τὸ γὰρ ἐγὼ προφερόμεθα κατὰ
τὴν πρώτην συλλαβὴν κατασπῶντες τὸ κάτω χεῖλος εἰς αὐτοὺς δει-
κτικῶς· ἀκολούθως δὲ τῇ τοῦ γενείου κινήσει καὶ ἐπὶ τὸ στῆθος νεύσει
173 καὶ τῇ τοιαύτῃ δείξει ἡ ἑξῆς συλλαβὴ παράκειται / οὐδὲν ἀποστηματικὸν
παρενσημαίνουσα, ὅπερ ἐπὶ τοῦ ἐκεῖνος συντέτευχεν.»
12 Διὰ ταύτης οὖν ἁπάσης τῆς ῥήσεως ὁ Χρύσιππος οὐδὲν μὲν
ἐπιστημονικὸν λῆμμα τοῦ τὴν ἀρχὴν τῆς ψυχῆς ὑπάρχειν ἐν καρδίᾳ
παραλαμβάνει, δύο δ' ἐς ταὐτὸν οὐκ οἰκεῖα τῷ προκειμένῳ συμπλέκει,
τὸ μὲν ἕτερον ἀπὸ τῆς ἐτυμολογίας, ὅτι τὴν ἐγὼ φωνὴν φθεγγόμενοι κατὰ
216 τὴν πρώτην συλλαβὴν τὴν ε̄ | λεγομένην τὸ στόμα κάτω που καὶ τὴν
γένυν ἀπάγομεν ὡς ἐπὶ τὰ στέρνα, τὸ δὲ ἕτερον, ὅτι καὶ τὴν χεῖρα συνεπι-
φέρομεν ἐνίοτε τοῖς στέρνοις ἡμᾶς αὐτοὺς δεικνύντες ἐν τῷ λέγειν «ἐμοὶ
13 τοῦτο προσήκει», «τοῦτο ἐγώ σοι λέγω». ὅτι δὲ καὶ τῆς ῥινὸς ἅπτονται
πολλάκις οἱ ἄνθρωποι λέγοντες «ἐμοὶ τοῦτο δός», «ἐμοὶ τοῦτο προσήκει»,
«τοῦτο ἐγώ σοι λέγω», παντελῶς ἐπιλέλησται. καίτοι κατά γε τὴν ἐγὼ
φωνὴν οὐκ ἐπελάθετο τῆς ἐκεῖνος οὐκ ἀπὸ παραπλησίας δή τινος, ἀλλ'
14 ἀπὸ τῆς αὐτῆς ἀκριβῶς συλλαβῆς ἀρχομένης, τῆς ε̄. ἐχρῆν δ', οἶμαι, /
174 καθάπερ ἐπὶ ταύτης ἐμνημόνευσε μέν, οὐκ ἔλυσε δὲ τὸ ἄτοπον, οὕτω
κἀπὶ τῆς ἐπὶ τοῦ στέρνου δείξεως ἐπιμνησθῆναι μὲν τῆς ἐπὶ τὴν ῥῖνα
φορᾶς τοῦ δακτύλου, μὴ μέντοι μηδ' ἐνταῦθα διαλύεσθαι τὸ προβληθέν,
εἰ μὴ ἄρα τις οἴεται τὴν ἀπόφασιν τοῦ Χρυσίππου ψιλὴν αὐτὴν μόνην
ῥηθεῖσαν ἀπόδειξιν ὑπάρχειν.
15 Τί γὰρ δὴ καί φησιν; «ἀκολούθως δὲ τῇ τοῦ γενείου κινήσει καὶ
ἐπὶ τὸ στῆθος νεύσει καὶ τῇ τοιαύτῃ δείξει ἡ ἑξῆς συλλαβὴ παράκειται
217 οὐδὲν ἀποστηματικὸν παρεμφαίνουσα, | ὅπερ ἐπὶ τοῦ ἐκεῖνος συντέ-
16 τευχεν.» ἐννοήσας γὰρ ὅτι καὶ ἡ ἐκεῖνος φωνὴ τὴν ἀρχὴν ἀπὸ τῆς αὐτῆς
ποιεῖται συλλαβῆς ὥσπερ καὶ ἡ ἐγώ, καὶ δεήσει καὶ ταύτην ἐνδείκνυσθαι
ταὐτὸν σημαινόμενον, εἰς τὴν τῶν ἐπιφερομένων συλλαβῶν διαφο-
17 ρὰν ἀναφέρει τὴν τοῦ ζητουμένου λύσιν. ἔστι δὲ τοιάδε· εἰπὼν τῆς
ἐγὼ φωνῆς τὴν δευτέραν συλλαβὴν τὴν γω̅ μηδὲν ἀποστηματικὸν ἐμ-
18 φαίνειν ἐπήγαγεν ἐπὶ [δὲ] τῆς ἐκεῖνος ἐμφαίνειν τὴν κει̅. τοῦτο δ' ἀπό-
175 φασίς ἐστι / ψιλὴ μηδεμίαν ἀπόδειξιν ἔχουσα, μὴ ὅτι βεβαίαν τε καὶ
ἐπιστημονικήν, ἀλλὰ μηδ' ἄχρι πιθανότητος ἢ ῥητορικῆς ἢ σοφιστικῆς

4–6] *cf. infra*, lin. 24–27

2 ὑπογραφομένην (ην *ex* ης *corr., ut vid.*) C κατὰ] καὶ C 3 αὐτοὺς M *Ald.* C: *corr. Kühn* 5 τῇ *om.* C 6 παρενσημαίνουσα] ἀπῆρεν σημαίνουσα M: παρεμφαίνουσα *Ald.* (*cf. infra, lin. 26*) 7 οὖν *om.* C 8 *post* ἐν *add.* τῇ *Ald.* 9 παραλαμβάνει] λα *in ras.* C δύος M 11 λεγομένην M *in textu Ald.*: λέγομεν M *in mg.* C κάτω ποῦ M *in textu Ald.*: κατασπῶντες M *in mg.* 14 προσῆκεν M *Ald.* τοῦτο[II] *om.* C 15 δός] δὲ M 17 δή] δέ *Ald.* C 18 ἀκριβῶς *om.* C 21 *post* ἐνταῦθα *add.* οἴεσθαι *Müller* 22 ὑψιλὴν M 25 τῇ *om.* C 26 ὅπερ] ὥσπερ M *Ald.* 27 καὶ ἡ] τὴν ἡ *Ald.*: ἡ C 30 ἔστι δὲ τοιάδε *om.* C εἰπὼν] ἐπὶ μὲν *Petersen*: εἰπὼν ἐπὶ μὲν *Wilamowitz* 31 γω̅] ἐγὼ *Ald.*: γε C 32 ἐπήγαγεν] δυνάμενος C: ἐξηγούμενος *vel* φάμενος *Petersen*: *del. Wilamowitz* ἐπιδεῖ *ex* ἐπιδὴ *mut.* M[2]: ἐπὶ δὲ *Ald.* C: *corr. Müller* τὴν] τῇ C 33 ἀπόδειξιν] ἀπόφασιν C

we say *egō* (I); indeed the very word *egō* (I) is of this description and its pronunciation is accompanied by the gesture next described. For 11
as we pronounce *egō* (I), at the first syllable we drop the lower lip in a way that points to ourselves, and in conformity with the movement of the chin, the nod toward the chest, and such gesturing, the next syllable is juxtaposed; and it gives no suggestion of distance, such as that produced by the second syllable of *ekeinos* (that person, he)."

Throughout this whole passage Chrysippus employs no scientific 12
premise for proving that the ruling part of the soul is in the heart, but he brings together two premises not appropriate to the problem at hand. One is from etymology, that in uttering the word *egō* (I) we somehow draw the mouth and jaw downward as though toward the chest when we pronounce the first syllable, *e*; the other is that we sometimes bring the hand also to the chest and point to ourselves as we say, "This suits me", "This I say to you". He completely forgot 13
that it also happens that men often touch their noses when they say "Give me this", "This suits me", "This I say to you". And yet when arguing from the word *egō* (I) he did not forget that *ekeinos* (he) begins not with some similar syllable, but with exactly the same syllable, *e*. But just as he mentioned the difficulty in the case of the 14
word but did not resolve it, so also, I think, along with the gesture of pointing to one's chest, he should have mentioned the movement of the finger to the nose, and there too the difficulty would not be resolved, unless indeed a person believes that Chrysippus' mere statement, alone and by itself, is scientific proof.

What in fact does he say? "In conformity with the movement of 15
the chin, the nod toward the chest, and such gesturing, the next syllable is juxtaposed; and it gives no indication of distance, such as that produced by the second syllable of *ekeinos* (he)." After noting 16
that the word *ekeinos* (he) begins with the same syllable as *egō* (I) and that this syllable will have to convey the same meaning, he shifts the resolution of the problem to the difference in the syllables that follow. This is his resolution: having said that in the word *egō* (I) the 17
second syllable, *gō*, gives no indication of distance, he added that the *kei* in *ekeinos* (he) does. This is mere assertion with no demonstration, 18
much less a secure and scientific (demonstration); indeed it does not even advance so far as rhetorical or sophistical plausibility. Should he 19

19 προϊοῦσα. διὰ τί γὰρ ἡ μὲν $\overline{\text{κει}}$ συλλαβὴ ἀποστηματικόν τι δηλώσει,
ἡ δὲ $\overline{\text{γω}}$ μή, οὐ προσθεῖναι δίκαιον ἦν αὐτὸν ἀπόδειξίν τινα; διὰ τί δὲ
τοῖς μὲν στέρνοις ἐπιφέροντες τὸν δάκτυλον ἐνδεικνύμεθα τὴν ἀρχὴν τῆς
20 ψυχῆς ἐνταῦθ' εἶναι, τῇ ῥινὶ δὲ ἐπιφέροντες οὐκ ἐνδεικνύμεθα; δίκαιον
γάρ, εἴπερ ἡ δεῖξις ἱκανὴ πίστις εἰς εὕρεσιν ἡγεμονικοῦ μορίου ψυχῆς,
οὐκ ἐπὶ μὲν τῶν στέρνων αὐτὴν ἱκανὴν ὑπάρχειν, ἀσθενῆ δὲ ἐπὶ τῆς ῥινός,
218 ἀλλὰ | κἀπὶ ταύτης ἰσχύειν ὁμοίως· ἢ εἴπερ οὐδ' ἐπὶ ταύτης, οὐδ' ἐπὶ
21 τῶν στέρνων. διὰ τί δὲ ἐν ταῖς συγκαταθέσεσιν ἐπινεύοντες τὴν κεφαλήν,
ἐφ' ὃ φέρομεν αὐτὴν μέρος, ἐν ἐκείνῳ τὴν ἀρχὴν τῆς ψυχῆς ὑπάρχειν
22 ἐνδεικνύμεθα μᾶλλον καὶ οὐκ ⟨ἐν⟩ αὐτῷ τῷ κινουμένῳ; τὸ γάρ τοι πρῶτον
176 κινούμενον ἐν ἡμῖν μόριον / ἐπινευόντων αὐτὸ δήπου πιθανώτερον ἔχειν
ἐστὶ τὴν ἀρχὴν τῆς ψυχῆς ἤπερ τι τῶν ἄλλων πρὸς ὃ φέρεται κινούμενον,
ἵνα μὴ νῦν ἐκείνων μνημονεύω τῶν ἀνθρώπων οἳ ταῖς κεφαλαῖς ἀνα-
νεύουσιν ἐπειδὰν συγκατατίθωνται· τάχα γὰρ φήσει τοὺς βαρβάρους,
ὥσπερ τἄλλα χείρους εἰσὶ καὶ ἀλογώτεροι τῶν Ἑλλήνων, οὕτω κἀν
23 τῷδε σφάλλεσθαι. πάντ' οὖν ὅσα τοιαῦτα τῶν ἐπιχειρημάτων ἐν τοῖς
Περὶ ἀποδείξεως ἐδείξαμεν οὐκ οἰκεῖα τῷ ζητουμένῳ πράγματι καὶ διὰ
τοῦτο νῦν οὐ χρὴ μηκύνειν περὶ αὐτῶν, ὥσπερ οὐδ' ἐπὶ τῶν ἐκ τῆς
ἐτυμολογίας ὁρμωμένων· εἴρηται γὰρ καὶ περὶ ἐκείνων αὐτάρκως ἐν
τοῖς Περὶ ὀνομάτων ὀρθότητος. |

219 3. Ἀλλὰ τίνα χρὴ ζητεῖν λήμματα τῷ προκειμένῳ προβλήματι προσ-
ήκοντά τε καὶ οἰκεῖα; γέγραπται μὲν δήπου καὶ περὶ τούτων ἐπὶ πλεῖ-
στον ἐν τοῖς περὶ ἀποδείξεως ὑπό τε τῶν παλαιῶν εἰρημένοις ἀσαφέστερόν
177 τε καὶ συντομώτερον / ὑπό τε ἡμῶν ἐξηγουμένων ἐκεῖνα σαφῶς τε ἅμα
2 καὶ διὰ πολλῶν. ἀρκέσει δὲ νῦν ἐξ αὐτῶν τὸ κεφάλαιον ἀναμνήσασι μόνον
3 ἐκείνῳ χρήσασθαι σκοπῷ εἰς τὴν τῶν κατὰ μέρος εὕρεσιν. ἦν δὲ τὸ κεφά-
λαιον ὡς ἀπ' αὐτῆς χρὴ τῆς οὐσίας τοῦ ζητουμένου πράγματος ἐξευρί-
σκειν τὰ προσήκοντά τε καὶ οἰκεῖα λήμματα, καθάπερ ἐν τούτοις ἐν οἷς
Χρύσιππος ἐπισκοπεῖται περὶ τοῦ τῆς ψυχῆς ἡγεμονικοῦ τὸν τῆς οὐσίας
λόγον εἰπόντας ὑπὲρ οὗ ζητοῦμεν πράγματος ἐκείνῳ χρῆσθαι κανόνι
τε καὶ σκοπῷ τῶν κατὰ μέρος ἁπάντων.

8–10] SVF II, p. 245 16–17] *cf. supra*, p. 102.25–27 19–20] *cf. supra*, p. 104.17–22 21–25] *cf.* Müller, Beweis, p. 50 n. 63

1 προιοῦσαν *Bas.* ἀποστηματικόν τι] -όν *ex* -ή *corr.* M: *om.* C 2 δὲ $\overline{\text{γω}}$] δἐγὼ M: δ' ἐγὼ C· μὴ οὐ· M: μὴ οὐ, *Ald.*: *corr. Kühn*: *om.* C αὐτὸν *om.* C 3 τοῖς *ex* τὸ *corr.* C ἐπιδεικνύμεθα M *Ald.* 5 *post* εὕρεσιν *add.* τοῦ *Müller* 7 κἐπὶ M ἢ *om.* C 8 *ante* ἐπινεύοντες *add.* οὐκ M 10 καὶ *om.* C ἐν *addidi* 14 συγκατατίθενται M *Ald.* φύσει M: φησὶ C 16 ὅσα] τὰ C τοιαῦτα] περὶ τὰ M *Ald.*: περιττὰ *Bas.* ἐγχειρημάτων M 17 τῷ ζητουμένῳ *om.* M *(spat. 10 litt. rel.)* 18 οὐδ'] δ' M *Ald.* *ante* τῶν *add.* τοῖς C 19 ἡρμωμένων M 21 τίνα] τί C λήμματα δὲ τῶ προκειμένω (πρ. *inser.*) προβλήματι M: τῶ προειρημένω λήμματι C 22 πλείστων M 23 εἰρημένοις] εἰρηκότων *Müller* ἀσφαλέστερόν M *Ald.* C: *corr. Müller* 26 εἰς] πρὸς *Petersen* 28 ἐν[II] *del. Müller* 29 *post* Χρύσιππος *add.* τε M *Ald.*

not have added some demonstration why the syllable *kei* indicates
separation and *gō* does not? Again, why is it that when we bring the
finger to the chest we imply that the rule of the soul is located there,
but when we bring it to the nose we do not? If the act of pointing is 20
sufficient evidence for discovering a governing part of the soul, it is
not right that it be sufficient in the case of the chest but inadequate in
the case of the nose. It should be just as valid for the latter too; or if it
does not hold for the nose, it ought not hold for the chest either. And 21
why is it that when we nod the head in assent we indicate that the
rule of the soul is rather in that member toward which we move the
head, and not in the member which is moved? For surely it is more 22
plausible that the member in us which is first moved when we nod is
itself the ruling part of the soul, rather than any of the other (members)
toward which its motion carries it. Let me not now mention those men
who nod the head upward in assent, for he will perhaps reply that as
the barbarians are inferior to the Greeks and less rational in all other
matters, so they are deceived in this matter too. Now all such argu- 23
ments we have shown in our work On Demonstration to be foreign to
the subject of the inquiry, and therefore it is not necessary to prolong
the present discussion of them; nor (need I discuss further) the argu-
ments derived from etymology, for enough was said about them in the
work On the Correctness of Names.

3. But what premises ought one seek as appropriate and proper
to the problem at hand? These have been discussed at length, both in
the rather unclear and brief statements made by the ancients about
demonstration, and in what we wrote in our clear and full explanation
of those statements. For the present it will be enough to recall from 2
them only the main point and use it as a guide for finding premises in
particular cases. The main point was that the appropriate and proper 3
premises must be found in the very essence of the matter under in-
vestigation. So in these (discussions) in which Chrysippus reflects
on the governing part of the soul, we should first state the definition
of the essence of the thing we are investigating, and then use it as a
standard and guide in all the particulars.

4 Ἔστι δὲ τὸ ἡγεμονικόν, ὡς καὶ αὐτοὶ βούλονται, τὸ κατάρχον αἰσθή-
5 σεώς τε καὶ ὁρμῆς. οὔκουν ἄλλοθεν χρὴ δεικνύναι τὴν καρδίαν ἐν αὐτῇ
τὸ ἡγεμονικὸν ἔχουσαν ἢ ἐκ τοῦ πάσης μὲν τῆς καθ' ὁρμὴν κινήσεως ἐξη-
220 γεῖσθαι | τοῖς ἄλλοις τοῦ ζῴου μορίοις, ἅπασαν δὲ αἴσθησιν εἰς αὐτὴν
6 ἀναφέρεσθαι. πόθεν οὖν τοῦτο δειχθήσεται; πόθεν δὴ ἄλλοθεν ἢ ἐκ τῶν
178 ἀνατομῶν; / εἰ γὰρ αὕτη τοῖς κατὰ μέρος ἅπασιν ἐπιπέμπει δύναμιν αἰ-
σθήσεώς τε ἅμα καὶ κινήσεως, ἀποπεφυκέναι τι πάντως ἀπ' αὐτῆς ἀγγεῖον
7 ἀναγκαῖόν ἐστιν εἰς τὴν αὐτῶν ὑπηρεσίαν. ὥστε ἐκ τῆς ἀποδεικτικῆς
μεθόδου πέφηνεν ὅτι τε χρησιμώτερον ἀνατέμνοντας τὰ ζῷα κατα-
σκέπτεσθαι τίνα καὶ πόσα γένη σωμάτων ἐκ τῆς καρδίας ἐκφυόμενα δια-
νέμεται τοῖς ἄλλοις τοῦ ζῴου μορίοις, ὅτι τε τούτων αὐτῶν ὄντων τοιού-
των καὶ τοσῶνδε τοῦτο μὲν αἴσθησιν ἢ κίνησιν ἢ ἄμφω παράγει, τοῦτο
δ' ἄλλο τι· καὶ οὕτως ἔχειν ἤδη τίνων ἐν τοῖς ζῴοις δυνάμεων ἡ καρδία
πηγή.
8 Ταύτης τῆς ὁδοῦ πᾶν ὅ τι περ ἂν ἔξω πίπτῃ, περιττόν τ' ἐστὶ καὶ
ἀλλότριον· καὶ ταύτῃ διήνεγκεν ἐπιστημονικὸν ἀποδείξεως λῆμμα ῥητο-
ρικοῦ τε καὶ γυμναστικοῦ καὶ σοφιστικοῦ, ὑπὲρ ὧν οὐδ' αὐτῶν οὐδεμίαν
ἐδίδαξαν ἡμᾶς οὔτε μέθοδον οὔτε γυμνασίαν οἵ γε περὶ τὸν Ζήνωνα
221 179 9 καὶ τὸν Χρύσιππον. ὅθεν ἀναμέμικται φύρδην ἐν τοῖς | βιβλίοις / αὐτῶν
ἐφεξῆς ἅπαντα τὰ λήμματα καὶ πολλάκις ἡγεῖται μέν, εἰ οὕτως ἔτυχε,
ῥητορικὸν ἐπιχείρημα, τούτῳ δ' ἕπεται γυμναστικόν τε καὶ διαλεκτικόν,
εἶθ' ἑξῆς ἐπιστημονικόν, εἶθ', οὕτως εἰ ἔτυχεν, σοφιστικὸν οὐκ εἰδότων
ὡς τὰ μὲν ἐπιστημονικὰ λήμματα πρὸς τὴν οὐσίαν ἀναφέρεται τοῦ
10 ζητουμένου καὶ τοῦτον ἔχει τὸν σκοπόν· τῶν δ' ἄλλων ἁπάντων ἔξωθεν
ὄντων, ὅσοις μὲν ὁ διαλεκτικὸς εἰς τὸ γυμνάσασθαι χρῆται καὶ σοφιστὰς
ἐξελέγξαι καὶ πεῖραν λαβεῖν κυήσεως μειρακίου καὶ μαιεύσασθαι
καὶ προσαγαγεῖν ἐπί τινος εὕρεσιν ἀπορῆσαί τε ποιῆσαι, ταυτὶ μὲν
ἅπαντα διαλεκτικά τε κάλει, εἰ βούλοιο, καὶ γυμναστικὰ καὶ τοπικά, τῶν
γὰρ ὀνομάτων οὐ φροντίζω, διορίζειν δὲ ταῦτα πειρῶ τῶν ἐπιστημο-
11 νικῶν· ὅσα δ' ἔτι τούτων ἀποκεχώρηκεν ἐξωτέρω καὶ μάλιστα διὰ παρα-
δειγμάτων ἐνδόξων τε καὶ πολιτικῶν ἐπαγωγῶν τέ τινων τοιούτων
180 ἢ μαρτύρων εἰς σύστασιν ἀφικνεῖται, ταῦτ' εἰ βού/λοιο πιθανά τε καὶ
222 ῥητορικὰ προσαγορεύειν, οὔ μοι μέλει τῆς κλήσεως, | γνωρίζειν δὲ αὐτῶν

1–2] *cf. infra*, p. 116.19–21; PHP 583.10–12; 649.6–8 Müller Müller, Beweis, p. 51 16–24] SVF II, pp. 76–77 28–29, 33] *cf. infra*, PHP 590.3 Müller

1 ὡς καὶ *om.* C, *inser.* C³: καὶ *om.* M *Ald.* 2 οὐκοῦν C αὐτῇ M *Ald.* C: *corr. Kühn* 3 ἢ] ὁ M 4 ἅπασαν] ἃ πασὶ M 5 οὖν *om.* M, *add.* M² δὴ] ἢ M: δὲ *Ald.*: δὲ ἢ C: *corr. Diels* 6 αὐτὴ C 7 *post* ἀποπεφυκέναι *add.* γὰρ C 8 αὐτὴν C 9 τε *del. Müller* ἀνατέμνονται C 11 τούτων] τῶν M ὄντων *om. Müller* 13 ἔχειν] ἔστιν ἰδεῖν *Müller* 15 πίπτει M 16 δείξεως *post lac. 3 litt.* M: δείξεως *Ald.* 17 ὧν] τῶν M 18 ἡμᾶς οὔτε] ἃς οὐ *e corr.* C οἵ] ἡ *Ald.* 19 τὸν *om.* C 20 ἔτυχε] ἔχει M *Ald.* 25 ὅσα M σοφιστικὰς C 26 μυήσεως M *Ald.* C: μαθήσεως *Kalbfleisch*: μαιεύσεως *Müller*: *correxi (cf. Plat. Theaet. 184 b 1–2)* μαιεύεσθαι C 27 προαγαγεῖν C 28 καλεῖν C καὶ τοπικά *om.* C 29 δὲ *om.* C 30 δ' ἔτι] δὲ τι C ἀποκεχώρηκε M *Ald.*: *corr.* p: ἀποκεχωρηκέναι C 31 ἐπαγωγῶν – τοιούτων *om.* C

The governing part (of the soul), as they too would have it, is the 4
source of sensation and conation. Therefore the demonstration that 5
the heart contains in itself the governing part must not proceed from
any other premise than that it initiates every voluntary motion in the
rest of the body, and every sensation is carried back to it. Now where 6
will the proof of this be found? Where else but from dissections? For if
this (organ) dispatches the power of sensation and movement to all the
individual members, then necessarily some vessel must grow out from
it to perform this service for them. So it has become evident from the 7
method of scientific proof that it would be more useful to dissect
animals and observe closely what and how many kinds of structures
grow out from the heart and spread to the other parts of the animal;
and, these very structures being of such and such kinds and so many
in number, (to observe) that this one transmits sensation or movement
or both, that one some other thing, and thus to reach the point where
one understands which powers in the body have the heart as their
source.

Everything which falls outside this course is superfluous and 8
irrelevant; and this is the way in which a scientific premise of a demon-
stration differs from one that is rhetorical, useful for training, or
sophistical. But even with regard to these (latter premises) Zeno and
Chrysippus taught us no method and gave us no training. For this 9
reason the premises are all jumbled together, one after another, in
their books. Often, as chance might have it, a rhetorical argument
leads the way, next comes one that is useful for training and dialectical,
then a scientific one, and after that, perhaps, a sophistical one. For
they do not know that scientific premises refer back to the essence of
the matter under investigation and have it as their guide. All others 10
are external. Some are used by the dialectician for practice, for refut-
ing sophists, for testing a young man's pregnancy, playing the midwife,
leading him to some discovery, and raising questions in his mind; all
of these, if you wish, you may call dialectical, gymnastic, and topical,
for I am not concerned about the names; but try to distinguish them
from scientific premises. Others are even more remote than these and 11
are constructed chiefly from generally accepted and every-day exam-
ples and from certain inductions of the same sort or from witnesses.
These you may call, if you wish, plausible and rhetorical, for I do not
care what name you give them; but you must try to learn their nature.

χρὴ πειρᾶσθαι τὴν φύσιν· ἔτι δὲ μᾶλλον ἀποκεχώρηκε τῆς οὐσίας τοῦ
ζητουμένου τὰ σοφιστικά.
12 Καὶ γέγραπται περὶ τούτων ἁπάντων τοῖς παλαιοῖς, ἐν μὲν τοῖς Σοφι-
στικοῖς ἐλέγχοις περὶ τῶν σοφιστικῶν – εἴτε προτάσεων ἐθέλοις ὀνομάζειν
εἴτε ἀξιωμάτων εἴτε λόγων, οὐδὲν γὰρ εἰς τὰ παρόντα διαφέρει –, κατὰ
δὲ τὰς 'Ρητορικὰς τέχνας ὑπὲρ τῶν ῥητορικῶν, ἐν δὲ τοῖς Τοπικοῖς ὑπὲρ
τῶν διαλεκτικῶν, ἐν δὲ τοῖς Περὶ ἀποδείξεως, ἃ δὴ καὶ Δεύτερα ἀναλυτικὰ
13 ἐπιγράφουσιν, ὑπὲρ τῶν ἐπιστημονικῶν. ὥστε ὅστις ὁτιοῦν ἀποδεικνύναι
πειρᾶται, πρῶτα μὲν χρὴ τοῦτον ἐγνωκέναι τὴν διαφορὰν τῶν λημμάτων
αὐτῶν, εἶθ' ἑξῆς χρόνῳ πολλῷ γεγυμνάσθαι, λέγοντος μὲν ἑτέρου γνωρί-
ζειν αὐτὰ ποίου γένους ἐστὶν ἐκ τῶν εἰρημένων, μὴ λέγοντος δὲ ἑτέρου
ταχέως ἐξευρίσκειν αὐτὸν εἰς ἕκαστον τῶν προβληθέντων· ἑνὶ δὲ λόγῳ,
181 14 καθάπερ ἐπὶ τοῦ λογίζεσθαι ποιοῦμεν, / οὕτω κἀνταῦθα πράττειν. εἰ
γάρ τις ἐθέλει γίγνεσθαι λογιστικός, οὗτος ἐκμανθάνει μὲν πρῶτον ἀριθ-
223 μοὺς ἅπαντας, οὓς ὀνομάζουσιν | ἐκεῖνοι τετραγώνους καὶ ἑτερομήκεις,
ἐφεξῆς δὲ γυμνάζεται χρόνῳ παμπόλλῳ πολλαπλασιάζειν καὶ μερίζειν,
εἶθ' ἑξῆς ἔτι μαθὼν ὀλιγίστας μεθόδους οὕτως ἤδη περὶ παντὸς τοῦ
προβληθέντος ἱκανὸς γίνεται λογίζεσθαι.
15 Καί μοι θαυμάζειν ἐπέρχεται τῆς τῶν πολλῶν δοξοσοφίας, εἰ προ-
βληθέντος μέν, ἂν οὕτω τύχῃ, τίς γίγνεται τόκος ἑκατοστὸς Ἀττικῶν
δισμυρίων πεντακισχιλίων ἑξακοσίων τριακονταεπτὰ μηνῶν τεσσα-
ρεσκαίδεκα, τοῖς λογιστικοῖς ἐπιτρέπουσιν εἰδότες, οἶμαι, σαφῶς ὡς αὐτοῖς
οὐ μέτεστιν ἐπιστήμη⟨ς⟩ οὐδεμιᾶ⟨ς⟩ τοῦ λογίζεσθαι τὰ τοιαῦτα, διότι
μήτ' ἤσκησαν αὐτὰ μήθ' ὅλως ἔμαθον, ἀποδείξει δὲ χρῆσθαι τολμῶσιν
εὖ εἰδότες ὡς οὔτε παρ' ἑτέρων ἔμαθον ὅλως οὐδὲν οὔτε αὐτοὶ καθ' ἑαυτοὺς
182 ἐξεῦρον, οἵ γε μηδὲ ἐζήτησαν, ὅπου γε / καὶ ἣν μεμαθήκεσαν ὁδὸν ἀπο-
δεικτικήν, οὐκ ἦν ἱκανόν, ἀλλ' ἐχρῆν, οἶμαι, πρότερον ἠσκῆσθαι κατ'
16 αὐτήν. οὐδὲ γὰρ τοῖς ῥήτορσιν ἀπόχρη μέθοδον ἐκμαθεῖν, ὡς χρὴ διαι-
ρεῖν ὑπόθεσιν ἅπασαν, ἀλλ' ἐπὶ τῇ γνώσει τῆς μεθόδου καὶ τὴν ἄσκησιν
224 17 ἐπάγουσιν. ἠβουλόμην ἂν οὖν | μοι καὶ τὸν ἀποδεικτικὸν εἶναι φάσκοντα
πρῶτον μὲν εἰπεῖν τὴν μέθοδον ᾗ χρῆται πρὸς τὰς ἀποδείξεις, εἶθ',
ὅπως ἤσκηται κατ' αὐτήν, ἐπιδείξασθαι.

5 οὐδὲν – διαφέρει] *cf. infra*, p. 134.18–19

1 ἀποκεχώρηκε *ex* -κα, *ut vid.*, *corr.* C 3 *ante* τοῖς[II] *add.* γὰρ C 3–4 Σοφιστικοῖς – περὶ *om.* C 4 ἐθέλεις *Ald.* 7 δὲ *om.* C, *add.* C[2? 3?] δευτέρων ἀναλυτικῶν C 8 ὥστε ὅστις] ὅσα θ' ὥς τις C 9 τοῦτ' *Ald.*: τούτων C 11 ἑτέρω M 12 ἐξευρίσκειν] *post lac. 7 litt.* σκειν M: ἐστὶν εὑρίσκειν *Ald.* 13 καθάπερ *om.* M, *lac. 6 litt. rel.* ἐπὶ τῶ λογίζεσθαι M *Ald.*: *corr. Müller*: ἐπιλογίζεσθαι C *post* οὕτω *add.* χρὴ *Müller* 13–14 εἰ γάρ] ἴσως *(sic) Ald.* 14 ἐθέλοι C μὲν ἐκμανθάνει M *Ald.* 16 παμπόλω M 17 ἔτι *om. Ald.* 18 *post* γίνεται *add.* μοι C 19 μοι *om.* C 20 τύχει M *Ald.* ἑκατοσταῖος ἀττικὸς C 21 τριάκοντα ἑπτὰ C τεσσαρισκαιδεκαταῖος C 22 ὡς αὐτοῖς *Wilamowitz*: ἑαυ[τ] M: ἑαυτοῖς R: ὡς ἑαυτῷ *Ald.*: οἷς C: ὡς ἑαυτοῖς *Müller* 23 ἐπιστήμη οὐδεμία M *Ald.* C: *corr. Petersen* 25 αὐτοὶ] αὐτόματοι C ἑαυτοὺς] αὐτοὺς C 26 ἣν] ἦν M C μεμαθήκασιν C 27–28 καθ' αὐτήν C

Sophistical (premises) depart still further from the essence of the
(matter) under investigation.

The ancients wrote about all these matters, in the Sophistical 12
Refutations about sophistical (premises) – you may call them premises
if you wish, or propositions or statements; it makes no difference for
our present purpose –, in the Rhetorics about rhetorical premises, in
the Topics about dialectical premises, and in the books On Demon-
stration, which are also called the Second Analytics, about scientific
premises. Anyone, therefore, who tries to demonstrate anything, must 13
first have learned the differences in the premises themselves; then he
must have undergone long training: when another is speaking, he must
recognize from what is said the kind of premises being used; and when
another is not speaking, he must find them quickly himself for every
problem. In a word, he must do here what he does in arithmetic. If a 14
person wishes to become an arithmetician, he first learns all the num-
bers which those people call 'square' and 'oblong'; then he undergoes
training in multiplication and division for a very long time; and then
finally, when he has also learned a very few methods, he is capable of
solving every problem.

I am moved to marvel at the conceit of wisdom in the majority 15
of men. If it so happened that the problem were posed, "What is the
interest on 25,637 Attic (drachmae) at one per-cent (a month) for
fourteen months?", they turn it over to the arithmeticians, being well
aware, I fancy, that they themselves have no share in the knowledge
how to reckon such sums, since they have neither practiced such things
nor learned them at all; yet they dare to use scientific demonstration,
knowing very well that they neither learned anything at all (about it)
from others nor discovered it by themselves, since they did not even
look for it; and in any case it would not be enough to have learned a
scientific method, but it would have been necessary, as I believe, to
have been trained in it beforehand. For rhetoricians, too, it is not 16
enough to learn the method for dividing every case, but to the knowl-
edge of method they add practice also. I would wish, therefore, that 17
the man who claims to be scientific first tell me the method he employs
for his scientific demonstrations and then show how he has been
trained in it.

18 Νυνὶ δὲ πῶς μὲν οἱ διὰ δύο τροπικῶν ἀναλύονται συλλογισμοὶ καὶ
πῶς οἱ ἀδιαφόρως περαίνοντες ἢ τινες ἄλλοι τοιοῦτοι τῷ πρώτῳ καὶ
δευτέρῳ θέματι προσχρώμενοι, πολλοῖς ἔστι συντυχεῖν ἀκριβῶς ἠσκη-
μένοις, ὥσπερ ἀμέλει καὶ ἄλλοις ἐφ' ὅσους διὰ τοῦ τρίτου θέματος ἢ
19 τετάρτου συλλογισμοὺς ἀναλύουσι. καίτοι τούτων τοὺς πλείστους
183 ἔνεστιν ἑτέρως ἀναλύειν συντομώτερον, ὡς / Ἀντίπατρος ἔγραψε,
πρὸς τῷ καὶ περιεργίαν εἶναι οὐ μικρὰν ἀχρήστου πράγματος ἅπασαν
τὴν τῶν τοιούτων συλλογισμῶν πλοκήν, ὡς αὐτὸς ὁ Χρύσιππος
ἔργῳ μαρτυρεῖ μηδαμόθι τῶν ἑαυτοῦ συγγραμμάτων εἰς ἀπόδειξιν
20 δόγματος ἐκείνων δεηθεὶς τῶν συλλογισμῶν. ὅπως δὲ χρὴ γνωρίζειν τε
καὶ διακρίνειν ἐπιστημονικὰ λήμματα διαλεκτικῶν τε καὶ ῥητορικῶν καὶ
σοφιστικῶν, οὐκέτι ἔγραψαν ἀξιόλογον οὐδὲν οἱ περὶ τὸν Χρύσιπ-
225 21 πον οὔτε φαίνονται χρώμενοι· ἀλλ' ὅτι τὰς χεῖρας ἐπιφέρομεν | τῷ
θώρακι δεικνύντες ἡμᾶς αὐτοὺς ἢ τῇ κεφαλῇ κάτω νεύομεν, εἰ τὴν ἐγὼ
φθεγγόμεθα φωνήν, εἰς ἔνδειξιν τοῦ τὴν καρδίαν εἶναι τὴν ἀρχὴν τῆς
ψυχῆς οὐκ αἰδοῦνται γράφοντες, ὧν ἡ μὲν δεῖξις οὐδὲν μᾶλλον ἐν τῇ
καρδίᾳ ἢ ἐν τῇ ῥινί τε καὶ τῷ μετώπῳ — καὶ γὰρ καὶ ταῦτα δείκνυται
184 πολλάκις ὑπὸ τῶν ἀνθρώπων — ἐμφαίνει τὸ / ἡγεμονοῦν εἶναι τῆς ψυχῆς,
ἡ δὲ ἐπίνευσις οὐδὲν μᾶλλον ἐν τοῖς κατὰ τὸν θώρακα ἢ ἐν τοῖς κατὰ τὴν
22 κεφαλήν. ἡ δὲ ε̅ φωνὴ πόσης ἀτοπίας ἔχεται, κατὰ τὸ δεύτερον ὑπέδειξα
τῶν Ὑπὲρ ὀνομάτων ὀρθότητος.

23 Εἴ τις οὖν καλῶς ἤσκηται τὰς διαφορὰς τῶν λημμάτων ἐξευρίσκειν τε
καὶ γνωρίζειν, οὐ δεήσομαι πρὸς αὐτὸν ἀντιλογίας μακροτέρας, ὥσπερ
24 οὐδὲ πρὸς τοὺς ἐκ τοῦ Περιπάτου. κατὰ γὰρ τὰς ἰδίας αὐτῶν διδασκα-
λίας ὁ λόγος ἔσται μοι πρὸς αὐτοὺς ὑπὲρ τοῦ τὴν τοῦ ἡγεμονικοῦ τῆς
ψυχῆς ἀρχὴν ἐν ἐγκεφάλῳ περιέχεσθαι, τῆς δὲ θυμοειδοῦς ἐν καρδίᾳ,
25 τῆς δ' ἐπιθυμητικῆς ἐν ἥπατι. πρὸς μέντοι τοὺς Στωϊκοὺς ἀναγκαῖόν
ἐστι μακρὸν ἀνύεσθαι λόγον, ἀνθρώπους ἐν μὲν τοῖς ἀχρήστοις τῆς |
226 λογικῆς θεωρίας ἱκανῶς γεγυμνασμένους, ἐν δὲ τοῖς χρησίμοις ἀγυμναστο-
τάτους τε ἅμα καὶ μοχθηραῖς ὁδοῖς ἐπιχειρημάτων ἐντεθραμμένους· ὥστε

1–13] SVF II, pp. 83–84 1–6] SVF III, pp. 248–249 10–13] *cf.* Prantl, Gesch. d. Logik I 570 n. 13–21] *cf. supra*, pp. 104.27–108.20 20–21] *cf. supra*, p. 104.20–22 27–30] SVF II, p. 84

1 *post* τροπικῶν *add.* τριῶν M *Ald.*, ἢ τριῶν *Ricci* 2 διαφόρως M C 3 ἔστι] ἔτι C 4 ἄλλοις ἐφ' *scripsi*: ἐπ' ἄλλοις M *Ald.* C: ἐν ἄλλοις *Müller* ὅσοις M *Ald.* C: *corr.* R *Müller* 5 συλλογισμοῦ C: *del. Müller* 6 ἑτέρων M 7 τῷ] τὸ M οὐ *om.* C 8 συλλογισμὸν C: *corr.* C[2] συμπλοκὴν *Ald.* 9 μηδαμόθεν M *Ald.* 10 δεήσειε C γνωρίζειν] γινώσκειν C 11–12 σοφιστικῶν καὶ ῥητορικῶν C 12 *post* οὐκέτι *add.* οὔτε *Müller* ἔγραψαν *ex* -εν *(?) corr.* C 14 κάτω νεύομεν] κατανεύομεν C εἰ] ἢ M *Ald.* 15 φωνὴν φθεγγόμεθα C *ante* τὴν[I] *add.* κατὰ C 16 μὲν *om.* M *Ald.* 17 *post* γὰρ *add. et del.* οὐδὲν μᾶλλο M 18 ἐμφαίνει] ἐμφαίνειν πολλάκις C 19 *post* μᾶλλον *add.* ἢ C 19–20 τὴν κεφαλὴν . . . τὸν θώρακα M *Ald.* C: *corr. Kalbfleisch* 20 ε̅] ἐγῶ̅ R[2]: *om.* C ἀτοπίας] ἀτόπου C 22 ἤσκησε C 23 μικροτέρας C 25–26 τοῦ[I] – ψυχῆς] τὴν τοῦ ἡγεμονικοῦ τῆς ψυχῆς M: ἡγεμονικοῦ καὶ ψυχῆς τὴν C: τοῦ τὴν τῆς μὲν ἡγεμονικῆς ψυχῆς *Kalbfleisch* 26 τῆς] τοῦ *Müller* 27 τοῦ δὲ ἐπιθυμητικοῦ *Müller* 28 ἀνίεσθαι M 30 ἐντεθραμμένοις C

Now you can find many persons expertly trained in the analysis 18
of syllogisms from two conditionals, or of tautologous arguments, or
of any others of this kind that employ the first and second transpo-
sition rules, just as you can find other persons (trained in) all the syllo-
gisms that are analyzed through the third rule or the fourth. And yet 19
it is possible to analyze most of these differently and more concisely,
as Antipater wrote; and besides, all the construction of such syllo-
gisms is no small amount of effort wasted on a useless task, as Chry-
sippus himself testifies by his practice, for nowhere in his own
writings did he need these syllogisms in order to prove a doctrine. And 20
Chrysippus and his school never went on to write anything worth
mentioning on the proper method of recognizing scientific premises
and distinguishing them from dialectical, rhetorical, and sophistic
ones; nor are they observed employing it. They are not ashamed, 21
however, to write that we bring our hands to our chest when pointing
to ourselves, or that we nod our head downward if we utter the word
egō (I), to indicate that the heart is the seat of the soul's rule. But the
pointing no more indicates that the governing part of the soul is in the
heart than in the nose or forehead – for people often point to these
also –, and the nodding no more indicates that it is in the region of the
chest than of the head. And throughout the second book of On the 22
Correctness of Names I have shown how absurd they are in their
remarks about the vowel *e*.

If then a person has been well trained in the discovery and 23
recognition of different kinds of premises, my answer to him need not
be long, no more than it need be in answering the Peripatetics. For 24
my argument with them will follow their own teachings, by which
I shall prove to them that the seat of the soul's governing part is
enclosed in the brain, that of its spirited part in the heart, and that of
its desiderative part in the liver. But a lengthy argument must be 25
employed against the Stoics, men adequately trained in the useless
parts of logic but completely unskilled in its useful parts and nurtured

ἀναγκαῖον εἶναι μὴ μόνον διδάσκειν αὐτοὺς ὅσον χρηστὸν ἀλλὰ πολὺ
185 26 πρότερον ἀπο/στῆσαι τοῦ μοχθηροῦ. τοῦτο δὲ χαλεπῶς μὲν ἂν ἴσως,
ἀνύσειν δ' ἠλπίσαμεν, εἴ τις αὐτῶν ὑπέμεινε τῇ Περὶ ἀποδείξεως πραγ-
ματείᾳ ἀκολουθήσας ἐπὶ πλέον ἐν αὐτῇ δοῦναί τε καὶ λαβεῖν λόγον ἐν
27 εὐμενέσιν ἐλέγχοις. ἐπεὶ δὲ οὐχ ὑπομένουσι μὲν τοῦτο, περὶ δὲ τοῦ προ-
τεθέντος ἀεὶ ζητοῦσι πρὶν ὅπως χρὴ ζητεῖν καταστήσασθαι, τίς ἂν
ἡμῖν ἐλπὶς ἔτι λείπαιτο τοῦ μεταστῆσαι τοὺς ἀνθρώπους ἀφ' ὧν ψευδῶς
ὑπειλήφασιν;

4. 'Αλλ' ἐπεὶ μὴ μόνον ἐκείνους πρόκειται πείθειν, ἀλλὰ καὶ τῶν
ἄλλων ἁπάντων ὅστις ἂν μήπω μοχθηροῖς ἔθεσι λόγων ἐντεθραμμένος
ἀνίατον ἔχῃ τὴν ἐν τῇ ψυχῇ διαστροφήν, ἄρξομαι πάλιν ἄνωθεν εἰς τὸ
προκείμενον σκέμμα δεικνύναι πῶς μὲν ἄν τις ἐπιστημονικὰ λαμβάνοι
227 λήμματα τὴν ἀληθινὴν ἀπόδειξιν συνιστάνοντα, πῶς δὲ ἂν | ταῦτα
186 διακρίνοι τις ἀπὸ τῶν ἄλλων λημμάτων, ἔτι τε πρὸς τούτοις / τῶν τὴν
φαινομένην ἀπόδειξιν οὐκ οὖσαν δὲ συνιστάντων λημμάτων ἐπιδείξω τὴν
2 φύσιν ἐπ' αὐτοῦ τοῦ νῦν ἡμῖν προκειμένου σκέμματος. ἥτις δὲ τούτων
αὐτῶν ἐστι πρὸς ἄλληλα διαφορά, καθόσον οἷός τ' εἰμί, σαφέστατα
περὶ πάντων ἐρῶ.

3 'Επεὶ τοίνυν πρόκειται σκέψασθαι περὶ τῆς καρδίας, εἰ τὸ τῆς
ψυχῆς ἡγεμονικόν ἐστιν ἐν αὐτῇ, τοῦτ' ἔστιν, εἰ κατάρχει πᾶσι τοῖς τοῦ
ζῴου μορίοις αἰσθήσεώς τε ἅμα καὶ τῆς καθ' ὁρμὴν κινήσεως, ἰστέον ὡς
ὅσα μὲν ἀπὸ τῶν ὑπαρχόντων αὐτῇ λαμβάνεται λήμματα, διττὴν ἕξει
τὴν διαφοράν· ἔσται γὰρ αὐτῶν τὰ μὲν κατ' αὐτὸ τὸ προκείμενόν τε καὶ
ζητούμενον ἐπιστημονικά, τὰ δ' ἄλλα πάντα γένους ἑτέρου δευτέρου
4 παρακειμένου τοῖς ἐπιστημονικοῖς· ὅσα δὲ ἀπὸ τῶν ἀνθρωπίνων δοξῶν
εἴτ' οὖν ἰδιωτῶν εἴτε ποιητῶν εἴτε φιλοσόφων εἴτε ἐξ ἐτυμολογίας τινὸς
εἴτε ἐκ νευμάτων, εἴτε ἐξ ἐπινευμάτων ἢ ἀνανευμάτων, εἴτε ἐξ ὁτουδή-
τινος ἑτέρου τοιούτου λαμβάνεται λήμματα, τοῦ τρίτου γένους ἔσται
187 228 ταῦτα, διττὴν μὲν ἀπόστασιν ἀφεστῶτα / τῶν ἐπιστημονικῶν, | οὐ
πολλῷ δέ τινι διαφέροντα τῶν σοφιστικῶν, ἅπερ ἐν ὁμωνυμίαις τέ τισι
καὶ τοῖς τῆς λέξεως σχήμασι μάλιστα συνίσταται.

5 'Αρκτέον οὖν ἀπὸ τῶν ὑπαρχόντων ἁπάντων τῇ καρδίᾳ καὶ λεκτέον
ἐφεξῆς ταῦτα πάντα, πρῶτον μὲν ἐν κεφαλαίοις τε καὶ κατὰ γένος, εἶθ'
6 οὕτως καὶ κατὰ μέρος τε καὶ κατ' εἶδος. ὑπάρχει δὴ τῇ καρδίᾳ θέσις καὶ
πηλικότης καὶ πλοκὴ καὶ διάπλασις καὶ διάθεσις καὶ κίνησις. ἀπὸ πρώ-

5–6] SVF II, p. 84 11–13] *cf.* Müller, Beweis, p. 49 20–21] *cf. supra*, p. 110.1–2 21–31] *cf. supra*, pp. 110.23–112.2 Prantl, Gesch. d. Logik I 570 n.

1 μὴ] μὲν M 3 ἀνύσσειν *Ald.* δ' *om.* C τῇ – πραγματείᾳ] εἰς τὴν περὶ ἀποδείξεως πραγματείαν C 4 ἐν αὐτῇ *del. Müller*, *def. Castiglioni* 10 μοχθηρῶν *Müller* 11 ἔχει *Ald.* C 12 μὲν *om. Ald.* λαμβάνει M 13 ταῦτα] αὐτὰ C 14 διακρίνῃ M *Ald.* C: *corr. Kühn* *ante* τῶν^II *add.* τε M 16 ἐπ'] ἀπ' C 18 περὶ *del. Müller* 20 ἐστιν ἐν αὐτῇ *om.* C τοῦτ' ἔστιν *om.* M *Ald.* εἰ] ὃ *Ald.*: ὁ M 25 δόξω C 27 εἴτε ἐκ νευμάτων *del. Kalbfleisch* εἴτε^II – ἀνανευμάτων *del. Müller* ἢ ἀνανευμάτων *om.* M *Ald.* 28 τοιούτου *om.* C ἐστὶ C 32 λεκτέων *Ald.* 33 πρῶτον] πρὶν τὸν C 34 καὶ^I *om.* C *ante* μέρος *add.* τὰ *Ald.* 35 πρώτου *Müller*

besides in unsound methods of reasoning. It is necessary, therefore, not only to teach them what is useful, but much more pressing is the necessity to make them give up what is bad. This would, perhaps, be 26
difficult; yet we would have hoped for success if any of them had had the patience to follow the argument of my treatise On Demonstration and to debate it at some length in friendly scrutiny. But since they do 27
not have the patience for this but make their investigation of any problem that is proposed before they have determined how the investigation should be conducted, what hope would we still have of freeing these men from their false assumptions?

4. But since our purpose is to persuade not the Stoics only but also all others who have been nurtured in fallacious habits of reasoning but whose minds are not yet incurably perverted, I shall begin again at the beginning and show, with reference to our present inquiry, how you may find scientific premises which produce a valid demonstration, and how you may distinguish these from all other premises. And in addition I shall exhibit, in this very problem now before us, the nature of those premises which yield a proof that appears scientific but is not really so. In every case I shall state as clearly as I can their 2
differences from one another.

Since our problem is to inquire about the heart, whether the govern- 3
ing part of the soul is in it, that is, whether it initiates perception and voluntary motion in all parts of the animal, you must know that the premises taken from its properties will be of two kinds: those which pertain to the subject of inquiry as such will be scientific; all the rest will belong to another class, the second, at one remove from the scientific premises. And all premises that are taken from men's 4
opinions, whether those of nonexperts or poets or philosophers, or from some etymology, or from nods, whether of assent or dissent, or from anything else of that kind, will belong to the third class. These premises are twice removed from the scientific and differ by no great amount from sophistical premises, which consist for the most part of certain homonyms and forms of expression.

We must begin, then, with all the properties of the heart; and 5
we must mention them all in turn, first by main heads and by genera, then also by parts and species. Now the heart has position, size, 6
texture, conformation, state, and motion. Let us first take up position,

της οὖν τῆς θέσεως ἀρκτέον ἐπιδεικνύντας ὅσαι προτάσεις ἀπ' αὐτῆς
7 συνίστανται. κεῖται δὲ ὡς πρὸς μὲν τὸν θώρακα μέση πως μᾶλλον· ἡ μὲν
γὰρ βάσις αὐτῆς ἀκριβῶς ἐστι μέση τοῦ θώρακος ἅπαντος, ἡ κορυφὴ δὲ καὶ
τὰ κάτω μέρη προήκει τοσοῦτον, ἡλίκον περ ἂν ᾖ τὸ μέγεθος τῆς καρδίας.
8 ὡς δὲ πρὸς ὅλον τὸ ζῷον ἀνωτέρω τῶν μέσων αὐτοῦ μερῶν τέτακται
τοσοῦτον ὅσον ἀπέχει τῶν κατὰ τὸν ὀμφαλὸν χωρίων· ἐκεῖνα γὰρ
ἀκριβέστατα τὰ μέσα. ἀλλὰ καὶ πρὸς τὴν φάρυγγα, δι' ἧς ἀναπνέομεν,
οὕτω πως ἔχει θέσεως, ὥστε διὰ μέσου τοῦ πνεύμονος αὐτῇ συνῆπται. /
188 229 9 κατὰ γὰρ τὴν ἀριστερὰν κοιλίαν τῆς καρδίας ἐκφύεταί τις | ἀρτηρία
φλεβώδης τὸ σῶμα, τὸ μὲν πρῶτον εἰς τοσαῦτα μόρια σχιζομένη,
ὅσοιπερ ἂν ὦσιν οἱ τοῦ πνεύμονος λοβοί· μετὰ ταῦτα δὲ ἤδη καθ'
ἕκαστον αὐτῶν ἑκάστη διανέμεται εἰς πολλὰ γιγνομένη μόρια, μέχρι περ
10 ἂν ἀναλωθῇ σύμπασα. τοῖς δὲ ἐσχάτοις αὐτῆς πέρασι παμπόλλοις
οὖσιν οἷόν περ δένδρου βλάσταις εἰς ταὐτὸν ἥκει τὰ τῆς τραχείας
ἀρτηρίας πέρατα τὸν αὐτὸν τρόπον εἰς ὅλον τὸ σπλάγχνον μερισθείσης
11 ὅνπερ ἡ φλεβώδης ἀρτηρία. καὶ μὲν δὴ καὶ πρὸς αὐτὸν τὸν πνεύμονα
θέσιν ἔχει τοιαύτην ὥστ' ἔξωθεν ὑπ' αὐτοῦ πανταχόθεν ἠμφιέσθαι.
12 Τὰ μὲν οὖν τῆς θέσεως ὧδε ἔχει τῇ καρδίᾳ καὶ δύναιτ' ἄν τις ἀπ'
αὐτῆς ἐπιχειρήματα ποιεῖσθαι τῇ μὲν ὡς πρὸς τὸ σύμπαν σῶμα, διότι
μέσον πως αὐτοῦ κεῖται δικαίας ἕνεκα νομῆς ὧν ἐπιπέμπει δυνάμεων
189 αὐτῷ, τῇ δὲ ὡς πρὸς τὴν τραχεῖαν ἀρτηρίαν, ὅτι τὴν φωνὴν / διὰ
13 ταύτης ἐκπέμπει. καὶ μὲν δὴ καὶ τὴν χρείαν τε καὶ τὴν ἐνέργειαν τῆς
ἀναπνοῆς συνάπτων αὐτῇ δύναιτ' ἄν τινα κἀντεῦθεν ἐπιχειρήματα
14 λαμβάνειν. κατὰ δὲ τὸν αὐτὸν τρόπον, ὅτι μέση τοῦ θώρακος, ἴσως ἂν
280 ἔχοι τι καὶ περὶ τούτου λαβεῖν ὁ βουλόμενος ἐκ | πάντων ἐπιχειρεῖν.
15 ἀλλ' οὔπω τούτων οὐδὲν ἐπιστημονικὸν οὐδὲ ἀποδεῖξαι τὸ προκείμενον
ἱκανόν, ἔστ' ἂν μηδέπω περαίνηται δι' αὐτῶν ὡς αἰσθήσεώς τε καὶ
κινήσεως τῆς κατὰ προαίρεσιν ἀρχὴ τοῖς ζῴοις ἐστὶν ἡ καρδία. οὐ γὰρ
ἐξ ἀνάγκης ἕπεται τῷ μέσην τῷ ζῴῳ κεῖσθαι τὸ πάντων ἀρχὴν ὑπάρχειν
16 αὐτήν. — καίτοι γε οὐδὲ αὐτὸ τοῦτο ἀληθές ἐστι, τὸ μέσην ἐν τοῖς ζῴοις
εἶναι τὴν καρδίαν· εἰ γὰρ ἀκριβῶς τις ἐξετάσειε, τὰ κατὰ τὸν ὀμφαλόν
ἐστι μέσα. — κατὰ δὲ τὸν αὐτὸν τρόπον οὐδὲ ὅτι μέση τοῦ θώρακος ἡ
καρδία, διὰ τοῦτ' ἀρχὴ τοῦ ζῴου παντός.

2] *cf.* Gal. UP vi. 2, 7: III 415–416, 433, 437 K. 2–3] *cf.* Gal. Anat. vii. 7: II 606 K. 9–13] *cf. supra*, p. 90.10–12 13–16] *cf.* Gal. UP vii. 3: III 520 K. 14–15] *cf. supra*, p. 90.13–18 16–17] *cf.* Gal. UP vi. 7: III 433 K. 31–32] *cf. supra*, lin. 6–7

3 ἀκριβὴς C ἅπαντα M 3–4 καὶ τὰ] καὶ τὰ καὶ τὰ M: εἰς τὰ C 4 προσήκει C ἡλίκο M 7 ἀκριβῶς C 8 αὐτὴ C συνῆπταν *Ald.* 10 φλεβώδης] φλεβώσεως M 11 μετὰ δὲ ταῦτα C 12 ἑκάστη *del. Müller* εἰς *om.* C 13 σύμπασα] πα M: σύμπα M[2] αὐτοῖς M *Ald.*: αὐτοῦ C: *corr. Bas. Corn.* παμπόλοις M 14 βλαστοῖς C 14–15 τῆς ἀρτηρίας τῆς τραχείας C 16 ὅπερ C 17 θέσιν] θέσι (-ει M[2]) γαρ M ἠμφίεσθαι M *Ald.*: *corr. Kühn*: ὑφίεσθαι C 18 δύνναιτ' *Ald.* 19 τῇ] τῆς *Müller* 19–20 ὅτι μέση *Müller* 21 τῇ δὲ] τοῖς δὲ C: τῆς δὲ *Müller* 25 περὶ] παρὰ C 27 μηδέποτε C 29 τῷ[I]] τὸ C *ante* τῷ[II] *add.* ἐν *Müller* τὸ] τῶ C 30 μέσον *Ald.* 33 τῷ ζῴῳ *Müller* *post* παντός *add.* ἐστιν *Müller*

pointing out how many premises are formed from it. It is situated 7
with respect to the thorax pretty well in the middle, for its base is at the exact middle of the whole thorax, and the apex and the parts
below it extend in proportion to the size of the heart. But with respect 8
to the whole animal, the heart has been placed above its middle point by as much as it is distant from the region of the navel, for that region is most precisely the middle. But also with respect to the windpipe through which we breathe, the heart is so placed that it is joined to
the windpipe through the lungs. For an artery, vein-like in body, 9
grows out from the left ventricle of the heart and first splits into as many parts as there are lobes of the lungs; the parts then spread through the lobes, one to each, and each (part) becomes many parts, until
the whole has been used up. Now the trachea is divided throughout 10
the whole organ in the same fashion as the vein-like artery, and its extreme ends meet the ends of that artery, which are very numerous
and resemble the branches of a tree. And indeed in relation to the 11
lungs themselves, the (heart's) position is such that it is enveloped by them externally on all sides.

These, then, are the facts about the heart's position, and a person 12
could argue from its position, in one way with regard to the whole body, that the heart lies in the middle of it for the sake of an even distribution of the powers the heart sends out to it, and in another way with regard to the trachea, that the heart sends the voice out through
it. Further, by connecting the heart with the use and activity of respi- 13
ration, one might also derive some arguments from that quarter.
Similarly, since it is in the middle of the thorax, a person who wishes 14
to use arguments from every source would perhaps be able to make
something of that also. But none of these (premises) is yet scientific or 15
sufficient to demonstrate the matter at hand, so long as one cannot yet infer from them that in animals the heart is the source of both sensation and voluntary motion. For it does not necessarily follow from its being situated in the middle of the animal that it is the source of
everything. – Indeed it is not even true that the heart is at the middle 16
point in animals; if you give a precise account, the region around the navel is the middle. – Similarly, there is no necessity either that because the heart is in the middle of the thorax, it is therefore the ruling part of the whole animal.

17 Οὐδὲ γὰρ ὅτι καθάπερ ἐν ἀκροπόλει τῇ κεφαλῇ δίκην μεγάλου
βασιλέως ὁ ἐγκέφαλος ἵδρυται, διὰ τοῦτ' ἐξ ἀνάγκης ἡ τῆς ψυχῆς ἀρχὴ
190 κατ' αὐτόν ἐστιν, οὐδὲ ὅτι καθάπερ τινὰς δο/ρυφόρους ἔχει τὰς αἰσθήσεις
περιῳκισμένας, οὐδ' εἴ γε καὶ τοῦτο λέγοι τις, ὅπερ οὐρανὸς ἐν ὅλῳ τῷ
κόσμῳ, τοῦτ' ἐν ἀνθρώποις εἶναι τὴν κεφαλὴν καὶ διὰ τοῦθ', ὥσπερ
ἐκεῖνος οἶκός ἐστι τῶν θεῶν, οὕτω τὸν ἐγκέφαλον οἶκον εἶναι τοῦ λογι-
231 18 σμοῦ. καὶ γὰρ τὰ τοιαῦτα πάντα καίπερ ὄντα πολὺ | [μὲν] πιθανώτερα
τῶν ἐπὶ τῆς καρδίας εἰρημένων, ὅμως οὐκ ἔστιν οὐδὲ αὐτὰ πιστὰ πρὸς
ἐπιστήμην ἀκριβῆ καθάπερ οὐδὲ ὅτι τῆς φωνῆς ἡ καρδία δημιουργός
ἐστιν.

19 Εἰ μὲν γὰρ ἀπόδειξίν τινα διδάσκειν ἡμᾶς ἔχουσιν, ἡδέως ἀκουσό-
μεθα· τὸ δὲ ἀπὸ τῆς θέσεως μόνης ὁρμᾶσθαι μοχθηρόν. οὕτω γάρ,
οἶμαι, καὶ τὸν πνεύμονα καὶ τὴν τραχεῖαν ἀρτηρίαν ἀρχὴν τῆς φωνῆς
ἐροῦμεν, ὡς ἐγγυτέρω γε ταῦτ' ἐστὶ τῆς καρδίας τοῖς φωνητικοῖς ὀργά-
νοις. αὐτὸ μὲν γὰρ τὸ πρῶτόν τε καὶ ἴδιον ὄργανον τῆς φωνῆς ὁ λάρυγξ
20 ἐστίν. εἰ γοῦν κατωτέρω τέμοις αὐτοῦ τὴν τραχεῖαν ἀρτηρίαν, οὐκέτ'
ἀκούσῃ φωνοῦντος τοῦ ζῴου, καίτοι γ' ἀναπνέον ἀκωλύτως ὄψει καὶ
191 νῦν αὐτό. καὶ / εἴπερ ἄνθρωπος εἴη τὸ οὕτω τρωθέν, ἐξέσται σοι κελεύειν
21 αὐτῷ φθέγξασθαί τι. προθυμηθήσεται μὲν γάρ, οὐδὲν δὲ ἀκούσῃ πλέον
ἐκπνοῆς ῥοιζώδους, ἣν ἡμεῖς ὀνομάζομεν ἐκφύσησιν· ἄνευ δὲ τοῦ προ-
θυμεῖσθαι φθέγξασθαι φέρεται μὲν ἔξω τὸ πνεῦμα κατὰ τὰς ἐκπνοάς,
22 οὐ μὴν σὺν ψόφῳ γέ τινι καὶ ἀθρόως. ὄψει δὲ καὶ τοὺς κατὰ τὸν θώρακα
232 μῦς | ἅμα τοῖς κατ' ἐπιγάστριον, ὅταν προθυμῆται φθέγγεσθαι τὸ
23 ζῷον, ἐντεινομένους σφοδρῶς. τούτους μέν γε καὶ πρὸ τοῦ τρωθῆναι τὴν
φάρυγγα σαφῶς ἔστιν ἰδεῖν τεινομένους, ἐπειδὰν βιαιότερον φωνῶμεν,
ἀλλ' ἐπί γε τετρωμένῃ τῇ φάρυγγι πονοῦσιν μάτην ὅσα γε πρὸς γένεσιν
24 φωνῆς. ἐκφύσησιν γὰρ μόνην ἐργάζονται διαφέρουσαν ἁπλῆς ἐκπνοῆς,
ὅτι μετὰ ψόφου τε ἅμα καὶ τάχους ἐκκενοῦται τὸ πνεῦμα.

25 Διττὸν οὖν ἁμαρτάνεται κἀνταῦθα ἁμάρτημα τοῖς τὴν φωνὴν ἐκ
τῆς καρδίας ἐκπέμπεσθαι νομίζουσιν, ὅτι πρῶτον μὲν ἀπὸ τῆς θέσεως
192 26 ἐπιχειροῦσιν, ἔπειτα δὲ οὐδὲ ἀπὸ ταύτης ὡς χρή. / τείνονται μὲν γὰρ οἵ
τε κατὰ τὸν θώρακα μύες ἅπαντες οἵ τε κατ' ἐπιγάστριον, ἐπειδὰν
θελήσῃ φωνῆσαι τὸ ζῷον, εἰς τάσιν δή τινα καὶ κίνησιν ἀγόμενοι, τῆς

1–12] *cf. infra*, p. 128.18–22 15–16] *cf. infra*, pp. 122.4–7; 124.5–6

3 δορυφόρους (δορ *e ras.*) τινὰς C **4** οὐδὲ *Müller*: οὔτ' M *Ald.* C *ante* ὅπερ *add.* ὅτι C οὐρανὸς *post* κόσμῳ *(lin. 5) trsp.* C **5** τοῦτ'] τοῦθ' C **6** εἶναι οἶκον M **7** καίπερ ὄντα] καὶ παρόντα C μὲν *del. Müller* **8** *post* ὅμως *add.* δὲ C **9** φωνῆς ἡ καρδία] καρδίας ἡ φωνὴ C **11** ἀκουσώμεθα C **14** τοῦτ' C **16** κατώτερον *Ald.*: κατ^{τρ}ω' M τραχ^{ττ}υ' M **17** ἀναπνέων *Ald.* **19** αὐτὸ M προθυμήσεται C: προμηθήσεται M δὲ] καὶ *Ald.* ἀκούσει C **20** ὑμεῖς C **21** φθέγγεσθαι C εἰσπνοάς C **23** προθυμεῖται *Ald.* **24** ἐκτεινομένους M *Ald.* *ante* τὴν *add.* τὴν τραχεῖαν ἀρτηρίαν M *Ald.* τὴν] τὸν *Ald.* **24–25** τὴν φάρυγγα *del. Ricci Corn.* **26** φάρυγγι] ἀρτηρίᾳ *Ald.* **30** πρῶτα M **31–32** οἵ τε κατὰ] εἴτε κἀπὸ (κ *expunxit* M^2) M **32** ἅπαντες *om.* C **33** θελήσει M στάσιν M: γρ τ$^{σιν'}$ *(ut vid.)* M^2 δή τινα] γρ δέ τινα M^2: δὲ C γρ ἄγονται M^2

Nor is it necessary that because the brain, like the Great King, 17
dwells in the head as in an acropolis, for that reason the ruling part of the soul is in the brain, or because the brain has the senses stationed around it like bodyguards, or even if one should go so far as to say that as heaven is to the whole universe, so the head is to man, and that therefore as the former is the home of the gods, so the brain is the home of the rational faculty. Although statements such as these are all 18
much more plausible than those others about the heart, yet one cannot rely even on these for accurate knowledge, any more than one can rely on the statement that the heart is the artisan of speech.

If they are able to give us some scientific proof, we shall gladly 19
listen; but it is fallacious to take location alone as one's starting-point. By this procedure, I fancy, we could say that the lungs and the trachea are the source of speech, on the ground that they are closer than the heart to the organs of speech. For the larynx is itself the primary and proper speech organ. Thus if you sever the trachea below it, you 20
will no longer hear the animal using its voice, yet you will see it even then breathing unhindered. And if the animal so wounded should be a man, you will be in a position to ask him to say something. He will try, 21
but you will hear nothing more than a whistling exhalation, which we call *ekphysēsis*. When he does not try to speak, his breath is expelled as he exhales, but not noisily or in a sudden burst. You will also see that 22
the muscles of the thorax together with those of the epigastrium are very tense when the animal tries to use its voice. Indeed, even before 23
the trachea is cut one may clearly see these muscles grow tense when we speak rather forcefully; but after the trachea has been cut their effort is to no effect, so far as the production of speech is concerned. For they produce only an expulsion of breath, which differs from 24
simple exhalation in that the air is emitted noisily and rapidly.

Therefore those who suppose that speech is sent out from the 25
heart are here also doubly mistaken: first, they argue from position; and second, they do not even do that as they should. For all the 26
muscles of the chest and epigastrium are tightened when the animal wishes to speak, being brought to a certain tension and motion; but

καρδίας οὐδεμίαν ἐν τούτῳ νεωτέραν ἐπικτωμένης ἐνέργειαν· οὐ μὴν ἤδη
γέ πω τὸ κάτωθεν ἀναφερόμενον πνεῦμα πρὶν ὑπὸ τοῦ λάρυγγος
ῥυθμισθῆναι φωνῆς ἔχει ἰδέαν, ἀλλ' ὡς εἴρηται πρόσθεν, ἐκφυσήσεως
233 27 μόνης, ὡς ἀπεδείξαμεν ἐν τῇ Περὶ φωνῆς πραγματείᾳ. | πληττομένη γὰρ
ὑπὸ τῶν κατὰ τὸν λάρυγγα χόνδρων οἷον ὑπὸ πλήκτρων τινῶν ἡ
28 ἐκφύσησις αὕτη φωνὴ γίνεται. σύγκειται δὲ ὁ λάρυγξ ἐκ τριῶν χόνδρων
ὑπὸ μυῶν πολλῶν κινουμένων. ὅστις δὲ ὁ τρόπος ἐστὶ τῆς τῶν χόνδρων
συστάσεως ἢ τῆς τῶν μυῶν κινήσεως, ἐμοὶ μὲν ἐν ταῖς περὶ τούτων
πραγματείαις οἰκείαις ἀκριβῶς εἴρηται· τοῖς δὲ ἀπὸ τῆς θέσεως μόνης
29 ἐπιχειροῦσιν οὐδὲν τῶν τοιούτων γιγνώσκεται. κἄπειτα θαυμάζουσιν
ἐξαίφνης ἀκούσαντες ἐξ ἐγκεφάλου γίγνεσθαι τὴν φωνήν· ἔτι δὲ μᾶλλον, /
193 ἐπειδὰν ἀκούσωσιν ὡς αἱ κατὰ προαίρεσιν ἅπασαι κινήσεις ὑπὸ μυῶν
ἐπιτελοῦνται, θαυμάζουσί τε καὶ παραδοξολόγους ἡμᾶς ἀποκαλοῦσι,
καίτοι γε ἡμεῖς ἅπερ ἐπαγγελλόμεθα λόγῳ ταῦτα ἐν ταῖς τῶν ζῴων
ἀνατομαῖς ἐπιδείκνυμεν, οἱ δ' οὐδὲν ἄλλο ἔχουσι λέγειν ἢ διότι πλησίον
ἐστὶν ἡ καρδία τῆς φάρυγγος, διὰ τοῦτ' ἐξ ἐκείνης ἄρχεσθαι τὴν φωνήν.
30 αἱροῦνται γάρ, οἶμαι, τὴν σύντομόν τε καὶ λείαν ὁδὸν ἐν τοῖς λόγοις
ἀντὶ τῆς τραχείας τε καὶ μακρᾶς, κἂν αὕτη μὲν ἀπάγῃ πρὸς τὸ ζητούμε-
234 νον, ἡ δὲ λεία τε καὶ ταχεῖα σφάλλῃ | τἀληθοῦς. οὐδ' ἔστιν ὅστις ἐμοί
ποθ' ὑπέμεινε δεικνύντι τοὺς μῦς ἅπαντας ὑφ' ὧν ἡ ἀναπνοή τε γίγνεται
31 καὶ φωνή. καίτοι γ' οὐκ ἐν τούτοις μόνοις ἐστὶ τὸ κῦρος τῆς ἀποδείξεως,
ἀλλ' ἡ τρίτη μοῖρα τοῦ λόγου παντός. οἱ μὲν γὰρ μύες ὄργανά τινα
κινοῦσιν ὑφ' ὧν ἀναπνοή τε καὶ φωνὴ γίγνεται, δέονται δ' αὐτοὶ πάλιν
ὅπως κινηθῶσι τῶν ἀπ' ἐγκεφάλου νεύρων, ὧν εἴ τι βρόχοις διαλάβοις
194 εἴτε τέμοις, ἀκίνητον / μὲν αὐτίκα μάλα ποιήσεις τὸν μῦν ἐκεῖνον, εἰς ὃν
τὸ νεῦρον ἐνέβαλεν, ἀκίνητον δὲ καὶ τοῦ ζῴου τὸ μέλος, ὃ πρότερον ὑπὸ
32 τοῦ μυὸς ἐκινεῖτο, πρὶν τμηθῆναι τὸ νεῦρον. ὅστις οὖν ὄντως ἀληθείας
ἐρᾷ, πρὸς ἡμᾶς ἡκέτω μαθησόμενος ἐναργῶς ἐπ' αὐτῶν τῶν ζῴων, εἰ
μόνον ἔχοι τὰς αἰσθήσεις ἀπηρώτους, ὑφ' ἑτέρων μὲν ὀργάνων τε καὶ
μυῶν καὶ νεύρων εἰσπνοὴν ἀβίαστον γιγνομένην, ὑφ' ἑτέρων δὲ τὴν μετὰ
33 βίας· ὀνομάζω δὲ ἀβίαστον μὲν τὴν τοῖς ὑγιαίνουσι καὶ μηδεμίαν ἰσχυρὰν
κίνησιν κινουμένοις ὑπάρχουσαν, βιαίαν δὲ τὴν ἔν τε πάθεσί τισι καὶ

1–10] Gal. De voce, test. 19: p. 8 Baumgarten 3–4] *cf. supra*, p. 120.19–20 17–19] *cf.* Hes. OD 288; 290–291 *infra*, p. 338.3 29–124.5] Rhazes, *al-Ḥāwī*, vol. III, p. 180.6–9 29–31] *cf.* Gal. Anat. viii. 2: II 657–659 K.; ix. 14: II, p. 22 Simon De loc. aff. ii. 8, iv. 7: VIII 102, 253 K. Baumgarten, 1962, pp. 183–184

2 τὸ *om.* C 3 ἔχειν C: ἔχον *Petersen* 4 ὡς *del. Petersen* ἀποδείξαμεν M: ἀπεδείξωμεν *Ald.* *ante* φωνῆς *add.* τῆς C 6 φωνῇ M δὲ *om.* M 7 τῆς *om.* M 9 οἰκείαις πραγματείαις C μόνοις M 11 ἐξ] ὑπ' C 13 τε] δὲ M *Ald.* C: *corr. Kühn* 14 ἐν ταῖς] ἐπὶ ταῖς M *Ald.*: ἐν ταῖς ἐπὶ C: *corr. Wilamowitz* 15 δι' ὅτι *Ald.*: δὴ ὅτι C 16 τὴν φωνήν *ex* τῆς φωνῆς *corr.* M[2] 18 αὕτη μὲν] αὐτὴ μὴ C ἀπάγει M *Ald.* 19 ἡ] εἰ M τραχεῖα M: βραχεῖα *Ald.* σφάλλει M *Ald.* C: *corr. Müller* τἀληθὲς C 20 ἡ *om.* C 21 οὐκ – μόνοις] ἐν τούτοις οὐ μόνον *Müller* 23 τε] τις *Ald.* φωνὴ] πνοὴ C πάλιν *om.* C 24 ὧν εἴ τι] ὃν εἴτε C: ὧν εἴτε τι *Müller* βρόγχοις C 25 μὲν *om. Ald.* 27 ὅστι M 29 ἀπειρώτους M C: *corr.* R[2] *Ald.* 30 *ante* εἰσπνοὴν *add.* τὴν *Müller* τὴν *om. Müller*

the heart meanwhile takes on no new activity. Nevertheless, the breath carried up from below, before it has been shaped by the larynx, does not yet have the form of speech, but only, as stated above, of expelled breath. This we demonstrated in our treatise On Speech. The expelled 27
breath becomes voice on being struck by the cartilages of the larynx as by a kind of pick. The larynx is composed of three cartilages moved 28
by many muscles. I gave an exact account of the consistency of the cartilages and the movement of the muscles in the treatises expressly dealing with these things; but such matters are quite unknown to those who argue from position alone. And then they marvel when 29
suddenly they hear that speech comes from the brain, and they marvel even more and call us posers of paradoxes when they hear that all voluntary movements are produced by muscles. And yet we demonstrate these claims of ours in dissections of animals, while they have nothing to say except that because the heart is near the windpipe, for that reason the voice begins from it. In my opinion they choose the 30
short and smooth road in their reasoning rather than the rough and long one, although the latter leads to the goal they seek, whereas the smooth and swift road misses the truth. And there is not one of them who ever heard me through when I pointed out all the muscles by which breathing and speech are generated. Yet these (muscles) are not 31
alone the crucial element in the proof; they are a third of the whole account. The muscles move certain organs which give rise to respiration and speech, but (the muscles) themselves in turn require for their motion the nerves from the brain; and if you block any of these (nerves) with a ligature, or cut it, you will immediately render motionless the muscle that the nerve entered, and you will also render motionless the member of the animal that was formerly moved by the muscle, before the nerve was cut. Then let everyone who really loves the truth 32
come to me and learn clearly from the animals themselves, if only his senses are unimpaired, that unforced inhalation is brought about by one set of organs, muscles and nerves, and forced inhalation by another set. I call unforced the inhalation of animals in good health and engaged 33
in no violent movement, and I call forced that which occurs in certain

235 τοῖς σφοδροῖς γυμνα|σίοις ἐπιτελουμένην, ἐφ' ἧς εὐθέως ὄψει συνεξαιρό-
μενα καὶ τὰ κατὰ τὰς ὠμοπλάτας ἅπαντα μόρια· καὶ δὴ κατὰ τὰς ἀνάλογον
αὐταῖς ἐκπνοὰς ὑφ' ἑτέρων μὲν ὀργάνων τε καὶ μυῶν καὶ νεύρων τὴν
ἀβίαστόν τε καὶ μικράν, ὑφ' ἑτέρων δὲ τὴν βίαιόν τε καὶ μεγάλην, ἣν
34 ὀνομάζειν ἔθος ἡμῖν ἐκφύσησιν. ἐπὶ δὲ τούτοις ἅπασιν ἑξῆς ὑποδείξομέν
195 σοι τὸ τῆς φωνῆς / ἴδιον ὄργανον, τὸν λάρυγγα, καὶ τοὺς κινοῦντας
αὐτὸν μῦς καὶ τὰ τῶν μυῶν ἐκείνων νεῦρα τὰ ἐξ ἐγκεφάλου καθήκοντα
καὶ μετὰ ταῦτα τὴν γλῶτταν, ἕτερον ὄργανον οὐ φωνῆς, ἀλλὰ διαλέκτου
τε καὶ διαλέξεως, ὁποτέρως ἂν ὀνομάζειν ἐθελήσῃς, καὶ τοὺς μῦς ἐπιδείξο-
35 μέν σοι καὶ τὰ νεῦρα τὰ ἐξ ἐγκεφάλου. καὶ δὴ καὶ ζῷα πλείω παρασκευά-
σαντες ἄλλην κατ' ἄλλο τῶν εἰρημένων ἐνεργειῶν ἐπιδείξομεν ἀπολ-
λυμένην ἐφ' ἑκάστου τῶν ἀπ' ἐγκεφάλου νεύρων τεμνομένου.
36 Τάχ' ἴσως ἐπιθυμεῖ τις ἀκοῦσαι τῶν εἰρημένων ἐνεργειῶν ἑκάστης
τὸ ἴδιον ὄργανον καὶ τοὺς κινοῦντας μῦς οἵτινές τέ εἰσι καὶ πόσοι τὸν
236 ἀριθμὸν ἥντινά τε θέσιν ἔχουσι καὶ πηλίκοι τὸ μέγεθος ὑπάρχουσι | καὶ
τίνα δέχονται νεῦρα καὶ πόσα καὶ πηλίκα καὶ κατὰ τί μάλιστα μέρος ἐξ
ἐγκεφάλου βλαστάνοντα τίς τε τοῖς ὑπ' αὐτῶν κινουμένοις ὀργάνοις
37 τρόπος ἐστὶ τῆς κινήσεως. ἐγὼ δὲ καὶ πρόσθεν εἶπον ὡς πολλάκις ὑπὲρ
196 τῶν αὐτῶν γράφειν οὐκ ἐπαινῶ, ἀλλ' εἴπερ ὄντως ἐστί τις / φιλομαθής,
ἑτέρας ὑπὲρ τούτων ἁπάντων ἔχει πραγματείας ἡμῖν γεγραμμένας,
πρῶτον μὲν τὴν Περὶ θώρακός τε καὶ πνεύμονος κινήσεως, ἔνθα δείκνυμεν
ὑπὸ τοῦ θώρακος κινούμενον τὸν πνεύμονα καὶ κατὰ μὲν τὰς διαστολὰς
διαστελλόμενον ἕλκειν τὸν ἔξωθεν ἀέρα καὶ τοῦτ' εἶναι τὴν εἰσπνοήν,
κατὰ δὲ τὰς συστολὰς συστελλόμενον ἐκθλίβειν τὸν ἐν αὐτῷ περιεχό-
μενον εἴς τε τὴν φάρυγγα καὶ τὸ στόμα καὶ διὰ τούτων ἐκπέμπειν ἔξω
38 καὶ τοῦτ' εἶναι τὴν ἐκπνοήν. ἑτέραν δ' ἔχει πραγματείαν ἐφεξῆς τῇδε
Περὶ τῶν τῆς ἀναπνοῆς αἰτίων, ἔνθα καὶ τοὺς μῦς ἅπαντας ἐδήλωσα καὶ
τὰ πρὸς αὐτῶν ὄργανα κινούμενα καὶ τὰ νεῦρα τὰ τοῖς μυσὶ τὴν ἐξ
39 ἐγκεφάλου παρέχοντα δύναμιν τὴν ψυχικήν. εἶτ' αὖθις ἄλλην ἑξῆς
ταῖσδε Περὶ τῆς φωνῆς ἔχει πραγματείαν ὑπέρ τε τῶν ⟨τῆς φωνῆς ὀργά-
237 νων γεγραμμένην καὶ τῶν⟩ ταῦτα | κινούντων μυῶν ἔτι τε τῶν εἰς τούτους
καθηκόντων ἐξ ἐγκεφάλου νεύρων.
40 Εἰς δέ γε τὰ παρόντα καὶ τοῦτ' ἀρκεῖ μοι μόνον εἰπεῖν, ὡς εἴπερ ἡ
197 φωνὴ τυπου/μένου πως τοῦ κατὰ τὸν πνεύμονα πνεύματος ὑπὸ τοῦ

4–5] *cf. supra*, p. 120.20   5–7] *cf.* Gal. Anat. xi. 1–5: II, pp. 61–80, 277–289 Simon   8–10] *cf.* Gal. Anat. x. 6–8, xi. 7: II, pp. 47–56, 85–88 Simon   29–32] Gal. De voce, test. 14 Baumgarten   33–126.3] SVF II, p. 244

1 ἐφ' ἧς] εὐθὺς M   συνεξαιρούμενα M   3 τε *om.* M *Ald.*   5 ἐπιδείξομέν *Kühn*   6 φάρυγγα *Ald.*   7 ἐκεῖνα M: δ' ἐκείνων C: *corr. Ald.*   9 τε *om.* C   ἐθελήσαις M *Ald.* C: *corr. Kalbfleisch et Herbst*   12 τεμνομένων M *Ald.* C: *corr. Kühn*   14 πόσοι] ὅσοι C   16 πόσα] πᾶσα, *ut vid.*, M   τί *om.* M, *lac. 2 litt. rel.*   17 βλαστάνονται *Ald.*   24 αὐτῷ M *Ald.* C: *corr. Kühn*   26 δὲ M *Ald.*   27 αἰτιῶν C   28 αὐτοὺς C   30 τῆς – 31 τῶν[I] *addidi*: *ante* ὑπέρ *add.* ἔνθα ἐπέδειξα ὑπέρ τε τῶν ἰδίων αὐτῆς ὀργάνων *Müller*, ἐ. ἐ. ὑ. τε τ. ἰδίων αὐτῆς τῆς φωνῆς ὀργάνων ἅμα καὶ τῶν τῆς διαλέξεως *Baumgarten*   33 ἡ *om.* C   34 *ante* τυπουμένου *add.* τοῦ C   ὑπὸ] ἀπὸ C

affections and in violent exercises; in the latter you will immediately see all the parts at the shoulder blades rising with (the intake of breath). Similarly in exhalation one set of organs and muscles and nerves causes unforced and light (breathing), another set the forced and heavy (expulsion of breath) that we customarily call *ekphysēsis*. After 34
all this we shall next point out to you the special organ of speech, the larynx, and the muscles that move it, and the nerves that come down to these muscles from the brain; and after that the tongue, another organ not of speech but of language and discourse – whichever name you choose to give it –; and we shall also show you its muscles and its nerves coming from the brain. Indeed we shall prepare several speci- 35
mens in advance, and by using a different specimen for each of the activities mentioned, we shall show how the activity is destroyed with the cutting of each of the nerves from the brain.

Perhaps someone may wish to learn about the organ proper to 36
each of the activities mentioned, the muscles that move it – which ones they are, how many, where located, and how large –, the nerves received by these muscles – their number and size, and the part of the brain from which they especially come –, and the nature of the motion in the organs moved by them. I said earlier that I do not approve of 37
writing many times about the same things, but anyone who is really a lover of learning has other works of mine written on all these matters. First, he has my work On the Motion of the Thorax and Lungs, where we show that when the lungs are moved by the thorax and distended as it expands, they draw the outside air in, and this is inhalation; but when they are contracted by its contractions, they force the air they contain into the windpipe and mouth and thus expel it, and that is exhalation. Next after this he has another treatise, On the Causes of 38
Respiration, in which I pointed out all the muscles, the organs moved by them, and the nerves that transmit the power of the mind from the brain to the muscles. Then after these he has still another treatise, On 39
Speech, in which I wrote about the organs of speech, the muscles that move these (organs), and the nerves that come down to these (muscles) from the brain.

For the present it is enough for me only to make this further state- 40
ment, that if speech were produced when pneuma in the lungs is

κατὰ τὴν καρδίαν ἐγίγνετο κἄπειθ' ἑαυτῷ τὸ κατὰ τὴν φάρυγγα
συντυποῦντος, οὐκ ἂν ἀπώλλυτο παραχρῆμα τμηθέντων νεύρων τινῶν
ἤτοι κατὰ τὸν τράχηλον ἢ τὴν κεφαλήν, ἔτι δὲ μᾶλλον οὐκ ἂν ἀπώλετο
θλιψάντων τὸν ἐγκέφαλον ἢ τρωσάντων ἄχρι κοιλίας ἢ διατεμόντων
41 τὸν νωτιαῖον μυελόν. τὸ μὲν γὰρ τῆς τραχείας ἀρτηρίας, ἥνπερ δὴ καὶ
φάρυγγα προσαγορεύομεν, ἢ τοῦ πνεύμονος ἢ τῆς καρδίας αὐτῆς βλα-
βείσης ἀπόλλυσθαι τὴν φωνὴν οὐδὲν ἂν ⟨ἦν⟩ οἶμαι θαυμαστόν, εἴπερ
ἐκ τῆς καρδίας ὡρμᾶτο· τὸ δὲ τοῦ ἐγκεφάλου θλιφθέντος ἤ τινος τῶν
ἐξ αὐτοῦ νεύρων τῶν εἰς τοὺς τοῦ λάρυγγος μῦς φερομένων ἄτοπόν τε
καὶ δεινῶς ἄλογον, εἴπερ γε μηδενὸς αὐτῶν ἡ τῆς φωνῆς γένεσις προσ-
42 δεῖται. καὶ μὴν ἔμπαλιν ἔχει τὸ φαινόμενον οὗ δοξάζουσιν ἐκεῖνοι. καρδίας
μὲν γὰρ γυμνωθείσης, ὡς κἀν τῷ πρὸ τούτου μοι λέλεκται γράμματι, |
238 καὶ κρατῶν καὶ θλίβων καὶ θλῶν οὔτε ἄπνουν οὔτε ἄφωνον οὔτε ἄλλην
198 τινὰ τῶν καθ' ὁρμὴν ἐνεργειῶν ἐμποδιζόμενον / ὄψει τὸ ζῷον· ἐγκέφαλον
δὲ γυμνώσας τῶν ὀστῶν ⟨καὶ τρώσας⟩ ἢ θλίψας ἡντινοῦν αὐτοῦ κοιλίαν
οὐκ ἄφωνον μόνον οὐδ' ἄπνουν εὐθύς, ἀλλὰ καὶ παντάπασιν ἀναίσθη-
τόν τε καὶ ἀκίνητον ἁπασῶν τῶν καθ' ὁρμὴν κινήσεων ἐργάσῃ τὸ ζῷον.
43 Εἴρηται δέ μοι καὶ πρόσθεν ὡς οὐ χρὴ συντιτράναι τοῦ θώρακος
44 οὐδετέραν κοιλότητα γυμνοῦντας τὴν καρδίαν. εἰ γὰρ δὴ τούτου τύχοι τις,
οὐ μόνον ἢ θλίβειν ἢ θλᾶν ἤ τι τοιοῦτον ἕτερον ἐργάζεσθαι βουληθεὶς δυνή-
σεται κατορθοῦν, ἀλλὰ καὶ βουληθεὶς ἀθρόως ὅλην ἐξελεῖν οὐκ ἀτυχήσει
45 τῆς χειρουργίας. γίγνεται μὲν οὖν τοῦτο καὶ κατὰ πολλὰς θυσίας ἐξ
ἔθους οὕτως ἐπιτελουμένας καὶ φαίνεται τὰ ζῷα τῆς καρδίας ἤδη κατὰ
τῶν βωμῶν ἐπικειμένης οὐκ ἀναπνέοντα μόνον ἢ κεκραγότα συντόνως,
46 ἀλλὰ καὶ φεύγοντα, μέχρι περ ἂν ὑπὸ τῆς αἱμορραγίας ἀποθάνῃ. τάχιστα
δὲ δήπουθεν αὐτῶν ἐκκενοῦται τὸ αἷμα τεττάρων μεγίστων ἀγγείων
239 διασπωμένων, ἀλλ' ἄχρι περ ἂν ἔτι ζῇ, | καὶ ἀναπνεῖ καὶ φωνεῖ καὶ
199 47 τρέχει. / τοὺς δέ γε κατὰ τὸν πρῶτον σπόνδυλον ὁσημέραι διατεμνο-
μένους ταύρους τὴν ἔκφυσιν τοῦ νωτιαίου μυελοῦ παραχρῆμα θεώμεθα
μὴ ὅτι δραμεῖν ἔτι δυναμένους, ἀλλὰ μηδ' ἐπ' ἐλάχιστον προβῆναι,
συναπόλλυται δ' αὐτοῖς ἅμα τῇ τομῇ καὶ ἡ ἀναπνοὴ καὶ ἡ φωνή· καὶ
48 γὰρ καὶ ταύταις ἄνωθέν ἐστιν ἡ ἀρχή. τὴν μέντοι καρδίαν ἐπὶ τῶν
οὕτω πληγέντων ταύρων ἔστιν ἰδεῖν ἄχρι πλείστου σφύζουσαν ἅμα

12–14] *v. supra*, p. 80.3–11 *cf. infra*, p. 210.20–26 18–22] libri primi test., *v. supra*, p. 70.13–17 23–25] *cf.* Maimonid. Aph. xxv. 71 28–31] *cf. supra*, p. 76.26–27 *infra*, PHP 607.1–3 Müller Orib. Coll. med. rel. xxiv. 3.6–8: CMG VI 2.1, p. 12.8–17

2 ἀπόλλυτο M *Ald.*: *corr. Chart.*: ἀπόλλοιτο C 4 κοι^λ C 6 φάρυγγκα *Ald.* αὐτῆς *om.* C 7 ἦν *add. Einarson (cf. infra, PHP 521.4 Müller)* 8 τὸ δὲ τοῦ] τοῦτο δὲ C θλιβέντος *Ald.* 11 οὗ] ἢ *Ald.* 12 μὲν *om.* C 15 γυμνάσας *Ald.* καὶ τρώσας *addidi* 18 ὡς οὐ χρὴ *om.* C 19 τύχῃ *Ald.* C 20 οὐ] οὗ M ἢ[I]] εἰ M *Ald.*: ἐὰν *Müller* θλᾶν] βοᾶν M ἐργάσασθαι C βουληθῇ M *Ald.*: *corr. Einarson*: *om.* C 21 κατορθοῦνται M: κατορθοῦται C ἀτυχήσεις C 22 οὖν τοῦτο] τοῦτο M *Ald.*: οὖν C: *corr. Müller* 24 μόνον *om.* C 25 ὑπὸ] ἀπὸ C ἀποθάνῃ] -ῃ *ex* -ει *corr.* M 27 ἀναπνεῖ] -πνεῖ *ex* -πνῇ *corr.* M 27–28 φωνῇ καὶ ἀναπνῇ καὶ τρέχῃ C 28 τοὺς] τοῦ C 28–29 διατεμνομένου ταύρου C 29 ἐκφύσησιν C

somehow shaped by the heart's pneuma and then imparts this shape to the pneuma in the windpipe, speech would not immediately be destroyed when certain nerves have been cut in the neck or head; and even less would it have been destroyed when we applied pressure to the brain or pierced it as far as a ventricle or cut through the spinal cord. It would not, I think, be at all surprising that injury to the 41
trachea, which we also call the *pharynx*, or to the lungs or the heart itself should destroy speech, if speech came from the heart; but it would be absurd and utterly irrational for speech to be destroyed by pressure on the brain or on one of the nerves that pass from the brain to the muscles of the larynx, if it were true that none of these is needed for the production of speech. But the observed facts are quite the 42
reverse of their doctrine. For when the heart has been exposed, as I mentioned also in the preceding book, if you lay hold of it and press or crush it, you will see that the animal is not deprived of breath or speech and is not prevented from performing any other of the activities that follow on conation; but when you have stripped the brain of its bones and have pierced or pressed any one of its ventricles, you will immediately deprive the animal not only of speech and breath, but of all sensation whatever, and of all the movements that follow on conation.

I also said earlier that when exposing the heart one must not at 43
the same time pierce either of the two chest cavities. If a person 44
should succeed in this, not only will he be able successfully to press or crush the heart or do anything else of the sort if he so wishes, but even if he wishes to remove the whole (heart) all at once he will not fail in his surgery. Now this very thing happens also in many sacrifices that 45
are customarily performed in this way, and animals whose heart already lies on the altar are observed not only to breathe and bellow vehemently, but also to flee, until they die from loss of blood. Of 46
course their blood empties out very quickly, as the four largest vessels have been torn away; but so long as the animals still live they breathe and cry out and run. But when we observe the bulls that are cut 47
every day at the first vertebra, where the spinal cord grows out (from the brain), we see immediately that they are no longer able to advance a single step, much less to run; and along with the incision they lose both breath and utterance, for these activities too are initiated from above. And yet we can see the heart of bulls thus cut pulsating for 48

ταῖς ἀρτηρίαις ἁπάσαις· οὐ γὰρ δὴ καὶ ταύταις γε παρ' ἐγκεφάλου τὸ
49 σφύζειν ἐστὶν ὥσπερ οὐδὲ αὐτῇ τῇ καρδίᾳ. ὡς γὰρ αἱ κινήσεις ἑτέρου
γένους εἰσίν, οὕτω καὶ τῶν ἀρχῶν οὐδετέρα προσδεῖται τῆς ἑτέρας, ἀλλ'
ἔστιν οὕτως ἥ τε καρδία πηγὴ τῆς κατὰ τοὺς σφυγμοὺς κινήσεως ὅ τ'
ἐγκέφαλος τῆς κατὰ προαίρεσιν οὐδ' ἔστιν οὐδεὶς λόγος ὃς ἀναγκάσει
μίαν ἀρχὴν ἁπασῶν εἶναι τῶν κατὰ τὸ ζῷον ἐνεργειῶν· οὔτε γὰρ ὡς
οὐκ ἐνδεχομένων εἶναι πολλῶν οὔθ' ὡς μὴ οὐχ οὕτως φαινομένων
ἐπιδείξει.
50 Ἀλλὰ περὶ μὲν τούτου κἀν τοῖς ἑξῆς ἐπὶ πλέον αὐτοῖς διαλέξομαι.
200 νυνὶ δ' ἐφ' ὅπερ ἔλεγον αὖθις / ἐπάνειμι, πρὸς τὸ μήτε τῆς ἀναπνευστικῆς
240 51 κινήσεως μήτε | τῆς φωνητικῆς δημιουργικὴν ἀρχὴν εἶναι τὴν καρδίαν. δι'
ἐκείνην μὲν γὰρ τὸ πλεῖστον, οὐ μὴν ὑπ' ἐκείνης γε τὴν ἀναπνοὴν γίγνε-
σθαι συμβέβηκεν, οὐ ταὐτὸν δ' ἐστὶν ὑπό του γίγνεσθαι καὶ διά τι. –
γέγραπται δὲ ἡμῖν ἐν βιβλίον ἰδίᾳ καθ' ἑαυτὸ Περὶ χρείας ἀναπνοῆς. –
5. Οἱ δ' ἡγούμενοι φωνὴν ἢ ἀναπνοὴν ὑπὸ τῆς καρδίας ἐπιτελεῖ-
σθαι πρὸς τῆς κατὰ τὴν θέσιν ἐγγύτητος ἠπατήθησαν οὐκ εἰδότες ὡς οὐ
πάντως εἴ τι πλησίον ἐστὶ μόριον ἐνεργείας ἡστινοσοῦν, ἐξ ἀνάγκης
2 τοῦτο καὶ ἀρχὴ τῆς ἐνεργείας ἐστίν. οὐδὲ γὰρ ὅσοι τὸν ἐγκέφαλον ὑπο-
λαμβάνουσιν ἀρχὴν εἶναι τῆς κατ' ὀφθαλμοὺς καὶ ὦτα καὶ ῥῖνας
αἰσθήσεως ὅτι πλησίον αὐτῶν ἐστιν, ὀρθῶς ἐπιχειροῦσιν, ἀλλὰ καὶ
τούτους ἡ θέσις ἔσφαλ⟨λ⟩ε, μᾶλλον δὲ οὐχ ἡ θέσις ἀλλ' ἡ περὶ τῆς
3 θέσεως δόξα. πάντως γὰρ δήπου τοιούτῳ τινὶ προσχρήσονται κατὰ τὰς
ἀποδείξεις ἀξιώματι· πᾶσι τοῖς ἐνεργοῦσιν ἐκ τῶν πλησίον ἐστὶν ἡ ἀρχή.
201 4 τούτου γὰρ ὑποτεθέν/τος ὡς ἀληθοῦς, εἶτ' ἐκ τοῦ φαίνεσθαι προσλη-
φθέντος ὡς ἐγκεφάλου ψαύει τὰ ὦτα, περαίνοιτ' ἂν ἤδη τὸ καὶ τὴν ἀρχὴν
241 5 αὐτοῖς τῆς ἐνεργείας ἐντεῦθεν ὑπάρχειν. | ἀλλ' οὔτε πρὸς αἴσθησιν οὔτε πρὸς
νόησιν ἐναργές ἐστιν ὡς πρῶτόν τε καὶ ἐξ ἑαυτοῦ πιστὸν εἶναι τὸ νῦν εἰρη-
μένον ἀξίωμα, τὸ πᾶσι τοῖς ἐνεργοῦσιν ἐκ τῶν πλησίον εἶναι τὴν ἀρχήν.
6 Οὔκουν οὔθ' ὅτι πλησίον ἐγκεφάλου τὰ ὦτα καὶ οἱ ὀφθαλμοὶ καὶ αἱ
ῥῖνες, ἐντεῦθεν αὐτοῖς ἡ τῆς αἰσθητικῆς δυνάμεώς ἐστιν ἀρχὴ οὔθ' ὅτι
πλησίον ἐστὶ καρδίας τὰ φωνητικά τε καὶ ἀναπνευστικὰ μόρια, διὰ τοῦτ'
7 ἐκ καρδίας αὐτοῖς ἡ ἀρχή. καὶ μὴν ὁ θαυμαζόμενος ὑπὸ τῶν Στωϊκῶν
λόγος ὁ Ζήνωνος, ὃν καὶ πρῶτον ἁπάντων ἔγραψεν ἐν τῷ Περὶ τοῦ τῆς
ψυχῆς ἡγεμονικοῦ Διογένης ὁ Βαβυλώνιος, οὐκ ἐξ ἄλλου τινὸς ἔχει

2–3] *cf. supra*, p. 80.14–15 *infra*, p. 150.3–6 5–6] *cf.* SVF II, p. 244 9] *cf. infra*, pp. 148.8–152.8 10] *cf. supra*, p. 120.9–10 14] Gal. De resp. usu: IV 470–511 K. *cf. infra*, PHP 718.8 Müller 18–22] *cf. supra*, p. 120.1–12 32–34] SVF III, p. 215 32–33] SVF I, p. 40

4 οὕτως] ὄντως C πληγή C 7 οὐχ *om. Ald.* 8 ἐπιδείξεις C 9 κἂν *Ald.* αὐτοῖς *secl. Müller* 10 τῆς *ex* τοῖς *corr.* M 13 γενέσθαι M 18 τούτω C 21 ἔσφαλε M *Ald.* C: *corr. Kühn* 22 θέσεως] αἰσθήσεως M *Ald.* 23 πλησίων M *Ald.* 24 ἀληθῶς M εἶτ' C 25 ἐγκέφαλον M *Ald.* περαίνειτ' M 26 αὐτοῖς *om.* C 27 ἑαυτοῦ] ἐγκεφάλου αὐτοῦ C 28 πλησίον] -ον *ex* -ων *corr.* M 29 Οὔκουν – 30 ἀρχὴ *om. lac. 5 vel 7 litt. rel.* M (λείπει *in mg.*) *Ald.* 31 *post* μόρια *add.* καὶ C 33 ἔγραψα C

a very long time, along with all the arteries; for the pulsation of the
arteries is not from the brain, nor is that of the heart itself. For as 49
the motions are different in kind, so also neither of the sources
has need of the other. This is true of the heart as source of motion
in the pulse, and the brain as source of voluntary motion, and there
is no argument that will make it necessary that there be a single
source for all the activities of the animal; for it will not be demonstrative either on the assumption that they cannot be many or that
they do not appear many.

I shall argue this point with them also in a subsequent passage at 50
greater length. Now I return to my earlier statement, that the heart
is not the source that shapes the movements either of respiration or of
speech. It happens that respiration takes place primarily on account 51
of the heart, but not by the agency of the heart, and taking place 'on
account of' something is not the same as 'by the agency of' something.
– I have written a special treatise, in one book, On the Use of Respiration. –

5. But those who suppose that speech or respiration comes about
by the agency of the heart have been deceived by proximity in
location, not being aware that even if some part is near an activity,
whatever it may be, there is no necessity at all that the part be also
the source of the activity. And those (philosophers) also use a fallacious 2
argument who take the brain to be the source of sensation in eyes,
ears, and nose, because it is close to them. They too were misled by
position, or rather, not by position, but by their opinion about position.
Obviously they will use some such premise as this in their proofs: All 3
things that are active have their source nearby. When this (premise) 4
has been accepted as true, and then the premise has been added from
observation, that the ears touch the brain, at that point the conclusion
would follow that the source of the ears' activity is from there. But 5
the proposition mentioned just now is evident neither to the senses
nor to the mind, so as to be primary and credible in itself, that 'All
things that are active have their source nearby'.

It does not follow, then, that because the ears, eyes, and nose are 6
near the brain, it is the source of their power of sensation, or that
because the vocal and respiratory parts are near the heart, their source
is therefore from the heart. And the argument of Zeno that amazes 7
the Stoics, which Diogenes of Babylon put at the very beginning
of his work On the Governing Part of the Soul, contains no cause for

8 τὸ θαυμάζεσθαι πλὴν οὗ νῦν εἶπον ἀξιώματος ἤδη. εἴσῃ δ' ἐναργέστερον
202 εἰ παραγράψαιμεν αὐτόν· ἔχει / γὰρ ὧδε· «Φωνὴ διὰ φάρυγγος χωρεῖ.
εἰ δὲ ἦν ἀπὸ τοῦ ἐγκεφάλου χωροῦσα, οὐκ ἂν διὰ φάρυγγος ἐχώρει.
ὅθεν δὲ λόγος, καὶ φωνὴ ἐκεῖθεν χωρεῖ. λόγος δὲ ἀπὸ διανοίας χωρεῖ, ὥστ'
οὐκ ἐν τῷ ἐγκεφάλῳ ἐστὶν ἡ διάνοια.»
9 Τὸν αὐτὸν δὴ τοῦτον λόγον Διογένης οὐ κατὰ τὴν αὐτὴν ἐρωτᾷ
λέξιν, ἀλλ' ὧδε· «Ὅθεν ἐκπέμπεται ἡ φωνή, καὶ ἡ ἔναρθρος, οὐκοῦν καὶ
ἡ σημαίνουσα ἔναρθρος φωνὴ ἐκεῖθεν, τοῦτο δὲ λόγος. καὶ λόγος ἄρα
242 10 ἐκεῖθεν | ἐκπέμπεται ὅθεν καὶ ἡ φωνή. ἡ δὲ φωνὴ οὐκ ἐκ τῶν κατὰ τὴν κεφα-
λὴν τόπων ἐκπέμπεται ἀλλὰ φανερῶς ἐκ τῶν κάτωθεν μᾶλλον. ἐκφανὴς
γοῦν ἐστι διὰ τῆς ἀρτηρίας διεξιοῦσα. καὶ ὁ λόγος ἄρα οὐκ ἐκ τῆς
11 κεφαλῆς ἐκπέμπεται, ἀλλὰ κάτωθεν μᾶλλον. ἀλλὰ μήν γε κἀκεῖνο ἀληθές,
τὸ τὸν λόγον ἐκ τῆς διανοίας ἐκπέμπεσθαι. ἔνιοι γοῦν καὶ ὁριζόμενοι
12 αὐτόν φασιν εἶναι φωνὴν σημαίνουσαν ἀπὸ διανοίας ἐκπεμπομένην. καὶ
203 ἄλλως δὲ πιθανὸν ὑπὸ τῶν ἐννοιῶν ἐνσεσημασμένον τῶν ἐν τῇ / διανοίᾳ
καὶ οἷον ἐκτετυπωμένον ἐκπέμπεσθαι τὸν λόγον καὶ παρεκτείνεσθαι τῷ
13 χρόνῳ κατά τε τὸ διανενοῆσθαι καὶ τὴν κατὰ τὸ λέγειν ἐνέργειαν. καὶ ἡ
διάνοια ἄρα οὐκ ἔστιν ἐν τῇ κεφαλῇ, ἀλλ' ἐν τοῖς κατωτέρω τόποις,
μάλιστά πως περὶ τὴν καρδίαν.»
14 Τοιοῦτος μέν σοι καὶ ὁ τοῦ Διογένους λόγος, ἔμπαλιν ἢ κατὰ τὸν
τοῦ Ζήνωνος εἰς μῆκος ῥήσεων ἐκτεταμένος, ὥστε ἐκείνῳ μὲν ἐλλείπειν
15 τινὰ τῶν ἀναγκαίων ἀξιωμάτων, πλεονάζειν δὲ τούτῳ. βούλομαι δὲ
πρὶν ἐλέγχειν αὐτοὺς ἔτι καὶ τὸν τοῦ Χρυσίππου παραθέσθαι τόνδε
τὸν τρόπον ἔχοντα· «Εὔλογον δὲ εἰς ὃ γίγνονται αἱ ἐν τούτῳ σημασίαι
243 16 καὶ ἐξ οὗ λόγος, ἐκεῖνο εἶναι τὸ | κυριεῦον τῆς ψυχῆς μέρος. οὐ γὰρ
ἄλλη μὲν ἡ πηγὴ λόγου ἐστὶν ἄλλη δὲ διανοίας, οὐδὲ ἄλλη μὲν φωνῆς
πηγὴ ἄλλη δὲ λόγου, οὐδὲ τὸ ὅλον ἁπλῶς ἄλλη φωνῆς πηγή ἐστιν
204 17 ἄλλο δὲ τὸ κυριεῦον τῆς ψυχῆς μέρος.» — τοιούτοις δὲ / καὶ τὴν διάνοιαν
18 συμφώνως ἀφοριζόμενοι λέγουσιν αὐτὴν πηγὴν εἶναι λόγου. — «τὸ γὰρ
ὅλον ὅθεν ὁ λόγος ἐκπέμπεται ἐκεῖσε δεῖ καὶ τὸν διαλογισμὸν γίγνεσθαι
19 καὶ τὰς διανοήσεις καὶ τὰς μελέτας τῶν ῥήσεων, καθάπερ ἔφην. ταῦτα
δὲ ἐκφανῶς περὶ τὴν καρδίαν γίγνεται, ἐκ τῆς καρδίας διὰ φάρυγγος καὶ
20 τῆς φωνῆς καὶ τοῦ λόγου ἐκπεμπομένων. πιθανὸν δὲ καὶ ἄλλως, εἰς ὃ

1–22] SVF III, pp. 215–216 1–5] SVF I, p. 40 7] *cf. infra*, p. 138.17 9–10] *cf. infra*, p. 138.17–19 14] *cf. infra*, p. 138.20 22–132.16] SVF II, p. 244 25] *cf. infra*, p. 138.24–25 28–29] *cf.* SVF II, p. 228.16–17 29–30] *cf. infra*, p. 138.27–29

1 εἴσῃ δ'] εἰσι μὲν M: εἰσί (η *supra*) δὲ C ἐνεργέστερον M 2 αὐτό C 6 δὴ *om.* C 8 *ante* λόγος[I] *et* λόγος[II] *add.* ὁ C 10 ἐμφανὴς *Ald.* 11 ἐστι διὰ] ἐστὶν ἐκ C 12 γε *om.* M *Ald.* 44 σημαίνουσαν – ἐκπεμπομένην *om.* C 15 ἐννοῶν C ἐνσεσημασμένων M: σεσημασμένον C 16 καὶ[I] *om.* C 17 χρόνῳ] λόγω C κατά] "*fortasse* παρά" *Müller* διανοεῖσθαι *Ald.* C 18 κατωτέροις C 21 ῥήσεως C ἐκεῖνος C 22 τοῦ' (τ *supra*) H C: τούτου M: *corr. Ald.* 23 αὐτοῦ C 24 μὲν H, *in* δὲ *corr.* H[2] αἱ *om.* C ἐν τούτῳ] ἐν τύπῳ *Corn.*: *secl. Müller* 25 λόγος] ὁ λόγος ἐκπέμπεται *Müller*: ὁ λόγος *v. Arnim*: sermo procedit *Andernacus* 26 ἡ *del. Müller* 27 ἁπλῶς *om.* C 28 τούτοις C *ante* καὶ *trsp.* συμφώνως *(lin. 29)* C 30 *ante* ὅλον *add.* καθόλου H, *expunxit* H[2] 32 *ante* γίγνεται *add.* οἷον C

amazement beyond that proposition of which I spoke just now. You 8
will see this more clearly if I transcribe it. It is as follows: "Speech
passes through the windpipe. If it were passing from the brain, it
would not pass through the windpipe. Speech passes from the same
region as discourse. Discourse passes from the mind. Therefore, the
mind is not in the brain."

Diogenes formulates this same argument, not in the same words, 9
but as follows: "The region from which articulate speech is sent out is
the same as that from which speech is sent out, and therefore meaning-
ful articulate speech also comes from that region; but meaningful
articulate speech is discourse. Therefore, the region from which
discourse is sent out is the same as that from which speech is sent out.
But speech is not sent out from the region of the head, but obviously 10
from a place lower down. Thus it clearly passes out through the
windpipe. Therefore, discourse also is not sent out from the head, but
from a place lower down. But certainly that too is true, that discourse 11
is sent out from the mind. Indeed some even define it as meaningful
speech sent out from the mind. And besides it is plausible that dis- 12
course is sent out imprinted and stamped, as it were, by the notions
in the mind, and that it is temporally coextensive with the occurrence
of the thought and the activity of speaking. The mind too, therefore, 13
is not in the head but in places lower down most surely (I think) in
the region of the heart."

Here you have Diogenes' argument also, the opposite of Zeno's 14
in the length to which it extends, so that the one lacks some of the
necessary propositions, the other has more than enough. But before 15
examining them I wish to set down Chrysippus' argument also; it is as
follows: "It is reasonable that that to which the meanings in this go and
out from which discourse comes is the sovereign part of the soul. For it is 16
not true that the source of discourse is other than the source of thought,
or that the source of speech is other than the source of discourse, or, to
state the whole matter simply, that the source of speech is other than the
sovereign part of the soul." – And their definition of thought is in 17
agreement with such (statements) as these; they say that it is the
source of discourse. – "For in general the region from which discourse 18
is sent out must be the region where reasoning and thinking and the
preparation of utterance take place, as I said. But these activities 19
manifestly take place about the heart, since both speech and discourse
are sent out from the heart through the windpipe. And it is credible 20
besides that utterances should receive their meaning from the place to

ἐνσημαίνεται τὰ λεγόμενα, καὶ σημαίνεσθαι ἐκεῖθεν καὶ τὰς φωνὰς ἀπ' ἐκείνου γίγνεσθαι κατὰ τὸν προειρημένον τρόπον.»

21 Ἅλις ἤδη μοι τῶν περὶ τῆς φωνῆς λόγων τῶν Στωϊκῶν· εἰ γὰρ
καὶ τοὺς ὑπὸ τῶν ἄλλων ἠρωτημένους ἐφεξῆς γράφοιμι σύμπαντας, εἰς
22 ἄμετρόν τι μῆκος ἐκπεσεῖται τὸ γράμμα. οὐ γὰρ ἂν οὐδὲ τῶν ὑπὸ
Χρυσίππου τε καὶ Διογένους εἰρημένων ἐμνημόνευσα λόγων, ἀλλ'
244 ἠρκέσθην ἐξετάσας τὸν τοῦ | Ζήνωνος μόνον, εἰ μὴ πρός τινα τῶν
Στωϊκῶν ἐγεγόνει μοί ποτε ἀμφισβήτησις ὑπὲρ τοῦ χωρεῖ ῥήματος,
205 ὃ παρέλαβεν ὁ Ζήνων ἐν τῷ λόγῳ γράψας / ὡδί· «φωνὴ διὰ φάρυγγος
23 χωρεῖ.» τὸ γὰρ χωρεῖ τοῦτο ῥῆμα ἐγὼ μὲν ἠξίουν ἀκούειν ἐν ἴσῳ τῷ
ἐξέρχεται ἢ ἐκπέμπεται. ὁ δὲ τούτων μὲν μηδέτερον ἔφη σημαίνεσθαι
24 πρὸς αὐτοῦ καὶ τρίτον ἄλλο παρὰ ταῦτα λέγειν οὐκ εἶχεν. ἠναγκάσθην
οὖν αὐτῷ τὰ τῶν ἄλλων Στωϊκῶν παραναγινώσκειν βιβλία μεταλαμ-
βανόντων τὴν λέξιν ἢ εἰς τὸ ἐξέρχεται ἢ εἰς τὸ ἐκπέμπεται, καθάπερ καὶ
νῦν ἀπέδειξα Χρύσιππόν τε καὶ Διογένην, μεθ' οὓς οὐκ ἀναγκαῖον
ἡγοῦμαι τὰς τῶν ἄλλων παραγράφειν ῥήσεις, ἀλλ' ἐπὶ τὴν ἐξέτασιν
αὐτῶν ἤδη τρέψομαι τὴν ἀρχὴν ἀπὸ τοῦ Ζήνωνος ποιησάμενος,
ὅσπερ δὴ καὶ πατήρ ἐστι τοῦ τε περὶ τῆς φωνῆς λόγου τοῦδε καὶ ἁπάσης
τῆς τῶν Στωϊκῶν αἱρέσεως.

25 Τὸ μὲν οὖν πρῶτον λῆμμα τῆς χωρεῖ φωνῆς μεταληφθείσης ἐπὶ τὸ
σαφέστερον ἔσται τοιόνδε· 'φωνὴ διὰ φάρυγγος ἐκπέμπεται', τὸ δὲ
ἐφεξῆς τούτῳ, τὸ δεύτερον, τοιοῦτον· 'εἰ δὲ ἦν ἀπ' ἐγκεφάλου ἐκπεμπο-
245 26 μένη, | οὐκ ἂν διὰ φάρυγγος ἐξεπέμπετο.' τοῦτό φημι τὸ λῆμμα μὴ ὅτι
206 τοῦ πρώτου γένους ἐκπεπτωκέ/ναι τῶν εἰς τὰς ἀποδείξεις ἐπιτηδείων,
ἀλλὰ καὶ τοῦ δευτέρου τε καὶ τρίτου, περιέχεσθαι δὲ ἐν τῷ τετάρτῳ
γένει τῶν σοφιστικῶν λημμάτων, εἴ γε δὴ σχῆμά τι λέξεως ὑποδύεται
πεπανουργημένον τε καὶ σεσοφισμένον πρὸς ἀμφιβολίαν, ἐκ ταύτης τὸν
27 ἔλεγχον ἐλπίζον ἀποδράσεσθαι. τὸ γὰρ «εἰ δ' ἦν ἀπὸ τοῦ ἐγκεφάλου
χωροῦσα, οὐκ ἂν διὰ φάρυγγος ἐχώρει» μοχθηρῶς ἔχει τὴν ἀπὸ πρό-
28 θεσιν ἐγκειμένην τῇ ῥήσει. δύο γάρ εἰσιν ἐν ἅπασι τοῖς τοιούτοις λόγοις
σαφεῖς προθέσεις, ἥ τε ὑπὸ καὶ ἡ ἐξ, ὧν οὐδεμίαν παρέλαβεν καίτοι
δυνάμενος εἰπεῖν 'εἰ δ' ἦν ἐκ τοῦ ἐγκεφάλου χωροῦσα, οὐκ ἂν διὰ φάρυγγος
ἐχώρει'· ἢ εἰ μὴ 'ἐκ τοῦ ἐγκεφάλου', 'ὑπὸ τοῦ ἐγκεφάλου' γε πάντως
29 ἐχρῆν εἰπεῖν αὐτόν. ἡ γὰρ διὰ τῆς φάρυγγος ἐκπεμπομένη φωνὴ ἔκ τινός
τε καὶ ὑπό τινος ἐκπέμπεται· ἔκ τινος μὲν ὡς ἀγγείου περιέχοντος, ὑπό
τινος δ' ὡς δυνάμεως κινούσης τὸ περιέχον· ὥσπερ ἀμέλει καὶ τὸ οὖρον
246 ἐξέρχεται μὲν διὰ τοῦ αἰδοίου, ἐκπέμπεται δ' | ἐξ ἀγγείου μὲν τῆς ὑπερκει-

9–10] *cf. supra*, p. 130.2 25–27] *cf. supra*, p. 116.29–31 *infra*, p. 136.34–36

3 τῶν^{II} *om.* C 4 γράφοι C 8 ἀμφισβήτησις ποτὲ C 9 ὅπερ ἔλαβεν H C: *corr. Müller* 10 ἠξίουν ἀκούειν] ἥξει συνακούειν C 13 παραγιγνώσκειν C 15 *post verbum* ἀπέδειξα *explicit* C, *incipit* L *(cf. supra, p. 31)* 21 φωνὴ *om.* H L: *sscr.* H^2 22 τούτων L 24 ἐκπέπτωκε L 27 πεπα. . . .μένω L σεσοφισμένω L 28 ἐλπίζων H L: *corr. Müller* ἀποδράσεσθαι] σε *e corr.* H: ἀποδράσασθαι M 30 λογισμοῖς L 33 ἐχώρει] ει *corr.* H^2 ὑπὸ τοῦ ἐγκεφάλου γε *inser.* H: γε L

which they convey meaning and that words should come from there in
the manner described."

I have now quoted enough of the Stoic arguments about speech. 21
If I should set down in order all the arguments formulated by the
rest of them, this book would extend to immoderate length. I would 22
not even have mentioned the arguments of Chrysippus and Dio-
genes, and I would have been content to examine that of Zeno alone,
if I had not once entered into a dispute with a certain member of the
Stoic school about the word "passes", which Zeno used in his
argument when he wrote, "Speech passes through the windpipe".
I thought that this word "passes" should be understood as the equi- 23
valent of "goes out" or "is sent out". But he denied that it had either
of these meanings, and yet he was unable to give a third other than
these. Therefore I was compelled to make a comparison with the books 24
of the other Stoics, who alter the expression either to "goes out" or
to "is sent out"; and I have now shown that Chrysippus and Dio-
genes do just that. After quoting them, I do not consider it necessary
to quote the others, but I shall now (at last) turn to my critical exami-
nation of them. I shall begin with Zeno, who is indeed the father of
this argument about speech and of the whole Stoic sect.

Now when the word 'passes' is replaced by a less obscure term, 25
the first premise will be: 'Speech is sent out through the windpipe';
the one that follows, the second, will be: 'If it were sent out from the
brain, it would not be sent out through the windpipe.' I say that this 26
premise not only falls outside the first class (of premises), those suit-
able for scientific proof, but even outside the second and third classes;
it belongs to the fourth class, the sophistical premises, since it hides
behind a verbal form that has been given a fraudulent and sophistical
ambiguity in the hope of thereby escaping refutation. For the state- 27
ment, "If it were passing from the brain, it would not pass through the
windpipe", is unsound because it contains the preposition 'from'. In 28
all such statements two prepositions are unambiguous: 'by' and 'out
of'. He used neither of these, although he could have said, 'If it were
passing out of the brain, it would not pass through the windpipe'; or
if he did not say 'out of the brain', he should at least have said, 'by
the brain'. For speech sent out through the windpipe is sent out of 29
something and also by something: out of something, as out of the
vessel that contains it; by something, as by the power which sets the
container in motion. It is exactly the same with urine: it goes out
through the genitals, and it is sent out of a vessel, the bladder that lies

207 μένης κύστεως, ὑπὸ δυνάμεως δὲ / τῆς τὴν κύστιν συστελλούσης εἰς
30 ἑαυτὴν ἵν' ἐκθλίψῃ τὸ οὖρον. ἡ δ' ἀπὸ πρόθεσις ἄδηλός ἐστιν εἴτ' ἀντὶ
τῆς ἐξ εἴτ' ἀντὶ τῆς ὑπὸ παρείληπται. εἰ μὲν οὖν ἀντὶ τῆς ἐξ, ἀληθής
ἐστιν ὁ λόγος, ἔσται γὰρ τοιοῦτος· 'εἰ δὲ ἦν ἐκ τοῦ ἐγκεφάλου ἐκπεμπομένη ἡ φωνή, οὐκ ἂν διὰ τῆς φάρυγγος ἐξεπέμπετο'· εἰ δὲ ἀντὶ τῆς ὑπό,
ψευδής, ἔσται γὰρ αὖ πάλιν τοιοῦτος· 'εἰ δὲ ἦν ὑπὸ τοῦ ἐγκεφάλου ἐκπεμπομένη, οὐκ ἂν διὰ τῆς φάρυγγος ἐξῄει'.

31 Ὅτι δ' οὐκ ἀληθής ἐστιν ὁ τοιοῦτος λόγος οὐκ ἐμὲ χρὴ κατασκευάζειν
ἀλλ' ἐκείνους αὐτοὺς ἀξιοῦν ἀποφήνασθαι προτέρους ὑπὲρ τοῦ τοιούτου
λόγου· 'τὸ οὖρον διὰ τοῦ αἰδοίου χωρεῖ· εἰ δὲ ἦν ὑπὸ τῆς καρδίας
ἐκπεμπόμενον, οὐκ ἂν διὰ τοῦ αἰδοίου ἐξῄει. καὶ μὴν ὑπὸ προαιρέσεώς
γε τῆς ἡμετέρας ἐκπέμπεται. οὐκ ἄρα ἐν τῇ καρδίᾳ ἐστὶν ἡ προαίρεσις.'
32 οὕτω δὲ καὶ περὶ διαχωρήματος ἐρωτᾶν ἐγχωρεῖ. καὶ γὰρ καὶ τοῦτο διὰ
μὲν τῆς ἕδρας, ὑπὸ μέντοι τῆς ἡμετέρας προαιρέσεως πρώτης κινούσης
208 ἐκπέμπεται, ἥτις οἶμαι καὶ τῶν πορρωτάτω κειμένων ἑαυτῆς δάκτυ/λον
247 ὁντινοῦν τῶν ἐν ποδὶ κινεῖ παραχρῆμα μηδὲν ἐκ τοῦ | διαστήματος
33 ἐμποδιζομένη πρὸς τὸ τάχος. εἴτε γὰρ ἐν ἐγκεφάλῳ θείης εἴτ' ἐν καρδίᾳ
τὴν προαίρεσιν ἢ διάνοιαν ἢ ὅ τί ποτε καὶ βούλει καλεῖν — οὐδὲν γὰρ
εἰς τὰ παρόντα διαφέρει —, χρόνος οὐδεὶς εὑρεθήσεται μεταξὺ γιγνόμενος
τοῦ τε βουληθῆναι κινῆσαι τὸν δάκτυλον καὶ τῆς ἐνεργείας αὐτοῦ, καθ-
34 άπερ οἶμαι κἀπὶ τῆς αἰσθήσεως ἔχει. οὐ γὰρ οὖν οὐδ' ἐπὶ ταύτης ἀναμεῖναι
δεῖ χρόνον τινὰ τοῦ νύξαντος ἢ τρώσαντος ἵν' αἴσθηται τὸ ζῷον ἀλλ'
35 ἅμα τε τὸ τέμνον τέμνει καὶ τὸ ζῷον αἰσθάνεται. καὶ τοῦτο βούλεταί γε
Ζήνων καὶ Χρύσιππος ἅμα τῷ σφετέρῳ χορῷ παντί, διαδίδοσθαι
τὴν ἐκ τοῦ προσπεσόντος ἔξωθεν ἐγγενομένην τῷ μορίῳ κίνησιν εἰς τὴν
36 ἀρχὴν τῆς ψυχῆς ἵν' αἴσθηται τὸ ζῷον. ὡς οὖν οὐδείς ἐστι χρόνος αἰσθητὸς ἐν τῷ μεταξὺ τοῦ τρωθῆναί τε τὸ μόριον αἰσθέσθαι τε τὸ ζῷον,
ὡσαύτως οὐδὲ τοῦ βουληθῆναι κάμψαι τὸν ἄνθρωπον δάκτυλον ἢ τὸν
209 πόδα καὶ αὐ/τῆς τῆς ἐνεργείας, οὕτως οὐδὲ τοῦ βουληθῆναι τὸ οὖρον
248 ἐκκρῖναι καὶ αὐτῆς τῆς ἐκκρίσεως, | ἀλλ' ἅμα τε τὸ τῆς ψυχῆς ἡγεμονικὸν
ἠβουλήθη καὶ τὰ τῆς ἐκκρίσεως ἐνήργησεν ὄργανα.

37 Πῶς οὖν λύσομεν ἐκεῖνον τὸν λόγον, ὦ σοφώτατοι, 'εἰ δὲ ἦν ὑπὸ τῆς
καρδίας ἐκπεμπόμενον τὸ οὖρον, οὐκ ἂν διὰ τοῦ αἰδοίου ἐξεκρίνετο';
38 ἣν γὰρ ἂν εἴπητε λύσιν, ἐξέσται δήπου καὶ ἡμᾶς αὐτῇ χρήσασθαι. κατὰ
μὲν δὴ τοὺς διαλόγους ἐκείνους ἀναγκάζειν χρὴ λύειν τὸν λόγον. ἐνταῦθα
δὲ οὐκ ἐγχωρεῖ ποιεῖν οὕτως ἀλλὰ χρὴ τὴν λύσιν αὐτοὺς εἰπεῖν οὐδὲν

19–29] *cf.* Nemes. De nat. hom. 6: p. 117.7–11 Matth. Jaeger, Nemesios, pp. 25–26 23–26] SVF I, p. 41; II, p. 236

1 τῆς *inser.* H συστελλούσης] συντελούσης H L *(ut vid.)*: *corr.* H[2] 4 ἐκ] ἀπὸ H L: *corr.* R[2] *in mg. Bas.* 7 τῆς] τοῦ L 9 ἀξιῶ R[2] *in mg.*: ἄξιον *Petersen* 10 αἰδοίου] ἰδίου L 11 αἱρέσεως L 14 μὲν *del.* H[3] μέντοι *om.* H πρώτου κινοῦντος *(ut. vid.)* L 15 τὸν πορρῶ (ττ supra) κείμενον L 16 ἐν ποδὶ] ἐμποδὼν L 20 ἐνεργείας] ας *e corr.* L αὐ(τ~ supra) L: αὐτῆς *Diels (cf. infra, lin. 29)* 25 προπεσόντος H: *corr.* H[2] ἐγγινομένην L 26 αἰσθάνηται L 27 τε[II] *om.* H L: *add.* H[2] *supra lin.* 31 ἐβουλήθη H ἐκκρίσεως] αἰσθήσεως H L: *corr. Einarson* 32 ἐκείνων L 35 ἐντεῦθεν L 36 δὲ] ὡς L

above them, but by a power, (the power) that causes the bladder to
contract in order to press out the urine. But the preposition 'from' is 30
unclear, as it may stand for either 'out of' or 'by'. If it has replaced
'out of', the statement is true, for it will be as follows: 'If speech were
sent out of the brain, it would not be sent out through the windpipe.'
But if it has replaced 'by', the statement is false, for then it will be,
'If speech were sent out by the brain, it would not go out through the
windpipe.'

I need not provide a proof that this statement is not true; I need 31
only ask that those men themselves first comment on the following
piece of reasoning: 'Urine passes through the genitals; if it were sent
out by the heart it would not go out through the genitals; but it is in
fact sent out by our choice; choice, therefore, is not in the heart.'
A syllogism about excrement may also be constructed in the same way. 32
Excrement is sent out through the fundament, but by our choice,
which first initiates the movement; and choice, I believe, even moves
instantaneously any one of the toes, which are furthest from it, the
distance presenting no obstacle to the speed. For whether you place 33
choice, or intellect, or whatever you wish to call it – it makes no differ-
ence for the present –, in the brain or in the heart, no time will be
found to elapse between the occurrence of the wish to move the toe and
the act of moving it; and the same, I believe, is true of sensation. For 34
in sensation too there is no need to wait a certain time after a prod or
wound so that the animal can feel it; the cut and the sensation are
simultaneous. Zeno and Chrysippus and all their company also 35
intend this, that the movement aroused in a member by a contact from
without be transmitted to the seat of the soul's rule so that the animal
may perceive it. As therefore there is no perceptible interval between 36
the wounding of the member and the animal's perceiving it, so also
there is none between a person's wishing to bend his toe or his foot and
the act itself, and similarly none between the wish to expel urine and
the actual expulsion; for the wish in the governing part of the soul and
the activity of the organs of expulsion were simultaneous.

How then, O ye sages, shall we answer that argument, 'If urine 37
were sent out by the heart, it would not be expelled through the
genitals'? Whatever answer you give, we can use it too. Now in dia- 38
logues one should compel one's opponents to answer the argument, but
that is not feasible here; rather, we must ourselves give an answer that

ἔχουσαν ἀποκεκρυμμένον ἢ μακρὸν ἢ χαλεπόν, ἀλλ' ἐκ προχείρου φαι-
39 νομένην. οὐδὲν γὰρ κωλύει, φήσομεν, ἐκ τῆς κύστεως ἐκκρίνεσθαι διὰ
τοῦ αἰδοίου τὸ οὖρον ἀρχὴν κινήσεως ἐπιπέμψαντος τοῦ ἡγεμονικοῦ ἵνα
40 συσταλῇ τὸ περιέχον ἀγγεῖον. λοιπὸν εἴτ' ἐγκέφαλός ἐστιν εἴτε καρδία
τὸ τῆς ψυχῆς ἡγεμονοῦν, οὐδὲν οἶμαι διαφέρειν εἴς γε τὴν τοῦ προκει-
41 μένου λόγου διάλυσιν. ἄν τε γὰρ ἐγκέφαλος ᾖ, τὴν ἀρχὴν τῆς κινήσεως
210 αὐτὸς ἐπιπέμψει καὶ τοῖς τὸ οὖρον / ἐκκρίνουσιν ὀργάνοις καὶ τοῖς τὸ
περίττωμα τῆς τροφῆς καὶ τοῖς τὸ σκέλος κινοῦσι καὶ τοῖς τὸν πόδα καὶ
249 42 τοὺς δακτύλους, ἄν θ' ἡ | καρδία, κατὰ τὸν αὐτὸν τρόπον. οὕτως
οἶμαι καὶ τῆς φωνῆς ἐκπεμπομένης διὰ φάρυγγος οὐδὲν κωλύει τὸν ἐγκέ-
φαλον αἴτιον ὑπάρχειν τῆς πρὸ τῆς φάρυγγος κινήσεως. ὥστε ἴσον ἔτι
μένει τὸ ζητούμενον ἐξ ἀρχῆς οὐδὲν ἔκ γε τοῦ φαινομένου πρὸς οὐδέτερον
43 τῶν δογμάτων ἐπικλῖναν. ὡς γὰρ ἐπὶ τῆς κατὰ τὴν κύστιν καὶ τὴν ἕδραν
κινήσεως ἄδηλον ὑπῆρχε πότερον ἐγκέφαλος ἢ καρδία τὴν ἀρχὴν ἔχει,
κατὰ τὸν αὐτὸν τρόπον ἐπί τε φωνῆς καὶ ἀναπνοῆς ὁμοίως ἔτ' ἄδηλον
ὁπότερον τῶν σπλάγχνων ἔχει τὴν ἡγεμονίαν.

44 Ἀλλ' ὡς εἴρηταί μοι καὶ πρόσθεν, ἡ τῆς θέσεως ἐγγύτης ἑκατέρους
ἐξαπατῶσα φαντασίαν ἀποτελεῖ τῶν λημμάτων ὡς ἐπιστημονικῶν τε
45 καὶ πρὸς ἀπόδειξιν ἐπιτηδείων· οὐ μὴν οὕτως γ' ἔχει τἀληθές. ὅ τε γὰρ
211 ἁπάντων ἀρχὴν ὑποτιθέμενος εἶναι τὴν καρδίαν οὐκ εὐλαβηθή/σεται τὴν
τῶν ὀφθαλμῶν ⟨οὐκ⟩ ἐγγύτητα, ὡς μὴ καὶ τούτους ἀπ' ἐκείνης ὥσπερ
πηγῆς τινος ἀρύεσθαι φάναι τὴν αἴσθησίν τε καὶ κίνησιν, ὅ τε τὸν ἐγ-
κέφαλον, οὐκ ἄλλο τι μόριόν φησιν ἀρχὴν εἶναι τῆς τῶν ἀναπνευστικῶν
250 τε καὶ φωνητικῶν ὀργάνων κινήσεως, | ἀλλ' ἐκεῖνον ὥσπερ τοῖς ἄλλοις
ἅπασιν ἐξηγεῖσθαι τῆς κατὰ προαίρεσιν κινήσεως, οὕτως καὶ τοῖσδε.

46 Ἅπερ οὖν ἐν ταῖς περὶ τῆς ἀποδείξεως μεθόδοις ἐδιδάχθημεν
καθόλου, ταῦθ' εὑρίσκεται κατὰ μέρος ἐπὶ πάσης ὕλης πραγμάτων
ἀληθεύοντα. χρὴ γὰρ οὐκ ἀπὸ πάντων τῶν ὑπαρχόντων τῷ προκει-
μένῳ πράγματι τἀληθὲς λαμβάνειν ἀλλ' ἀπὸ μόνου τοῦ συνημμένου τῷ
47 προβλήματι. Ζήνων δὲ καὶ Χρύσιππος καὶ Διογένης οἵ τ' ἄλλοι
Στωϊκοὶ κἂν μυριάκις ἐπὶ τῷ λόγῳ θαρρῶσιν, οὐχ ἕξουσιν ἀπολογήσα-
48 σθαι περὶ τῶν ἁμαρτημάτων αὐτοῦ. τὸ γάρ τοι δεύτερον λῆμμα τὸ κατ'
αὐτὸν εἰ μὲν ἀκριβῶς τε ἅμα καὶ σαφῶς καὶ διωρισμένως εἴρητο, τῶν ἐκ
δευτέρου γένους ἓν ἂν ἐφωράθη πάντως ὑπάρχον· ἐπεὶ δὲ κατὰ τὸ τῆς
212 λέξεως σχῆμα πεπανουργημέ/νην ἀμφιβολίαν ἐπεσπάσατο, τοῦ τετάρ-
49 του γένους ἐν τούτῳ μετέσχεν. εἰ μὲν οὖν γινώσκων αὐτοῦ τὴν πανουρ-

26–27] *cf. supra*, pp. 102.25–28; 110.23–112.2 32–36] *cf. supra*, p. 132.21–28
32–33] *cf. supra*, p. 130.3

1 ἀποκεκρυμμένον] αὐτῶ κεκρυμμένον L φαινόμενον H L: *corr.* H[2] 2 κωλύειν L φήσομεν *ex* φήσαιμι *(?) corr.* H 4 καρδία] καὶ διὰ L 7 ἐπιπέμψει αὐτὸς L 10 *post* διὰ *add.* τοῦ L, τῆς *Müller* 11 πρὸ τῆς] . . .της τοῦ L: πρώτης τῆς *Müller* 12 μένειν L 13 τὴν[I] *om.* H 20 εὐλαβηθήσεται] εὐλαβὴς ἔσται L 21 οὐκ *add. Müller (adprobat Wifstrand)*, ἐγκεφάλου *Troost*, πρὸς τὸν ἐγκέφαλον *Petersen* *aut* τούτων *aut* τούτοις *in* τούτους *corr.* L 24 ἐκείνων L 25 καὶ] κἂν L 29 τἀληθὲς] τὰ λήμματα *coni. Schöne* 33 αὐτὸν *ex* αὐτῶν *corr.* H[2] 34 ἂν *om.* L 36 ἐν τούτῳ *secl. Müller*

contains nothing obscure or remote or difficult, but is at hand and evident. We shall say that nothing prevents the expulsion of urine out 39
of the bladder through the genitals, when the governing part has transmitted a beginning of motion in order that the containing vessel should contract. And whether the brain or the heart is the governing 40
part of the soul makes no difference, I believe, for the refutation of the argument before us. If it is the brain, then the brain will itself 41
transmit the beginning of motion to the organs that expel urine and to those that expel the residue from food and to those that move the leg and the foot and the toes; and so also if it is the heart. Similarly, 42
I think, when speech is sent out through the windpipe, nothing prevents the brain from being the cause of the motion prior to that of the windpipe. Therefore the answer to our original question remains evenly balanced; it does not incline at all toward either view as a result of the observation. For as in the motion of the bladder and the 43
fundament it was unclear whether the brain or the heart is the source, so also in speech and breathing it is not yet clear which of the two inner organs is in command.

As I said before, proximity in position, deceiving both (parties), 44
makes the premises look scientific and suitable for demonstration; but the truth is otherwise. The person who supposes that the heart is 45
the source of everything will not be deterred by the non-proximity of the eyes from asserting that they too draw sensation and motion from the heart as from a spring; and the person who says that it is the brain holds that no other member is the source of motion in the organs of breath and speech, but the brain initiates voluntary motion in these as in all else.

Those universal propositions, then, that we were taught with 46
reference to the methods of proof are found to be true in particular cases in every subject-matter. For it is not the truth about all the properties of the object before us that must be used as a premise, but only about the property that is pertinent to the problem. And Zeno, 47
Chrysippus, Diogenes, and all the other Stoics, though they are ten thousand times confident of their argument, will be unable to defend its errors. For the second premise in the argument, if it were 48
stated accurately and clearly and with the proper distinctions, would be detected as surely a premise of the second class; but since it has acquired a fraudulent ambiguity in its verbal form, it thereby partakes of the fourth class. Now if Zeno was aware of this fraud and made use 49

γίαν ὁ Ζήνων ἑκὼν παρεχρήσατο, σοφιστὴς ἂν εἴη τις, οὐ φιλόσοφος·
50 εἰ δὲ ἀγνοήσας ἄκων ἐχρήσατο, λογικῆς θεωρίας ἀγύμναστος. ἀλλ' ἡμεῖς
251 γε μήθ' ἑκόντες ποτὲ τοιούτοις | χρησαίμεθα λόγοις, ἐχθροῦ γὰρ ἀληθείας ἀνδρὸς τὸ πανούργημα, μήτ' ἄκοντες ὑπὸ ἀμαθίας τε ἅμα καὶ ἀγυμνασίας ἐμπίπτοιμεν εἰς αὐτούς.
51 Ὁμοίαν δὲ ἔχει τῷ δευτέρῳ λήμματι καὶ τὸ τέταρτον ἀτοπίαν, ἐν
52 ᾧ φησιν «ὁ λόγος ἀπὸ διανοίας χωρεῖ». ὁ γάρ τοι λόγος οὗτος, ἡ σημαίνουσα φωνή, ὑπὸ μὲν τῆς διανοίας ἐκπέμπεται, καθάπερ καὶ τἆλλα πάντα τὰ κατὰ προαίρεσιν ἐνεργούμενα, οὐ μὴν ἐκ τῆς διανοίας γε, ἀλλὰ ἐκ
53 τοῦ λάρυγγος. ἔμπροσθεν δὲ οὐδέπω φωνὴ τὸ ἀναφερόμενόν ἐστιν, ἀλλ' ὡς ἔφαμεν ὕλη τις οἰκεία φωνῆς, ἣν ὀνομάζομεν ἐκφύσησιν. ἐκπέμπεται δὲ ἐκ τῶν κατὰ πνεύμονα τραχειῶν ἀρτηριῶν, ὧν οὐδεμία τῆς καρδίας ἅπτεται.
213 54 Ὁ μὲν / οὖν Ζήνων εἴτε ἄκων εἴτε ἑκὼν ἀσαφεῖ τῇ λέξει χρησάμενος εἰς τὸ τέταρτον εἶδος ἐμπέπτωκε τῶν λημμάτων, ὁ Διογένης δὲ τὰ
55 πολλὰ μὲν εἰς τὸ δεύτερον, ἅπαξ δέ που καὶ αὐτὸς εἰς τὸ τέταρτον. ὅταν μὲν γὰρ λέγῃ «ὅθεν ἡ φωνὴ ἐκπέμπεται» καὶ ὅταν «ἡ δὲ φωνὴ οὐκ ἐκ τῶν κατὰ τὴν κεφαλὴν τόπων ἐκπέμπεται, ἀλλὰ φανερῶς ἐκ τῶν κάτω μᾶλ-
252 λον», | ἐκ τοῦ δευτέρου γένους τῶν ἐπιχειρημάτων χρῆται τοῖς λήμμασιν· ὅταν δὲ φῇ τὸν λόγον ἀπὸ διανοίας ἐκπέμπεσθαι, δέον ὑπὸ διανοίας
56 φάναι, τῷ τετάρτῳ χρῆται γένει τῶν ἐπιχειρημάτων. ὁ δὲ ἔλεγχος καὶ τῶν τούτου σφαλμάτων ὁ αὐτὸς τῷ προγεγραμμένῳ κατὰ τὸν τοῦ Ζήνωνος λόγον.
57 Οὕτω δὲ καὶ ὁ Χρύσιππος ἐπειδὰν μὲν λέγῃ «καὶ ἐξ οὗ ὁ λόγος ἐκπέμπεται, ἐκεῖνο εἶναι τὸ κυριεῦον τῆς ψυχῆς μέρος» ἀντιληψόμεθα τοῦ λόγου καὶ φήσομεν, ὑφ' οὗ μὲν ὁ λόγος ἐκπέμπεται τὸ κυριεῦον
58 ὑπάρχειν, οὐ μὴν ἐξ οὗ γε. κατὰ δὲ τὸν αὐτὸν τρόπον κἀπειδὰν εἴπῃ «τὸ γὰρ ὅλον ὅθεν ὁ λόγος ἐκπέμπεται, ἐκεῖσε δεῖ καὶ τὸν διαλογισμὸν γίνε-
214 σθαι» οὐχ ὅθεν / φήσομεν, ἀλλ' ὑφ' οὗ μέρους ὁ λόγος ἐκπέμπεται, καὶ τὸ
59 λογίζεσθαι κατ' ἐκεῖνό τε καὶ ἐν ἐκείνῳ γίγνεσθαι. δῆλον γὰρ δὴ ὅτι τὸ ἐκεῖσε ἀντὶ τοῦ ἐκεῖ ὁ Χρύσιππος εἴρηκεν, ὅπερ ἴσον δύναται τῷ ἐν ἐκείνῳ τῷ μέρει τοῦ σώματος. οὐ γὰρ δὴ τό γε εἰς ἐκεῖνο τὸ μόριον ἡγητέον αὐτὸν βούλεσθαι δηλοῦν ἐν τῷ λέγειν ἐκεῖσε, κἂν ὅτι μάλιστα
253 60 τὸ μὲν ἐκεῖσε εἰς τόπον ᾖ δηλοῦν, τὸ δὲ ἐκεῖ ἐν | τόπῳ. σολοικίζειν γὰρ μᾶλλον ὑποληπτέον ἐν τῇ φωνῇ τὸν Χρύσιππον ἤπερ οὕτω προφανῶς ἀδιανόητα λέγειν· τὸ μὲν γὰρ ἱκανῶς σύνηθες αὐτῷ καὶ μόνον οὐ

7] *cf. supra*, p. 130.4 7–8] *cf. supra*, p. 130.13–14 11] *cf. supra*, pp. 120.19–20; 122.1–4 17] *cf. supra*, p. 130.7 17–19] *cf. supra*, p.130.9–10 20] *cf. supra*, p. 130.14 24–25] *cf. supra*, p. 130.25 27–29] *cf. supra*, p. 130.29–30 30–140.3] SVF II, pp. 244–245

1 οὐ *scr. Petersen*: ἢ H L: μᾶλλον ἢ *Ald.* 2 *ante* ἄκων *add.* τί L 4 πανούργευμα L 7 οὗτος *om.* L 9 τὰ *om.* L 11 τῆς οἰκείας L 14 ἑκών, *ut vid.*, L, *ex* ἐκτὸς *corr.* H 15 ἐκπέπτωκε L 17 ἐκπέμπεται ἡ φωνή *Müller (cf. supra, p. 130.7)* οὐκ *inser.* H 18 κάτωθεν *Müller (cf. supra, p. 130.10)* 20 φησι L 21 χρῆται *bis scr.* L 24 ἐξ] ε *ex* κ *corr.* H 26 λόγου] λεγομένου L 32 ἐν – τῷ] ἐκείνω τοῦ L 33 δηλοῦν] δῆλον αὐτὸν L 35 ἐν *del. Cobet* εἴπερ H L: *corr.* H² p 36 λ^ε' H: λέγει L: *corr.* p *Ald.*

of it intentionally, he would be a sophist, not a philosopher; if he used
it in ignorance and unintentionally, his training in logic was deficient.
May I never willingly use such arguments, for the fraud is the mark 50
of a man who hates the truth; and may I never fall into them un-
intentionally through lack of study and training!

The fourth premise, in which he says that "discourse passes from 51
the mind", has the same absurdity as the second. For this discourse, 52
'speech conveying meaning', is sent out by the mind, like every other
voluntary act; and yet it is not sent out of the mind, but out of the
larynx. Before (it reaches the larynx), what is carried up is not yet 53
speech but, as we said, matter suitable for speech, which we call expel-
led breath. It is sent out from the tracheal arteries in the lungs; and
none of these touches the heart.

Zeno, then, by using an unclear expression either voluntarily or 54
involuntarily, has fallen into the fourth kind of premises; Diogenes
for the most part uses the second kind, although on one occasion he too
falls into the fourth. For when he says "the place from which speech is 55
sent out" and "But speech is not sent out from the region of the head,
but obviously from a place lower down", he is using premises from the
second class of arguments; but when he says that discourse is sent out
'from the mind', when he should have said 'by the mind', he is using
an argument of the fourth class. And the refutation of Diogenes' 56
errors is the same as that which was presented earlier in reply to
Zeno's argument.

So also when Chrysippus says, "and that out from which 57
discourse is sent is the sovereign part of the soul", we shall reject his
statement and say that that 'by' which discourse is sent out is the
sovereign part, not that 'out from' which. And in the same way when 58
he says, "For in general the region from which discourse is sent out
must be the region where reasoning takes place", we shall reply that
not the part 'from' which but 'by' which discourse is sent out must be
the part at which and in which reasoning takes place. It is clear that 59
Chrysippus used the word *ekeise* (thither) instead of *ekei* (there),
which is equivalent to 'in that part of the body'. We must not suppose
that he meant 'to that part' when he said *ekeise* (thither), even though
ekeise most certainly means 'to a place', and *ekei* 'in a place'. We must 60
sooner assume that Chrysippus commits a solecism in his use of the
word than that he says something so obviously unintelligible. For the
one thing is habitual enough with him and is found in almost every

61 καθ' ἑκάστην ῥῆσιν γινόμενον, τὸ δ' ἀδιανόητα λέγειν οὐδαμῶς. ἐνίοτε
γάρ που καὶ ψευδῆ λέγει, καθάπερ καὶ κατὰ τοῦτον τὸν λόγον, ἀλλ'
οὐκ ἀδιανόητά γε· διαφέρει γὰρ πάμπολυ τὸ ψεῦδος τοῦ ἀδιανοήτου.
62 ἐπεὶ τοίνυν τὸ ἐκεῖσε ἀντὶ τοῦ ἐκεῖ πιθανώτερόν ἐστιν εἰρῆσθαι πρὸς
τοῦ Χρυσίππου, γένοιτ' ἂν ἡ ῥῆσις εἰς τὴν τῶν Ἑλλήνων διάλεκτον
215 μεταληφθεῖσα τοιάδε· «ὅθεν ὁ λόγος ἐκπέμπεται, ἐκεῖ / δεῖ καὶ τὸν δια-
63 λογισμὸν γίγνεσθαι, τουτέστιν ⟨ἐν⟩ ἐκείνῳ τῷ μορίῳ.» τοῦτο δὲ φήσομεν
ἄντικρυς εἶναι ψεῦδος. οὐ γάρ, εἴ τι κατὰ προαίρεσιν ἔκ τινος ἐκπέμπεται,
κατ' ἐκεῖνο τὸ μόριον δείκνυται τὴν διάνοιαν ὑπάρχειν, καθάπερ οὐδὲ
τὸ οὖρον οὐδὲ τὸ πτύελον οὐδὲ ἡ κόρυζα οὐδὲ τὸ ἀποπάτημα.
64 Φαίνεται τοίνυν τοῦτο σφῆλαν τόν τε Ζήνωνα πρῶτον καὶ μάλιστα
254 καὶ μετ' αὐτὸν ἤδη τοὺς ἄλλους Στωϊκούς, οὐχ | ἥκιστα δὲ καὶ τὸν
Χρύσιππον, ὅσον γε ἐπὶ τῇ προγεγραμμένῃ ῥήσει. κατὰ μὲν γὰρ ἄλλην
τινὰ μετ' οὐ πάνυ πολὺ ταύτης γεγραμμένην ἠναγκάσθη τὸ ἀληθὲς
65 ὁμολογῆσαι. ἀναγκασθῆναι δὲ εἶπον αὐτόν, ὅτι λόγον ἕτερον ἀνατρέψαι
βουλόμενος ὡς οὐκ ἀληθῆ κἄπειτα τὸ τῆς ἀντιλογίας εἶδος αἰσθόμενος
οὐδὲν ἧττον ἐπιστρέφον καὶ καθ' ἑαυτοῦ συνανατρέψαι καὶ τὸν ἴδιον
66 οὐκ ὤκνησε τῷ τῶν ἑτεροδόξων. ἐχρῆν δ' αὐτὸν ἢ μὴ ταῦτα γράφειν
216 ἢ μὴ ἐκεῖνα καὶ μάλιστα πλη/σίον οὕτως ἀλλήλων. εἰ μὲν γὰρ ἀληθὴς
οὗτος ὁ λόγος, οὐκ ἀληθὴς ἐκεῖνος, εἰ δ' ἐκεῖνος ὑγιής, κίβδηλος οὗτος.
67 ἡμεῖς μὲν οὖν ἐπιστημονικαῖς μεθόδοις γεγυμνασμένοι γνωρίζειν τε καὶ
διακρίνειν δυνάμεθα τόν τε ἀληθῆ καὶ τὸν ψευδῆ· τοῖς δ' ἀγυμνάστοις οὐ
σμικρὸν ἂν εἴη ζήτημα πότερον αὐτῶν ἕλωνται.
68 Παραγράψω δὴ καὶ τὴν ῥῆσιν αὐτὴν ἐν ᾗ δείκνυσιν ὁ Χρύσιππος
69 ὡς οὐκ ἔστιν ὁ προγεγραμμένος λόγος ἀποδεικτικός. ἔστι δὲ τοιάδε· «ἔχει
δ'.ὡς ἔφην πλείονα αὐτοῖς ἐπὶ πᾶσι, μή ποτ' εἰ καὶ τοῦτο δοθείη, καθ-
255 άπερ ἐπιπορεύονται, ἀπὸ τῆς κεφαλῆς εἶναι τὴν | ἀρχὴν ἐπὶ τὰ εἰρη-
70 μένα μέρη. ἐπιζητήσωμεν· σχεδὸν γάρ, οἷα ἄν τινα λέγοιεν περὶ τοῦ
τὴν φωνὴν ἐκ τοῦ στήθους φέρεσθαι διὰ τῆς φάρυγγος, ἀπὸ τῆς κεφαλῆς
ποιᾶς τινος καταρχῆς γιγνομένης, τοιαῦτ' ἔξεστι λέγειν, ἐν τῇ καρδίᾳ
217 μὲν / τοῦ ἡγεμονικοῦ ὄντος, τῆς δὲ τῶν κινήσεων ἀρχῆς ἀπὸ τῆς κε-
71 φαλῆς οὔσης.» [οἷον] ὃ γὰρ δὴ βούλεται λέγειν ὁ Χρύσιππος ἐν τῇδε
τῇ ῥήσει, τοιοῦτόν ἐστιν· εἰ καὶ συγχωρήσειέ τις ἀρχὴν εἶναι νεύρων
τὴν κεφαλήν, οὐ πάντως ἐν αὐτῇ συγχωρήσει[ε] καὶ τὸ ἡγεμονικὸν

13–18] SVF II, p. 246 24–142.5] SVF II, pp. 246–247

1 γενόμενον *Cobet* ἀνόητα H [δι] 2 λέγει *ex* -ειν *corr.* H 3 γε] λ[ε'] L 4 ἐκεῖ] ἐκεῖνο H: ἐκεινω H[2] 7 ἐν *add. Ald.* 8 οὐ] εἰ L 10 οὐδὲ[II]] ἡ δὲ L 11 τοίνυν *om.* L τε *om.* L 14 μετ' οὐ] μετὰ τοῦ L ταύτην L 17 ἐπιστρέψον L 18 τῷ *om.* L αὐτὸν] αὖ H L: *suppl. Müller* 21 γυμνασάμενοι H 24 δὴ] δὲ *Ald.* 26 *post* αὐτοῖς *add.* ἀντειπεῖν *v. Arnim (SVF II, p. 260.33)* 26–27 καθάπερ – κεφαλῆς] ὅτι τὰ νεῦρα καθάπερ ἀπὸ πηγῆς πορεύονται τῆς κεφαλῆς, ἐνταῦθα *Müller* 28 μέρη] μετρίως L ἐπιζητήσομεν H: ζητήσωμεν *Müller* οἷα ἄν τινα λέγοιε H: εἰ ἀντιλέγοιεν L: *corr. Müller* 29 τῆς[I]] τοῦ L 30 *post* λέγειν *add.* περὶ τῶν νεύρων *Müller* 31 κινήσεων] νεύρων *Müller* *post* ἀρχῆς *add.* καὶ L 32 οἷον *secl. Ald.* ὃ δὴ γὰρ H: γὰρ δὴ L: *corr. Müller* 33 συγχωρήσειέ] χ *ex* γ, ω *ex* ν *corr.* H 34 *post* πάντως *add.* ἂν *Müller* συγχωρήσειε H L: *corr. Kühn* καὶ *ex* τὸ *corr.* H[2]: *om.* L

sentence, but it is not his habit to talk unintelligibly. Sometimes, no 61
doubt, his statements are false, as in the argument before us, but they are not unintelligible; for there is a very great difference between the false and the unintelligible. Since then it is more credible that Chry- 6
sippus used *ekeise* (thither) instead of *ekei* (there), his statement, translated into Greek, is as follows: "The region from which discourse is sent out must be the region where – that is, in that part (of the body) – reasoning takes place." And this, we say, is obviously false. 63
For if something is sent out from something by choice, this does not prove that the mind resides in that part, and this holds for urine, saliva, nasal mucus, and excrement.

It is apparent that Zeno erred here, first and foremost, and after 64
him the other Stoics, and Chrysippus himself not the least of them, at any rate in the passage quoted above. In another (passage) written not much later he was compelled to acknowledge the truth. I say he was compelled, because when he wished to refute another line 65
of reasoning as untrue and then perceived that the form of refutation turned no less against himself, he did not hesitate to overturn his own (position) along with that of his opponents. Either he should not have 66
written this later passage, or not that earlier one, and especially not so close together. For if the later reasoning is true, the earlier is not; and if the earlier is sound, the later is false. Now we who have been 67
trained in scientific methods can identify and distinguish true (reasoning) from false; but for the untrained it is no small question which to choose.

I shall now transcribe the actual passage in which Chrysippus 68
shows that the earlier argument is not demonstrative. It is as follows: 69
"But as I said, it is more important for them on all counts if perhaps this too should be granted, that according as they travel about, the source is from the head to the parts mentioned. Let us examine (the 70
matter) further. Surely the same sort of statement that they might make about speech, that it is carried out of the chest through the windpipe with an initiation of some kind coming from the head, can be made if the governing part is in the heart but the beginning of the movements is from the head." What Chrysippus means in this 71
passage is this: even if a person should concede that the head is the source of nerves, he will not necessarily concede that the governing

72 ὑπάρχειν. ἃ γὰρ ἐκεῖνοι δύνανται λέγειν ὑπὲρ τοῦ τὴν φωνὴν ἐκ τοῦ
στήθους διὰ τῆς φάρυγγος ἐκφέρεσθαι τὴν ἀρχὴν τῆς ἐνεργείας τοῖς
μορίοις ἐπιπεμπούσης τῆς κεφαλῆς, τοιαῦτ' ἔξεστι λέγειν ὑπὲρ τῶν νεύρων
ἡμῖν, ὡς ἐκ μὲν τῆς κεφαλῆς ἀρχομένων, ἀπὸ δὲ τῆς καρδίας τὴν ἐνέργειαν
73 ἐχόντων. ὥσθ' ὅτι δυνατόν ἐστιν ἐκ τοῦ στήθους τε καὶ διὰ τῆς φάρυγ-
γος ἐκπέμπεσθαι τὴν φωνήν, ἀρχὴν τῆς κινήσεως τοῖς ἐνταῦθα μορίοις
παρεχούσης τῆς κεφαλῆς, αὐτὸς ὁ Χρύσιππος ὡμολόγησεν.
74 Οὔκουν χρηστέον ἐστὶν ὡς ἀποδεικτικῷ τῷ λόγῳ, καθάπερ οἱ
256 πλεῖστοι | τῶν Στωϊκῶν ὑπειλήφασιν. ἐπιχειρεῖται γὰρ ὡς εἶπον ἀπὸ /
218 τῆς κατὰ τὴν θέσιν ἐγγύτητος, ὅθεν καὶ λείπειν ἡγητέον τῷ τοῦ Ζή-
75 νωνος λόγῳ λήμματα πρὸς τὸ τελέως ἠρωτῆσθαι. δειχθείη δὲ ἂν ἐν-
αργέστερον τοῦτο τῶν λημμάτων μεταληφθέντων ἐπὶ τὸ σαφέστερον,
ὡς εἶναι τὸν λόγον τοιόνδε· 'φωνὴ διὰ φάρυγγος ἐκπέμπεται. εἰ δὲ ἦν
ἐκ τοῦ ἐγκεφάλου ἐκπεμπομένη, οὐκ ἂν διὰ φάρυγγος ἐξεπέμπετο. ὅθεν
δὲ λόγος, καὶ φωνὴ ἐκεῖθεν ἐκπέμπεται. λόγος δὲ ἐκ διανοίας ἐκπέμπεται.
76 ὥστ' οὐκ ἔστιν ἐν τῷ ἐγκεφάλῳ ἡ διάνοια.' τὸ μὲν οὖν πρῶτον λῆμμα τῶν
πρὸς αἴσθησιν ἐναργῶν ἐστιν, ὥστ' οὐδ' ἀποδείξεως αὐτὸ δεῖται· πιστὰ γὰρ
ἐξ αὑτῶν ὑπάρχει πάντα τὰ πρὸς αἴσθησιν ἐναργῆ. τὸ δὲ δεύτερον οὔτε τῶν
πρὸς αἴσθησιν οὔτε τῶν πρὸς νόησιν ἐναργῶν ἐστι· τὴν ἀρχὴν γὰρ οὐδὲ
ἐκ τῶν πρώτων ἀξιωμάτων ὑπάρχει· ἀλλ' ἐχρῆν ὧδέ πως ἐρωτηθῆναι
τὸν λόγον, εἴπερ ἐκ τῶν πρώτων τε καὶ ἀποδεικτικῶν ἤμελλεν ἄρχε-
77 σθαι. «φωνὴ διὰ φάρυγγος ἐκπέμπεται. πᾶν δὲ τὸ διά τινος ἐκπεμπό-
257 219 μενον ἐκ τῶν συνεχῶν αὐτῷ μορίων ἐκπέμπεται. | οὐκ ἔστι / δὲ ἐγκέφαλος
78 τῇ φάρυγγι συνεχής· οὐκ ἄρα ἐξ ἐγκεφάλου ἐκπέμπεται.» μετὰ δὲ τοῦτον
τὸν λόγον αὖθις ἕτερον ἐχρῆν ἐρωτᾶσθαι τὸ συμπέρασμα λῆμμα ποι-
ησάμενον, ὡς εἶναι τοιόνδε τι· «ὅθεν ἡ φωνὴ ἐκπέμπεται, ἐκεῖθεν καὶ
ἡ σημαίνουσα φωνή, τουτέστιν ὁ λόγος. ἐκ δὲ διανοίας ὁ λόγος ἐκπέμ-
πεται, ἀλλ' οὐκ ἐκ τοῦ ἐγκεφάλου· οὐκ ἄρα ἐν τῷ ἐγκεφάλῳ ἐστὶν ἡ
διάνοια.»
79 Οὕτω μὲν ἐχρῆν ἠρωτῆσθαι τοὺς λόγους ὑπὸ τοῦ Ζήνωνος, εἰ
μηδὲν τῶν λημμάτων ἤμελλεν μήτε παραλειφθήσεσθαι μήτε ἐκ περιττοῦ
παραληφθήσεσθαι. ἔνεστι δὲ καὶ συντομώτερον ἔτι κατὰ τόνδε τὸν
80 τρόπον ἐρωτῆσαι συνθέντα τοὺς λόγους ἀμφοτέρους ἐς ταὐτόν· «ὁ λόγος
διὰ φάρυγγος ἐκπέμπεται. πᾶν δὲ τὸ διά τινος ἐκπεμπόμενον ἐκ τῶν
συνεχῶν αὐτῷ μορίων ἐκπέμπεται. ὥστε καὶ ὁ λόγος ἐκ τῶν συνεχῶν τῇ

13] *cf. supra*, p. 132.21 13–14] *cf. supra*, p. 134.4–5 15] *cf. supra*, p. 138.6–10 25] *cf.* Gal. UP i. 16: III 45 K. 26–27] *cf. supra*, p. 130.13–14

1 ἃ *ex* οἷα *corr.* H[2] *(cf. supra, p. 140.28)* 2 τῆς[I]] τοῦ L 5 ἐστιν *om.* L τῆς] τοῦ L 6 *ante* ἀρχὴν *add.* τὴν *Müller* 8 οὐκοῦν L χρηστέον] δεικτέον L ἀποδεικτικωτάτω H L: *corr.* H[2] 11 ἐναργέστερον] ἐν *ex* ἀν *corr.* L 14 ἐκ τοῦ *bis scr.* H: *corr.* H[2] *ante* φάρυγγος *add.* τοῦ L 18 αὑτῶν H L: ἑαυτῶν p: *corr. Müller* 22 *post* φωνὴ *add.* γὰρ L πᾶν] πάλιν L 23 αὐτὸ L 24 τῇ *ex* τὸ *(?) corr.* L 25 συμπέρασμα τὸ λῆμμα L 26 τι] τὸ H L: *corr. Diels* 28 ἀλλ'] ἀλλὰ καὶ L 31 παραληφθήσεσθαι L 33 συνθετά L 35 αὐτῷ] ω *ex* ο *corr.* L τῇ] τῷ L

part is also in the head. For the kind of statements that those others 72
can make about speech being carried out of the chest through the windpipe while the head sends the beginning of action to the parts, may be made to us about the nerves, that they start from the head
but receive their activity from the heart. Thus Chrysippus himself 73
conceded that it is possible that speech be sent out of the chest and through the windpipe, while the head supplies the beginning of motion to the parts in that region.

The argument therefore must not be considered demonstrative, 74
as most of the Stoics have supposed. For it proceeds, as I said, from proximity of position; and therefore we must hold that Zeno's argument lacks some of the premises required for a complete formu-
lation. This would be more evident if the premises were rephrased 75
for greater clarity, so that the argument would have the following form: 'Speech is sent out through the windpipe. If it were sent out of the brain, it would not be sent out through the windpipe. But speech is sent out of the same region as discourse. Discourse is sent out of the
mind. Therefore, the mind is not in the brain.' Now the first premise 76
is of the type evident to sense-perception, so that it needs no proof itself; for all things evident to the senses are credible in themselves. But the second is of the type evident neither to sense-perception nor to thought; for obviously it is not one of the first axioms. The argument should have been formulated as follows, if it was to begin from primary
and scientific premises: "Speech is sent out through the windpipe. All 77
that is sent out through something is sent out of the parts continuous with it. The brain is not continuous with the windpipe. Therefore,
(speech) is not sent out of the brain." And after this argument still 78
another should have been formulated, using the conclusion as a premise, something like this: "From the region from which speech is sent out, meaningful speech is sent out, that is, discourse. Discourse is sent out of the mind, but not out of the brain. Therefore, the mind is not in the brain."

This is how the arguments should have been formulated by Zeno, 79
if no premise was to be omitted and none was to be added superfluously. It is also possible to make the formulation even shorter by
combining both arguments in this way: "Discourse is sent out through 80
the windpipe. All that is sent out through something is sent out of the parts continuous with it. Therefore discourse too is sent out of the

φάρυγγι μορίων ἐκπέμπεται. ἐγκέφαλος δὲ οὐκ ἔστι συνεχὴς τῇ φάρυγγι·
οὐκ ἄρα ἐξ ἐγκεφάλου λόγος ἐκπέμπεται· ἀλλὰ καὶ ἐκ τῆς διανοίας ἐκ-
81 πέμπεται· οὐκ ἄρα ἐν ἐγκεφάλῳ ἐστὶν ἡ διάνοια.» — ἔξεστι δὲ δηλονότι
220 258 καὶ τὸ κυριεῦον /| εἰπεῖν ἀντὶ τοῦ τῆς διανοίας ὀνόματος, ὡσαύτως δὲ
καὶ τὸ ἡγεμονικὸν καὶ τὸ ἡγεμονοῦν καὶ τὸ ἡγούμενον καὶ τὸ δεσπόζον
καὶ τὸ ἄρχον καὶ τὸ λογιζόμενον καὶ τὸ νοοῦν καὶ τὸ φρονοῦν· οὐδὲν
γὰρ διαφέρειν ἡγητέον ὅπως ἄν τις ὀνομάζειν ἐθέλῃ ταὐτὸ φυλάττων
τὸ ὑποκείμενον πρᾶγμα. —
82 Εἰ οὕτως ἅπαντες ἠρωτήκεσαν τὸν λόγον καὶ μὴ τὸ ἀναγκαι-
ότατον τῶν λημμάτων παραλελοίπεσαν, ἐν ᾧ δηλοῦται τὸ πᾶν τὸ
διά τινος ἐκπεμπόμενον ἐκ τῶν συνεχῶν αὐτῷ μορίων ἐκπέμπεσθαι,
τὰ δὲ οὐκ ἀναγκαῖα μὴ μάτην προσετεθήκεσαν, εὐφώρατος ἂν ἦν ὁ
λόγος ἀπό τε τῆς ἀπὸ προθέσεως ἐπιχειρεῖν ὡρμημένος οὐκ ἀπο-
83 δεικνύς τε τὸ προκείμενον. εἰ μὲν γὰρ ἡ ἐξ πρόθεσις ἐγκέοιτο κατὰ τὸ
λῆμμα τὸ λέγον ἀπὸ τῆς διανοίας ἐκπέμπεσθαι τὸν λόγον, ψευδὲς εἶναι
φήσομεν αὐτό· μὴ γὰρ ἐκ τῆς διανοίας ἀλλ' ὑπὸ τῆς διανοίας αὐτὸν ἐκ-
221 84 πέμπεσθαι· / εἰ δὲ τὴν ὑπὸ πρόθεσιν ἐκ τῆς ἀπὸ δηλουμένην νομίζομεν,
ὡς εἶναι τὸ λῆμμα τοιοῦτον· 'ὁ λόγος ὑπὸ τῆς διανοίας ἐκπέμπεται',
τὸ μὲν λῆμμα φήσομεν ἀληθὲς ὑπάρχειν, ἀπέραντον δὲ εἶναι τὸν λόγον,
259 ὡς ἂν μηκέτι πάντων τῶν λημμάτων ὁμοίως ἠρωτη|μένων, ἀλλὰ τῶν
85 μὲν τὴν ἐξ, τῶν δὲ τὴν ὑπὸ πρόθεσιν ἐχόντων. εἰ δέ γε πάνθ' ὁμοίως
ἐρωτηθείη, κατὰ μὲν τὴν ἐξ πρόθεσιν ἐν τῷ προτέρῳ λήμματι γενήσεται
τὸ ψεῦδος, κατὰ δὲ τὴν ὑπὸ τουτὶ μὲν ἀληθὲς ἔσται, τὸ καθόλου δὲ
τὸ παραλελειμμένον ὑπ' αὐτῶν, ὡσαύτως δὲ καὶ τὸ κατὰ μέρος, ἄμφω
86 ψευδῆ. τὸ μὲν γὰρ καθόλου γενήσεται τοιοῦτον· 'ἅπαν τὸ διά τινος
ἐκπεμπόμενον ὑπὸ τῶν συνεχῶν αὐτῷ μορίων ἐκπέμπεται', τὸ δὲ κατὰ
μέρος· 'ὁ λόγος ὑπὸ τῶν συνεχῶν τῇ φάρυγγι μορίων ἐκπέμπεται'. οὐ
γὰρ ὑπὸ τῶν συνεχῶν, ἀλλ' ἐκ τῶν συνεχῶν ἀληθῶς ἂν λέγοιτο.
222 87 δέδεικται τοίνυν ἤδη σαφῶς τὸ / κυριώτατον τῶν λημμάτων παραλε-
λειμμένον αὐτοῖς ἢ ἑκοῦσι σοφιστικῶς ἢ ἄκουσιν ὑπὸ ἀγυμνασίας τῆς
88 μεθόδου. διὸ καὶ παρακρούονται τὸν ἀκροατὴν οὐ δυνάμενον ἀκριβῶς

25–27] *cf. supra*, p. 142.34–144.1 *infra*, pp. 146.10–13

1 ἐγκέφαλος] γ *inser.* H τῇ] τῷ L 2 *ante* λόγος *add.* ὁ L καὶ *om.* *Ald.* ἐκπέμπεται *secl. Müller* 4 κυριεῦον εἰπεῖν] εὖον εἰ *in ras.* L 6 νοῦν L 7 ὅπως ἄν τις ὀνομάζειν] οὕτως ἀντονομάζειν L ἐθέλοι H L: *corr. Kalbfleisch* ταὐτὸ *om.* L φυλάττων] ω *ex* ο *corr.* H 8 τὸ *om.* L 9 μὴ τὸ] μὴν L 10 λημμάτων H²: λοιπῶν H L 11 αὐτὸ L 12 μὴ *om.* L προσετεθείκεσαν L: προσετεθήκεισαν H: *corr. Ald.* εὐφώρατος] ω *ex* ο *corr.* H²: εὐφορωττ' L: εὐφωρατότατος *Müller* ἦν *om.* L 13 ἀπō προθέσεως H: θέσεως H²: προθέσεως L ἐπιχειρεῖν ὡρμημένος] ἐπιχειρούμενος L 13–14 ἀποδεικνύς τε] ἀποδείκνυσθαι L 14 μὲν γὰρ] μὴ L 15 ἀπὸ] ἐκ H L: *corr. Corn.* ψεῦδος L 16 αὐτό *e corr.* H ἀλλ' — αὐτὸν *inser.* H αὐτὸν — 18 διανοίας *om.* L 17 νομίζοιμεν *Müller* 19 *ante* τὸ *add.* ἤδη L μὲν *om.* L ἀπέραντον] ἀπεράντω· ψευδῆ L 20 τῶν^{I} *om.* L ἠρωμένω L 21 τὴν^{I} *om.* L ὑπὸ *om.* L 22 ἐν — λήμματι *secl. Müller* γενήσεται *ex* γε κινήσεται *corr.* H³ 23 τοῦτο H τὸ^{II} *om.* L 27 ὁ λόγος *om.* L *post* λόγος *add.* τῶν H, *del.* H² συνεχῶν τῷ φάρυγγι L: ἐν τῇ φάρυγγι H: ἐν τῇ φ. συνεχῶν H²: *corr. Müller* *post* μορίων *add.* ἡ φωνὴ L 28 γὰρ ὑπὸ] μὴν ἐκ L ἐκ *ex* ὑπὸ (?) *corr.* H συνεχῶν^{II}] συνεχῶς L

parts continuous with the windpipe. But the brain is not continuous with the windpipe. Therefore discourse is not sent out of the brain. But also, discourse is sent out of the mind. Therefore, the mind is not in the brain." – Obviously one may say 'sovereign part' instead of 81
'mind', and also the part that governs, guides, leads, dominates, rules, calculates, thinks, reasons. We must recognize that it makes no difference what name a person wishes to use, so long as he keeps the reference to the same thing. –

If all of them had formulated the argument in this way and had 82
not omitted the most essential premise, that which states that all that is sent out through something is sent out of the parts continuous with it, and had not added unnecessary premises that serve no purpose, then it would have been easy to detect that their argument sets out from the preposition 'from' and does not prove the point. For if the preposition 'out of' should be inserted in the premise 83
that says 'Discourse is sent from the mind', we shall say that the premise is false, for it is not sent out of the mind, but by the mind. But if we suppose that the preposition 'from' means 'by', so that 84
the premise is of this kind: 'Discourse is sent out by the mind', we shall say that the premise is true but the reasoning inconclusive, for all the premises would no longer be formulated in the same way; some would contain the preposition 'out of', others the preposition 'by'. But if all are formulated alike, the preposition 'out of' in the 85
prior premise will result in a false statement; and with the preposition 'by' that (premise) will be true but the universal that they omitted, and also the particular, will both be false. The universal 86
will be, 'All that is sent out through something is sent out by the parts continuous with it'; and the particular, 'Discourse is sent out by the parts continuous with the windpipe'. For it would not be correct to say 'by' the continuous parts, but 'out of' them. Now it 87
has already been clearly shown that they omitted the most important premise, whether with intentional sophistry, or unintentionally from lack of training in method. Therefore they also mislead the 88
listener who is unable to determine accurately which formulation

διελέσθαι πότερον τῶν λημμάτων ἐστὶν ἀληθές, εἴτε τὸ κατὰ τὴν ἐξ πρό-
θεσιν ἠρωτημένον εἴτε τὸ κατὰ τὴν ὑπό· τὴν ἀρχὴν μὲν γὰρ οὐδὲ λέ-
γουσιν αὐτὸ κατά γε τὴν λέξιν, εἰς δέ γε τὴν σύστασιν τοῦ λόγου παντὸς
260 89 ὡς εἰρηκότες προσχρῶνται. | τὸ γὰρ εἰ δ' ἦν ἀπὸ τοῦ ἐγκεφάλου
ἐκπεμπομένη, οὐκ ἂν διὰ φάρυγγος ἐξεπέμπετο, κατὰ τὴν τοῦ παραλε-
λειμμένου λήμματος δύναμιν ἀληθὲς εἶναι φαντάζεται.
90 Πᾶσιν οὖν τοῖς ἁμαρτήμασιν ὁ τοῦ Ζήνωνος λόγος ὑπεύθυνός
ἐστι κατὰ τὸ δεύτερον τῶν λημμάτων τὸ νυνί μοι λελεγμένον· πρῶτον
μὲν ὅτι τὴν ἀπὸ πρόθεσιν ἐν αὐτῷ παρέλαβεν δέον ἤτοι τὴν ἐξ ἢ τὴν
ὑπό· δεύτερον δ' ὅτι τὰ κυριώτατα παρέλιπε, τό τε καθόλου, τὸ 'πᾶν
δὲ τὸ διά τινος ἐκπεμπόμενον ἐκ τῶν συνεχῶν μορίων αὐτῷ ἐκπέμπεται',
223 τό τε κατὰ / μέρος, ὅτι ἡ φωνὴ καὶ ὁ λόγος ἐκ τῶν συνεχῶν τῇ φάρυγγι
91 μορίων ἐκπεμφθήσεται. τούτων γὰρ οὕτω διορισθέντων εἰ μὲν κατὰ
τὴν ἐξ πρόθεσιν ἅπαντα ἐρωτηθείη τὰ λήμματα, ψεῦδος ἔσται τὸ τὸν
λόγον ἐκ τῆς διανοίας ἐκπέμπεσθαι· εἰ δὲ κατὰ τὴν ὑπό, τό τε καθόλου
τὸ νυνὶ λελεγμένον μοι, τὸ πᾶν τὸ διά τινος ἐκπεμπόμενον ὑπὸ τῶν
συνεχῶν ἐκπέμπεσθαι, καὶ τὸ κατὰ μέρος, τὸ τὸν λόγον ὑπὸ τῶν ⟨συν-
92 εχῶν⟩ τῇ φάρυγγι μορίων ἐκπέμπεσθαι. εἰ δὲ μικτῶς ἐρωτηθείη κατά
261 τινα μὲν λήμματα τῆς ἐξ προθέ|σεως ἀκριβῶς παραλαμβανομένης, καθ'
ἕτερα δὲ τῆς ὑπό, καθάπερ κἂν τῷ τὸν λόγον ὑπὸ τῆς διανοίας ἐκπέμ-
πεσθαι, τῶν μὲν λημμάτων οὐδὲν μεμψόμεθα, τὸν ὅλον δὲ λόγον
ἀπέραντον ὑπάρχειν ἐροῦμεν· οὐ γὰρ ἔτι συναφθήσονται πρὸς ἀλλήλας
93 αἱ κύριαι τοῦ συμπεράσματος προτάσεις. ἔστι γὰρ αὐτῶν ἡ μὲν ἑτέρα
τοιαύτη· «ὁ λόγος ὑπὸ τῆς διανοίας ἐκπέμπεται», ἡ δὲ ἑτέρα «ὁ λόγος
224 ἐκ τοῦ ἐγκεφάλου οὐκ ἐκπέμπεται». ἐχρῆν δέ γ' / ἀμφοτέρας ἤτοι κατὰ
τὴν ὑπὸ πρόθεσιν ἢ κατὰ τὴν ἐξ ἠρωτῆσθαι, ἵν' ἐπιφέρηταί τι κοινὸν
αὐταῖς συμπέρασμα.
94 Τάχ' ἂν ἔτι πλείω λέγειν ὑπὲρ τῆς τοῦ λόγου μοχθηρίας ἐπειρώμην,
εἰ μὴ καὶ ὁ Χρύσιππος ἐγνώκει τε τὴν ἀτοπίαν αὐτοῦ καὶ τὸν τρόπον
τῆς ἀντιλήψεως αὐτὸς ἐγεγράφει δι' ἧς ὀλίγον ἔμπροσθεν παρεθέμην
ῥήσεως ἐγχωρεῖν φάσκων ἐκ τῶν κατὰ τὰ στήθη μερῶν ἐκπέμπεσθαι
τὸν λόγον τὴν ἀρχὴν τῆς κινήσεως ἐπιπεμπούσης τῆς κεφαλῆς, ὥσπερ
γε καὶ τὰ νεῦρα πάντα τὴν ἔκφυσιν ἐκ τῆς κεφαλῆς ἔχοντα τὴν ἀρχὴν
262 95 τῆς δυνάμεως ἀπὸ τῆς καρδίας λαμβάνειν. ταῦτα μὲν οὖν ὀρθῶς | εἴρηται
τῷ Χρυσίππῳ καὶ διὰ τοῦτ' ἄν τις αὐτῷ καὶ μᾶλλον μέμψαιτο, διότι καὶ
κατιδὼν τὸ ἀληθὲς ὅμως οὐ χρῆται· τὰ δὲ ἀπὸ τῆς θέσεως ἐπικεχειρημένα

4–5] *cf. supra*, pp. 130.3; 132.22–23, 28–34; 134.3–7; 142.13–14 30–31] *cf. supra*, p. 140.25–32 34–148.2] SVF II, p. 247

1 τὸ *om.* L 2 ἠρωτημένον] ἠ *ex* ἐ *corr.* H: ἐρωτώμενον L τὸ *om.* L τὴν^{II} *om.* L 3 δέ] μέν L 7 *ante* οὖν *add.* μὲν L 11 αὐτῷ μορίων *Müller* 12 ἡ φωνὴ *om.* L τῇ] τῶ L 16 λεγόμενόν H 17 τὸ^{II}] τῶ L συνεχῶν *add.* *Müller* 18 *ante* τῇ *add.* ἐν H *post* ἐκπέμπεσθαι *add.* ἄμφω ψευδῆ *Müller* 20 ἑκάτερα H L: *corr. Corn.* τῆς^{II} *inser.* H 24 ὑπὸ – λόγος^{II} *om.* L 25 οὐκ *inser.* H, *om.* L, *ante* ἐκ *ponendum censet Petersen* ἀμφότερα H L: *corr. Müller* 28 λόγου] κόσμου L 30 ἀπολήψεως H ἐγεγράφη H 31 στάθη L 32 τῆς κινήσεως τὴν ἀρχήν L 35 ἄν] ἂν εἰ L 36 ἐπικεχειρημένα] κεχωρισμένα L

of the premise is true, that with the preposition 'out of', or that with 'by'; for they do not put it into words at all but use it for the construction of the whole argument as if they had said it. And the proposition, 89
'If it were sent out from the brain, it would not be sent out through the windpipe', has a semblance of truth by virtue of the missing premise.

Zeno's argument, then, is chargeable with all these errors in 90
the second of its premises, which I have just now quoted: first, because he used the preposition 'from' in it when he should have used either 'out of' or 'by', and second, because he omitted the most important (premises), both the universal, 'All that is sent out through something is sent out of the parts continuous with it', and the particular, that speech and discourse will be sent out of the parts continuous with the windpipe. When these (premises) have been thus 91
distinguished, then if all the premises should be formulated with the preposition 'out of', the premise that states, 'Discourse is sent out of the mind', will be false; if with 'by', both the universal that I just mentioned, 'All that is sent out through something is sent out by the continuous parts', and the particular, 'Discourse is sent out by the parts continuous with the windpipe', will be false. And if the formu- 92
lation is mixed, some premises using accurately the preposition 'out of', others 'by', as in the premise, 'Discourse is sent out by the mind', we will not find fault with any of the premises but will say that the reasoning as a whole is inconclusive; for the propositions that control the conclusion will no longer combine with each other. The one of 93
them is "Discourse is sent out by the mind"; the other, "Discourse is not sent out of the brain". Both would have to be formulated either with 'by' or with 'out of', in order that a conclusion common to both might be drawn.

I would perhaps attempt to say yet more about the fallacy of 94
the argument, if Chrysippus had not also recognized its absurdity and had not himself written down the method of refutation in the passage that I quoted a little earlier, where he said that it is possible for discourse to be sent out of the parts in the chest while the head conveys the source of movement, just as it is possible that the nerves all have their growth out of the head but receive their source of power from the heart. Now Chrysippus was correct in saying this, and 95
therefore one might blame him the more, because even though he sees the truth he does not use it; but what he said about arguments

καὶ τούτων ὅσα μᾶλλον ποιηταὶ μαρτυροῦσιν ἢ οἱ πολλοὶ τῶν ἀνθρώ-
96 πων ἢ ἐτυμολογία τις ἤ τι τοιοῦτον ἕτερον, οὐκ ὀρθῶς. κάλλιον γὰρ
225 ἦν ἐπιμείναντα τοῖς κατὰ τὴν ἀποδεικτικὴν μέθοδον / ὑποβαλλομένοις
97 λήμμασιν ἐξετάσαι τε καὶ κρῖναι διὰ τῆς αἰσθήσεως. αὐτὸς δὲ ὥσπερ
οὐ κατ' ἐπιστήμην, ἀλλὰ κατὰ τύχην εἰρηκὼς τὸ ἀληθὲς ἀπεχώρησέ
τε τῆς ζητήσεως αὐτοῦ καὶ ποιητὰς ἐπάγεται μάρτυρας.

6. Ὅπερ οὖν ὁ Χρύσιππος ἐθεάσατο μὲν οὐκ ἐπεξῆλθε δὲ τῷ λόγῳ,
2 τοῦτ' ἐγώ μοι δοκῶ προσθήσειν. ἐπειδὴ γὰρ ἐγχωρεῖ, κἂν ὅτι μάλιστα
πάντων τῶν νεύρων ἐγκέφαλος ἀρχὴ φαίνηται, τὴν καρδίαν ἐπιπέμπειν
αὐτῷ δύναμιν αἰσθητικήν τε καὶ προαιρετικήν, ὡσαύτως δὲ κἂν ἐκ
τῶν κατὰ τὸν θώρακα μορίων ὁ λόγος ἐκπέμπηται, τὴν ἀρχὴν τῆς
κινήσεως αὐτῶν ἀπ' ἐγκεφάλου καταφέρεσθαι, ζητητέον ἐφεξῆς ἐστι
268 πότερον οὐδέτερον οὐδετέρῳ μεταδίδωσιν | οὐδεμιᾶς δυνάμεως ἢ τὸ
3 ἕτερον τῷ ἑτέρῳ. γένοιτο δ' ἂν ἡ ζήτησις ὧδε. τὰ συνάπτοντα τὴν
καρδίαν ἐγκεφάλῳ διασκέψασθαι χρὴ κατὰ τὰς τῶν ζῴων ἀνατομὰς
ὁπόσα τ' ἐστὶ καὶ ὁποῖα, κἄπειτα κατὰ τὸν τράχηλον ἕκαστον αὐτῶν ἢ
226 τέμνειν ἢ θλᾶν ἢ βρόχοις διαλαμβάνειν, εἶτ' ἐπισκέπτεσθαι τίνα / κατα-
4 λαμβάνει τὸ ζῷον παθήματα. συνάπτει δὲ καρδίαν ἐγκεφάλῳ τὰ τρία
γένη τῶν ἀγγείων, ἅπερ δὴ καὶ παντὸς τοῦ σώματος ὑπάρχει κοινά,
φλέβες καὶ ἀρτηρίαι καὶ νεῦρα, φλέβες μὲν αἱ σφαγίτιδες ὀνομαζόμεναι,
ἀρτηρίαι δὲ αἱ καρωτίδες, νεῦρα μὴν τὰ ταύταις ταῖς ἀρτηρίαις παρα-
5 πεφυκότα. τὰς μὲν δὴ σφαγίτιδας φλέβας ἢ τὰς καρωτίδας ἀρτηρίας οὐχ
ἁπλῶς χρὴ τέμνειν, ὥσπερ τὰ νεῦρα, τεθνήξεται γὰρ εὐθέως τὸ ζῷον αἱμορ-
ραγίᾳ λάβρῳ συσχεθέν, ἀλλ' ἄμεινον βρόχοις ἰσχυροῖς διαλαβόντα
πρῶτον ἔν τε τοῖς ἄνω καὶ κάτω μέρεσι τοῦ τραχήλου τὸ μέσον τῶν
6 βρόχων διατέμνειν, ὡς μηδεμίαν αἱμορραγίαν ἀκολουθῆσαι· τὰ νεῦρα
δὲ εἴτε θλᾶν εἴτε διαλαμβάνειν ἐθέλοις βρόχοις τισὶν ἢ τοῖς αὐτοῦ δα-
264 κτύλοις εἴτε τέμνειν, ἐφ' | ἅπασι τούτοις τοῖς παθήμασιν ἓν καὶ ταὐτὸν
ἀκολουθήσει σύμπτωμα τῷ ζῴῳ· ἄφωνον ἔσται παραχρῆμα, τῶν δὲ
ἄλλων ἐνεργειῶν οὐδεμίαν οὔτ' ἐν τῷ παραυτίκα βεβλαμμένον οὔτ'
227 7 ἐξ ὑστέρου φανεῖται. τῶν ἀρτη/ριῶν δέ γε βρόχοις διαληφθεισῶν ἢ ὡς
εἴρηται τμηθεισῶν ἄφωνον μὲν ἢ καρῶδες, ὡς οἱ πλεῖστοι τῶν μεθ'
Ἱπποκράτην κακῶς ἀνατεμόντων ἔγραψαν, οὐκ ἔσται τὸ ζῷον, αἱ
δὲ ἀνωτέρω τῶν τρωθεισῶν ἀρτηριῶν ἅπασαι τελέως ἄσφυκτοι γενήσον-

4–6] SVF II, p. 247 24–26] Rhazes, *al-Ḥāwī*, vol. XII, pp. 217.12–218.2 29–31] *cf.* Gal. Anat. viii. 5: II 675 K.

1 ποιεῖται L 3 *post* ἦν *add.* ἢ L 4 αὐτὸς] καὶ αὐτὰ L 6 αὐτοῦ] ἑαυτοῦ L: *secl. v. Arnim* 9 φαίνεται H L: *corr. Müller* 10 τε καὶ προαιρετικὴν *om. Müller* *post* ὡσαύτως *add.* εἰ L 12 αὐτοῦ H 14 ἦδε L τὴν *om.* L 15 *ante* χρὴ *add.* πρῶτον L 18 δὲ *om.* L 19 ὑπάρχει *om.* L κοιναὶ L 21 μὴν] δὲ L 24 λάβρως L 25 πρῶτον] πρότερον L 25–26 τῶν βρόχων] τῶ τὸν βρόχον L 27 ἐθέλοι L *ante* βρόχοις *add.* ἢ L αὐτοῦ H L: *corr. Müller*: σαυτοῦ *Chart.* 28 ἓν καὶ ταὐτὸν] ἐν ταυτῶ L 29 τὸ ζῷον L 30 οὐδεμία H οὔτ' ἐν τῷ] οὐδὲν τῶν L βεβλαμμένη H: βεβλαμμένην L: *corr. Einarson* οὔτ'II] εἴτ' L 31 φανεῖται] αI *ex* ω *corr.* H 33 ἱπποκτ' H: ἱπποκράτη L: *corr.* R *Ald.* ἔγγρα/ L ἔστι L 34 ἄφυκτοι H

from position, and about those among them that rest for the greater part on the evidence of poets, or the majority of mankind, or an etymology, or something else of that kind, was not correct. He would 96
have done better to remain with the premises supplied by the scientific method, and to examine and judge them through sense-perception. It is as if he had spoken the truth not from knowledge but by 97
chance; of his own accord he abandoned the investigation of it and brings in poets as his witnesses.

6. I have decided therefore to add an account of this matter that Chrysippus saw but did not fully discuss. Since it is possible, even 2
if one grant that the brain is clearly the source of all the nerves, that the heart may convey to it the power of perception and choice, and similarly, (since it is possible) that even though discourse is sent out of the parts in the chest, the source of their movement may descend from the brain, we must next inquire whether the brain and heart do or do not transmit power to each other. The inquiry 3
would be conducted in the following way. One must determine in one's dissection of animals the number and nature of the structures that connect the heart with the brain; next one must cut or crush or stop with ligatures each of these (structures) at the neck and then observe what the effects are on the animal. The heart and brain are 4
connected by the three kinds of vessels that are common to the whole body, veins, arteries, and nerves: the veins are the so-called jugular veins, the arteries, the carotid arteries, and the nerves the ones that lie beside these arteries. You must not simply cut the 5
jugular veins or the carotid arteries, as you do the nerves, for the animal will suffer a violent hemorrhage and quickly die; it is better first to intercept them with strong ligatures in the upper and lower parts of the neck, then to cut between the ligatures, so that no hemorrhage ensues. As for the nerves, whether you wish to crush them, 6
or intercept them with ligatures or with your fingers, or cut them, all of these operations will have one and the same effect on the animal: it will immediately be voiceless, but it will show no impairment of any other activity, either at the moment or later on. When the 7
arteries have been intercepted by ligatures or cut in the manner described, the animal will not be voiceless or stupefied, as the majority of Hippocrates' successors have written because of their faulty dissection, but all the arteries above the injury will become

8 ται. τὰς δὲ φλέβας οὔτε βρόχοις διαλαμβάνων οὔθ' ὡς εἴρηται τέμνων
ὄψει τινὰ σαφῶς ἐνέργειαν ἀπολλυμένην.
9 Ἐκ τούτων τῶν φαινομένων ἕτοιμόν ἐστι συλλογίσασθαι μήτε
τὴν καρδίαν εἰς τὴν τῶν σφυγμῶν κίνησιν ἐγκεφάλου τι προσδεῖσθαι
μήτε τὸν ἐγκέφαλον καρδίας, ἵν' αἰσθάνηταί τε καὶ κατὰ προαίρεσιν
10 ἐνεργῇ τὸ ζῷον. ὅτι μὲν γὰρ οὐδὲν ἡ καρδία πρὸς τὴν οἰκείαν κίνησιν
ἐγκεφάλου δεῖται, δῆλόν ἐστιν ἐκ τοῦ καὶ τῶν φλεβῶν καὶ τῶν ἀρτηριῶν
καὶ τῶν νεύρων τῶν προειρημένων βρόχοις διαληφθέντων ὁμοίως ἔτι
265 σφύζειν αὐτὴν καὶ τὰς καθ' ὅλον τὸ ζῷον ἀρτηρίας· | αἱ γὰρ ἀνωτέρω
τῶν βρόχων μόναι παντάπασιν ἄσφυκτοι γίγνονται τοῦ συνεχοῦς
228 αὐτῶν μέρους τοῦ μέχρι καρδίας / ὡσαύτως ταῖς ἄλλαις σφύζοντος.
11 ὅτι δὲ οὐ τῶν ἐξ ἐγκεφάλου δυνάμεων ἡ καρδία τὴν πρώτην ἀρχὴν ἔχει,
μάθοις ἂν ἐκ τοῦ πάντων τῶν εἰρημένων νεύρων ἤτοι τμηθέντων ἢ
βρόχοις διαληφθέντων ἄφωνον μόνον γίγνεσθαι τὸ ζῷον, εἰσπνεῖν μέντοι
καὶ ἐκπνεῖν ἀκωλύτως κατ' ἀμφοτέρας τὰς διαφορὰς τῶν ἔμπροσθεν
εἰρημένων εἰσπνοῶν τε καὶ ἐκπνοῶν, οὕτω δὲ κἂν τοῖς τέσσαρσι κώλοις
ἔτι καὶ νῦν ἐνεργεῖν, καὶ καθάπερ καὶ πρόσθεν ἀκούειν τε καὶ βλέπειν
12 καὶ πᾶσαν αἴσθησιν αἰσθάνεσθαι. μόνη γάρ, ὡς εἴρηται, φωνὴ διαφθεί-
ρεται τοῦ ζῴου τμηθέντων τῶν παρὰ ταῖς ἀρτηρίαις νεύρων.
13 Ὅσοι δὲ τῶν ἰατρῶν τε καὶ φιλοσόφων ἐπὶ ταῖς εἰρημέναις ἀρτηρί-
αις ἤτοι τμηθείσαις ἢ ὡς εἴρηται διαληφθείσαις ᾤοντο καροῦσθαι τὸ
ζῷον, εἶτ' ἐκ τούτου συνελογίζοντο τὴν καρδίαν ἐγκεφάλῳ χορηγεῖν
αἴσθησίν τε καὶ κίνησιν, ἐσφάλθαι μὲν αὐτοὺς ὑποληπτέον ἐν τῇ περὶ
266 τὸ φαινόμενον ἐμπειρίᾳ, τὸ δ' ἐξ ὑποθέσεως ἀκολουθοῦν | ἀκριβῶς ἑωρα-
229 14 κέναι· εἴπερ γὰρ / ὄντως ἐγίγνετο καρῶδες τὸ ζῷον, ὅπερ αὐτοῖς ὄνομα
βούλεται σημαίνειν τὸ ἀναίσθητόν τε καὶ ἀκίνητον, ἐξ ἀνάγκης ἂν
ἀκολουθεῖν τὸ τὴν καρδίαν ἐπιπέμπειν ἐγκεφάλῳ τὴν πρώτην ἀρχὴν
αἰσθήσεώς τε καὶ κινήσεως, ἣν αὐτὸς ἅπαντι τῷ σώματι διὰ νεύρων
χορηγεῖ, ὥστ' εἶναι δευτέραν τινὰ ἀρχὴν αὐτόν, οὐκ ἀκριβῶς πρώτην,
15 ἀνάλογον ὑπάρχῳ μεγάλου βασιλέως. ἀποδεδειγμένου γὰρ ἐν τοῖς
ἔμπροσθεν ὡς ἡ μὲν καρδία τῶν ἀρτηριῶν ὁ δ' ἐγκέφαλος τῶν νεύρων
ἐστὶν ἀρχή, περαίνοιτ' ἄν, εἴπερ ἀληθὲς ἦν τὸ λεγόμενον, ὡς ἡ καρδία
16 διὰ τῶν ἀρτηριῶν ἐγκεφάλῳ χορηγεῖ δύναμιν ψυχικήν. οὐ μὴν ἀληθές
γ' ἐστίν, ἀλλὰ κατεψεύσαντο τοῦ φαινομένου κατὰ τὰς ἀνατομάς. καρῶδες
μὲν γὰρ οὐδ' ἐπὶ τοῖς νεύροις τμηθεῖσι γίγνεται τὸ ζῷον, μήτι γε δὴ
ταῖς ἀρτηρίαις· ἄφωνον δὲ τῶν νεύρων μὲν βλαβέντων γίγνεται, τῶν

1–2] *cf. infra*, PHP 508.2–6 Müller 3–6] *cf. supra*, pp. 80.14–15; 128.2–5 25–26] *cf.* Gal. De loc. aff. iv. 3: VIII 231–232 K.

3 ἐστι] εἶναι H L: *corr. Kühn*: "*fortasse eiciendum*" *Müller* 7 προσδεῖται L 10 ἄφυκτοι H 11 αὐτοῖς L 12 οὐ τῶν ἐξ] οὐκ ἐκ τῶν H L: οὐκ ἔτι τῶν *Ricci*: οὐ τῶν *Müller*: *correxi* 14 εἰσπνεῖ H 15 ἐκπνεῖ H 16 τέτταρσι L κώλοις] οὐ κωλύσει H: κωλύσοι L: *corr.* H^2 17 καὶ^{II} *om.* H 22 καρδίαν] κ *ex* α *corr.* H 25 αὐτοῖς, ὅπερ L 27 ἠκολούθει *Müller* τὸ *om.* L τῇ πρώτῃ ἀρχῇ H: *corr.* H^2 28 ἧς L 29 αὐτῶν L 30 ὑπάρχον L ἀποδεδειγμένον *et* -μένων H: ἀποδεδειγμένον L: *corr. Müller* 33 διὰ *inser.* H δυνάμεως L ψυχικὴν *ex* τῇ ψυχῇ *corr.* H: ψυχικῆς L 34 γ' *om.* L 35 οὐδ' ἐπὶ] οὐδέν τι L μήτι *in* μήτοι *mut.* H^2

completely pulseless. But neither when you intercept the veins with 8 ligatures nor when you cut them in the manner described will you see any activity clearly destroyed.

From these observations, therefore, one may readily conclude 9 that the heart needs no help from the brain to move the pulse, and the brain needs none from the heart for the animal to have sensation and act in accordance with choice. That the heart has no need of the 10 brain for its proper motion is clear from the fact that even after the above-mentioned veins, arteries and nerves have been intercepted by ligatures the heart and the arteries throughout the whole body pulsate as before; only the arteries above the ligatures become entirely pulseless, while the portion of them that extends in unbroken continuity as far as the heart pulsates like the rest. That the heart 11 does not have the first source of the powers from the brain you would learn from the fact that when all the above-mentioned nerves have either been cut or intercepted by ligatures, the animal only becomes voiceless; it breathes in and out without hindrance in both forms of inhalation and exhalation that were mentioned above and, similarly, has even now activity in its four limbs, and hears and sees and uses all its senses as before. For as we said, only the voice of the animal 12 is destroyed when the nerves (that lie) alongside the arteries are cut.

All of those physicians and philosophers who supposed that the 13 animal became stupefied when the arteries mentioned were cut or intercepted in the manner described, and who then inferred from this that the heart supplies sensation and motion to the brain, must be assumed to have erred in their experience of the phenomenon but to have seen clearly the conclusion that follows from their assumption. For if the animal really became stupefied – a term that to them 14 means lack of sensation and motion –, it would necessarily follow (as they saw) that the heart sends to the brain the first beginning of sensation and motion, which the brain itself supplies through the nerves to the whole body, so that the brain is a kind of second source, not strictly the first, but comparable to a satrap of the Great King. For 15 as it was demonstrated earlier that the heart is the source of the arteries, and the brain of the nerves, the conclusion would follow, if their statement were true, that the heart through the arteries supplies the brain with psychic power. But it is not true; for they were mistaken 16 about what appears in dissections. The animal does not become stupefied even after you cut the nerves, much less the arteries. It becomes voiceless when the nerves have been damaged, but not when the

17 ἀρτηριῶν δ' οὐ γίγνεται καὶ πολὺ δὲ μᾶλλον ἔτι τῶν φλεβῶν. ἀλλ' οἱ
πλεῖστοι τῶν ἰατρῶν τε καὶ φιλοσόφων ἅμα ταῖς ἀρτηρίαις τὰ νεῦρα
230 267 τοῖς βρόχοις διαλαμβάνοντες, εἶτα ἄφωνον ὁρῶντες / αὐτίκα τὸ | ζῷον
γιγνόμενον ἀρτηριῶν τὸ πάθος ᾠήθησαν ὑπάρχειν καὶ κάρον ὠνό-
μασαν — οὐκ ὀρθῶς, οἶμαι, εἰ μή τι ἄρα τὴν ἀφωνίαν ἐθέλουσιν ὀνομά-
ζειν κάρον· οὕτω γὰρ ⟨ἂν⟩ ὀνόματι μόνον σφάλλοιντο κατά γε τοῦτο,
περὶ δὲ τὸ πρᾶγμα αὐτὸ ἁμαρτάνοιεν, εἴπερ ἐπὶ ταῖς ἀρτηρίαις ὑπολαμ-
βάνοιεν ἄφωνον γίγνεσθαι τὸ ζῷον.
7. Ἐγὼ μὲν δή μοι δοκῶ τὸ κελευσθὲν ὑπὸ τοῦ Χρυσίππου πε-
πραχέναι ζητήσας εἴτ' ἀπὸ καρδίας ἐγκεφάλῳ δύναμίς τις εἴτ' ἀπ'
2 ἐγκεφάλου τῇ καρδίᾳ χορηγεῖται. Χρύσιππος δ' αὐτὸς ὀλιγώρως
ἐσχηκέναι φαίνεται περὶ τὴν τοῦ πράγματος ἔρευναν ἰδὼν μὲν τὴν ὁδὸν
3 ᾗ χρὴ τὸ ζητούμενον ἁλῶναι, μὴ χρησάμενος δὲ αὐτῇ. μέμφομαι δ'
αὐτῷ καὶ διότι καθ' ἓν βιβλίον ἐναντία λέγειν ὑπέμεινεν οὐκ ἀπὸ μακροῦ
διαστήματος ἀλλήλων, ἔμπροσθεν μὲν ὡς ἀποδεικτικὸν γράψας τὸν
τοῦ Ζήνωνος λόγον, ἐπὶ προήκοντι δὲ τῷ συγγράμματι δεικνὺς αὐτοῦ
231 4 τὴν λύσιν. εὑρίσκω δ' οὐχ ἥκιστα τὸν Χρύ/σιππον καὶ ἄλλας τινὰς
ἐναντιολογίας ἐν αὐτῷ τούτῳ τῷ λόγῳ περὶ τοῦ τῆς ψυχῆς ἡγεμονικοῦ |
268 5 πεποιημένον. ἐν ἀρχῇ γὰρ προειπὼν ὡς τὰ μὲν ἄλλα μέρη τῆς ψυχῆς
ἐν οἷς ἐστι τοῦ ζῴου μορίοις ὁμολογεῖται, περὶ δὲ τοῦ ἡγεμονικοῦ μόνου
ζητεῖται διὰ τὸ μήτε αἴσθησιν ἐκφανῆ μηδεμίαν εἶναι αὐτοῦ μήτ' ἐναρ-
γές τι τεκμήριον, ὀλίγον ὕστερον ὡς περὶ φαινομένου τοῦ μέρους δια-
6 λέγεται. ἔχουσι δὲ αἱ ῥήσεις αὐτοῦ τόνδε τὸν τρόπον· «οὕτω φαίνεται
διαφεύγειν ὁ τόπος ἡμᾶς οὔτε αἰσθήσεως ἐκφανοῦς γιγνομένης, ὅπερ
ἐπὶ τῶν λοιπῶν συντέτευχεν, οὔτε τῶν τεκμηρίων δι' ὧν ἄν τις συλλογί-
σαιτο τοῦτο· οὐδὲ γὰρ ἂν οὐδ' ἐπὶ τοσοῦτον ἀντιλογία προῆλθεν
7 ἰατροῖς τε καὶ φιλοσόφοις.» ταῦτα προειπὼν ὁ Χρύσιππος ἐφεξῆς
φησιν ὡς ἅπαντες ἄνθρωποι τῶν τῆς διανοίας παθῶν αἰσθάνονται κατά
8 τε τὸν θώρακα καὶ τὴν καρδίαν. ἔχει δὲ καὶ ἥδε ἡ ῥῆσις ὧδε· «κοινῇ
232 δέ μοι δοκοῦσιν οἱ πολλοὶ φέρεσθαι ἐπὶ τοῦθ' ὡσανεὶ αἰσθανό/μενοι
περὶ τὸν θώρακα αὐτοῖς τῶν κατὰ τὴν διάνοιαν παθῶν γιγνομένων
καὶ μάλιστα καθ' ὃν ἡ καρδία τέτακται τόπον, οἷον μάλιστα ἐπὶ τῶν
φόβων καὶ τῶν λυπῶν λέγω καὶ ἐπὶ τῆς ὀργῆς καὶ μάλιστα τοῦ θυμοῦ.»
269 9 κατὰ τήνδε τὴν ῥῆσιν, εἰ καὶ μηδὲν | ἄλλο, τὸ γοῦν ὡσανεὶ προσέθηκεν
οὐ τολμήσας ἄντικρυς εἰπεῖν αἰσθάνεσθαι τοὺς ἀνθρώπους τῶν κατὰ

4–5] *cf. supra*, p. 86.27–30 Gal. In Hipp. Epid. II comm. iv: CMG V 10.1, p. 331 9–11] *cf. supra*, p. 148.7–14 13–17] SVF II, p. 247 17–154.14] SVF II, pp. 240–241 23–27] *cf. infra*, pp. 170.23–27; 220.5–9 29–33] *cf. infra*, p. 172.20–24

5 οἶμαι] εἶναι L 6 ἂν *add. Kühn* μόνον] μὲν L σφάλοιντο L 7 αὐτῶν L 10 εἴτ'[II] *ex* εἴ τις *corr.* H 12 ἰδὼν] εἰδὼς L ὁδὸν H[2]: ὄψιν H 16 τοῦ *om.* L λόγον *ex* -ου *corr.* H[2] 21 αἰσθήσεσιν L 24 ὅπερ] ὥσπερ L 25 τις *om.* L συλλογήσαιτο H 26 ἂν οὐδ' *om.* L: ἂν *Müller* ἀντιλογίας H: ἀντιλο^γ' L: ἡ ἀντιλογία *Müller (cf. infra, p. 170.26)* προῆλ^θ L: προῆλθε καὶ ἐν *Müller* 27 τε καὶ] καὶ ἐν *Müller* ἑξῆς L 29 τε] γε H κοινοὶ L 33 λοιπῶν L λέγω *del. Müller* 35 ἄντικρυς εἰπεῖν] ι, υ, ει *e corr.* L

arteries, and still less when the veins have been damaged. But most 17
physicians and philosophers, who intercepted the nerves along with
the arteries by their ligatures and then saw the animal immediately
become voiceless, thought that the effect was the work of the arteries
and called it stupor – wrongly, in my opinion, unless perhaps they
mean to give the name stupor to voicelessness. In that case their error
here would be only in the name; but they would be mistaken about
the reality itself if they should suppose that the animal becomes voice-
less when the arteries are intercepted.

7. By inquiring whether a power is supplied from heart to brain
or from brain to heart, I believe that I have done what Chrysippus
indicated. Chrysippus himself appears to have scorned the investi- 2
gation of the matter; he saw the method by which the answer must
be found, but he did not pursue it. And I blame him also for permit- 3
ting himself to make contradictory statements in a single book at
no great distance from each other, writing first that Zeno's argu-
ment is apodeictic, but later on in the treatise showing how it is re-
futed. Not the least of my findings is that Chrysippus involved him- 4
self in certain other contradictions also in this very discussion of the
governing part of the soul. At the beginning he said that there is 5
agreement on the members of the animal in which the other parts
of the soul reside, and that the seat of the governing part alone is in
doubt, since there is neither clear perception of it nor any manifest
sign; yet a little later he speaks of the member as of something evi-
dent. His words are as follows: "Thus the place seems to elude us, 6
since we have neither a clear perception of it, as was the case with the
others, nor signs from which this matter might be inferred; otherwise,
disagreement among physicians and philosophers would not have grown
so great." After this earlier statement Chrysippus goes on to say that 7
all men perceive the affections of the mind in the chest and heart. Again 8
I quote the passage in his own words: "The multitude of men seem
to me to be brought together to this view since they perceive, as it
were, the affections of the mind happening to them in the region of
the chest and especially in the place assigned to the heart. I mean
especially in fear and distress, in anger, and inflamed anger most of
all." He qualified this statement, if in no other way, at least by add- 9
ing 'as it were', not venturing to state outright that men perceive

τὴν διάνοιαν παθῶν ἐν τῷ θώρακι γιγνομένων· «ὡσανεὶ» γὰρ ἔφη «συν-
10 αισθανόμενοι». μικρὸν δ' ὕστερον καὶ τὸ ὡσανεὶ περιελὼν οὑτωσὶ
γράφει· «ἡ γὰρ περὶ τὴν διάνοιαν γιγνομένη ταραχὴ καθ' ἕκαστον
11 τούτων αἰσθητῶς περὶ τοὺς θώρακάς ἐστιν.» εἶτ' ἐφεξῆς· «τῆς μὲν γὰρ
ὀργῆς γιγνομένης ἐνταῦθα εὔλογον καὶ τὰς λοιπὰς ἐπιθυμίας ἐνταῦθα
εἶναι», καὶ πάλιν ἐν τοῖς ἑξῆς τοῦ συγγράμματος «καὶ τὰ τῶν ὀργιζο-
μένων δὲ πάθη» φησὶ «φαίνεται περὶ τὸν θώρακα γιγνόμενα καὶ τὰ
τῶν ἐρώντων», καὶ λοιπὸν οὐκέτι παύεται περὶ τῶν παθῶν διαλεγό-
μενος ὡς ἔν τε τῷ θώρακι καὶ περὶ τὴν καρδίαν μάλιστα συνίστασθαι
233 12 φαινομένων. ὥστ' ἔγωγε θαυ/μάζω τἀνδρός, ὅπως τὸ κατ' ἀρχὰς ὑφ'
ἑαυτοῦ γραφόμενον οὐκ ἐξήλειψεν, ἔνθα φησὶν οὔτ' αἴσθησιν οὐδεμίαν
ἐκφανῆ γίγνεσθαι ποῦ τὸ κύριον τῆς ψυχῆς μέρος, οὔτε τεκμήριον· οὐ
γὰρ ⟨ἂν⟩ ἐπὶ τοσοῦτον διενεχθῆναι πρὸς ἀλλήλους ἰατρούς τε καὶ φιλο-
13 σόφους. ἢ εἴπερ ἀρέσκεται τῷδε τῷ λόγῳ, πῶς οὐκ ᾐδέσθη πάλιν ἐν
270 τοῖς ἑξῆς αἰσθήσει τε κρίνων τὸ δόγμα καὶ «φαίνεται» | λέγων;
14 Ἐγὼ δή μοι δοκῶ, καθάπερ ὀλίγον ἔμπροσθεν ἔπραξα τὸν ἀληθέ-
στερον ἑλόμενος λόγον ὃν ὁ Χρύσιππος ἔγραψε πρὸς ἑαυτὸν ἐναντιο-
15 λογούμενος, οὕτω καὶ νῦν ποιήσειν. οὐδεμία γὰρ αἴσθησις ἡμῖν γίγνεται
τοῦ τῆς ψυχῆς ἡγεμονικοῦ κατὰ τὴν καρδίαν ἢ τὸν θώρακα περιεχο-
μένου καὶ διὰ τοῦτ' ἐπαινῶ μὲν τὰ πρῶτα τοῦ Χρυσίππου, δι' ὧν
ὁμολογεῖ τὸ ἀληθές, οὐκ ἐπαινῶ δὲ ἐν οἷς καταψεύδεται τῆς αἰσθή-
16 σεως. οὐ γὰρ ἓν ἔτ' ἐνταῦθα δοκεῖ μοι σφάλλεσθαι κατὰ τὸν λόγον,
234 ἀλλὰ δύο μεγάλα· πρῶτον μέν, / ὅτι παντὸς τοῦ σώματος ἐν τοῖς τῆς
ψυχῆς πάθεσιν ἐναργῶς ἀλλοιουμένου καὶ ποτὲ μὲν ὠχριῶντός τε καὶ
καταψυχομένου καὶ τρέμοντος, ὡς ἐν τοῖς φόβοις φαίνεται γιγνόμενον,
ἔστιν ὅτε δ' ἐρυθριῶντός τε καὶ θερμαινομένου καὶ σφοδρῶς ἐντεινομένου,
καθάπερ ἐν τοῖς θυμοῖς, οὐδενὸς μὲν ἄλλου μέμνηται μορίου, μόνων δὲ
17 τῶν κατὰ τὸν θώρακα· ἔπειτα δ' ὅτι κἂν συγχωρηθῇ μειζόνως ἡ καρδία
τῶν ἄλλων τοῦ ζῴου μορίων ἐξισταμένη τοῦ κατὰ φύσιν ἐν φόβοις τε
καὶ λύπαις ἀγωνίαις τε καὶ θυμοῖς ἅπασί τε τοῖς ἄλλοις πάθεσιν, οὐ
271 τὸ λογιζόμενον τῆς ψυχῆς, | ἀλλὰ τὸ θυμούμενον ἢ ἐπιθυμοῦν ἐνταῦθα
ὑπάρχειν ἐνδείξεται· ὥστε πλέον θάτερον ἢ ὅπερ αὐτὸς βούλεται πε-
18 ραίνεσθαι διὰ τοῦ λόγου. εἰ γὰρ ἐν μὲν τῷ διανοεῖσθαί τε καὶ μανθά-
νειν ἢ διδάσκειν οὐδεμία κίνησις ἐξαίρετος ἐμφαίνεται κατὰ τὴν καρδίαν,

6–8] *cf. infra*, p. 218.19–20 11–14] *cf. supra*, p. 152.23–27 15] *cf. supra*, lin. 7 16] *cf. supra*, p. 146.28–35 23–24] *cf.* Gal. De sympt. caus. ii. 5: VII 191–194 K. Nemes. De nat. hom. 20: p. 232.6 Matth. Domański, 1900, p. 124

1–2 ἔφησεν αἰσθανόμενοι *coniecerit Einarson* 2 ὕστερον δὲ L 4 τὸν θώρακά *Müller* γὰρ] οὖν *Müller* 7 δὲ *om. Ald.* 8 λοιπὸν] ὁ *ex* ῶ *corr.* L 9 μάλιστα] μόλις L 10 ὅπως *(?) in* ὅτε *mut.* H²: ὅτι *Kühn* 10–11 τὰ ... γραφό(μν,) L 12 ἐμφανῆ H L *(ut vid.)*: *corr. Müller* που τὸ H: *corr. Kühn*: τοῦτο L 13 ἂν *hic add. Müller, post* διενεχθῆναι *Kühn* τοσοῦτο L 15 τε] γὲ *Ald.* 16 δή] δέ *Ald.* 18 οὕτω] ἑαυτῷ L 20 ἐπαινῶ μὲν] ἐπαινοῦμεν L 21 τἀληθὲς L 22 ἓν *om.* L 26 καὶ^{II} – ἐντεινομένου *om.* L 29 ἐξισταμένου L τε *om.* L 32 ὥστε] ἅτε L ἢ ὅπερ] ἥπερ L

the affections of the mind happening in the chest; for he said, "since
they have, as it were, an inner awareness". But a little later he even 10
cuts out the 'as it were' and writes: "For the disturbance of mind that
arises in each of these (affections) is perceptibly in the region of
the chest." Then he continues: "For since anger arises there, it is 11
reasonable that the other desires are there also"; and again later in
the book he says: "The affections of angry men are observed to arise
in the region of the chest, and also those of lovers"; and in the rest
he never stops speaking of the affections as appearing to be in the
chest and especially in the region of the heart. Therefore I marvel at 12
the man, how it was that he did not expunge what he had first written,
in which he said that there arises neither a clear perception of the place
occupied by the sovereign part of the soul, nor a sign of it, for other-
wise physicians and philosophers would not have disagreed with each
other to such an extent. Or if he is satisfied with this initial reasoning, 13
how was it that he felt no shame when he subsequently rested his
opinion on sense-perception and said, "are observed"?

I think I shall now do what I did a short time ago, when I chose 14
from Chrysippus' self-contradictory statements the one that came
closer to the truth. (The truth is that) we have no perception of the 15
governing part of the soul as enclosed in the heart or chest, and there-
fore I praise Chrysippus' initial statement, in which he acknowl-
edges the truth, but I do not praise the one in which he gives a false
account of sense-perception. His reasoning there seems to me no 16
longer to contain one error only, but two major errors. The first is
that although the whole body is clearly altered in the affections of
the soul, at one time turning pale and cold and trembling, as we see
happening in fear, at another growing red and hot and very tense,
as in inflamed anger, yet Chrysippus mentions no parts (of the body)
other than those in the chest. The second is that even if we concede 17
that the heart departs further from its natural state than any of the
living being's other members in times of fear, distress, anxiety,
inflamed anger, and all the other affections, this fact will not indicate
that the reasoning part of the soul is there, but rather the spirited
or desiderative part; so that his argument leads to the other con-
clusion more than to the one he intended. For if no special motion 18
of the heart is evident in the act of thinking and learning or teaching,

ἐν ἅπασι δὲ τοῖς πάθεσιν ἐναργῶς φαίνεται, δῆλον οἶμαι γίγνεται τὸ
μὲν λογιζόμενον τῆς ψυχῆς οὐκ εἶναι κατὰ τὴν καρδίαν, τὸ δ' ἀλόγιστόν τε
235 καὶ παθητικὸν ὀνομαζόμενον ἐν αὐτῇ περιέ/χεσθαι· εἰ δ' ἔνθα τὸ πάσχον
ἐνταῦθά φησι καὶ τὸ λογιζόμενον ὑπάρχειν, αὐτὸ τὸ ζητούμενον ἀπ'
19 ἀρχῆς ἐξ ἑτοίμου λήψεται. πολλῷ δ' ἦν ἄμεινον ἀπόδειξίν τινα ἡμᾶς
διδάξαι τοῦ λαβεῖν ἐκ προχείρου τὸ ζητούμενον· ἀλλ' οὔτ' ἐν τούτῳ τῷ
βιβλίῳ τῷ πρώτῳ Περὶ ψυχῆς οὔτ' ἐν τοῖς Περὶ παθῶν ἀπόδειξίν τινα
εἶπε τοῦ χρῆναι πάντως, ἔνθ' ἄ⟨ν⟩ ᾖ τὸ ἄλογον, ἐνταῦθ' εἶναι καὶ τὸ
λογιζόμενον, ἀλλ' ἑτοίμως τε κἀκ προχείρου πανταχοῦ λαμβάνει, καίτοι
Πλάτωνος ἐνίας μὲν ἀποδείξεις ἐν τῷ τετάρτῳ τῆς Πολιτείας γρά-
ψαντος, ἐνίας δ' αὖθις ἐρεῖν ἀναβαλομένου περὶ ὧν ἐνδείκνυται κατὰ
272 τὸν | Τίμαιον, ἃς κἀγὼ διὰ τῶν ἑξῆς ὑπομνημάτων ἁπάσας γράψω.
20 νυνὶ δ' οὔπω μοι πρόκειται τοῦτο δεικνύειν ἀλλ' ὅτι τὸ λογιζόμενον τῆς
ψυχῆς, ὃ δὴ καὶ ἡγεμονικόν τε καὶ διάνοιαν καὶ κύριον αὐτὸς ὁ Χρύσιπ-
21 πος ὀνομάζει, κατὰ τὸν ἐγκέφαλόν ἐστι. τούτου γὰρ ἀποδειχθέντος,
ἐάν τις ἑτέρα δύναμις ἐν τῇ καρδίᾳ φαίνηται περιεχομένη μηδαμόθεν
236 ἑτέρωθεν / ὁρμωμένη, τὰς δύο μὲν ἀρχὰς ἤδη σαφῶς ἕξομεν, ἐφεξῆς δὲ
καὶ τὴν τρίτην ὁμοίως ἐξευρήσομεν. ἀλλὰ τοῦτο μὲν εἰς τὸν μέλλοντα
λόγον ἀναβεβλήσθω.

22 Νυνὶ δ' ἐπανέλθωμεν αὖθις ἐπ' ἐκεῖνον τὸν λόγον ὅθεν εἰς τοῦτον
ἐξέβημεν, ὡς ἄρα ὁ Χρύσιππος ἐναντιολογούμενος ἑαυτῷ παρὰ
πόδας οὐκ αἰσθάνεται, καθάπερ ἐπεδείξαμεν, διά τε τοῦ περὶ τῆς φωνῆς
λόγου καὶ τοῦ φάσκειν ἐνίοτε μὲν οὐδεμίαν αἴσθησιν ἡμῖν γίγνεσθαι
τοῦ περιέχοντος τόπου τὸ ἡγεμονικόν, ἐνίοτε δὲ φαίνεσθαι λέγειν αὐτόν.
ἀλλὰ γὰρ οὐδὲ τοῦτ' αὐτὸ πρόκειταί μοι νῦν ἀποδεικνύειν, ὅτι μὴ πάρ-
εργον. |

273 8. Ἀλλ' ἦν ἐξ ἀρχῆς τὸ προκείμενον ἐν τούτῳ τῷ γράμματι τὰς
2 τέτταρας διαφορὰς ἐπιδεῖξαι τῶν λημμάτων. ἐκάλουν δὲ τὸ μὲν πρῶτον
γένος αὐτῶν ἐπιστημονικόν τε καὶ ἀποδεικτικόν, τὸ δὲ δεύτερον γυμνα-
στικόν τε καὶ ὡς ⟨ἂν⟩ Ἀριστοτέλης ὀνομάσειε διαλεκτικόν, τὸ δὲ τρίτον
πιθανόν τε καὶ ῥητορικόν, τὸ δὲ τέταρτον σοφιστικόν, ἐπεδείκνυόν τε τὰ
μὲν ἀπὸ τῶν ὑπαρχόντων τε καὶ συμβαινόντων τῇ καρδίᾳ συνιστά-
237 μενα κατὰ μὲν αὐτὸ τὸ ζητού/μενον πρᾶγμα τῶν ἐπιστημονικῶν εἶναι
λημμάτων, τὰ δ' ἄλλα σύμπαντα διαλεκτικά, τὰ δ' ἀπὸ τῶν ἔξωθεν

3–5] *cf. supra*, p. 152.30–33 *infra*, pp. 176.17–18, 23–28; 234.16–20; PHP 652.4–8 Müller   6–9] SVF II, p. 241   11–12] *cf. infra*, p. 338.1–7   27–158.2] *cf.* Prantl, Gesch. d. Logik I 570 n.   28–158.2] *cf. supra*, pp. 110.23–112.2; 116.23–31 *infra*, p. 168.14–20

6 τούτῳ *om.* H   8 ἔνθ' ἂν *scripsi*: ἔνθα H L: ἔνθα ἂν *Müller*   ᾖ τὸ ἄλογον] τὸ ἄλογον ἐστὶν H   9 ἕτοιμον L   11 ἀναβαλλομένου L   13 οὔπω] οὕτω L   16 τις] τις οὖν L: ἡτισοῦν *Müller*   22 οὐκ αἰσθάνεται] ἐπαισθάνεται L   ἀπεδεί-ξαμεν L   23 αἴσθησιν] αἰσθητικὴν L   24 ἐνίοτε] τ *ex* ντ *corr.* H   25 αὐτὸ] αὖθις L   30 *ante* καὶ *add.* καὶ ἀγύμναστον L   ἂν *hic add. Schöne, post* Ἀριστ. *Diels*   31 τὸ δὲ τέταρτον] ...τε...ρτον H   σοφιστικόν] σοφι.... H   32 ἀπὸ τῶν] ἀπ.. H: ὑπὸ τῶν L   .παρχόντων H: ἀρχόντων L   33 *ante* μὲν *add.* μόνον H   μὲν *del.* H^3?

but such a motion is clearly evident in all the affections, then it becomes clear, I think, that the reasoning part of the soul is not in the heart, but the part which is called irrational and affective is enclosed in it. And if he says that where the affective part is, there the rational is also, then he will be making a ready assumption of the very matter that has been under investigation from the start. It 19
would have been much better to give us some demonstration than to take for granted the point at issue. But neither in the first book On the Soul nor in the books On the Affections did he offer any proof that the rational part must by all means be where the irrational is; everywhere he takes this to be ready and at hand. Plato, however, gave some proofs in the fourth book of the Republic and postponed some, which he presented in the Timaeus. I shall give all of these proofs later on in this treatise. It is not my plan to prove that point 20
at this time, but to prove that the rational part of the soul, which Chrysippus himself terms 'governing part', 'mind', and 'sovereign part', is in the brain. When this has been proved, then if any other 21
power is seen to be contained in the heart and to arise from no other source, we shall have got clear possession of two of the first principles, and subsequently we shall find the third in the same way; but let that (inquiry) be postponed to the next book.

Let us now go back to the argument from which this digression 22
began, that Chrysippus in fact fails to notice that he contradicts himself straight away, as we pointed out, through his account of speech and through his asserting at one time that we have no perception of the place that contains the governing part, but at another that it is manifest. But it is not my purpose at this time to prove this point either, except incidentally.

8. From the beginning my object in this book has been to exhibit the four kinds of premises. I called the first kind of them scien- 2
tific and demonstrative, the second useful for training and, as Aristotle would say, dialectical, the third persuasive and rhetorical, and the fourth sophistical; and I showed that of the premises based on the properties and attributes of the heart, those that are pertinent to the very matter under investigation belong to the class of scientific premises, and all the rest are dialectical, that (premises) taken from

μαρτύρων ῥητορικά, τὰ δ' ὁμωνυμίαις τισὶν ἢ τοῖς τῆς λέξεως σχήμασι
πεπανουργημένα σοφιστικά.
3 Τὰ μὲν οὖν ἐπιστημονικὰ καθ' ἕκαστον πρᾶγμα παντάπασιν ὀλίγα
τε καὶ εὐαρίθμητ' ἐστί, τὰ δὲ γυμναστικὰ πάμπολλα· καθ' ἕκαστον γὰρ
4 τῶν ὑπαρχόντων τε καὶ συμβαινόντων τῷ πράγματι συνίσταται. τὸν
γοῦν ἀπὸ τῆς φωνῆς ἐρωτώμενον λόγον ἐκ τῆς θέσεως ὁρμώμενον
ἐπέδειξα· οὕτω δὲ καὶ τὸν ἀπὸ τῆς εἰσπνοῆς τε καὶ ἐκπνοῆς· ὡσαύτως
274 δ' ἔχοντα | εὑρήσεις καὶ τὸν ἀπὸ τῆς ἐν ταῖς λύπαις δήξεως· ἐναργῶς μὲν
⟨γὰρ⟩ ἡ δῆξίς ἐστιν ἐν τῷ στόματι τῆς γαστρός, οἱ δ' ἐς τὴν καρδίαν
5 ἀναφέρουσιν αὐτήν. εἰ μὲν οὖν ὅτι πλησίον ἡ καρδία τέτακται τῷ στόματι
τῆς γαστρός, διὰ τοῦτ' ἀπ' ἐκείνης ἄρχεσθαι νομίζουσι τὸ πάθος, ἀπὸ
τῆς θέσεως ἐπιχειροῦσιν· εἰ δ' αὐτὴν ὄντως οἴονται τὴν καρδίαν δάκνε-
238 6 σθαι, πάμπολυ / σφάλλονται. κάτω μὲν γὰρ τοῦ θώρακος ἡ δῆξίς ἐστιν
ὑπὸ τῷ κατὰ τὸ στέρνον χόνδρῳ, ἡ καρδία δ' ἐν μέσῳ τέτακται τῷ
θώρακι· καὶ οὐδεὶς ᾔσθετο πώποτε τῆς καρδίας αὐτῆς δακνομένης οὔτ'
ἐν λύπαις οὔτ' ἐν ἄλλῳ πάθει ψυχῆς ἢ σώματος.
7 Οὐ μὴν οὐδ' ἡ καρδιαλγία τοὔνομα τὴν ἐν τῷ θώρακι περιεχομένην
καρδίαν ὀδυνᾶσθαι δηλοῖ, ἀλλ' ἔστιν ὁμωνυμία τις οὐδένα λανθάνουσα
8 τῶν ὡμιληκότων ἀρχαίων γράμμασι. ὥσπερ γὰρ τὸ κατὰ τὸν θώρακα
σπλάγχνον, οὕτω καὶ τὸ τῆς γαστρὸς στόμα καρδίαν ὀνομάζουσιν οἱ
9 παλαιοὶ καὶ πάμπολύ γε τοὔνομά ἐστι παρ' αὐτοῖς. ἀλλ' ἐγὼ δυοῖν ἢ
τριῶν ἐπιμνησθήσομαι τῶν παραδειγμάτων ὑπὲρ τοῦ σαφῶς ἐνδείξασθαι |
275 10 τὸ σημαινόμενον ἐκ τῆς λέξεως. ὁ μὲν δὴ Νίκανδρος ὧδέ πώς φησιν·

«ἦν κραδίην ἐπιδόρπιον, οἱ δὲ δοχαίην
κλείουσι στομάχοιο.»

239 11 Θουκυδίδης δ' ὧδε· «καὶ ὁπότε εἰς τὴν καρδίαν στηρίξειεν, / ἀνέτρεπέ
τε αὐτὴν καὶ ἀποκαθάρσεις χολῆς πᾶσαι ὅσαι ὑπὸ τῶν ἰατρῶν ὠνομα-
12 σμέναι ἐπῆεσαν»· ὁ δ' Ἱπποκράτης· «γυνὴ ἐκαρδιήλγεε καὶ οὐδὲν
καθίστη· πάλην ἐς ῥοιῆς χυλὸν ἀλφίτων ἐπιπάσσουσα καὶ μονοσιτίη
ἤρκεσε καὶ ⟨οὐκ⟩ ἀνήμεεν οἷα τὰ Χαιρίωνος.»

8–160.8] *cf.* Müller, Beweis, pp. 56–57 13–15] *cf.* Nemes. De nat. hom. 20: p. 232.15–233.1 Matth. 24–25] Nicand. Alexipharm. 21–22 *cf.* A. S. F. Gow, A. F. Scholfield, Nicander, Cantab. 1953, pp. 94, 191 26–28] Thuc. ii. 49.3 28–30] Hipp. Epid. ii. 2.1: V 84 L. *cf.* Gal. De alim. fac. ii. 24: CMG V 4.2, p. 294 In Hipp. Epid. II comm. i: CMG V 10.1, pp. 198–199

1 ἢ τοῖς] ἤτοι L 2 πεπανουργευμένα L 4 πάμπολα H 6 ἐκ] . . H 7 καὶ ἐκπνοῆς] . . .κπνοῆς H 8 λοιπαῖς L δή. .ως H: δείξεως L ἐναργὴς L 9 γὰρ *add. Bas.* δεῖξις L 12 οἴονται] οἷον τε L 13 δεῖξις L 17 καρδιαλ.:α H: καρδία ἀλγεῖ L 18 τοῖς οὐδύνα L λανθάνουσα *ex* λανθάνει *(?) corr.* H: λανθάνουσι L 19 ἀρχαίοις L τὸ] τὸν L 20 γαστρὸς] καρδίας L 21 γε] τε L 22 . . .μνησθήσομαι H 24 ἦν] ἣν L καρδίην H δοχέην L 26 Θοικυδίδης H στηρί. . .εν H: στηρίξαιεν M *Ald.*: στήριξεν L: *ex Thuc. corr. Kühn* ἀνέπρεπέ L 27 τῶν *om.* L 28 ἐκραδιήλγεε L: ἐκαρδιάλγεε *Müller, Beweis, p. 57* οὐδὲ L 29 πάλην] πλὴν H: πλὴν L: *ex Hipp. corr. Müller* ῥυῆς L ἄλφιτον H L: *ex Hipp. corr. Müller* μονοσιτεῖν H: μονοσίτην L: *ex Hipp. corr. Müller* 30 οὐκ *ex Hipp. add. Corn.* ἀνήμεεν *ex* ἀνήεμεν *corr.* H[3] Χαιρίωνος] κηρίωνος H L: *ex Hipp. corr. Diels*: Χαρίωνος *Corn.*

external witnesses are rhetorical, and those that fraudulently exploit
certain homonyms or forms of expression are sophistical.

Now the scientific (premises) pertaining to any matter are very 3
few and easily enumerated, but those that are useful for training
are many, for they are formed from every property and attribute
of a thing. Thus I pointed out that the argument based on speech 4
starts from position, and this is true also of the argument based on
inhalation and exhalation. And you will find that it is the same with
the argument from the pain that accompanies distress of mind; for
the pain is clearly at the mouth of the stomach, but they refer it to
the heart. Now if they hold that because the heart is placed close 5
to the mouth of the stomach, therefore the affection begins from
the heart, they are arguing from position; but if they think that the
pain is actually in the heart itself, they are quite mistaken. For the 6
pain is below the thorax under the cartilage of the sternum, whereas
the heart is placed in the middle of the thorax; and no one has ever
perceived the heart itself suffering pain either in distress or in any other
disorder of soul or body.

Nor does the term 'heartburn' signify that the heart enclosed 7
in the thorax suffers pain; there is here an identity of names that
deceives no one who is familiar with the writings of the ancients.
For the ancients called not only the organ in the chest but also the 8
mouth of the stomach the 'heart', and they often used the word in
this meaning. I shall cite two or three examples in order to show this 9
meaning clearly through the wording of the texts. Nicander speaks 10
as follows:

"which some call the digestive 'heart', others
the gullet's receptacle;"

and Thucydides says, "and when it settled in the 'heart' it upset 11
it, and all the discharges of bile that have been named by the physi-
cians ensued". Hippocrates (also writes), "A woman suffered heart- 12
burn and nothing relieved her; sprinkling the finest barley meal into
pomegranate juice and eating once a day, she warded it off; and she
did not vomit as Chairion did."

13 Ἅπαντες οὗτοι δηλοῦσιν ἐναργῶς τὸ στόμα τῆς γαστρὸς ὀνομά-
ζεσθαι καρδίαν. ὥστε ταύτης μὲν τῆς καρδίας εἴη ἄν τι πάθος ἡ καρδιαλ-
γία, τοῦ σπλάγχνου δ' ὑπὲρ οὗ πρόκειται σκοπεῖν, εἰ τὸ κυριεῦον τῆς
ψυχῆς μόριον ἐν ἑαυτῷ περιέχει, τοιοῦτον πάθος οὐδέποτε γίγνεται.
14 οὐδὲ γὰρ οὐδ' αὐτοῦ τοῦ στόματος τῆς γαστρὸς ἅπαν ἄλγημα
καρδιαλγίαν προσαγορεύουσιν, ἀλλὰ μόνον ἐπειδὰν ὑπὸ δριμέων ὑγρῶν
15 ἐρεθίζηταί τε καὶ ἀναδάκνηται. τοῦτο δ' αὐτῷ συμβαίνει ἐν ταῖς λύπαις·
276 240 διὸ | καὶ χολὴν / ἐμοῦσιν οἱ λυπηθέντες, ἐν οἷς δ' ὑπέρχεται κάτω καὶ ἡ
16 γαστὴρ αὐτοῖς ἄκρατα χολώδη διαχωρεῖ. συμβαίνει δὲ οὐ μόνον τοῖς
λυπηθεῖσιν ἀλλὰ καὶ τῶν ἐπὶ πλέον ἀσιτησάντων οὐκ ὀλίγοις δάκνεσθαι
τὸ τῆς γαστρὸς στόμα καὶ μᾶλλον εἰ σφοδρῶς προγεγυμνασμένοι μὴ
17 προσενέγκοιντο σιτία. τοῖς τε γὰρ λυπηθεῖσι καὶ τοῖς γυμνασαμένοις
εὐτονώτερον εἰς τὴν γαστέρα συρρεῖ χολὴ ξανθή· πρὸς ταύτης οὖν
18 δακνόμενοι καρδιαλγοῦσιν. οὐδ' ἐστὶν ἀναγκαῖον ἐν τῷδε τῷ λόγῳ τὴν
αἰτίαν ἐπισκέπτεσθαι δι' ἣν τοῦτο συμβαίνει· μόνον γάρ μοι πρόκειται
δεῖξαι κατά γε τὸ παρὸν ὡς οὐκ ἔστι τῆς καρδίας τοῦ σπλάγχνου τὸ
πάθος ἡ καρδιαλγία, καθάπερ οὐδὲ τὸ δάκνεσθαι κατὰ τὰς λύπας,
ἀλλὰ τὸ μὲν σύμπτωμα τοῦ στόματος τῆς γαστρός, ἐπικεχείρηται δὲ
ἀπὸ τῆς κατὰ τὴν θέσιν ἐγγύτητος, ὥσπερ γε καὶ τὸ πάλλεσθαι τὴν
καρδίαν ἐν τοῖς φόβοις ἀπὸ συμβεβηκότος ἐπιχειρεῖται, ὧν ἑκάτερον οὐκ
19 ἔστιν ἐπιστημονικόν. εἰ δὲ συγχωρηθείη τοιοῦτον ὑπάρχειν, οὐ Στωϊ-
241 κοῖς καὶ Περιπατητικοῖς, ἀλλ' Ἱπποκράτει / καὶ Πλάτωνι
277 μαρτυρεῖ, καθάπερ καὶ ὁπόσα τοῖς θυμουμένοις ὁ | Χρύσιππος γράφει
20 συμπίπτειν ἔν τε τῷ θώρακι παντὶ καὶ κατὰ τὴν καρδίαν. ἄχρι γὰρ
ἂν ἐν μὲν τῷ διδάσκειν τε καὶ μανθάνειν καὶ ὅλως κινεῖσθαι τὴν ψυχὴν
κατ' ἐπιστήμην τινὰ μηδὲν ἐπιδεικνύωσι συμβαῖνον τῇ καρδίᾳ, κατὰ
δὲ τὰ πάθη δεικνύωσιν, οὐ μόνον οὐκ ἀνατρέπουσι τὸν παλαιὸν λόγον
ἀλλὰ καὶ κατασκευάζουσιν.
21 Τὰ μὲν δὴ τοιαῦτα τῶν ἐπιχειρημάτων ἐκ τοῦ δευτέρου γένους ἐστὶ
τῶν λημμάτων, ὥσπερ οἶμαι καὶ τὸ πρώτην ἁπάντων τῶν μορίων τοῦ
22 ζῴου διαπλάττεσθαι τὴν καρδίαν. οὐ γὰρ τὴν κατὰ δύναμιν ἀρχὴν
ἐνδείκνυται τοῦτο συγχωρηθὲν ὑπὲρ ἧς νῦν ζητοῦμεν, ἀλλὰ τὴν κατὰ
γένεσιν. — εἴρηται δέ μοι καὶ διώρισται σαφῶς ὑπὲρ τῆς διαφορᾶς τῶν
23 ἀρχῶν ἐν τῷ πρόσθεν λόγῳ. — τὸ μέντοι πρώτην μὲν ἁπάντων ἄρχε-
σθαι κινεῖσθαι τῶν τοῦ ζῴου μορίων αὐτήν, ὑστάτην δὲ παύεσθαι τῶν
24 ἀποδεικτικῶν ἐστι λημμάτων. ἐνδείκνυται γὰρ ἀρχὴν εἶναι κινήσεως αὐ-
242 τήν, οὐ μὴν ἁπάσης γε, ἀλλὰ μόνης τῆς κατὰ τοὺς σφυγμούς, / ἥτις

31–34] libri primi test., *v. supra*, p. 66.27–29 *cf. infra*, PHP 543.12–14 Müller

1 γαστρὸς *ex* καρδίας *corr.* L 3 δ' *om.* L 6 καρδιαλγίαν *ex* καρδίαν *corr.* H[3] 7 αὐτὸ L 8 ἐν οἷς *in* ἐνίοις *mut.* H[3] δ' *om.* L καὶ[II] *om.* L 9 ἄκρατα] ἄκρα τὰ H 13 εὐτονώτερον] εὐ *in* ἐν *mut.* L[2] 15 προὔκειτο L 16 τῇ καρ[δ'] L 21 *post* δὲ *add.* καὶ *Müller* 23 καθ. .ερ H 24 τῷ] . . H 25 ἂν *om.* L 26 ἐπιδεικνύουσι H : ἐπιδείκνυσι L : *corr. Kühn* συμβαίνειν L 26–27 κατὰ δὲ] καὶ τάδε L 27 δεικνύουσιν H L : *corr. Kühn* 37 *ante* τῆς *add.* γε L ἥτις] ἡ τῆς L

All these (passages) clearly reveal that the mouth of the stomach 13
was called the 'heart'. Heartburn would thus be an affection of this
'heart'; but the organ that we are now investigating, in order to deter-
mine whether it contains in itself the sovereign part of the soul,
never experiences anything of the kind. Furthermore, not even the 14
mouth of the stomach is said to suffer heartburn at every pain,
but only when it is disturbed and irritated by acrid fluids. This is 15
what happens to it in distress of mind, and this is why distressed per-
sons vomit bile; but in some the bile goes downward, and their stom-
ach passes unmixed bilious excrement. And not only the distressed, 16
but also many who have fasted excessively experience an irritation
at the mouth of the stomach, and even more if they do not eat after
violent exercise. For yellow bile collects in the stomachs of persons 17
who are distressed or have exercised too strenuously; and being irri-
tated by it, they suffer heartburn. My present argument does not 18
require that I investigate the reason why this happens; for my only
purpose at present is to show that neither heartburn nor the irri-
tation in distress is an affection of the heart – the internal organ –,
but that the symptom is in the mouth of the stomach and the argu-
ment is from proximity in position, and similarly, that the argument
from the palpitation of the heart in fear is from an attribute; and neither
of them is scientific. And if one should grant that this latter argument 19
is scientific, it does not support the Stoics and Peripatetics, but
Hippocrates and Plato; and the same is true of all the symptoms
that Chrysippus writes about in the whole thorax and in the re-
gion of the heart when a person is inflamed with anger. For as long as 20
they do not show something happening to the heart when the soul is
teaching and learning and generally moving in accordance with
some science, but only show something happening to it in the affec-
tions, not only do they not refute the ancient view, they even con-
firm it.

Arguments of this kind are from the second class of premises, 21
and with them, I think, the argument that the heart is the first of
all the parts of the animal to take form. For this (premise), if granted, 22
does not point to the beginning that pertains to power, which is what
we are now looking for, but that which pertains to origin. – In the
preceding book I discussed and clearly distinguished the different
kinds of beginnings. – But it is a scientific premise that the heart 23
is the first of all the parts of the animal to begin to move, and the
last to stop; for it indicates that the heart is a beginning of motion, 24
not, indeed, of all motion, but only of the motion of the pulse, which

ἑτέρου γένους ἐστὶ τῆς κατὰ προαίρεσιν· ἐκείνης δ' οὔτ' ἄρχεσθαι πρώ-
278 25 την οὔθ' ὑστάτην | παύεσθαι τὴν καρδίαν ἔχει τις δεῖξαι. περαίνοιτ' ἂν
οὖν κἀκ τούτου τοῦ λήμματος οὐχ ὅπερ Ἀριστοτέλης τε καὶ Χρύ-
σιππος ὑπολαμβάνουσιν, ἀλλ' ὃ Πλάτωνι καὶ Ἱπποκράτει δοκεῖ,
τῆς μὲν κατὰ προαίρεσιν ἐν ἡμῖν κινήσεως ἀρχὴν εἶναι τὸν ἐγκέφαλον,
ἑτέρας δέ τινος ἀπροαιρέτου τὴν καρδίαν.
26 Ἦν μὲν οὖν καὶ ταῦθ' ἱκανὰ πρὸς ἀπόδειξιν τῶν προκειμένων, ἀλλ'
ἐπειδὴ προὐθέμην ἐν τῷδε τῷ βιβλίῳ τὰ λήμματα ἐπελθεῖν ἅπαντα τὰ
λαμβανόμενα ἐκ τῶν ὑπαρχόντων τῇ καρδίᾳ, προσθεὶς ἔτι τὰ ὑπόλοιπα
27 καταπαύσω τὸν λόγον. ἐπ' αὐτοῖς δ' ἐστὶ καὶ τὸ τοῦ Ἀριστοτέλους
λῆμμα, περὶ οὗ κατὰ τὴν τελευτὴν τοῦ πρώτου βιβλίου διῆλθον, ἐκ τῶν
ὑπαρχόντων τῇ καρδίᾳ· πλῆθος γάρ τι νεύρων ἐν αὐτῇ φαίνεσθαί φησιν.
28 ἐδείχθη δ' ὑφ' ἡμῶν ὡς νευρώδη μέν τινα σώματα κατὰ τὴν καρδίαν εἴη,
243 νεῦρα δ' οὐκ εἴη, καὶ ὡς τὰ μὲν νευρώδη τῇ τοῦ σώ/ματος ἰδέᾳ μόνον ἔοικε
τοῖς νεύροις, οὐκ ἐνεργείᾳ τε καὶ χρείᾳ, κρίνεσθαι δὲ προσήκει τὴν ἐν τοῖς
ὀργάνοις ἑτερότητα καὶ ταὐτότητα ταῖς ἐνεργείαις καὶ ταῖς χρείαις αὐτῶν.
279 29 ὥστ' οὐδὲν ἔτι περὶ τῶν | αὐτῶν δέομαι διέρχεσθαι, μεταβήσομαι δ' ἐπί τι
τῶν ὑπολοίπων, οὗ σχεδὸν ἅπαντες μεμνημονεύκασιν οἷς ἡ καρδία
30 πασῶν τῶν δυνάμεων ἀρχὴ τῶν ἐν τοῖς ζῴοις ὑπείληπται. λέγουσι γὰρ
ὅθεν ἡ τοῦ τρέφεσθαι τοῖς ζῴοις ἀρχή, κατ' ἐκεῖνο τὸ μόριον εἶναι καὶ τὸ
λογιζόμενον τῆς ψυχῆς· ἐν καρδίᾳ δ' εἶναι τὴν τοῦ τρέφεσθαι τοῖς ζῴοις
ἀρχήν, ὥστε καὶ τὸ λογιζόμενόν τε καὶ διανοούμενον ὑπάρχειν ἐν αὐτῇ.
31 ψεύδονται δ' ἐν ἀμφοτέροις τοῖς λήμμασιν. οὔτε γὰρ ἐν καρδίᾳ τὴν ἀρχὴν
τοῦ τρέφεσθαι τοῖς ζῴοις εἶναι συγχωροῦμεν — ἀλλ' ἕν τι καὶ τοῦτ' ἔστι
τῶν ἐν τῇδε τῇ πραγματείᾳ προκειμένων εἰς τὴν σκέψιν, οὐ χρὴ δὲ τὸ
ζητούμενον ὡς ὁμολογούμενον λαμβάνειν —, οὔτε τὸ μίαν ἀρχὴν ἀμφοτέρων
ὑπάρχειν τῶν δυνάμεων, ἀλλὰ καὶ τούτου τὸ ἐναντίον ἡμεῖς ἀποδείκνυμεν.
244 32 θαυμάζω τοίνυν / κἀνταῦθα τῶν ἀνδρῶν, εἰ ἄμφω τὰ ζητούμενα προχείρως
λαμβάνουσιν οὐδεμίαν ἀπόδειξιν προστιθέντες.
33 Ὅμοιον δέ τι ποιοῦσι κἀπειδὰν ὅθεν ἡ ἀρχὴ τῆς τροφῆς ἐστιν
ἐνταῦθ' εἶναι φάσκωσι καὶ τὸ ἡγεμονικόν, εἶθ' ἑξῆς προσλαμβάνωσιν
280 34 ὡς ἐν τῇ | καρδίᾳ τῆς τροφῆς ἐστιν ἀρχή. οὔτε γὰρ τοῦτ' ἀληθές· «ἀρχὴ»
γὰρ «τροφῆς καὶ ὑγρᾶς καὶ ξηρᾶς στόμα, στόμαχος, κοιλίη» φησὶν
Ἱπποκράτης, οὔτ' εἰ καὶ παντὸς μᾶλλον, ἂν ἐξ ἀνάγκης ἠκολούθει,
καθ' ὃ μόριον ἡ ἀρχὴ τῆς τροφῆς ἐστι, κατὰ τοῦτο ὑπάρχειν τὸν λογι-

12] *cf. supra*, p. 92.2–3 13–14] *cf. supra*, p. 92.21–22 15–16] *cf. supra*, p. 92.23–25 17–22] SVF II, p. 241 32–33] Hipp. De alim. 30: CMG I 1, p. 82.11–12 = p. 144.12–13 Joly

1 ἑτερογενοῦς L 4 ἀλλ' ὃ] ἀλλὰ L 10 ἐπ'] ἐν *Müller* 11 οὗ] ὧν H L: *corr. Ald.* 12 ἑαυτῇ L 14 τῇ *om.* H 16 *post* ἑτερότητα *add.* τε L 17 τι] τὸ L 18 οἷς] ἧς L 19 ἀρχὴ *ex* ἄρχει *corr.* H³ τοῖς *om.* L γὰρ *om.* L 22 *ante* διανοούμενον *add.* τὸ L 23 ἐν ἀμφοτέροις] ἀμφότεροι L 24 τούτων L 29 προτιθέντες H 31 φάσκουσι L προσλαμβάνουσιν H L: *corr. Kühn* 32 τοῦτ' ἀληθές] τἀληθές L 33 στόμα *om.* L κοιλίη] κοινῇ L 34 *post* μᾶλλον *add.* ἀληθὲς ἦν, οὐδ' οὕτως *Schöne* *post* ἂν *add.* ἡ L ἠκολούθει ἐξ ἀνάγκης H 35 ἡ *om.* L

differs in kind from voluntary motion. No one can show that the heart is the first to begin voluntary motion, or the last to stop it.
This premise too, therefore, does not prove the supposition made by 25
Aristotle and Chrysippus, but rather the view of Plato and Hippocrates, that the brain is the beginning of voluntary motion in us, while the heart (is the beginning) of some other motion, which is not voluntary.

Now these (considerations) would be sufficient to prove what I 26
set out to prove; but since I proposed to review in this book all the premises taken from the properties of the heart, I shall add those
that remain and then bring the book to a close. In addition, the 27
premise of Aristotle that I discussed at the end of the first book is also from the properties of the heart; for he says that a certain quan-
tity of nerves is observed in it. We pointed out that there are some 28
nerve-like bodies in the heart, but they are not nerves, and also that these nerve-like bodies are like nerves in bodily form only, not in activity and use, and the difference and sameness of organs are properly
judged in terms of their activities and uses. There is therefore no 29
need for me to go over the same material again, and I shall pass to one of the remaining arguments, which almost everyone has mentioned who supposed that the heart is the source of all the powers in animals.
They say that the member from which comes the source of nourish- 30
ment for animals contains also the reasoning part of the soul; the source of nourishment for animals is in the heart; therefore, the part
of the soul that reasons and thinks is in it also. But they are mistaken 31
in both (their) premises. We concede neither that nourishment begins for animals in the heart – this too is one of the things that we propose to investigate in this treatise, and a matter that is being inquired into must not be taken as agreed upon –, nor that both powers have a single source; we even demonstrate that the opposite of this is true.
So here again I marvel at the men, if they readily assume both of 32
the matters in question without adding any proof.

They do something similar also when they assert that the member 33
from which comes the source of nutriment also contains the governing part, then add as a further premise that the source of nutriment is in
the heart. This added premise is not true, for, in Hippocrates' 34
words, "The source of nutriment, both wet and dry, is the mouth, the gullet, the belly"; and even if it were truest of all, it would not necessarily follow that the member in which the source of nutriment is should also have in it the reasoning faculty, for that is one of the

35 σμόν· τοῦτο γὰρ ἕν τι τῶν ζητουμένων ἐστί. τὸ δ' ἕτερον τῶν ζητουμένων
ψεῦδος. ἡ μὲν γὰρ πρώτη τῆς τροφῆς ἀρχὴ «στόμα, στόμαχος, κοιλίη», ἡ
δευτέρα δ' αἱ ἐξ ἥπατος εἰς κοιλίην καθήκουσαι φλέβες, ἐν αἷς πρώταις
αἷμα γίγνεται, ἡ τρίτη δὲ τὸ ἧπαρ αὐτό, ἡ τετάρτη δὲ μετὰ τὸ ἧπαρ ἡ
κοίλη φλέψ, ἐν ᾗ πρώτῃ καθαρὸν τῶν περιττωμάτων ἀπολείπεται τὸ /
245 αἷμα, παρὰ ταύτης δ' ἤδη τῆς φλεβός, ὥσπερ τἆλλα τοῦ ζῴου μόρια
πάντα, κατὰ τὸν αὐτὸν τρόπον καὶ ἡ καρδία λαμβάνει τὴν τροφήν.
36 Οὐ μὴν οὐδ' ὅταν εἴπωσιν ὅθεν ἡ χορηγία τοῦ πνεύματος, ἐνταῦθ'
εἶναι τὸ ἡγεμονικόν, εἶτ' ἐπ' αὐτῷ προσλαμβάνωσιν ἐκ τῆς καρδίας
37 χορηγεῖσθαι τὸ πνεῦμα, συγχωρητέον αὐτοῖς. καὶ γὰρ κἀνταῦθα πάλιν,
281 εἰ μὲν τὸ ψυχικὸν πνεῦμά φασιν ἐκ τῆς καρδίας ἄρχεσθαι, | τὸ ζητούμενον
αὐτὸ λαμβάνουσιν· εἰ δὲ τὸ ζωτικόν, οὐκ ἐξ ἀνάγκης ἀκολουθήσει τὴν
38 αὐτὴν ἀρχὴν ἀμφοτέροις ὑπάρχειν. Ἐρασίστρατος γοῦν οὐχ ἁπλῶς,
ὥσπερ οὗτοι, τὸ ζητούμενον λαμβάνων ἀλλὰ μετὰ κατασκευῆς λόγων
οὐκ ὀλίγων ἐκ μὲν τῆς κεφαλῆς φησι τὸ ψυχικόν, ἐκ δὲ τῆς καρδίας τὸ
39 ζωτικὸν ὁρμᾶσθαι πνεῦμα. εἰ δ' οὐδέτερον μὲν τούτων τῶν πνευμάτων
ἠρωτῆσθαι κατὰ τὸν λόγον ἐροῦσι, τὸ δὲ ἀνάλογον τῇ ξηρᾷ καὶ ὑγρᾷ
τροφῇ, τὸ προσαγορευόμενον ὑλικόν, ἀκούσονται καὶ περὶ τοῦδε παρ'
246 Ἱπποκράτους· / «ἀρχὴ τροφῆς πνεύματος στόμα, ῥῖνες, βρόγχος,
40 πνεύμων, καὶ ἡ ἄλλη διαπνοή.» οὔκουν οὔτε τούτων τῶν λόγων ἰσχυρὸς
οὐδεὶς οὔθ' ὅταν ὁ Διογένης εἴπῃ «ὃ πρῶτον τροφῆς καὶ πνεύματος
ἀρύεται, ἐν τούτῳ ὑπάρχει τὸ ἡγεμονικόν, ὃ δὲ πρῶτον τροφῆς καὶ
41 πνεύματος ἀρύεται, ἡ καρδία». τὸ γὰρ πρῶτον ἐρωτήσομεν ὅπως λέγει.
εἰ μὲν γὰρ ὡς ὄργανον πρῶτον, οὐδαμῶς ἡ καρδία τροφῆς καὶ πνεύματος
282 ἀρύεται πρώτη, ἀλλὰ τροφῆς μὲν «στόμα, | στόμαχος, κοιλίη», πνεύματος
42 δὲ «στόμα, ῥῖνες, βρόγχος, πνεύμων»· εἰ δ' ὡς ὅθεν ἡ ἀρχὴ τῆς κινήσεώς
ἐστι τοῖς ἀρυομένοις, ἀληθὲς μὲν τὸ πρότερον λῆμμα, τοῦ δευτέρου δ'
ἀντιληψόμεθα φάσκοντες αὐτὸ τὸ ζητούμενον ἑτοίμως λαμβάνειν αὐτόν.
43 ἡμεῖς μὲν γὰρ ἀπὸ κεφαλῆς πεμφθήσεσθαι τὴν ἀρχὴν ὁμολογοῦμεν τῆς
κινήσεως, ἐπειδὰν ἐσθίειν ἢ πίνειν ἢ ἀναπνεῖν βουλώμεθα. ὁ Διογένης
247 δὲ τοῦτο λαβὼν χωρὶς ἀποδείξεως ἀμφισβήτησιν πεποίη/κεν ἰδίαν.
44 κατὰ τὸν αὐτὸν δὲ τρόπον καθ' ἑαυτοῦ τοῖς λόγοις ἐχρήσατο. «τό» φησι

8–10] SVF II, p. 241   13–16] *cf. supra*, p. 78.24–26   19–20] Hipp. De alim. 30: CMG I 1, p. 82.10–11 = p. 144.11–12 Joly   19] Gal. De respir. usu 5: IV 504 K.   20–23] SVF III, p. 216   25] *cf. supra*, p. 162.33   26] *cf. supra*, lin. 19–20   32–166.7] SVF III, p. 216 *cf.* F. L. Ganter, Philologus 53 (1894), p. 475

1 ἑτέρα *(ut vid.)* L   2 στόμα *om.* L   3 αἱ *om.* L   4 αἷμα] ἅμα L   7 καὶ *om.* H   8 ὅθεν *ex* ὅταν *corr.* H³   9 εἶτ'] εἴτε L   προσλαμβάνουσιν H: *corr. Kühn*: προσλάβωσιν L   13 *ante* ἀμφοτέροις *add.* ἐν H   γοῦν] γὰρ L   15 ὀλίγων] ὀλίγης ἀλλ' L   18 προσαγόμενον L   20 τῶν λόγων τούτων L   22 ἀρρύεται L   ἐν – 23 ἀρύεται *om.* L   23 ἐρωτήσωμεν H L: *corr. Chart.*   25 ἀρρύεται L   τροφὴ L   27 ἀρυομένοις] ἀρχομένοις L   *ante* δευτέρου *add. et del.* δε H   δ' *om.* L   29 πεμφθήσεσθαι – 166.4 εἶναι *om.* L, *lac. fere 170 litt. rel.*   ὁμολογοῦμεν – 166.3 τρέφον *om.* H, *lac. fere 365 litt. rel.*, *suppl.* H⁸, *post* τρέφον *spat. fere 75 litt. rel.*   31 ἀμβισβήτησιν H⁸: *corr. Ald.*   32 καθ'] καὶ H⁸: *corr. Müller*   φησι] φύσει H⁸: *corr. Ricci Al. Just.*

matters for inquiry. But the premise that is different from the ques- 35
tions at issue is false, for the first source of nutriment is "the mouth,
the gullet, the belly"; the second is the veins descending from the
liver to the belly, in which nutriment first becomes blood; third is
the liver itself; fourth after the liver is the vena cava, where first
the blood is rendered free of impurities; and when that stage is
reached, the heart, like all the other parts of the animal, draws from
this vein its nutriment.

We must not agree with them either when they say that the 36
ruling part is in the member from which the supply of pneuma
comes, then add to this the premise that pneuma is supplied from the
heart. For here again, if they say that the psychic pneuma begins 37
from the heart, they are assuming the very matter that is under
investigation; if (they say) vital pneuma, it will not necessarily follow
that both (pneumas) have the same source. Thus Erasistratus 38
does not simply assume the matter in question, as they do, but sup-
ports with no few arguments his assertion that psychic (pneuma)
starts from the head, and vital pneuma from the heart. And if they 39
say that neither of these pneumas is meant in the argument, but
rather the so-called material pneuma, which is analogous to dry and
moist nutriment, they will learn about this too from Hippocrates:
"The source of the nourishment of pneuma is mouth, nostrils, wind-
pipe, lungs, and breathing generally." None of these arguments, 40
then, is valid, nor is that in which Diogenes says, "The governing
part is the member which first draws in nutriment and pneuma;
and the member which first draws in nutriment and pneuma is the
heart." For we shall ask what he means by first. If he means the 41
first instrument, the heart is by no means the first to draw in nutri-
ment and pneuma; for nutriment it is "mouth, gullet, belly", and for
pneuma, "mouth, nostrils, windpipe, lungs". But if by 'first' he means 42
that from which comes the beginning of motion in the parts that
draw them in, then his first premise is true, but we shall challenge
the second on the ground that he is readily assuming the very matter
that is under investigation. For we assent to the view that the be- 43
ginning of motion will be sent from the head whenever we wish
to eat or drink or breathe; and Diogenes, by making his assumption
without demonstration, has created a private controversy. In the 44
same way he also used arguments against himself. He says: "That

«κινοῦν τὸν ἄνθρωπον τὰς κατὰ προαίρεσιν κινήσεις ψυχική τίς ἐστιν ἀναθυμίασις, πᾶσα δὲ ἀναθυμίασις ἐκ τῆς τροφῆς ἀνάγεται, ὥστε τὸ κινοῦν πρῶτον τὰς κατὰ προαίρεσιν κινήσεις καὶ τὸ τρέφον ἡμᾶς ἀνάγκη ἓν καὶ ταὐτὸν εἶναι.»

45 Ὅταν ταῦτα ὁ Διογένης γράφῃ περὶ μὲν τοῦ τὴν οὐσίαν εἶναι τῆς ψυχῆς ἀναθυμίασιν, εἴτ' οὖν ἐκ τροφῆς εἴτ' ἐκ πνεύματος, οὐδὲν ἔν γε τῷ παρόντι φήσομεν ἀμφισβητεῖν, ἵνα μὴ τὰ πάντα λυπῶμεν τὸν ἄνδρα,
283 περὶ δὲ τοῦ ταὐτὸν εἶναι τὸ κινοῦν | πρῶτον ἡμᾶς τὰς κατὰ προαίρεσιν
46 κινήσεις καὶ τὸ τρέφον ἀντιληψόμεθα. τοὐναντίον γὰρ ἅπαν ἐξ ὧν ὑπέθετο περαίνεσθαι φήσομεν, ἐξ αἵματος μὲν ὁμολογοῦντες ⟨. . .⟩.
248 47 καὶ αὐτὸς ἐπιλανθανόμενος / τῶν οἰκείων δογμάτων αἷμά φησιν εἶναι
48 τὴν ψυχήν, ὡς Ἐμπεδοκλῆς καὶ Κριτίας ὑπέλαβον. εἰ δέ γε ἕποιτο Κλεάνθει καὶ Χρυσίππῳ καὶ Ζήνωνι τρέφεσθαι μὲν ἐξ αἵματος φήσαντι τὴν ψυχήν, οὐσίαν δ' αὐτῆς ὑπάρχειν τὸ πνεῦμα, πῶς ἔτι ταὐτὸν ἔσται
49 τὸ τρέφον τε καὶ κινοῦν εἴπερ τρέφει μὲν τὸ αἷμα κινεῖ δὲ τὸ πνεῦμα; ὥστε πρὸς τοῖς ἄλλοις ἀτόποις καὶ ἀπέραντός ἐστιν ὁ τοῦ Διογένους λόγος.
50 ὃ γὰρ ἐπιφέρει τοῖς ὑποτεθεῖσι λήμμασιν, οὐκ ἐξ ἀνάγκης ἕπεται. δειχθήσεται δὲ ἐπὶ πλέον ὑπὲρ αὐτοῦ διὰ τῶν ἐξῆς ὑπομνημάτων. ἐν μὲν γὰρ τῷ παρόντι δοκῶ μοι καιρὸν εἶναι καταπαύειν ἐνταῦθα τὸ βιβλίον.
51 ὑποσχόμενος γὰρ περὶ τῶν ἐναργῶς φαινομένων ὑπάρχειν τῇ καρδίᾳ
284 τὸν λόγον ἐν τῷδε τῷ γράμματι ποιήσασθαι, | τί ἂν ἔτι δεοίμην ἐφάπτεσθαι τοιούτων ἐπιχειρημάτων ὧν δόγματα μᾶλλον, οὐ τὸ φαινόμενον ἐκ τῆς ἀνατομῆς, ἡ ἀρχὴ τῆς συστάσεώς ἐστιν; /||

11–15] SVF III, p. 216 12–14] SVF I, pp. 38, 117–118

1 *post* κινοῦν *add.* πρῶτον *Müller* ψυχικῆς H[s]: *corr. Chart.* 5 *post* μὲν *add.* οὖν H 6 ἐκ[II] *om.* L 10 *post* ὁμολογοῦντες *spatium fere 150 litt. reliquit* H, *in quo loco* οὐ λείπ(ει) *scripsit* H[s]. *Supplenda autem huiusmodi quaedam:* τρέφεσθαι τὸν ἄνθρωπον, ὑπ' ἀναθυμιάσεως δὲ κινεῖσθαι τὰς κατὰ προαίρεσιν κινήσεις, ἐκ τούτων δὲ περαίνοντες ὅτι τὸ τρέφον ἐξ ἀνάγκης ἕτερόν ἐστι τοῦ κινοῦντος. 11 καὶ — 19 βιβλίον *om.* L, *lac. 95 litt. rel.* 13 κλεαν[θ]' H: *corr.* R[2] *Ald.* φήσαν[τ] H: *corr.* F[2]: φήσασι *Wachsmuth* 15 τε καὶ] καὶ τὸ *v. Arnim* 20 περὶ] ὑπὸ L ὑπαρχόντων L 23 τῆς[II] *om.* L γα(ληνοῦ) περὶ τῶν ἱπποκράτ(ους) καὶ πλάτ(ω)ν(ος) δογμάτων δεύτερον (δεύτ. *non habet* H) *subscr.* H L

which causes a man to make voluntary movements is a certain psychic
vaporization; but every vaporization arises from nutriment; there-
fore, that which first causes voluntary movements and that which
nourishes us is necessarily one and the same."

When Diogenes writes this, we shall say that for the moment 45
we do not challenge his saying that the substance of the soul is a
vaporization, whether from nutriment or from pneuma, lest we cause
him complete distress; but we shall contest the statement that what
first causes us to make voluntary movements and what nourishes
us are the same. For we shall say that the conclusion to be drawn 46
from the premises he posited is the very opposite; we agree that +man
is nourished+ from blood +and performs voluntary movements through
the agency of vaporization, but from this we conclude that what
nourishes us is necessarily different from what moves us+[1]. And he 47
himself forgot the doctrines of his own school when he said that the
soul is blood, as Empedocles and Critias had supposed. But if he 48
should follow Cleanthes, Chrysippus and Zeno, who say that
the soul is nourished from blood, but its substance is the pneuma,
how will the source of nourishment and the cause of motion remain
the same, since it is the blood that nourishes and the pneuma that
causes motion? So in addition to his other absurdities, Diogenes' 49
reasoning is invalid; for the conclusion that he draws from the prem-
ises he posits does not necessarily follow from them. His argument 50
will be examined at greater length in the books that follow. For the
present, I think it is time to end this book here. I promised to give in it 51
an account of the clearly observable properties of the heart; why,
then, must I be further concerned with arguments such as these,
that rather take opinions, not anatomical observations, as their start-
ing-point?

[1] +man – nourished+ ... +and – us+: These words translate a proposed restoration. See the app. crit.

ΓΑΛΗΝΟΥ

ΠΕΡΙ ΤΩΝ ΙΠΠΟΚΡΑΤΟΥΣ ΚΑΙ ΠΛΑΤΩΝΟΣ ΔΟΓΜΑΤΩΝ

ΒΙΒΛΙΟΝ ΤΡΙΤΟΝ

249 285 1. Ὅτι μὲν ἀναγκαῖόν ἐστιν οὐ φιλοσόφοις μόνον ἀλλὰ καὶ ἰατροῖς
ὅσοι γε μὴ ἀλογίστως ἅπτονται τῆς τέχνης, ἐσκέφθαι περὶ τῶν διοικου-
σῶν ἡμᾶς δυνάμεων ὁπόσαι τέ εἰσι κατὰ γένος ὁποία τέ τις ἑκάστη κατ'
εἶδος ἐν τίνι τε μάλιστα τοῦ ζῴου μορίῳ καθίδρυται, διὰ τοῦ πρώτου
2 δέδεικται λόγου, ὅτι δ' οἱ κάλλιστα περὶ αὐτῶν ἀποφηνάμενοι Πλάτων
286 τε καὶ Ἱπποκράτης εἰσίν, ἐρρέθη | μὲν οὐκ ὀλίγα καὶ διὰ τοῦ πρώτου
βιβλίου, τελεώτατα δὲ ἐπεξῆλθον τῷ λόγῳ κατὰ τὸ δεύτερον γράμμα
τὰς διαφορὰς ἁπάντων τῶν λημμάτων ἐκθέμενος οἷς ἐχρήσαντο περὶ τοῦ
3 προκειμένου δόγματος οἱ ἐπιφανέστατοι τῶν φιλοσόφων. ἀναγκαῖον δέ
250 μοι δοκεῖ καὶ / νῦν ἔτι περὶ αὐτῶν ἀναμνήσαντι περαίνειν οὕτω τὸν
4 ὑπόλοιπον λόγον. τέτταρας ἔλεγον εἶναι τὰς πάσας διαφορὰς τῶν λημ-
μάτων· ἔνια μὲν γὰρ αὐτῶν ἀπὸ τῶν ὑπαρχόντων τῷ μορίῳ λαμβάνεσθαι
κατὰ τὴν τοῦ προβλήματος οὐσίαν, ἔνια δὲ ἀπὸ τῶν ὑπαρχόντων μὲν
οὐ μὴν κατὰ τὸ προβεβλημένον τε καὶ ζητούμενον, ἕτερα δὲ ἀπὸ τῶν
ἔξωθεν μαρτύρων, πρὸς τούτοις δὲ καὶ τέταρτον τὸ [ἀπὸ] τῶν σοφιστι-
κῶν λημμάτων τοῖς τῆς λέξεως σχήμασι πρὸς ἀμφιβολίαν πεπανουργη-
μένων.

5 Οὐκ ὀλίγα δὲ ἔγραψα παραδείγματα ἀφ' ὧν ἕκαστον τῶν λημμάτων
ἐφευρίσκεται γένος, αὐτὰ τὰ ῥήματα τῶν χρωμένων αὐτοῖς προτιθέμενος.
6 καὶ δὴ τοὺς λόγους αὐτῶν ἀνατρέπων ἱκανῶς βέλτιον ἐγνώκειν ἐν αὐτῷ
τῷ τρίτῳ γράμματι τόν τ' ἀριθμὸν καὶ τὰς οὐσίας τῶν ἀρετῶν διδάσκειν·|
287 κατὰ δὲ τὸν αὐτὸν τρόπον ἐπέρχεταί μοι τῶν ἀρετῶν μνημονεύσαντι
7 [τὸ] λέγειν τὸν ἀριθμὸν καὶ τὰς διαφορὰς τῶν συμβεβηκότων· καί⟨τοι⟩
251 τίς γε τῶν ἐπιφανεστάτων σοφιστῶν / μοι φήσας ὡς οὐ δυνατὸν ἀνα-
τρέπειν ὅσαπερ ὁ Χρύσιππος ἔγραψεν περὶ τοῦ τὴν καρδίαν μόνην
ἐν τῷ σώματι τοῦ ζῴου ἀρχὴν εἶναι τοῦ ἡγεμονικοῦ, κατὰ τοῦτο τὸ

4–8] libri primi test., *v. supra*, p. 64.26–30 14–20] *cf. supra*, pp. 110.23–112.2 Prantl, Gesch. d. Logik I 570 n.

1–3 γαληνοῦ περὶ τῶν ἱπποκράτους καὶ πλάτωνος δογμάτων, τρίτον H L 8 δέδεικται] δεδήλωται L 9 ἐρέθη H 11 ἐκτιθέμενος L αἷς H L: *corr. Ald.* 12 δέ *om.* L 15 τῷ – 170.29 γὰρ *om.* L 17 ἕτερα – 170.12 ἀρτηρίαν *om.* H *spat. rel., suppl.* H[s] 18 τὸ τέταρτον H[s]: *corr. Wilamowitz* ἀπὸ *del. Müller* 19 πεπανουργημένον H[s]: *corr. Petersen* 25 ἐπέρχεσθαί H[s]: ὑπέρχεταί *Ald.*: *corr. Kühn* μνημονεύσαν τί H[s]: *corr.* M *Ald.* 26 τὸ *del. Müller* καίτοι] καί H[s]: *supplevi* 27 μοι] μὴ H[s]: *corr. Corn.* 29 ἡγεμονοῦντος *Müller*

GALEN

ON THE DOCTRINES OF HIPPOCRATES AND PLATO

BOOK III

1. In the first book I pointed out that it is necessary not only for philosophers, but also for all physicians who approach the art rationally, to have inquired about the powers that govern us, how many they are in kind, what is the specific nature of each, and in what part of the animal each power mainly resides. I also spoke at some 2
length in the first book on the point that the men who gave the best account of these (things) were Plato and Hippocrates; and in the second book I made a complete review of the matter, after (first) giving a classification of all the premises that the most eminent philosophers employed (in their treatment) of the doctrine in question. It seems necessary to me to mention them again at this time, before 3
proceeding to the remainder of my account. I said that there are four 4
kinds of premises in all. Some of them are taken from those of the part's properties that pertain to the essence of the problem, some from properties that do not pertain to the problem and the inquiry; others are from outside witnesses; and fourth, in addition to these, is the class of sophistical premises, made ambiguous by a fraudulent use of figures of speech.

I cited many examples from which each kind of premise is discov- 5
ered, quoting the very words of the men who use them. And as I 6
gave an adequate refutation of their arguments, I decided that it would be better in this very third book to explain the number and the essences of the virtues; and it occurs to me that after having made mention of the virtues, I might enumerate and differentiate their properties in the same way. But when one of the most eminent soph- 7
ists said to me that it was not possible to refute all that Chrysippus had written to prove that the heart alone in the body of an animal is the source of the governing part, he forced me to present

τρίτον ὑπόμνημα ἐπεξελθεῖν με τῷ λόγῳ τά γ' ἐλλείποντα παρεβία-
8 σεν. ἴσως μὲν οὖν τοῦτο αἴτιον αὐτὸ γενήσεται τοῦ ἐπαίνου, ἐπεί τοι οἱ
μνημονεύοντες τῶν εἰρημένων ἐν τῷ δευτέρῳ λόγῳ γινώσκουσιν ἡμᾶς τὸ
ἰσχυρόν τε καὶ γενναῖον ὧν ὁ Χρύσιππος εἶπεν ἀνατρέποντας ἐάσαντάς
τε τὸ ἀσθενέστατον ἐπιδεικνύειν αὐτοῦ τὰ σφάλματα.
9 Λέγω δὴ ὅτι ὁ Χρύσιππος κατὰ τὸ⟨ν⟩ πρῶτον αὐτοῦ Περὶ ψυχῆς
λόγον τῶν μερῶν αὐτῆς τοῦ ἡγεμονικοῦ μνημονεύειν ἀρχόμενος, ἔνθα δὴ
δεικνύναι πειρᾶται τὴν ἀρχὴν τῆς ψυχῆς ἐν τῇ καρδίᾳ μόνῃ περιέχεσθαι
10 οὑτωσὶ λέγει· «ἡ ψυχὴ πνεῦμά ἐστι σύμφυτον ἡμῖν συνεχὲς παντὶ τῷ
11 σώματι διῆκον ἔστ' ἂν ἡ τῆς ζωῆς εὔπνοια παρῇ ἐν τῷ σώματι. ταύτης
252 288 οὖν τῶν μερῶν ἑκάστῳ διατε/ταγμένων μορίῳ τὸ | διῆκον αὐτῶν εἰς τὴν
τραχεῖαν ἀρτηρίαν φωνὴν εἶναι, τὸ δὲ εἰς ὀφθαλμοὺς ὄψιν, τὸ δὲ εἰς ὦτα
ἀκοήν, τὸ δ' εἰς ῥῖνας ὄσφρησιν, τὸ δ' εἰς γλῶτταν γεῦσιν, τὸ δ' εἰς ὅλην
τὴν σάρκα ἁφὴν καὶ τὸ εἰς ὄρχεις ἕτερόν τιν' ἔχον τοιοῦτον λόγον,
σπερματικόν, εἰς ὃ δὲ συμβαίνει πάντα ταῦτα ἐν τῇ καρδίᾳ εἶναι, μέρος
12 ὂν αὐτῆς τὸ ἡγεμονικόν. οὕτω δὲ ἐχόντων αὐτῶν τὰ μὲν λοιπὰ συμφω-
νεῖται, περὶ δὲ τοῦ ἡγεμονικοῦ μέρους τῆς ψυχῆς διαφωνοῦσιν ἄλλοι ἐν
ἄλλοις λέγοντες αὐτὸ εἶναι τόποις. οἱ μὲν γὰρ περὶ τὸν θώρακά φασιν
13 εἶναι αὐτό, οἱ δὲ περὶ τὴν κεφαλήν. κατὰ τὰ αὐτὰ δὲ ταῦτα διαφωνοῦσι,
ποῦ τῆς κεφαλῆς καὶ τοῦ θώρακός ἐστιν, οὐ συμφωνοῦντες αὐτοῖς.
14 Πλάτων δὲ καὶ τριμερῆ τὴν ψυχὴν φήσας εἶναι τὸ μὲν λογιστικὸν
ἔλεγεν ἐν τῇ κεφαλῇ εἶναι, τὸ δὲ θυμοειδὲς περὶ τὸν θώρακα, τὸ δὲ
253 15 ἐπιθυμητικὸν περὶ τὸν ὀμφαλόν. οὕτω φαίνε/ται διαφεύγειν ὁ τόπος
ἡμᾶς οὔτ' αἰσθήσεως ἐκφανοῦς γενομένης, ὅπερ ἐπὶ τῶν λοιπῶν συντε-
τύχηκεν, οὔτε [τῶ] τῶν τεκμηρίων δι' ὧν ἄν τις συλλογίσαιτο τοῦτο· |
289 οὐδὲ γὰρ ἂν ἀντιλογία ἐπὶ τοσοῦτον προῆλθεν καὶ ἐν ἰατροῖς καὶ ἐν
φιλοσόφοις.»
16 Αὕτη πρώτη ῥῆσις γέγραπται ὑπὸ Χρυσίππου περὶ ἡγεμονικοῦ
κατὰ τὸ πρότερον Περὶ ψυχῆς. τὸ μὲν γὰρ ἥμισυ μέρος αὐτῷ τῆς βίβλου
17 τὸ πρότερον ὑπὲρ οὐσίας ψυχῆς ἔχει τὴν σκέψιν. κατὰ δὲ τὸ ἐφεξῆς
ἥμισυ τὸ ἀπὸ τῆς γεγραμμένης ῥήσεως ἀρχόμενον ἐπιδεικνύναι πειρᾶται
18 τὸ τῆς ψυχῆς ἡγεμονοῦν ἐν καρδίᾳ περιέχεσθαι. τὴν μὲν οὖν ἀρχὴν τοῦ
λόγου δίκαιον ἀγάσασθαι· σαφῶς τε γὰρ ἅμα καὶ ἀκριβῶς, ὡς ἐχρῆν
εἰπεῖν ἀρχόμενον ἄνδρα τηλικούτου δόγματος, εἴρηται Χρυσίππῳ.

6–34] SVF II, pp. 238–239 9] *cf.* Gal. In Hipp. Epid. VI comm. v. 5: CMG V 10.2.2, p. 273 21–23] Plat. Tim. 69d–70a, 70d–e *cf. infra*, p. 234.27–29; PHP 652.8–10 Müller 23–27] *cf. supra*, p. 152.23–27 *infra*, p. 220.5–9

1 με] μὲν *(supra lin.)* H^{s}: *corr. Kühn* 2 τοι] γ' [οι] *Petersen* 4 ἐάσας τάς H^{s}: ἐάσαντές *Ald.*: *corr. Chart.* 5 τὸ ἀσθενέτα H^{s}: *corr.* M: τὰ ἀσθενέστατα *Ald.* ἐπιδεικνύον H^{s}: *corr. Ald.* 6 τὸν] τὸ H^{s}: *corr. Kühn* αὐτοῦ *Kühn* Περὶ] π' H^{s}: *corr. Ald.* 7 δή, *ut vid.*, H^{s}: *om. Ald.* 8 πέχεσ H^{s}: *corr. Ald.* 10 εὔπνοια] εὐτονία *Ilberg* 11 αὐτῆς *Ald.* 12 *post* φωνὴν *add.* φαμεν *Müller* τὸ^{II}] τὰ H: *corr.* R^{2} 13 τὸ^{I}] τὰ H: *corr. Müller* 14 ἔχον *ex* ἔχοντα *corr.* H^{3} 20 αὐτοῖς H: *corr. Kühn* 25 τῶ τῶν H: *corr. Ald.*: τοιούτων *v. Arnim* 30 ἔχει ψυχῆς L 33 ὡς *om.* L

in this third book a full discussion of the things I had passed over.
Perhaps this very thing will become a reason for praise, since those 8
who remember what I said in the second book know that I exposed
Chrysippus' errors by overturning what was strong and noble in
his arguments and disregarding the weakest part of them.

I say that as Chrysippus in the first book of his treatise On 9
the Soul begins to mention among its divisions the governing part,
in the passage where he tries to prove that the ruling power of the
soul is contained in the heart alone, he speaks as follows: "The 10
soul is pneuma connate with us, extending as a continuum through
the whole body as long as the free-flowing breath of life is present
in the body. Now of the parts of the soul that have been assigned to 11
the several parts (of the body), that of them which extends to the
trachea is the voice; that to the eyes, sight; that to the ears, hearing;
that to the nostrils, smell; that to the tongue, taste; that to the entire
flesh, touch; and that which extends to the testicles, possessing an-
other such *logos*, is seminal. That part where all these meet is in the
heart, being the governing part of the soul. This being so, there is 12
agreement about all other parts, but about the governing part of
the soul there is disagreement, some placing it in one region, others
in another. For some say it is located in the chest, others in the head.
And there are differences even within these locations, as they do not 13
agree among themselves where in the head or chest it is located.
Plato, who said that the soul has three parts, placed the rational 14
part in the head, the spirited in the region of the chest, and the
desiderative in the region of the navel. Thus the place seems to elude 15
us, since we have neither a clear perception (of it), as we had with
the others, nor sure signs from which this matter might be inferred;
otherwise disagreement among physicians and philosophers would
not have grown so great."

This is the first passage that Chrysippus wrote about the 16
governing part in the first of his two books On the Soul; for the first
half of the book contains his inquiry into the substance of the soul.
In the second half, which begins with the passage I have quoted, he 17
tries to show that the governing part of the soul is situated in the
heart. Now the beginning of his discourse deserves to be admired, 18
for Chrysippus spoke both with clarity and precision, as a man
should when he begins a doctrine of such magnitude. Indeed (he 19

19 καὶ γὰρ ὅτι Πλάτων τρία μέρη τῆς ψυχῆς ἐτίθετο καὶ ἅτινα ταῦτα
254 εἴρηκε / καὶ καθ' οὕστινας τόπους ἐν τοῖς ζῴοις καθιδρυμένα καὶ ὅτι
λόγῳ χρὴ διασκέψασθαι περὶ τοῦ δόγματος ἐκφυγόντος τὰς αἰσθήσεις.
20 τὰ δ' ἐφεξῆς οὐκέθ' ὁμοίως ἔχει. δίκαιον γὰρ ἦν, οἶμαι, πρῶτον μὲν
εἰπεῖν ὑπὸ τίνων πιθανῶν ἀναπεισθεὶς ὁ Πλάτων οὕτως ἐδόξαζεν,
ἔπειτα δὲ ἐξελέγξαι καὶ διαβαλεῖν αὐτὰ κἀπὶ τούτῳ τὴν ἑαυτοῦ κατα-
290 σκευάσαι δόξαν, | οὐκ ἐκ πιθανῶν ἐπιχειρημάτων οἷοις ἔθος ἐστὶ χρῆσθαι
σοφισταῖς τε καὶ ῥήτορσιν, ἀλλ' ἐξ ἐπιστημονικῶν τε καὶ ἀποδεικτικῶν,
ἃ δὴ μεταχειρίζεσθαι πρέπει φιλοσόφοις ἀνδράσιν ἀλήθειαν σπουδά-
21 ζουσιν. ἆρ' οὖν οὕτως ὁ Χρύσιππος ἔπραξεν, ἢ πᾶν τοὐναντίον
ἐπελάθετο μὲν ὡς μηδὲ προειρηκὼς ὅλως τι περὶ τῆς τοῦ Πλάτωνος
δόξης, ἄρχεται δ' ἐπιχειρεῖν ἀπὸ τοῦ γένους τῶν λημμάτων ὃ κατὰ
μαρτύρων δόξαν ἢ πλήθους, οὐ κατὰ τὴν τοῦ πράγματος φύσιν ἄξιον
255 22 πιστεύεσθαι; παραγράψω δὲ καὶ τὴν ῥῆσιν αὐτὴν / ὧδέ πως ἔχουσαν·
«περὶ ὧν ἑξῆς ζητήσομεν παραπλησίως ἀπὸ τῆς κοινῆς ὁρμώμενοι φορᾶς
23 καὶ τῶν κατὰ ταύτην εἰρημένων λόγων·» 'κοινὴν' ἐνταῦθα 'φορὰν' ὁ
Χρύσιππος εἴρηκε τὸ κοινῇ πᾶσιν ἀνθρώποις δοκοῦν. εἶτ' ἐπιφέρων
φησί· «καὶ ἐπὶ τούτων ἱκανῶς φαίνονται ἐνηνέχθαι ἀπ' ἀρχῆς εἰς τὸ εἶναι
24 τὸ ἡγεμονικὸν ἡμῶν ἐν τῇ καρδίᾳ.» εἶτ' ἐφεξῆς τούτων ἁπτόμενος ἤδη
25 τῶν ἐπιχειρημάτων αὐτῶν ὧδέ πως γράφει κατὰ λέξιν· «κοινῇ δέ μοι
291 δοκοῦσιν οἱ πολλοὶ φέρεσθαι ἐπὶ τοῦτο ὡσανεὶ συναισθα|νόμενοι περὶ
τὸν θώρακα αὐτοῖς τῶν κατὰ τὴν διάνοιαν παθῶν γιγνομένων καὶ
μάλιστα καθ' ὃν ἡ καρδία τέτακται τόπον, οἷον μάλιστα ἐπὶ τῶν λυπῶν
καὶ τῶν φόβων καὶ ἐπὶ τῆς ὀργῆς καὶ μάλιστα τοῦ θυμοῦ· ⟨ὡσανεὶ γὰρ⟩
ἐκ τῆς καρδίας ἀναθυμιωμένου καὶ ὠθουμένου ἐκτὸς ἐπί τινα καὶ ἐμ-
φυσῶντος τὸ πρόσωπον καὶ τὰς χεῖρας γίγνεσθαι ἡμῖν ἐμφάσεις.»
256 26 Ἐν τούτοις / ἤδη πάνυ σφόδρα θαυμάζω τοῦ Χρυσίππου πάνθ'
27 ἅμα συγχέοντός τε καὶ συνταράττοντος. εἰρηκώς τε γὰρ ὀλίγον ἔμπρο-
σθεν ὡς ὁ Πλάτων ἐν τοῖς περὶ τὸν θώρακα τόποις ὑπολαμβάνει τὸ
θυμοειδὲς ὑπάρχειν, εἶτ' ἀφ' ὧν κινηθεὶς ἐπὶ τοῦθ' ἧκεν ὑπερβὰς εἰπεῖν,
ὑπερβὰς δὲ καὶ τὸ διαβαλεῖν αὐτά, κατασκευάζειν εὐθὺς ἄρχεται τὰ
δοκοῦντα αὐτῷ πρώτου πάντων τῶν ἐπιχειρημάτων μνημονεύων δι' οὗ
28 δείκνυται τὸ θυμοειδὲς ἐν τοῖς κατὰ τὸν θώρακα τόποις ὑπάρχον. οὐ γὰρ

4–7] SVF II, p. 239 4–6] *cf. infra*, pp. 346.19–20; 348.23–25; PHP 652.11–14 Müller 12–24] SVF II, pp. 239–240 20–24] *cf. supra*, pp. 152.29–33; 154.1–2 24–26] *cf. infra*, p. 174.3–5 28–33] *cf.* PHP 652.11–16 Müller

4 οὐκέθ'] κ *ex* θ *corr.* H 5 ὑπὸ τίνων *in mg. deperdita* L 7 οὐκ] οὔτ' L 9 πρέπει] ει *e corr.* L 12 γένυος L δ] οὐ L 13 πλῆθος L 15 ζητήσωμεν L 16 ἔνθα L 18 *post* καὶ *add.* γὰρ *v. Arnim* φαίνονται *ex* φέρονται *corr.* H 20 κοινοὶ L 21 πολλοὶ *scr. Ricci*: λοιποὶ H L 22 αὐτοῖς H L: *corr. Einarson* 24 ὡσανεὶ γὰρ *add. Müller (cf. infra, p. 174.3)* 25 ἀναθυμιωμένου *om.* L: ἀναθυμιωμένου τοῦ θυμοῦ *post* γὰρ *inser. Müller (cf. infra, p. 174.3)* καὶ[II] *om.* L ἐκφυσσῶντος L 26 γίγνεται *Ald.* ἐμφάσεις, *ut vid.*, L: ἔμφασις H 28 συνταράττον. . L: ταράττοντος H τε[II] *om. Müller* 30 εἶτα ὑφ' *Müller* ὑπερβὰς] ὑπὲρ μιᾶς L 31 ὑπερβὰς] β *ex* δ *corr.* H 32 δ...ῦντα H: δοκ...τ' L αὐτῶ H L: *corr. Einarson* παντὸς H L: *corr. Ald.*

said) that Plato posited three parts of the soul, and he told us what
these are and what places in animals they occupy, and that one must
use reason when investigating a doctrine that eludes the senses. But 20
what comes next is no longer the same. First, in my opinion, he should
have stated the plausible arguments by which Plato was persuaded
to adopt this view, then he should refute and discredit them, and
after that establish his own position, not from the kind of plausi-
bilities that sophists and rhetoricians are wont to employ, but from
scientific and demonstrative arguments, the use of which is proper
for philosophical men who earnestly seek the truth. Is this what 21
Chrysippus did, or did he, quite the contrary, forget, as though
he had earlier said nothing at all about Plato's view, and begin
to argue from the kind of premises that deserve credit as being in
accord with the opinion of witnesses or of the multitude, but not
with the nature of the thing (itself)? I shall quote the actual passage 22
in his own words: "We shall next inquire about these (matters),
starting out in the same way from the common tendency and the
expressions that are in accord with it;" here by 'common tendency' 23
Chrysippus means a view that is held by all people in common.
Then he continues: "And in these matters it is sufficiently clear
that people have been brought from the outset to the view that our
governing part is in our heart." Immediately thereafter, as he now 24
begins the actual argumentation, he writes these words: "The multi- 25
tude of men seem to me to be brought together to this view since
they have, as it were, an inner awareness of the affections of the mind
happening to them in the region of the chest and especially the place
assigned to the heart. This is especially so in distress and fear, in
anger and inflamed anger most of all; for impressions arise in us as
if it were vaporized from the heart and were pushing out against
someone and were blowing into the face and hands."

At this point I am quite overcome with amazement at Chry- 26
sippus' both confounding and confusing everything. Having said a 27
little earlier that Plato supposes the spirited part to be in the region
of the chest, then neglecting to mention the considerations which
moved Plato to accept this view and neglecting to discredit them,
he begins immediately to establish his own position, mentioning
first from all his arguments that by which the spirited part is shown
to be in the region of the chest! Indeed there are no observations 28

δὴ ἐξ ἄλλων πραγμάτων φαινομένων ἢ ἐξ ὧν εἴρηκεν ὁ Χρύσιππος
νῦν ἐναργέστερον ἄν τις ἀποδείξειεν ἐκ θώρακός τε καὶ καρδίας ὁρμᾶσθαι
29 τὸν θυμόν. «ὡσανεὶ γάρ», φησίν, «ἀναθυμιωμένου» τοῦ θυμοῦ «ἐκ τῆς
292 καρδίας καὶ ὠθουμένου ἐκ|τὸς ἐπί τινα καὶ ἐμφυσῶντος, τὸ πρόσωπόν τε
30 καὶ τὰς χεῖρας γίγνεσθαι ἐμφάσεις.» ἐν ταύτῃ τῇ ῥήσει συγχωρεῖν
257 ἔοικεν ὁ Χρύσιππος τῷ παλαιῷ λόγῳ ζέσιν τινὰ τῆς ἐμφύτου / θερμότητος ὑπολαμβάνοντι γίγνεσθαι κατὰ τὴν καρδίαν ἐν τοῖς θυμοῖς, ᾗ ζέσει τό τε διαφυσᾶσθαι τὸ πρόσωπον ἕπεται καὶ σύμπαν ἐρεύθειν τε καὶ θερμαίνεσθαι τὸ σῶμα καὶ σφοδρῶς πηδᾶν τὴν καρδίαν σὺν ταῖς κατὰ
31 τὸ ζῷον ἁπάσαις ἀρτηρίαις. ἆρ' οὖν ὁ Πλάτων ἕτερόν τί φησιν, ἐπειδὰν ἐν Τιμαίῳ γράφῃ· «τὴν δὲ δὴ καρδίαν ἅμ⟨μ⟩α τῶν φλεβῶν καὶ πηγὴν τοῦ περιφερομένου κατὰ πάντα τὰ μέλη σφοδρῶς αἵματος εἰς τὴν δορυφορικὴν οἴκησιν κατέστησαν ἵν' ὅτε ζέσειε τὸ τοῦ θυμοῦ μένος, τοῦ λόγου παραγγείλαντος ὥς τις ἄδικος περὶ αὐτὰ γίγνεται πρᾶξις ἔξωθεν ἢ καί τις ἀπὸ τῶν ἔνδοθεν ἐπιθυμιῶν, ὀξέως διὰ πάντων τῶν στενωπῶν πᾶν ὅσον αἰσθητικὸν ἐν τῷ σώματι τῶν τε παρακελεύσεων καὶ ἀπειλῶν
32 αἰσθανόμενον γίγνοιτο ἐπήκοον.» ἔτι δὲ τούτοις ἐφεξῆς καὶ τάδε γράφει·
258 «τῇ δὲ δὴ πηδήσει τῆς καρδίας ἐν / τῇ τῶν δεινῶν προσδοκίᾳ καὶ τῇ τοῦ
293 θυμοῦ ἐγέρσει προγιγνώσκοντες ὅτι [οἷα] διὰ πυρός γε | ἡ τοιαύτη πᾶσα ἔμελλεν οἴδησις γίγνεσθαι τῶν θυμουμένων, ἐπικουρίαν αὐτῇ
33 μηχανώμενοι τὴν τοῦ πνεύμονος ἰδέαν ἐνεφύτευσαν.» ὥστε ὦ φίλτατε Χρύσιππε, τὰ Πλάτωνος δόγματα γράφεις, ἐπειδὰν ἐκ τῆς καρδίας ἀναθυμιᾶσθαί τε καὶ πρὸς τὸ ἐκτὸς ὠθεῖσθαι καὶ τὸ πρόσωπον ἐμφυσᾶν λέγῃς τὸν θυμόν.

2. Οὐ μὴν τοῦτό γ' ἦν σοι τὸ ἀμφισβητούμενον, εἰ τὸ θυμούμενον τῆς ψυχῆς ἐν καρδίᾳ κατῴκισται, ἀλλ' εἰ τὸ λογιζόμενον, ὅπερ ἐχρῆν ἀποδείξαντα μὴ πολλὰ κάμνειν ὑπὲρ τοῦ θυμουμένου μηδ' ἐμπιπλάναι τὸ βιβλίον ἐπῶν ποιητικῶν ὧν ἐφεξῆς γράφεις ὡδί·

3–5] *cf. supra*, p. 172.24–26 6–7] *cf. infra*, PHP 577.1–3 Müller 9 πηδᾶν τὴν καρδίαν] *cf.* Arist. De respir. 20: 479 b 17 – 480 a 15 11–17] Plat. Tim. 70a 7 – b 8 *cf. infra*, PHP 575.9–576.2 Müller 11–13] *cf.* Gal. De foet. form. 3: IV 671–672 K. Brenner, Prim. Czern., p. 81 n. 1 18–21] Plat. Tim. 70c 1–5 *cf. infra*, PHP 721.9–13 Müller 25–176.16] SVF II, pp. 241–242

3 ἀναθυμιουμένου L 4 ἐμφυσῶντα L 5 γίγνεται L ἔμφασις H L: *correxi (cf. supra, p. 172.26)* 9 θερμαίνεσθαι] συμπεραίνεσθαι L σὺν *om.* L 11 γράφῃ] η *ex* ει *corr.* L δὴ *om.* H ἅμα H L: *corr.* H[2] 13 *ante* τὸ *add.* τε L μένος] μέγεθος L 14 ὥς τις] ὅταν H 16 ἐν τῷ σώματι *ex* ἐντὸς *(?)* σωμάτων *corr.* H[2?]: ἐν τῷ ἴσω L τε *om.* L 17 γίγνεται H L: *ex Plat. corr. Müller* ἔτι] ἐπὶ *Schöne* 18 δὲ δὴ] δ' εἴσω L 19 ἐγέρσει] ἐνεργείᾳ L ὅτε L οἷα *ex Plat. del. Müller* διάπυρός γε ἡ H: *corr.* F R: πρὸς γῇ L γε *ex Plat. del. Müller* 20 πάσας ἔμελλον L οἴκησις H: οἰκήσεις L: *corr. Müller (cf. infra, PHP 721.11 Müller)* τοῦ θυμουμένου H 21 ἐφύτευσαν L 24 τὸν – 25 τοῦτό *deperdita in* L 26 ἐν *om.* H κατῳκεῖσθαι L 27 ἀποδείξαντα μὴ *deperdita in* L

other than those mentioned by Chrysippus which give a clearer
proof that inflamed anger arises from the chest and heart. "For im- 29
pressions arise in us", he says, "as if" the inflamed anger "were va-
porized from the heart and were pushing out against someone and
were blowing into the face and hands." In this passage Chrysippus 30
seems to agree with the ancient account which held that a kind of
boiling of innate heat arises in the heart in times of inflamed anger,
and from this boiling the face is inflated, the whole body grows red
and hot, and the heart pounds violently along with all the arteries
in the body. Does Plato say anything other than this when he writes 31
in the Timaeus: "The heart, knot of the veins and fountainhead of
the blood that courses violently through all the limbs, they set in the
guardroom, so that when the strength of anger boils on receiving
a message from reason that some unjust act is taking place in the
limbs, whether from without or from the desires within, every sentient
part of the body, quickly perceiving the commands and threats through
all the narrow channels, might be obedient"? Next after this he writes: 32
"And for the leaping of the heart in anticipation of danger and in
the rising of passion, since they knew beforehand that all such swel-
ling in angry persons would arise through fire, they devised as an aid
to it the form of the lungs and implanted it." So then, my dear Chry- 33
sippus, you are expressing Plato's view when you say that in-
flamed anger rises as a vapor from the heart and pushes its way to
the outside and inflates the face.

2. The question before you, however, was not whether the passionate part of the soul resides in the heart, but whether the reasoning part resides there; and you should have proved that and not have expended great effort on the passionate part or filled your book with lines from the poets, which you quote one after another, as follows:

2 «ὅς τε πολὺ γλυκίων μέλιτος καταλειβομένοιο
ἀνδρῶν ἐν[ὶ] στήθεσσιν ἀέξεται ἠΰτε καπνός.»
καὶ πάλιν /
259 «ὁ θυμὸς αὐτὸν τῶν φρενῶν ἐξῆρ' ἄνω.»
καὶ πάλιν
«πηδῶν δ' ὁ θυμὸς ἔνδοθεν μαντεύεται.» |
294 3 καὶ μυρία ἕτερα τοιαῦτα παρ' ὅλον τὸ γράμμα κατασκευάζοντα τὸ
θυμούμενον ὑπάρχειν ἐν τῇ καρδίᾳ, δέον μὴ τοῦτο δεικνύειν, ἀλλὰ
τὸ λογιζόμενον ἢ νὴ Δία, εἴπερ ἀδύνατος ἦν ἄντικρυς ἐπιδεικνύναι
τοῦτο, πειραθῆναι γοῦν [ἐπιχειρῆσαι] δεῖξαι καθ' ἓν τοῦτο τὸ μόριον
4 εἶναι τό τε θυμούμενον τῆς ψυχῆς καὶ τὸ λογιζόμενον. ὁ δέ γε τουτὶ μὲν
οὐδ' ἐπεχείρησε πρᾶξαι κατ' οὐδὲν μέρος τοῦ βιβλίου, χρῆται δ' αὐτῷ
5 διὰ παντὸς ἐξ ἑτοίμου λαμβάνων· εὐθὺς γοῦν ἐν τοῖς ἐφεξῆς οὕτω γράφει·
«τῆς μὲν ὀργῆς γιγνομένης ἐνταῦθα εὔλογον καὶ τὰς λοιπὰς ἐπιθυμίας
ἐνταῦθ' εἶναι καὶ νὴ Δία καὶ τὰ λοιπὰ πάθη καὶ τοὺς διαλογισμοὺς καὶ
6 ὅσον τούτοις ἐστὶ παραπλήσιον.» οὐδὲν γὰρ ἀναγκαῖον ἔνθα τὰ πάθη
260 καὶ τοὺς διαλογισμοὺς ἐνταῦθ' ὑπάρχειν, ὡς, εἴ γε τοῦτ' ἐκ / προχείρου
τις ἀξιώσειε λαμβάνειν, αὐτὸ τὸ ζητούμενον λήψεται.
7 Πλάτωνος μὲν γὰρ λέγοντος οὐκ ἐκ ταὐτοῦ μέρους ὁρμᾶσθαι
λογισμόν τε καὶ θυμὸν καὶ ἐπιθυμίαν, Ζήνωνος δὲ ἐν καρδίᾳ καθιδρύον-
τος ἅπαντα, προσῆκον ἦν, οἶμαι, καὶ Χρυσίππῳ καὶ παντὶ τῷ μετὰ |
295 Πλάτωνα καὶ Ζήνωνα κρίνοντι τὰ δόγματα τῶν ἀνδρῶν προσθεῖναι
8 θατέρῳ μὲν αὐτῶν ἀπόδειξιν, θατέρῳ δ' ἔλεγχόν τινα. τὸ δὲ χωρὶς
ἀποδείξεως ἀποφήνασθαι, καθάπερ ὁ Χρύσιππος ἐποίησεν, ὡς ἔνθ'
ἂν ᾖ τὸ παθητικὸν τῆς ψυχῆς, ἐνταῦθα καὶ τὸ λογιστικὸν ὑπάρχει[ν],
τοσούτου δεῖ φιλοσόφῳ προσήκειν ὥστ' οὐδ' οἱ ῥήτορες οὐδ' οἱ σοφισταὶ
πράττουσιν αὐτό· πειρῶνται γοῦν κἀκεῖνοι πίστεσί τισι πιθαναῖς
9 χρῆσθαι. τὸ δὲ ἕκαστον τῶν ζητουμένων ἐξ ἑτοίμου λαμβάνειν οὔτε
σοφισταῖς οὔτε ῥήτορσιν οὔτε διαλεκτικοῖς οὔτ' ἀποδεικτικοῖς οὐδ' ὅλως
οὐδενὶ τῶν πάντων προσήκει.

1–2] Hom. Il. xviii. 109–110 *cf. infra*, pp. 178.25–26; 236.14–15 4] Nauck, TGF, p. 875 (Adespota 175) 6] Nauck, TGF, p. 876 (Adespota 176) 11–13] *cf. infra*, PHP 652.14–16 Müller 14–16] *cf. infra*, p. 200.21–24 23–28] *cf. supra*, p. 156.3–5 *infra*, p. 234.16–20; PHP 652.4–8 Müller

1 ὅς γε H: ὥστ. L: *ex Hom. corr. Müller* πολὺ *deperditum in* L γλυκίων] ι *ex* ει *corr.* H[2] 2 ἐνὶ H L: *ex Hom. corr. Müller* . . .θεσσιν L: στήθεσιν H *hic et passim in versibus Homericis* 4 αὐτῶν L ἐξῆρεν H (ἐξῆρ *tantum exstat in* L): *corr. Valckenaer* 4–5 ἄνω. καὶ πάλιν *deperdita in* L 8 ὑπάρχειν ἐν *deperdita in* L 10 ἐπιχειρῆσαι *del. Müller* 11–12 μὲν οὐδ' *deperdita in* L 12 δ' αὐτῷ *om.* H 14 *post* μὲν *add.* οὖν *Müller (cf. infra, p. 200.21)* 15 ἐντεῦθεν L καὶ[II] *om.* H 16 ὅσα . . . παραπλήσια *Müller (cf. infra, p. 200.23–24)* οὐδὲν *deperditum in* L 17 *post* διαλογισμοὺς *add.* καὶ ὅσον τούτοις ἐστὶν παραπλήσιον L 18 αὐτὰ L 19 οὐκ *inser.* H[3] 21 ἦν] οὖν L καὶ[II] *om.* L 22 τὰ *om.* L 23 ἀπόδειξιν] ει *ex* ε *corr.* H 25 ὑπάρχειν H L: *corr. Schöne* 26 δεῖ] δὲ L προσήκει L 27 πίστεσί – 28 ἕκαστον] καθέκαστον *(ex* καθ' ἕκαστον *corr.)* L

"Far sweeter than dripping honey it 2
rises up like smoke in men's breasts."

and again,

"Rage lifted him above his wits."

and again,

"Rage, leaping from within, forebodes."

and thousands of other verses of this sort throughout the whole book, 3 which go to prove that the passionate part (of the soul) is in the heart, though what ought to be demonstrated is not that the passionate, but that the reasoning part is in the heart; or indeed if he was unable to show it outright, then at least he should have tried to prove the presence of the passionate and the reasoning parts of the soul in this one member. And yet he did not attempt to do that in any part of 4 his book, but he takes it for granted and uses it throughout. Thus 5 in the very next passage he writes these words: "Since anger arises here, it is reasonable that the other desires are here too, and indeed the remaining affections, and deliberations, and whatever resembles these things." There is no necessity that 'deliberations' should be 6 where the affections are; therefore anyone who thinks it right to assume this out of hand will be assuming the very point under investigation.

For since Plato says that reason, anger, and desire do not come 7 from the same member, but Zeno places them all in the heart, then in my opinion it is incumbent upon Chrysippus and everyone who comes after Plato and Zeno and passes judgment on their views to provide a proof for the one and to give some refutation of the other. But to assert without proof, as Chrysippus did, that 'where the 8 affective part of the soul is, there the reasoning part is also,' is so unbecoming to a philosopher that even rhetoricians and sophists do not do it; even they try to use some plausible arguments. But the ready 9 assumption of each matter under investigation is not proper conduct for sophists, rhetoricians, dialecticians, scientific reasoners, or anyone at all.

10 Κάλλιον οὖν ἦν, οἶμαι, καθάπερ ὁ Πλάτων ἀποδεῖξαι προὐθυμήθη
261 τὸ ἑαυτοῦ / δόγμα, καὶ τὸν Χρύσιππον οὕτω πειραθῆναι τὸ τοῦ Ζήνωνος ἀποδεῖξαι καὶ μὴ πλῆθος ἐπῶν παραγράφειν ἐξ ἁπάντων τῶν ποιητῶν ἐκλέγοντα δεικνύντων ὀργὴν καὶ θυμὸν καὶ φόβον καὶ δειλίαν καὶ θράσος καὶ θάρσος καὶ καρτερίαν ὅσα τ' ἄλλα τοιαῦτα τὰ μὲν ἐνεργείας
296 11 τινὰς εἶναι, | τὰ δὲ παθήματα τῆς καρδίας. τί γὰρ αὐτῷ βούλεται ταυτὶ τὰ ἔπη τὰ ἐξ Ὁμήρου συνειλεγμένα;

«κραδίη δέ οἱ ἔνδον ὑλάκτει.»

καὶ

«στῆθος δὲ πλήξας κραδίην ἠν[ε]ίπαπε μύθῳ·
τέτλαθι δὴ κραδίη· καὶ κύντερον ἄλλο ποτ' ἔτλης.»

καὶ

«ὣς πυκίν' ἐν στήθεσσιν ἀναστενάχιζ' Ἀγαμέμνων
νειόθεν ἐκ κραδίης, περὶ γὰρ δίε νηυσὶν Ἀχαιῶν.»

καὶ

«ἀλλά μοι οἰδάνεται κραδίη χόλῳ.» /

262 καὶ

«Ἥρῃ δ' οὐκ ἔχαδε στῆθος χόλον, ἀλλὰ προσηύδα.»

καὶ

«ἀλλά τε καὶ μετόπισθεν ἔχει κότον, ὄφρα τελέσ⟨σ⟩ῃ
ἐν στήθεσσιν ἑοῖσιν.»

297 12 ἐν ἅπασι γὰρ τούτοις οὐ τὸ λογιστικόν, ἀλλὰ τὸ θυμοει|δὲς ἐν τῇ καρδίᾳ περιέχεσθαι δηλοῦται, ὥσπερ οἶμαι κἀν τοῖσδε·

«καὶ χόλος ὅς τ' ἐφέηκε πολύφρονά περ χαλεπῆναι,
ὅς τε πολὺ γλυκίων μέλιτος καταλειβομένοιο
ἀνδρῶν ἐν στήθεσσιν ἀέξεται ἠΰτε καπνός.»

καὶ

«καρδίῃ ἄλ⟨λ⟩ηκτον πολεμίζειν ἠδὲ μάχεσθαι.»

13 καὶ πρὸς τούτοις ἔτι

«καί οἱ μυίης θάρσος ἐνὶ στήθεσσιν ἔθηκε.»

1–182.20] SVF II, pp. 252–254 1–2] *cf. supra*, p. 156.9–12 8] Hom. Od. xx. 13 *cf. infra*, p. 186.19 10–11] Hom. Od. xx. 17–18 *cf. infra*, pp. 184.18–19; 186.23–24 13–14] *cf.* Hom. Il. x. 9–10; ix. 433; xi. 557 16] Hom. Il. ix. 646 *cf.* [Plut.] De vita et poesi Homeri ii. 129 18] Hom. Il. iv. 24 *cf. infra*, pp. 222.16; 236.11, 27 20–21] Hom. Il. i. 82–83 24–26] Hom. Il. xviii. 108–110 *cf. infra*, p. 236.13–15 24] *cf. infra*, p. 222.18 25–26] *cf. supra*, p. 176.1–2 28] Hom. Il. ii. 452; xi. 12 *cf.* [Plut.] Hom. ii. 130 30] Hom. Il. xvii. 570 *cf.* [Plut.] Hom. ii. 85

1 οὖν ἦν] οὐ μὴν L 2 τὸ τοῦ] καὶ L 3 μὴ *deperditum in* L παραγραφὴν L τῶν *om.* L 5 θράσος] σ *ex* γ *corr.* H τἆλλα L 8 καρδίη H *hic et (praeter lin. 16; p. 180.25) passim in versibus Homericis* 10 ἠνείπαπε H L: *ex Hom. corr. Chart.* μύθῳ] θυμῷ H 11 καὶ – ἔτλης *om.* L 13 ὡς L πυκίναις H ἀναστεναχίζων L 14 νειόθεν *in* νειόθε *mut.* H³ δῖε L: *corr. Greenhill*: δὴ ἐν H 16 ἀλλά H L: *corr.* H³ οἰδύνεται *(?)* H: ὀηδάνεται H³ 20 ἀλλά H τελέσῃ H L: *ex Hom. corr. Chart.* 25 καταλιβομένοιο H, *in* καταλειβομένοιο *corr.* L 26 ἐνὶ H ἤΰτοι L 28 ἄληκτον H L: *ex Hom. corr. Greenhill* *ante* πολεμίζειν *add.* πόλεμον H 30 μυίης] γύοισι H: μύης L: *ex Hom. corr. Greenhill*

It would have been better in my opinion, just as Plato was in- 10
tent on proving his own doctrine, so for Chrysippus also to have
attempted to prove Zeno's doctrine, and not to quote a multitude
of verses culled from all the poets, which show that anger, rage, fear,
cowardice, boldness, courage, endurance, and all such things, are
some of them activities, others affections of the heart. Of what use 11
to him are these verses collected from Homer?

"His heart within him howled."

and

"Striking his breast, he rebuked his heart with words:
Endure, my heart; you once put up with a thing more shameful."

and

"Thus Agamemnon heaved repeated sighs in his breast,
from deep in his heart, for he feared for the ships of the Achaians."

and

"But my heart swells with bitter anger."

and

"But Hera's breast could not contain her bitter anger, and she spoke out."

and

"Yet he retains a rankling in his breast,
until it gains its end."

In all these (lines) it is not the rational but the spirited part whose 12
presence is revealed in the heart; and the same is true, I take it, of
the following:

"And bitter anger, which drives even the very wise to harshness;
far sweeter than dripping honey,
it rises in men's breasts like smoke."

and

"(The goddess put strength in each man's)
heart to engage unceasingly in war and battle."

and again, in addition to these, 13

"And she put the boldness of a fly in his heart."

καὶ

«δύη ἄχος κραδίην Λαερτιάδεω Ὀδυσῆος.» /

263 καὶ

«ἐν δ' ἄρα οἱ στήθεσσι μένος πατρώϊον ἧκε.»

καὶ

«αὐτὰρ Ἀχιλλεὺς
δεινὸν ἐνὶ στήθεσσιν ἔχει μεγαλήτορα θυμόν.» |

298 καὶ

«σοὶ δ' ἄλ⟨λ⟩ηκτόν τε κακόν τε
θυμὸν ἐνὶ στήθεσσι θεοὶ θέσαν εἵνεκα κούρης.»

καὶ

«ὣς Αἰνείᾳ θυμὸς ἐνὶ στήθεσσι γεγήθει.»

καὶ

«πρῆσεν ἐνὶ στήθεσσιν ἐρισθενέος Διὸς ἀλκὴν
γνώμεναι.»

14 καὶ πρὸς τούτοις ἔτι

«καὶ δέ μοι αὐτῷ θυμὸς ἐνὶ στήθεσσι φίλοισι
μᾶλλον ἐφορμᾶται πολεμίζειν ἠδὲ μάχεσθαι.»

καὶ

«σεῖσ', ἐπὶ δ' αὐτὸς ἄϋσε μάλα μέγα, τοῖσι δὲ θυμὸν /
264 ἐν[ὶ] στήθεσσιν ἔθελξε, φόβου δ' ἐμνήσαθ' ἕκαστος.»

καὶ

«Νέστορ, ἔμ' ὀτρύνει κραδίη καὶ θυμὸς ἀγήνωρ.»

καὶ

«οὗ πέρι μὲν πρόφρων κραδίη καὶ θυμὸς ἀγήνωρ.» |

299 καὶ

«ὦ γέρον, εἴθ', ὡς θυμὸς ἐνὶ στήθεσσι φίλοισιν,
ὥς τοι γούναθ' ἕποιτο.»

15 καὶ

«οἶσθα γὰρ οἷος θυμὸς ἐνὶ στήθεσσι γυναικός.»

καὶ

«σὸν δὲ φίλον κῆρ
τετλάτω ἐν στήθεσσι κακῶς πάσχοντος ἐμεῖο.»

2] Hom. Od. xx. 286 4] *cf.* Hom. Il. v. 125 6–7] *cf.* Hom. Il. ix. 628–629 9–10] Hom. Il. ix. 636–637 12] Hom. Il. xiii. 494 14–15] Versus heroici, XII, ed. Allen 17–18] Hom. Il. xiii. 73–74 21–22] *cf.* Hom. Il. xv. 321–322 23] Hom. Il. x. 220 25] Hom. Il. x. 244 27–28] Hom. Il. iv. 313–314 30] Hom. Od. xv. 20 *cf.* Stob.: IV, p. 552 Hense 32–33] Hom. Od. xvi. 274–275 *cf.* Plut. Mor. 31 D

2 δύη] δύε δ' H λαερτιάδαω (δα *ex* δη ? *corr.*) H ὀδυσσῆος L 4 στήθεσι *ex* στῆθος *corr.* H 6 ἀτὰρ L 9 ἄληκτόν H L: *ex Hom. correxi* 10 στήθεσσι] στ *e corr.* L θεοὶ *om.* L 14 προῆσεν L 15 *ante* γνώμεναι *lac. suspicatus est Müller* 17 δ' ἐμοὶ *ex Hom. Müller* 20 σεῖσ', ἐπὶ] σεῖός τε ἐπι H: σεῖο τε ἐπὶ L: *ex Hom. corr. Müller* μέγα] μετὰ L θυμὸν] μῦθον L 21 ἐνὶ H L: *corr. Ald.* ἕκαστος] ἕκτωρ H 23 νέστορ' ἔμ' L: νέστωρέ μ' H: *corr. Chart.* ἀγήνωρ *deperditum in* L 24 καὶ – 25 ἀγήνωρ *om.* L 25 οὗ] οἱ H: *ex Hom. corr. Müller* περὶ H: *ex Hom. correxi* 27 φίλοισι H 28 γύναθ' H 30 γυναικός *deperditum in* L 33 ἐμοῖο H

and

"That pain might enter the heart of Odysseus, son
of Laertes."

and

"She put his father's strength in his breast."

and

"But the proud
spirit in Achilles' breast is hard."

and

"The gods put an evil and unrelenting
spirit in your breast because of a girl."

and

"Just so Aeneas' spirit rejoiced in his breast."

and

"He blew in his breast strength from almighty Zeus
for men to see."

and in addition, 14

"As for me, the spirit in my breast
arouses me even more to war and battle."

and

"He shook the aegis, and himself gave a loud cry
besides, and he confounded the spirit
in their breasts, and each man turned his mind to flight."

and

"Nestor, my heart and manly spirit urge me on."

and

"Whose heart and manly spirit are exceedingly zealous."

and

"Old man, if only your knees might follow
the spirit in your breast."

and 15

"For you know what sort of spirit dwells in a woman's
breast."

and

"Let your heart
in your breast endure the wrongs that I suffer."

καὶ

«ὢς φάτο, τοῖσι δὲ θυμὸν ἐνὶ στήθεσσιν ὄρινε.»

καὶ

«Τηλέμαχος δ' ἐν μὲν κραδίῃ μέγα πένθος ἄεξεν.»

καὶ /

265 «ὢς φάτ' ἐνὶ στήθεσσι καθαπτόμενος φίλον ἦτορ·

[καὶ]

τῷ δὲ μάλ' ἐν πείσῃ κραδίη μένε τετληυῖα.»

300 16 πάντα μὲν γὰρ ταῦτα τὰ ἔπη καὶ πρὸς τούτοις ἔτι μυρία | ἕτερα τὸ πλῆθος ὧν Χρύσιππος παρατίθεται τὸ θυμοειδὲς ἐν τῇ καρδίᾳ φησὶν ὑπάρχειν. ἐγὼ δὲ εἰ πάντα παραγράφοιμι, πληρώσω τὸ βιβλίον, ὥσπερ καὶ ὁ Χρύσιππος ἐπλήρωσεν.

17 Ἀλλ' ἐξ Ὁμήρου μὲν ἱκανὰ καὶ ταῦτα· τῶν δ' ἐξ Ἡσιόδου παραγραφέντων ὑπὸ Χρυσίππου παμπόλλων καὶ αὐτῶν ὄντων ἀρκέσει μοι δυοῖν ἢ τριῶν ἐπιμνησθῆναι παραδειγμάτων ἕνεκα·

«τοῦ[δε] γὰρ ἀέξετο θυμὸς ἐνὶ στήθεσσι φίλοισι.»

καὶ

«οἷον ἐνὶ στήθεσσι χόλον θυμαλγέ' ἔχουσα.»

καὶ

«πάντων ἐν[ὶ] στήθεσσιν ἀέξετο θυμὸς ἀγήνωρ.»

18 Ἐν οἷς ἐγὼ μὲν ἐκπλήττομαι τῆς μεγαλοψυχίας τὸν Χρύσιππον. / 266 δέον γὰρ ὡς ἄνθρωπον ἀνεγνωκότα τοσούτους ποιητὰς καὶ γιγνώσκοντα σαφῶς ἅπασι τοῖς δόγμασιν αὐτοὺς μαρτυροῦντας ἄλλοτε κατ' ἄλλα τῶν ἐπῶν, ὥσπερ καὶ Πλούταρχος ἐπέδειξεν ἐν τοῖς τῶν Ὁμηρικῶν μελετῶν, ἐκλέγειν μὲν ἐξ αὐτῶν ὅσα μαρτυρεῖ τῷ σπουδαζομένῳ πρὸς | 301 αὐτοῦ δόγματι, παραλείπειν δὲ τὰ μαχόμενα καὶ πᾶν ἐνίοτε κατα-
19 σκευάζοντα τοὐναντίον· ὁ δ' ὁμοίως ἑξῆς ἁπάντων μέμνηται. τὰ μὲν γὰρ τοιαῦτα τῶν ἐπῶν ἅπαντ' ἐχρῆν ὑπ' αὐτοῦ παραλελεῖφθαι, δι' ὧν δὲ νοῦν καὶ φρένας καὶ διάνοιαν καὶ λογισμὸν εἰπέ τις ποιητὴς ἐν καρδίᾳ περιέχεσθαι, συνάγειν ἔδει, καθάπερ ἔχει καὶ τὰ τοιαῦτα·

«καὶ τότε δὴ στηθέων Ἀθάμα φρένας ἐξέλετο Ζεύς.»

2] Hom. Il. ii. 142 *cf.* Hom. Od. xvii. 150 4] Hom. Od. xvii. 489 6 *et* 8] Hom. Od. xx. 22–23 *cf.* [Plut.] Hom. ii. 129 6] *cf. infra*, p. 186.28 8] *cf.* Plut. Mor. 506 B 16] Hes. fr. 317 Merkelbach-West 18] Hes. fr. 318 Merkelbach-West 20] Hes. Theog. 641 21–26] Plut. fr. 125 Sandbach 27–184.6] SVF II, p. 254 31] Hes. fr. dub. 69 Merkelbach-West

2 ὄρινε] ὠ. . . . L 4 ἐν μὲν] ἐμὸς L ἔαξε L 6 ἐν L 7 καὶ *del. Müller* 8 μάλ' *deperditum in* L ἐνεπίσῃ H: ἐν πίσῃ, *ut vid.*, L: *ex Hom. corr. Müller* μένε τετληυῖα] σημαίνετε τληυῖα H: σήμαινε τετληυία L: *ex Hom. corr. Müller* 9 ταῦτα μὲν γὰρ L τὸ *om.* L 14 παμπόλων H 15 παραδείγματος *Müller* 16 τοῦδε H L: *corr. Nauck Müller* ἀέξετο *in* ἄξετο *mut.* H²: ἀσσ.τ. L 18 ἔχουσι L 20 ἐνὶ H L: *corr. Ald.* 21 τῇ μεγαλοψυχίᾳ *Müller* τοῦ χρυσίππου L 23 αὐτοῦ H L: *corr. Müller* ἄλλοτε κατ' ἄλλα] ἄλλως τε καὶ τἄλλα L 25 ἐκλέγει H 26 παραλείπει H παρασκευάζοντα L 27 ὁ δ' H L: *corr. Kühn*: *del. Müller* 28 δὲ *om.* L 29 νοῦν] ν[II] *ex* ς *corr.* L 30 συνάγειν ἔδει *om.* L 31 ἀθ' ἅμα H: ἀθ' ἅμα L: *corr.* H² *Wilamowitz*

and

"Thus he spoke, and he aroused the spirit in their breasts."

and

"Telemachus fostered great grief in his heart."

and

"Thus he spoke, upbraiding his heart in his breast,
and his heart remained steadfast in obedience."

Now all these verses and in addition to them still others, numbering 16
in the thousands, from among those that Chrysippus cites say that the spirited part (of the soul) is in the heart. If I were to copy them all I would fill my book with them, just as Chrysippus filled his.

But these are enough from Homer. Chrysippus' citations 17
from Hesiod are also very numerous; I shall be content to mention two or three as examples:

"For his anger rose up in his breast."

and

"Having such bitter anger in her breast, that pains the spirit."

and

"A manly spirit arose in every breast."

In these citations I am amazed at Chrysippus' loftiness of 18
mind. Being a person familiar with the work of so many poets and knowing perfectly well that sooner or later, in some verse or other, they are witnesses to all doctrines, as Plutarch also showed in his Homeric Studies, Chrysippus should have selected from them whatever supports the doctrine he favors and omitted lines that disagree and at times prove the contrary view; but he quotes all alike,
one after another. He should have omitted all the contrary verses and 19
collected the ones in which some poet has stated that mind, intelligence, thought, and reason reside in the heart, such lines as these:

"Then Zeus removed the wits from the breast of Athamas."

καὶ

«ἔγνως, Ἐννοσίγαιε, ἐμὴν ἐν στήθεσι βουλήν.»

καὶ /

267 «αἰεί τοι τοιοῦτον ἐνὶ στήθεσσι νόημα.»

καὶ

«οὔ μοι τοιοῦτον ἐνὶ στήθεσσι νόημα.»

20 ὥσπερ γὰρ τοῦ προτέρου γένους τῶν ἐπῶν, δι' ὧν ἐν τῇ καρδίᾳ δεί-
κνυται τὰ τῆς ψυχῆς πάθη, παμπόλλη τις ἀφθονία παρὰ τοῖς ποιηταῖς
ἐστιν, οὕτως οὐδὲ θάτερον ὀλίγον, ἐν οἷς τὸ λογιζόμενον ἐν τῇ καρδίᾳ
τις, ὅσον ἐπὶ τοῖς ποιηταῖς, ἐπιδεῖξαι δυνήσεται. |

302 3. Ταῦτ' οὖν ἐχρῆν ἐκλέγειν μόνα τὸν Χρύσιππον, εἴπερ ὅλως
2 κατὰ μάρτυρας ἐγνώκει διαιρεῖν τὸν ἀγῶνα. τὸ δὲ πλείω μὲν ἐκεῖνα,
ταυτὶ δ' ἐλάττω γράψαι τῷ μὲν τὸ ἀληθὲς τῆς ἱστορίας ἐπιδεικνύντι
καλῶς ⟨ἂν⟩ γίγνοιτο· πλείω γὰρ ὄντως ἐστὶν ἐκεῖνα· τῷ δ' ὅπερ ὁ Χρύ-
σιππος σπουδάζει κατασκευάζειν ἐπιχειροῦντι πρὸς ἐναντιώματος ἂν
εἴη, καὶ μάλισθ' ὅσα φανερῶς ἐπιτιμῶντα[ι] ποιεῖ τὸν λογισμὸν τῷ
θυμῷ, καθάπερ καὶ τάδε· /

268 «στῆθος δὲ πλήξας κραδίην ἠν[ε]ίπαπε μύθῳ·
τέτλαθι δὴ κραδίη· καὶ κύντερον ἄλλο ποτ' ἔτλης.»

3 ταυτὶ γὰρ Ὅμηρος ἐποίησε τὸν Ὀδυσσέα λέγοντα πρὸς ἑαυτὸν
ἡνίκ' ἐφ' οἷς ἑώρα κατὰ τὴν οἰκίαν πραττομένοις ὑπὸ τῶν θεραπαινῶν
ἀνέζεσέ τε τὸ κατὰ τὴν καρδίαν αὐτοῦ θερμὸν ἔμελλέ τε νικήσας ὁ θυμὸς
4 τὸν λογισμὸν ἐπ' ἄκαιρον κόλασιν ἄξειν αὐτὸν τῶν γυναικῶν. ὃν γὰρ
ἱππεὺς πρὸς ἵππον ἢ κυνηγέτης πρὸς κύνα λόγον ἔχουσιν, τοῦτον ὁ
303 5 λογισμὸς πρὸς θυμόν. ἄρχειν μὲν γὰρ ἐν | ἅπασι καὶ κρατεῖν ἐστι δικαιό-
τερον τὸ φύσει κρεῖττον, ἱππεὺς μὲν ἵππου, κυνηγέτης δὲ κυνός, λογισμὸς
δὲ θυμοῦ, συμβαίνει δ' οὐκ ἀεὶ νόμῳ φύσεως διοικεῖσθαι τὴν συζυγίαν,
ἀλλ' ἵππος μὲν ἐνίοτε δυσπειθὴς οὐ κατὰ κόσμον ἐκφερόμενος συναπ-
ήνεγκεν αὑτῷ τὸν ἀναβάτην ἀρρωστίᾳ δυνάμεως ἢ ἐπιστήμης ἱππικῆς
ἀμαθίᾳ νικηθέντα, θυμὸς δὲ ἰσχυρὸς ἐπὶ τιμωρίαν ἄκαιρον ἐξορμήσας
269 σφοδρότερον ἔστιν ὅτε συνεπεσπάσατο λογι/σμὸν ἄρρωστον ἢ ἀμαθῆ.
6 εἰ μὲν γὰρ καὶ ῥώμην καὶ ἐπιστήμην ἔχοι, κρατήσει πάντως ὅ τε λογισμὸς
τοῦ θυμοῦ καὶ ὁ ἡνίοχος τοῦ ἵππου· εἰ δ' ἤτοι θατέρου τούτων ἢ ἀμφοῖν
στεροῖτο, κίνδυνος ἐνταῦθα τοῦ φύσει κρείττονος ἐπικρατῆσαι τὸ χεῖρον,

2] Hom. Il. xx. 20 *cf.* [Plut.] De vita et poesi Homeri ii. 115 4] Hom. Od. xiii. 330 6] *cf.* Hom. Od. xvii. 403 12–19] SVF III, p. 254 18–19] Hom. Od. xx. 17–18 *cf. supra*, p. 178.10–11 *infra*, p. 186.23–24 22–23] *cf. infra*, PHP 577.1–3 Müller

2 ἐνοσίγαιε L ἐνὶ L 6 οὔ μοι] οἴμοι L: οὔ τοι *Hom.* 8 παμπόλη H 9 θατέρου ὀλίγα *Bas.*: θατέρων ὀλίγη *Petersen* ἐν τῇ καρδίᾳ] τὸ H, *del. et* ἐν καρδία *sscr.* H² 10 τις] τοῖς L 12 τὸ] τοῦ L 13 τὸ *om.* L 14 ἂν *add. Kühn* ἐστὶν ἐκεῖνα *in ras.* L 16 ἐπιτιμῶνται H L: *corr. Corn.* ποιεῖ τὸν] ποιητῶν L 18 ἠνείπαπε H L: *corr. Kühn* 19 ποτ'] τ' H 20 ταῦτα L 22 αὐτῶ L θυμὸς] μ *ex* ρ *corr.* H 23 ὃν γὰρ] ὅνπερ L 24 λόγον ἔχουσιν] λέγουσι L 25 γὰρ *om.* L 27 ἀεὶ *ex* αἰεὶ *corr.* H 29 αὐτῶ L ἐπιστήμη L *(teste Müller)* 30 *ante* ἐπὶ *add.* καὶ H τιμωρίαν] τι μόριον L 31 συνα-πεσπάσατο L *(teste Müller)* 34 κίνδυνος] καιρὸς L

and

"You know, Earth-shaker, the design in my breast."

and

"Such a thought is always in your heart."

and

"No such thought is in my heart."

For just as there is in the poets a very great abundance of verses of 20
the former sort, by which the passions of the soul are shown to be in the heart, so this second class is by no means small, (the class of verses) in which one can show, so far as it depends on the poets, that reason is in the heart.

3. Now Chrysippus should have selected only this (latter kind), if his intention had been simply to decide the contest by witnesses.
Quoting more of the former and less of the latter would be an excel- 2
lent procedure for a person who is presenting the true state of the record, as the former are in fact more numerous; but for one who is endeavoring to make a case for the view that Chrysippus favors it would be perverse to cite them, especially the passages that clearly portray reason censuring passion, such as these:

"Striking his breast, he rebuked his heart with words:
Endure, my heart; you once put up with a thing more shameful."

This is what Homer had Odysseus say to himself when the heat 3
boiled up in his heart at the sight of the things being done in his house by the serving girls, and inflamed anger was about to overpower reason and lead him to an untimely punishment of the women.
For as a horseman is to a horse or a hunter to a hound, so reason is 4
to anger. For with greater justice the naturally superior rules and 5
prevails in all things, the horseman over the horse, the hunter over the hound, reason over anger; but it does not always happen that the union is governed by the law of nature. Sometimes a disobedient horse, running in wild disorder, has carried along his rider, defeated through weakness or ignorance of horsemanship; and a powerful anger, starting violently toward an untimely punishment, has sometimes dragged with it a reason that is weak or ignorant. If they have 6
strength and knowledge, reason will always rule over anger, and the charioteer over the horse; but if they lack either or both of these, then there is risk that the worse will overpower what is naturally

ὥσπερ ἐν Σκύθαις τε καὶ Γαλάταις καὶ πολλοῖς ἄλλοις βαρβάροις
ἔθνεσιν ὁ θυμὸς κρείττων τοῦ λογισμοῦ, παρ' ἡμῖν δὲ ἔν τε παισὶ καὶ
7 τοῖς ἀπαιδεύτοις ἀνθρώποις. Ὅμηρος δὲ δὴ τοῦτ' αὐτὸ ἐπιδεῖξαι βου-
λόμενος Ἕκτορα μὲν καὶ Ἀχιλλέα καί τινας ἑτέρους τοιούτους θυμῷ |
804 δουλεύοντας ὑποτίθεται νεανίσκους· Ὀδυσσέα δὲ καὶ Πολυδάμαντα
καὶ Νέστορα τῷ λογισμῷ κρατοῦντας τοῦ θυμοῦ, πολλάκις μὲν οὕτως
ἰσχυρῶς ὡς μηδ' ἐξορμῆσαι πρὸς ἄλογόν τινα πρᾶξιν τὸν θυμόν, ἔστιν
ὅτε δ' ὁρμῶντα μέν, ἀλλ' ὑπὸ τοῦ λογισμοῦ κατεχόμενον, ὥσπερ κἀν
8 τοῖσδε τοῖς ἔπεσιν Ὀδυσσέα πεποίηκεν· ἅπαντα δ' ἐφεξῆς αὐτὰ παρα-
γράψω·

«ἔνθ' Ὀδυσεὺς μνηστῆρσι κακὰ φρονέων ἐνὶ θυμῷ
κεῖτ' ἐγρηγορόων· ταὶ δ' ἐκ μεγάροιο γυναῖκες /
270 ἤϊσαν, αἳ μνηστῆρσιν ἐμι⟨σ⟩γέσκοντο πάροιθεν,
ἀλλήλοισι γέλω[τά] τε καὶ εὐφροσύνην παρέχουσαι.
τοῦ δ' ὠρίνετο θυμὸς ἐνὶ στήθεσσι φίλοισι·
πολλὰ δὲ μερμήριζε κατὰ φρένα καὶ κατὰ θυμόν,
ἠὲ μεταΐξας θάνατον τεύξειεν ἑκάστῃ,
ἦ ἔτ' ἐῷ μνηστῆρσιν ὑπερφιάλοισι μιγῆναι
ὕστατα καὶ πύματα· κραδίη δέ οἱ ἔνδον ὑλάκτει
[ἀγαζομένου κακὰ ἔργα].
9 ὡς δὲ κύων ἀμαλῇσι περὶ σκυλάκεσ⟨σ⟩ι βεβῶσα
ἄνδρ' ἀγνοιήσασ' ὑλάει μέμονέν τε μάχεσθαι, |
805 ὥς ῥα τοῦ ἔνδον ὑλάκτει ⟨ἀγαζομένου κακὰ ἔργα·⟩
στῆθος δὲ πλήξας κραδίην ἠν[ε]ίπαπε μύθῳ·
τέτλαθι δή, κραδίη· καὶ κύντερον ἄλλο ποτ' ἔτλης
ἤματι τῷ, ὅτε τοι μένος ἄσχετος ἤσθιε Κύκλωψ
ἰφθίμους ἑτάρους, σὺ δ' ἐτόλμας, ὄφρα σε μῆτις /
271 ἐξάγαγ' ἐξ ἄντροιο οἰόμενον θανέεσθαι.
ὣς ἔφατ' ἐν στήθεσσι καθαπτόμενος φίλον ἦτορ.»

1–3] *cf.* Maimonid. Aph. xxiv. 56 M. Etziony, Bull. Hist. Med. 35 (1961), 163–168 1 Σκύθαις] *cf.* Plat. Resp. 435 e 6 2–3] *cf.* Plat. Resp. 441 a 7–9 11–28] Hom. Od. xx. 5–22 19] *cf. supra*, p. 178.8 Plut. Mor. 506 B [Plut.] Hom. ii. 130 20–21] *cf.* Plut. Mor. 494 D 20] *cf.* [Plut.] Hom. ii. 86 23–24] *cf. supra*, pp. 178.10–11; 184.18–19 Plat. Resp. 390 d 4–5 Phaed. 94 d 8 – e 1 Heracl. Quaest. Hom. 18 23] *cf. infra*, p. 356.2, 21 24] *cf.* [Plut.] Hom. ii. 129 28] *cf. supra*, p. 182.6

1 *ante* ἐν *add.* γὰρ H 2 παισὶ *ex* πᾶσι *corr.* H 3 δὲ δὴ] δή μοι L 7 τινα πρᾶξιν *deperdita in* L 11 ὀδοσσεὺς H: ὀδυσσεὺς L: *corr. Ald.* 12 δ' ἐκ *deperdita in* L 13 ἦσαν L ἐμιγέσκοντο H L: *corr. Kühn* 14 ἀλλήλῃσι *ex Hom. Müller* γέλωτά τε H: γέλωτα L: *ex Hom. correxi* 15 τοῦ δ' *deperdita in* L 16 πολλὰ *ex* πολα *(?) corr.* H μερμέριζε H 17 θανάτου L 18 ἐτεῷ H: *corr. Ald.*: ἐτεὸν L 19 ὕστατα *ex* ὦστ' *(?) corr.* L ἀγαζομένου κακὰ ἔργα H: ἀγεομένου *(?)* κα.ὰ ἔργα στῆθος δὲ πλήξας L: *del. Ald.* 20 ὁμαλῇσι L: *ex Hom. corr. Müller*: ἀπαλῇσι *(ex -οῖσι corr.)* H σκυλάκεσι H L: *corr. Ald.* 21 ἀγνοιήσας H μέμηνέ H L: μέμονέ *Ald.*: *ex Hom. corr. Chart.* 22 ἀγαζομένου κακὰ ἔργα *suppl. Ald.* *(cf. lin. 19)* 23 ἠνείπαπε H L: *corr. Chart.* 25 τοι μένος] ἤμενος L 26 δὲ ἐτόλμας L: δὲ ἔτλης H ὄφρά H L: *corr. Chart.* μήτις H L: *corr. Chart.* 27 ἐξάγαγ' ἐξ] ἐξαγάγετ' L

superior. Indeed among the Scythians and Gauls and many other barbaric peoples, anger is stronger than reason; and among us this is the case with the young and the uneducated. Homer, wishing to 7
portray this very thing, represents Hector, Achilles, and some others of the same kind, as young men enslaved to anger; but he represents Odysseus and Polydamas and Nestor as overcoming anger with reason, often with such power that the anger does not even set out toward some irrational act; and when on occasion it does set out, it is restrained by reason, as Homer has portrayed Odysseus in the following verses. I shall quote the whole passage 8
in order:

"Then Odysseus lay awake, planning evil in his spirit against the suitors;
and the women came out of the great hall,
the women who in times past had been lying with the suitors,
providing each other with laughter and merriment.
His spirit stirred in his breast,
and he debated much in his mind and spirit,
whether he should rush upon the women and devise death for each of them,
or allow them to lie with the proud suitors
this last and final time; and his heart within him howled.
As a bitch, standing by her young pups, 9
barks at a man she does not recognize and is eager to fight,
just so his heart within him howled in indignation at their evil deeds.
And striking his breast he rebuked his heart with words:
Endure, my heart; you once put up with a thing more shameful,
on that day when the Cyclops with unbridled passion ate
your mighty companions; yet you endured until your craft
led you from the cave where you thought you would die.
Thus he spoke, upbraiding his heart in his breast."

10 εἰ μὴ σαφῶς ἐν τούτοις Ὅμηρος ἐκδιηγεῖται μάχην θυμοῦ πρὸς λογι-
σμὸν ἐν ἀνδρὶ φρονίμῳ καὶ νίκην μὲν τοῦ λογισμοῦ, τοῦ θυμοῦ δ' εὐπεί-
θειαν πρὸς αὐτόν, οὐδ' ἄλλ' οὐδὲν ἄν τις ἡμῖν συγχωρήσειε μανθάνειν
11 τοῦ ποιητοῦ. τῶν γὰρ οὕτως ἐναργῶς λεγομένων εἰς ἀμφιβολίαν ἀ-
χθέντων οὐδὲ τοῖς ἄλλοις ἂν ἔχοι τις ὅ τι χρήσαιτο. τὰς γὰρ θεραπαίνας
ἁμαρτανούσας ὁρῶν Ὀδυσσεὺς ὑπὸ μὲν τοῦ θυμοῦ βιαίως εἵλκετο πρὸς
τὴν τιμωρίαν αὐτῶν, ὑπὸ δὲ τοῦ λογισμοῦ κατείχετο τὴν ἀκαιρίαν ἐκ-
12 διδάσκοντος. ἐπεὶ δ' οὐκ ἠδύνατο ῥᾳδίως πείθειν ὁ λογισμὸς τὸν θυμὸν
306 ἀνα|βάλλεσθαι τὴν τιμωρίαν εἰς ἐπιτηδειότερον καιρόν, σφοδρότερον
αὐτῷ προσφέρεται, καθάπερ ἵππον ἐκφερόμενον ἡνίοχος ἀντισπῶν βιαίως
ἰσχυρῷ χαλινῷ, καὶ δὴ καὶ ταῦτά φησι πρὸς αὐτόν· 'καρτέρει κατὰ
272 τὸ παρόν, ὦ γενναιοτάτη καρδία, καθάπερ / που καὶ πρότερον ἐκαρ-
τέρησας ἐπὶ Κύκλωπος, ὁρῶσα τοὺς ἑταίρους ὑπ' αὐτοῦ διαφθει-
ρομένους.'

13 Ἐμοὶ μὲν δὴ τούτων τῶν ἐπῶν εὐκαιρότατα μὲν ὁ Πλάτων δοκεῖ
μνημονεύειν ἐν τετάρτῳ Πολιτείας, ἀκαιρότατα δ' ὁ Χρύσιππος, ἔτι
δὲ μᾶλλον ὧν Εὐριπίδης ἐποίησε λέγουσαν τὴν Μήδειαν, ἡνίκα καὶ
14 κατὰ τὴν ἐκείνης ψυχὴν ὁ λογισμὸς ἐστασίαζε πρὸς τὸν θυμόν. ᾔδει μὲν
γὰρ ὡς ἀνόσιόν τι καὶ δεινὸν ἔργον ἐργάζοιτο τῇ τῶν παίδων ἐπι-
χειροῦσα σφαγῇ, καὶ διὰ τοῦτ' ὤκνει τε καὶ ἀνεβάλλετο καὶ οὐκ εὐθὺς ὁρ-
15 μήσασα ἔπραξε τοὔργον. αὖθις δ' αὐτὴν ὁ θυμὸς ὥσπερ τις ἵππος δυσπει-
θὴς νικήσας τὸν ἡνίοχον ἐπὶ τοὺς παῖδας εἷλκε βίᾳ καὶ ἔπειτα πάλιν ὁ
λογισμὸς ἀντέσπα τε καὶ ἀπῆγεν, εἶτ' αὖθις ἀνθεῖλκεν ὁ θυμός, εἶτ'
16 αὖθις ὁ λογισμός. ὥστε πολλάκις ἄνω καὶ κάτω πρὸς ἀμφοῖν ἀγομένη,
307 ὡς συνεχώ|ρησε τῷ θυμῷ, τηνικαῦτα ποιεῖ λέγουσαν ὁ Εὐριπίδης
αὐτήν· /

273 «καὶ μανθάνω μὲν οἷα δρᾶν μέλλω κακά,
θυμὸς δὲ κρείττων τῶν ἐμῶν βουλευμάτων.»

17 μανθάνει μὲν δήπου τὸ μέγεθος ὧν μέλλει δράσειν κακῶν ὑπὸ τοῦ λογι-
σμοῦ διδασκομένη, κρείττονα δ' εἶναί φησιν αὐτοῦ τὸν θυμὸν καὶ διὰ
τοῦθ' ὑπ' ἐκείνου πρὸς τοὔργον ἀπάγεσθαι βιαίως ἔμπαλιν Ὀδυσσεῖ
18 τῷ λογισμῷ τὸν θυμὸν ἐπισχόντι. βαρβάρων μὲν γὰρ καὶ ἀπαιδεύτων
ἀνθρώπων ἔθετο παράδειγμα τὴν Μήδειαν Εὐριπίδης, οἷς ὁ θυμὸς
ἰσχυρότερος τοῦ λογισμοῦ· Ἑλλήνων δὲ καὶ πεπαιδευμένων, οἷόν περ
αὖ πάλιν ὁ ποιητὴς ὑπέθετο τὸν Ὀδυσσέα, κρείττων ὁ λογισμὸς τοῦ

15–18] SVF II, p. 255 16] Plat. Resp. iv: 441 b–c *cf. infra*, p. 356,2
27–28] Eur. Medea 1078–1079 *cf. infra*, pp. 244.2–5; 274.13–14

2 ἐν *om.* H 3 ἄν] ἣν L συγχωρήσει ἐκμανθάνειν H *post* μανθάνειν *add.* παρὰ *Diels* 4 λεγομένων] φαινομένων L ἀχθέντων] λεχθέντων L 5 οὐδὲ] οὔτε L ἄλλοι H γὰρ *om.* L 6 *post* ὁρῶν *add.* δ' L 11 αὐτὸν *in* αὐτὸν *mut.* L 13 ἐπὶ κύκλω$^{\pi}$ H: ὑπὸ τοῦ κύκλωπος L ὑπ' αὐτοῦ *om.* L 15 εὐκαιρο$^{\tau\tau}$' H: ἐνκαιρο$^{\tau\tau}$' L: εὐκαιρότατος R: *corr. Ald.* 16 τετάρτῳ] τῷ τετάρτω τῆς L ἀκαιρο$^{\tau\tau}$' H L: ἀκαιρότατος R: *corr. Ald.* 17 τὴν *ex* τῆς *corr.* L 20 ἀνεβάλετο L 21 *post* δ' *add.* ἂν L 25 τηνικαῦτα ποιεῖ] τοιαῦτα ποιεῖ τηνικαῦτα L: τηνικαῦτα ποιεῖ τοιαῦτα *Müller* 33 οἷς] ὡς L

If Homer is not clearly describing in these (verses) a battle of anger 10
against reason in a prudent man, the victory of reason and the obe-
dience of anger to it, then there is nothing else that anyone would
concede that I understand in the poet. For when the meaning of such 11
clear statements is brought into dispute, then a person cannot do
anything with the rest either. Odysseus, seeing the misconduct
of the maidservants, was drawn forcibly by anger to their punishment
but was checked by reason, which pointed out that the time was not
right. But since reason could not easily persuade anger to postpone 12
punishment to a more suitable occasion, it attacked with greater
vehemence, like a charioteer forcibly checking a runaway horse by a
pull on a strong bit; and reason addressed these words to it: 'Be patient
for the present, my gallant heart, even as you were patient before
in the Cyclops' cave, when you saw your comrades destroyed by
him.'

Plato, I think, recalls these words most opportunely in the 13
fourth (book) of the Republic, but Chrysippus most inopportunely;
and even less apposite is his quotation of the lines which Euripides
had Medea speak, when in her soul, too, reason was contending
with anger. She knew what an unholy and terrible thing she was 14
doing, when she set out to kill her children, and therefore she hesi-
tated and delayed and did not immediately carry out the act she
had started to do. Then anger dragged her again to the children by 15
force, like some disobedient horse that has overpowered the chario-
teer; then reason in turn drew her back and led her away, then anger
again exerted an opposite pull, and then again reason. Consequently, 16
being repeatedly driven up and down by the two of them, when she
has yielded to anger, at that time Euripides has her say:

> "I understand the evils I am going to do,
> but anger prevails over my counsels."

Of course she knows the magnitude of the evils she is going to do, 17
being instructed by reason; but she says that her anger overpowers
her reason, and therefore she is forcibly led by anger to the deed,
quite the opposite of Odysseus, who checked his anger with reason.
Euripides has made Medea an example of barbarians and unedu- 18
cated persons, in whom anger is stronger than reason; but among
Greeks and educated people, such as Odysseus, as the poet presents

19 θυμοῦ. πολλάκις μὲν οὖν ὁ λογισμὸς εἰς τοσοῦτον τοῦ θυμοειδοῦς μέρους
τῆς ψυχῆς κρείττων ἐστίν, ὡς μηδέποτε μάχην αὐτοῖς γίγνεσθαι πρὸς
ἀλλήλους, ἀλλὰ τὸν μὲν ἄρχειν, τὸν δὲ ἄρχεσθαι, καὶ τοῦτο μὲν τοῖς
20 εἰς τέλος ἥκουσι φιλοσοφίας ὑπάρχει· πολλάκις δ' ὁ θυμὸς τοῦ λογισμοῦ
808 κρατεῖ τοσοῦτον ὡς | ἄρχειν τε καὶ ἡγεῖσθαι διὰ παντός, ὁρᾶται δ' ἔν
274 τε πολλοῖς τῶν βαρβάρων τοῦτο / καὶ τῶν παίδων τοῖς φύσει θυμικοῖς,
21 ἔτι δὲ θηρίων οὐκ ὀλίγοις καὶ ἀνθρώπων τοῖς θηριώδεσιν· ἔστιν ὅτε δὲ
οὐδέτερον εἰς τοσοῦτον ἰσχυρότερόν ἐστιν ὡς ἐφέλκεσθαι παραχρῆμα
θάτερον, ἀλλ' ἐναντιοῦταί τε πρὸς ἄλληλα καὶ διαμάχεται καὶ νικᾷ τῷ
χρόνῳ θάτερον — ἐπ' Ὀδυσσέως μὲν ὁ λογισμός, ἐπὶ Μηδείας δ' ὁ
θυμός —, ὡς δύο ὄντα αὐτὰ μόρια τῆς ψυχῆς ἢ εἰ μὴ μόρια, πάντως γε
22 δυνάμεις τινές. ὁ δὲ Χρύσιππος οὔτε μόρια ψυχῆς ταῦτ' εἶναι νομίζων
οὔτε δυνάμεις ἀλόγους ἑτέρας τῆς λογικῆς ὅμως οὐκ ὀκνεῖ τῶν Ὀδυσσέως
τε καὶ Μηδείας ἐπῶν μνημονεύειν ἐναργῶς καταβαλ⟨λ⟩όντων τὴν δόξαν
αὐτοῦ.

23 Πῶς ἂν οὖν τις ἔτι διαλέγοιτο τοιούτοις ἀνδράσι μήτε τῶν ἐναργῶς
φαινομένων φροντίζουσιν, ὡς ἤδη πολλάκις ἔδειξα, καὶ τῶν ἐξελεγχόν-
24 των τὰ δόγματ' αὐτῶν ὡς μαρτυρούντων μνημονεύουσιν; ἐμπέπλησται
γὰρ ὁ περὶ ἡγεμονικοῦ λόγος ὑπὸ Χρυσίππου γεγραμμένος ἐπῶν
309 ποιητικῶν ἤτοι τὰ πάθη περὶ τὸν θώρακά τε καὶ τὴν καρδίαν | συνί-
275 στασθαι μαρτυρούντων ἢ δύο εἶναι τῆς ψυχῆς / δυνάμεις ὅλῳ τῷ γένει
25 διαφερούσας ἀλλήλων, τὴν μὲν ἄλογον, τὴν δὲ λογικήν. ὥσπερ γὰρ
ἐξ Ὁμήρου καὶ Ἡσιόδου βραχέα παρεθέμην ὀλίγῳ πρόσθεν ὧν ὁ
Χρύσιππος ἔγραψεν, οὕτως ἐξ Ὀρφέως καὶ Ἐμπεδοκλέους καὶ
Τυρταίου καὶ Στησιχόρου καὶ Εὐριπίδου καὶ ἑτέρων ποιητῶν
ἐπῶν μνημονεύει παμπόλ⟨λ⟩ων ὁμοίαν ἐχόντων ἀτοπίαν, οἷον καὶ ὅταν
εἴπῃ Τυρταῖον λέγοντα

«αἴθωνος δὲ λέοντος ἔχων ἐν στήθεσι θυμόν.»

26 ὅτι μὲν γὰρ ἔχει ὁ λέων θυμόν, ἀκριβῶς ἅπαντες ἄνθρωποι καὶ πρὶν
ἀκοῦσαι Τυρταίου γιγνώσκομεν, οὐ μὴν Χρυσίππῳ γ' ἔπρεπε πα-
27 ραθέσθαι τὸ ἔπος ἀφαιρουμένῳ τοὺς λέοντας τὸν θυμόν. οὐδὲν γάρ, ὡς
οἴεται, τῶν ἀλόγων ζῴων οὔτε τὸ θυμοειδὲς οὔτε τὸ ἐπιθυμητικὸν οὔτε
τὸ λογιστικὸν ἔχει ἀλλ' ὡς εἴρηταί μοι καὶ κατὰ τὸ πρῶτον γράμμα,
παρὰ πᾶσαν τὴν ἐνάργειαν ἀφαιροῦνται τῶν εἰρημένων ἁπάντων αὐτὰ
810 *276* 28 σχεδὸν ἅπαντες οἱ Στωϊκοί. Τυρταῖος δέ γε, | καθάπερ / οὖν καὶ
Ὅμηρος καὶ Ἡσίοδος καὶ ἁπλῶς εἰπεῖν ἅπαντες οἱ ποιηταί, σφο-
δρότατον ἔχειν φησὶ τοὺς λέοντας τὸν θυμόν, ὥστε καὶ τῶν ἀνθρώπων
ὅστις ἂν ᾖ θυμοειδέστατος, εἰκάζουσι λέοντι· καὶ χωρὶς δὲ τῶν ποιητῶν
29 ἅπαντες ἄνθρωποι τοὺς θυμικωτάτους λέοντας ὀνομάζουσιν, [οὕτως]

12–15] SVF II, p. 255 18–35] SVF II, p. 255 28] Tyrt. fr. 10 Diehl 31–35] libri primi test., *v. supra*, p. 70.6–9 *cf. supra*, p. 102.23–24

1 τοῦτο L 3 τὸν[II] *in* τὸ *correxerit Einarson* 5–6 ἔν τε] ἐν τοῖς L: ἔν τε τοῖς *Müller* 7 οὐκ – 306.17 τοιαῦτα *om.* L 14 καταβαλόντων H: *corr. Ald.* 23 Ὁμήρου] ηρ *e corr.* H 26 παμπόλων H: *corr. Ald.* 27 εἴπῃ] ἐπαινῇ *Müller* 29 ὁ *del. Petersen* 34 ἐνάργειαν] ἐνέργειαν H: *corr. Cobet* 37 φασὶ H: *corr. Einarson* 39–192.1 οὕτως . . . οὕτως H: *prius del. Schöne, posterius Müller*

him, reason prevails over anger. In many instances reason is so much 19
stronger than the spirited part of the soul that a conflict never arises
between them; the one rules, the other is ruled. This is the case with
persons who have reached the ultimate goal of philosophy. In many 20
other instances anger is so much more powerful than reason that it
rules and governs everywhere; this is seen in many barbarians, in
children who are naturally inclined to anger, and in no few beasts
and beastlike men. There are times when neither of the two is so 21
much stronger that it immediately pulls the other its way, but they
oppose each other and fight it out, and eventually one of them pre-
vails – reason in Odysseus, anger in Medea –, inasmuch as they are
two parts of the soul or, if not parts, then certainly powers. But 22
Chrysippus, who holds that they are not parts of the soul, and
that the soul has no irrational powers separate from reason, neverthe-
less does not hesitate to mention the lines spoken by Odysseus
and Medea that clearly refute his doctrine.

How can you still talk to such men, who pay no attention to 23
evident facts, as I have often pointed out before now, and who intro-
duce evidence refuting their views as attesting them? For the account 24
of the governing part that Chrysippus wrote is filled with lines of
verse which testify either that the affections arise in the region of
the chest and heart, or that there are in the soul two powers entirely
different in kind, the one irrational, the other rational. And just as I 25
gave a brief review a short time ago of the excerpts that Chrysippus
took from Homer and Hesiod, so also he cites very many lines
from Orpheus, Empedocles, Tyrtaeus, Stesichorus, Euri-
pides, and other poets, with the same ineptness, as when he speaks
of Tyrtaeus as saying:

"With a tawny lion's spirit in his breast."

We all know very well that a lion has spirit, even before hearing it 26
from Tyrtaeus; and yet it was not appropriate for Chrysippus to
cite the line, since Chrysippus denies spirit to lions. He holds that 27
none of the irrational animals has the spirited or desiderative or
rational part; as I said also in the first book, every Stoic, so far as
I know, contrary to all clear evidence deprives them of all these
(parts). But Tyrtaeus, like Homer and Hesiod, and, in short, 28
all poets, says that lions have the most violent spirit, and that is
why they compare the most spirited persons to lions. And quite
apart from the poets, all men speak of very high-spirited persons as

οὐδὲ τοῖς ἀθληταῖς παύονται καθ' ἑκάστην ἡμέραν οὕτως ἐγκελευόμενοι. καὶ τοὐναντίον ἔοικεν ἅπαν ἢ βούλεται συμπίπτειν τῷ Χρυσίππῳ. τῶν γὰρ ἀπὸ τῆς φύσεως αὐτοῦ τοῦ ζητουμένου πράγματος ἐπιχειρημάτων ἀποχωρῶν ἑκάστοτε καὶ ῥητορικῶς μᾶλλον ἢ φιλοσόφως ἐν πλήθει μαρτύρων τὸ νικᾶν θέμενος ὑπ' αὐτῶν ὧν ἐπικαλεῖται προ[παρα]δίδοται.

4. Καὶ γὰρ οὖν ὅταν εἴπῃ διὰ τοῦτο λέγεσθαί τινας ἀκαρδίους, ὅτι πεπιστεύκασιν ἅπαντες ἄνθρωποι τὸ ἡγεμονικὸν τῆς ψυχῆς ἐν τῇ καρδίᾳ περιέχεσθαι, θαυμάζειν ἄξιον τἀνδρός, εἰ μὴ ἄχρι τοσούτου παρακολουθεῖ τοῖς λεγομένοις ὡς γνωρίζειν ὅτι μηδένα τῶν ἀνοήτων τε
311 καὶ ἀσυνέτων ἀκάρδιον ὀνομάζουσιν, ἀλλ' ἐκείνους μὲν ἅπαντας | ἐπει-
277 δὰν σκώπτωσιν οὐκ ἔχειν ἐγκέφαλόν φασι, τοὺς ἀτόλμους δὲ καὶ / δει-
2 λοὺς ἀκαρδίους ὀνομάζουσιν. ἐξελέγχεται τοίνυν κἀνταῦθα τὸ τοῦ Χρυσίππου δόγμα πρὸς αὐτῶν ὧν ἐπικαλεῖται μαρτύρων ἐν ἐγκεφάλῳ μὲν ὑπολαμβανόντων εἶναι τὸ λογιζόμενον, ἐν καρδίᾳ δὲ τὸ θυμο-
3 ειδές. ἀλλὰ νὴ Δία θαυμασίως ὅπως ἐξηγεῖται τοὔνομα τὸ[ν] ἀκάρδιον ᾗτινι διανοίᾳ λέγουσιν οἱ πολλοί, συνάπτων εὐθὺς αὐτῷ καὶ τὸν ἄ-
4 σπλαγχνον· ἔχει δὲ ἡ ῥῆσις ὧδε· «παραβάλλουσι δὲ τοῖς εἰρημένοις καὶ τὰ τοιαῦτα τῶν λεγομένων, οἷον τοὺς ἀσπλάγχνους, καθ' ὅ φαμεν μὴ ἔχειν τινὰς ἐγκέφαλον καὶ ἔχειν, οὕτως ἡμᾶς ὑπονοοῦντες λέγειν καὶ μὴ ἔχειν καρδίαν τινὰς καὶ ἔχειν κατὰ τὰ προειρημένα, τῶν μὲν ἀσπλάγχνων τάχα λαμβανομένων κατὰ τὸ μηδὲν ἔχειν ἔνδον συναλγοῦν κατὰ τὰ ἐναντία καὶ ἀπὸ τῆς καρδίας οὕτως αὐτῶν κοινότερον λεγομένων, τοῦ δ' ἐγκεφάλου λαμβανομένου ἤτοι κατὰ τὰ αὐτὰ ὁμοίου τινὸς ὄντος ἢ διὰ
278 5 τὸ καὶ τοῦτον ἔχειν τινὰ κυρίαν τοῖς σπλάγχνοις ὁμοίαν.» ἡ / μὲν ῥῆσις
312 αὕτη· χρὴ δ' αὐτὴν ἀναγνῶναί τινα καὶ τρὶς καὶ τετράκις | ἐπὶ σχολῇ πολλῇ ἀκριβῶς προσέχοντα τὸν νοῦν τοῖς λεγομένοις. οὕτως γὰρ μόνως οἶμαι πεισθήσεσθαι τὸ κατὰ τὴν παροιμίαν λεγόμενον ὑπάρχειν
6 αὐτῇ, τὸ «λαβὲ μηδὲν καὶ κράτει καλῶς». ἔγωγ' οὖν ἐν πολλοῖς πολλάκις βιβλίοις ἀνεγνωκὼς ῥήσεις ἐν αἷς ὀνόματα καὶ ῥήματα συνάπτεται μηδεμίαν ἔχοντα διάνοιαν, οὐδαμόθι τοῦτ' ἀκριβούμενον εἶδον οὕτως ὡς
7 κατὰ τήνδε τὴν νῦν ἡμῖν προγεγραμμένην λέξιν. αἴνιγμα γάρ ἐστιν ὁ λόγος τοῦ Χρυσίππου θαυμαστῇ τινι καταπεπλεγμένον ἀσαφείᾳ μετὰ συντομίας ἀκαίρου. καίτοι τήν γε συντομίαν οὐδὲ καθ' ἕνα τῶν ἑαυτοῦ λόγων ἐζήλωκεν, ἀλλ' οὕτω μακρός ἐστιν ὡς πολλάκις ἐν ὅλῳ βιβλίῳ πολυειδῶς ὑπὲρ τῶν αὐτῶν ἄνω τε καὶ κάτω τοὺς λόγους ἐλίτ-
8 τειν. τὸ μὲν δὴ τῆς ἀσαφείας αὐτῷ σύνηθες ἀσθενείᾳ τῆς ἑρμηνευτικῆς

3–5] *cf. supra*, p. 110.22–24, 30–33 4 ἀποχωρῶν] *cf. infra*, PHP 578.4 Müller 7–9] SVF II, p. 249 16–29] SVF II, p. 249 29] *cf.* Erasmus, Adagia, chil. IV, centur. VII, prov. XXIV 34–194.1] SVF II, p. 249 36] *cf. infra*, p. 258.27–28 Plat. Theaet. 195 c 2–3

6 προπαραδίδοται H: *corr. Cobet Schöne* 16 ἐξηγῆται H: *corr. Ald.* τὸν H: *corr. Ald.* 19 καθὸ H: *corr.* R *Ald.* 29 ἐγώ γ' H: *corr. Kühn* 31 οὐδαμό' (θ superscr.) H: οὐδαμόθεν M *Ald.*: *corr. Müller* 36 ἐλίττειν H: *corr. Bas.* 37 αὐτῶν H: *corr. Ald.*

lions, and every day without end they urge athletes on in this way. 29
The outcome seems to be the exact opposite of what Chrysippus
intends. In every case he withdraws from arguments based on the 30
nature of the thing itself that is under investigation; and placing
victory in an abundance of witnesses, more like a rhetorician than a
philosopher, he is betrayed by the very witnesses he invokes.

4. When Chrysippus says that the reason why some people
are called 'heartless' is that everyone believes that the governing part
of the soul is enclosed in the heart, I must marvel at the man, if he
does not understand common usage well enough to recognize that
in no case do people speak of unintelligent and stupid persons as
'heartless'; all such persons, they say when they mock them, have
no brain. It is the timid and cowardly that they call heartless. Here, 2
too, the doctrine of Chrysippus is refuted by the very witnesses he
calls upon, since they suppose reason to be in the brain and the
spirited part in the heart. But it is indeed amazing how he explains 3
the meaning that common usage gives to the word 'heartless', from
which he immediately passes to the person who 'has no internal
organ'. The passage is as follows: "And people set beside the expres- 4
sions mentioned such expressions as the following, for example, 'those
who have no internal organ', in virtue of which mode of speech we
say that this or that person 'has no brain' or 'has (a brain)'; they do
so with the notion that in this sense we also say that this or that
person 'has no heart' or 'has (a heart)', in the meaning that accords
with what we said earlier. Here perhaps the expression 'those who
have no internal organ' gets its meaning in virtue of their having
nothing inside that shares pain, these persons being also more usually
described by a negative reference to the heart, the 'brain' being taken
either in the same sense, since it is something similar (to the heart),
or else because the brain too has some role (in these matters) like
that of the internal organs." This is the passage. You must read it 5
three or four times over, taking plenty of time, and giving close atten-
tion to what is said. For this is the only way, I believe, that you will
be persuaded that the words of the proverb apply to it: "Take nothing
and guard it well." For my part, I have read many passages in many 6
books, in which nouns and verbs were strung together without any
meaning, but I have never seen this done with such skill as in the
passage I have just now quoted. For Chrysippus' argument is a 7
riddle, contrived in amazing obscurity along with ill-timed brevity.
Yet he showed no strong desire for brevity in a single one of his
works; on the contrary, he is so longwinded that often for a whole
book he twists his arguments up and down, in many forms, about the
same subjects. Lack of clarity, to be sure, is habitual with him, being 8
the result of a deficiency in his ability to express himself; and it seems

δυνάμεως ἑπόμενον, καί μοι δοκεῖ καὶ αὐτὸς αἰσθανόμενος αὐτῆς τρὶς
279 καὶ τετράκις ὑπὲρ τῶν αὐτῶν ἐπὶ πλεῖ/στον ἐκτείνειν τοὺς λόγους οὐκ
9 ὀκνεῖ· τὸ δὲ τῆς βραχυλογίας ἀηθές τε καὶ σπανίως ὑπ' αὐτοῦ γιγνό-
813 μενον, ἐν οἷς ἂν μάλιστα | λόγοις ἄφυκτον αἰσθάνηται τὸ σφάλμα τῶν
ἑαυτοῦ δογμάτων. βούλεται γὰρ οἶμαι παρατρέχειν αὐτὸ διὰ ταχέων,
10 ἀλλ⟨ως⟩ ὑπομένων ἐξελέγχεσθαι. καί μοι δοκεῖ, καθάπερ ἐν τοῖς ἄλλοις
λόγοις ἀγωνίζεται σαφῶς ἑρμηνεύειν, οὕτως ἐν οἷς ἐξελέγχεται συγκρύ-
πτειν τὸν λόγον ἀσαφείᾳ μετὰ βραχυλογίας ἵνα δηλαδὴ δοκῇ μὲν ἀπολε-
λογῆσθαι πρὸς τοὔγκλημα καὶ μὴ παρεληλυθέναι τελέως αὐτό, μηδὲν δὲ
ἡμεῖς ἔχωμεν ἀντιλέγειν τοῖς εἰρημένοις, ὧν οὐδ' ὅλως μανθάνομεν.

11 Αὐτίκα γέ τοι κατὰ τὴν προγεγραμμένην ῥῆσιν, ἐν ᾗ τὸ ἄσπλαγ-
χνον καὶ τὸ μὴ ἔχειν ἐγκέφαλον ὅπως οἱ πολλοὶ λέγουσιν ἐξηγεῖται,
ἐμοὶ μὲν δοκεῖ τοιόνδε τι δηλοῦν· ἀσπλάγχνους μὲν καλοῦσιν ἐνίους ἐν
ἴσῳ τῷ ἀκαρδίους, ἐπειδὴ σπλάγχνον ἡ καρδία, τὸ δ' ἐγκέφαλον μὴ
ἔχειν ἐν ἴσῳ τῷ ἄσπλαγχνον εἶναι λέγουσιν, ἐπειδὴ καὶ οὗτος σπλάγχνον
280 12 τ' ἐστὶ καὶ κύριον. οὐ μὴν προσίενταί γε πάντες οἱ / Στωϊκοὶ τὴν τοι-
αύτην ἐξήγησιν ἀλλ' ἕτερον μέν τι λέγεσθαί φασιν, οὐ δηλοῦσι δὲ αὐτό,
τῶν ἐσωτερικῶν ὑπάρχον δηλονότι, καὶ ἐπιτιμῶσιν ἡμῖν εὐθέως ὡς προ-
814 πετῶς | ἀντιλέγουσι πρὶν γνῶναι τὸ λεγόμενον· οἱ δὲ καὶ λοιδοροῦντες
σφοδρότερον ἀνεισάκτους τε καὶ φιλονείκους ἀποκαλοῦσιν οὔ φασί τε
13 διδάξειν τὸ λεγόμενον ἀπαιδεύτους ἀνθρώπους. καίτοι τά γ' ἄλλα καὶ
μὴ βουλομένων ἡμῶν διεξέρχονται μακρῶς, ἀλλ' ὅταν ὡς εἶπον ἐπί τι
τοιοῦτον ἀφίκωνται μηδεμίαν ἔχον εὐπορίαν φλυαρίας, οἱ μὲν γράφοντες
τὰ βιβλία ταχέως θ' ἅμα καὶ ⟨ἀ⟩σαφῶς παρατρέχουσιν, οἱ δ' ἐξηγούμενοι
τὰ τούτων συγγράμματα φθόνου μᾶλλον ὑπόνοιαν εἰς τοὺς ἀκούοντας
ἐκπέμπειν ἕτοιμοι γίγνονται προσποιούμενοι μὴ βούλεσθαι διδάσκειν
ἡμᾶς ἤπερ ὁμολογοῦντες νενικῆσθαι.

14 Ἀλλὰ τοὺς μὲν ἀσπλάγχνους τε καὶ ἀνεγκεφάλους ἤδη παρέλθωμεν,
ἵνα μὴ λυπῶμεν ἐπὶ πλέον τοὺς περὶ τὸν Χρύσιππον ἐναργῶς κατα-
281 μαρτυρουμένους ὑφ' ὧν ἐπικαλοῦνται μαρτύρων· ὅθεν δ' / ἀπελείπομεν
15 ἐκεῖσε πάλιν ἐπανέλθωμεν. ἐμπλήσας ὁ Χρύσιππος ὅλον τὸ βιβλίον
ἐπῶν Ὁμηρικῶν καὶ Ἡσιοδείων καὶ Στησιχορείων Ἐμπεδο-
κλείων τε καὶ Ὀρφικῶν, ἔτι δὲ πρὸς τούτοις ἐκ τῆς τραγῳδίας καὶ παρὰ
815 Τυρταίου καὶ τῶν | ἄλλων ποιητῶν οὐκ ὀλίγα παραθέμενος, εἶτα
[μὴ] συνεὶς τῆς θαυμαστῆς δὴ ταύτης ἀπεραντολογίας — τοῦτο γὰρ
αὐτῇ μᾶλλον ἡγοῦμαι προσήκειν τοὔνομα —, ταῦτα κατὰ λέξιν ἐπι-

3–5] SVF II, p. 249 5–6] *cf. infra*, p. 228.31 8–30] SVF II, pp. 249–250 18 προπετῶς] *cf. infra*, PHP 655.17 Müller 31–196.3] SVF II, p. 255 *cf.* Usener, Epicurea, p. 342

3 ὀκνεῖν *Müller (cf. Kalbfleisch, 1892, p. 24)* 4 αἰσθάνεται H: *corr. Kühn* 6 ἄλλως] ἀλλ' H: *corr. Müller*: ἄλλο *Ricci* (aliud *Andernacus)* 9 παρεληλυθέναι] λη *ex* ρη *corr.* H 10 οὐδὲν *Diels, sed cf. infra, p. 202.9* 17 μὲν *inser.* H 20 τε^{I} *om.* R: ἡμᾶς p 23 ἀπορίαν H: *corr. Ricci (*occasio *Andernacus)* 24 σαφῶς H: *corr. Müller* 26 εἰσπέμπειν *Müller* 27 ὁμολογοῦσι *Müller* 30 ἀπελίπομεν *Chart.* 31 ἐκεῖθεν H: *corr. Kühn* 35 μὴ *del. Müller*: μὴν R: μόνον οὐ *Usener*

to me that because he was himself aware of this (deficiency) he did not
hesitate to discuss the same subject three or four times, extending his
remarks to an inordinate length. But brevity was not his custom; he 9
used it rarely, for the most part in arguments where he perceived that
there was no escape from the error of his own doctrines. For as I think, 10
he wants to pass over the matter quickly, for otherwise he would be
subjected to refutation. And I also think that just as he struggles in
his other arguments to express himself clearly, so when he is open to
refutation he tries to veil his argument in obscurity and brevity, his
aim obviously being that he should appear to have answered the charge
and not to have evaded it completely, and that we should have no
reply to his words, which we do not even understand.

In the passage before us, at any rate, where he explains what people 11
mean by the expressions 'having no internal organ' and 'having no
brain', it seems to me that he is saying something like this: people use
the expression 'having no internal organ' as equivalent to 'heartless',
since the heart is an internal organ; and they use 'having no brain' as
equivalent to 'having no internal organ', since the brain too is an inter-
nal organ and has authority. Yet not all the Stoics accept an inter- 12
pretation to this effect. They say that something else is meant, but
they do not disclose it, as it is evidently one of their secret doctrines;
then they proceed at once to blame us for hastily disagreeing before we
understand what is meant. And those who go further in their abuse
call (us) uninformed and contentious and say that they will not reveal
the meaning to uneducated persons. And yet they explain everything 13
else (to us) at great length, even against our will; but when, as I said,
they come to something like this, which provides no opening for non-
sense, those who write the books pass over it hastily and obscurely,
while those who interpret their writings would sooner spread among
the audience a suspicion that they are ungenerous by pretending un-
willingness to teach us, than concede the point and suffer defeat.

It is time to dismiss those (people) without inner organs and 14
without brains, lest we give even greater pain to Chrysippus and his
followers, who are clearly convicted by their own witnesses. Let us
return to the point from which we digressed. Chrysippus filled his 15
whole book with lines from Homer, Hesiod, Stesichorus, Empe-
docles and Orpheus, and cited in addition to these no few lines from
tragedy, from Tyrtaeus, and other poets; then on becoming aware
of this amazing flow of endless talk – I consider that a more appro-
priate name for it –, he concludes with these words: "They will say 16

16 φέρει· «ταυτὶ μὲν φήσουσιν ἀδολεσχίαν εἶναι γραώδη, τυχὸν δὲ καὶ
γραμμάτων διδασκάλου βουλομένου στίχους ὅτι πλείστους ὑπὸ τὸ αὐτὸ
17 διανόημα τάξαι.» καλῶς εἶπες ὦ Χρύσιππε ταῦτα, κάλλιον δ' ἦν εἰ
μὴ μόνον εἶπες ἀλλὰ καὶ παντάπασιν ἐφυλάξω τὴν γραώδη ταύτην
18 ἀδολεσχίαν. τί γὰρ ἂν εἴη γραωδέστερον ἢ ἀδολεσχότερον ἢ γραμμα-
τιστῇ πρεπωδέστερον ἢ πόρρω μᾶλλον ἀπεληλαμένον ἀποδείξεως προσ-
ηκούσης ἀνδρὶ φιλοσόφῳ τοῦ μνημονεύσαντα κατ' ἀρχὰς εὐθὺς τοῦ
Πλάτωνος δόγματος ἐᾶσαι μὲν τοῦτο καὶ ἀπορρῖψαι παντάπασιν οὐδ'
282 ὡς ὑπὸ τῶν μετ' αὐτὸν κατεσκεύασται προ⟨σ⟩γράψαντα, / παρελθεῖν
δὲ καὶ τὴν πρὸς τοὺς ἠρωτημένους ὑπὸ τῶν ἀνδρῶν λόγους ἀντιλογίαν
τε καὶ λύσιν, ἐφ' ᾗ δίκαιον ἦν αὐτὸν ἀποδείξεσι χρησάμενον ἐπιστημο-
νικαῖς ἐμπεδῶσαι τὸ ἑαυτοῦ δόγμα, ποιητῶν δὲ μεμνῆσθαι καὶ πλῆθος
816 ἰδιωτῶν καλεῖν μαρτυρῆσον καὶ τί | λέγουσιν αἱ γυναῖκες γράφειν, οὐδ'
οὖν οὐδὲ ἐν αὐτοῖς οἷς καλεῖ μάρτυσιν εὐτυχοῦντα;
19 Καὶ γὰρ οἱ ποιηταὶ κατ' αὐτοῦ λέγουσιν ἅπαντες τὰ πλείω καὶ
οἱ ἰδιῶται. τίς γοῦν οὐκ ἔγραψε ποιητὴς ἐπιθυμεῖν τε καὶ θυμοῦσθαι
20 πολλὰ τῶν ζῴων ἀνθρώπου σφοδρότερον; τίς δ' ἰδιώτης οὐχ οὕτω
χρῆται τοῖς ὀνόμασιν ὡς τὸ Πλάτωνος βούλεται δόγμα, τὸν μὲν
ἀκάρδιον ἐν ἴσῳ τῷ δειλὸν καὶ ἄτολμον καὶ ἄνανδρον ὀνομάζων,
καρδίαν δὲ λαβεῖν ἐγκελευόμενος ἐπειδὰν εἰς ἀνδρείαν πρᾶξιν ἐπε-
γείρῃ τὸν πέλας, ἐπεγγελῶν δὲ τοῖς ἀνόητον εἰποῦσί τι, κενεγκε-
φάλους καὶ ἀσυνέτους ὀνομάζων αὐτούς, ἑτέρους δ' ἀγχίνους καὶ ἔν-
νους φάσκων, οὓς ἂν ὡς συνετοὺς ἐπαινῇ, ἀσπλάγχνους δὲ ἀπο-
283 καλῶν τοὺς μὴ / ἐλεοῦντας μηδένα μήτε φιλοῦντας μήθ' ὅλως φρον-
τίζοντας ἢ ἐπαινούντων ἢ ψεγόντων ἢ ἀδικούντων ἢ ὠφελούντων, ἀλλ'
21 ὥσπερ λίθους ἀναισθήτους ὑπάρχοντας; οὓς γὰρ ἂν εἰς ἀναισθησίαν
παντελῆ σκῶψαι βουληθῶσιν, ἀσπλάγχνους ὀνομάζουσιν, ὥσπερ τοὺς
22 ἀνάνδρους μὲν ἀκαρδίους, ἀνεγκεφάλους δὲ τοὺς ἄφρονας. ἐπεὶ δ' ἐστὶ
817 καὶ τρίτον τι | σπλάγχνον τὸ ἧπαρ ἐν ᾧ τὸ ἐπιθυμητικὸν ἵδρυται τῆς
ψυχῆς, καὶ χρὴ καὶ τούτῳ συμμετρίαν τινὰ τῶν οἰκείων ὑπάρχειν κινή-
σεων εἰ μέλλοι τελέως κεκοσμῆσθαι τὴν ψυχὴν ὁ ἄνθρωπος, εἴη ἂν καὶ
ὁ κατὰ τοῦτ' ἀναίσθητος, ὡς ἐπὶ τοῖς ἄλλοις τοῖς δύο, καὶ μοχθηρῶς δια-
23 κείμενος ἄσπλαγχνος ὀρθῶς ὀνομαζόμενος. ὁ δ' ἐναντίος αὐτῷ μεγαλό-
σπλαγχνος λέγεται, καθάπερ ὁ Εὐριπίδης εἰσάγει τὴν Μήδειαν ὄντως
μεγαλόσπλαγχνον, ἁπάσας τὰς τῶν τριῶν σπλάγχνων δυνάμεις τε
καὶ κινήσεις ἰσχυρὰς ἔχουσαν. ἐπιθυμητικωτάτην μὲν γὰρ προτίθεται
24 τὴν γυναῖκα καὶ θυμ[ητ]ικωτάτην ἅμα καὶ λογίσασθαι δεινήν. ἱκανὰ δὲ

1–3] *cf. infra*, p. 214.33–216.2 12–14] *cf. supra*, p. 104.8–15 *infra*, p. 232.17–20; PHP 578.3–9 Müller 34–35] *cf. infra*, p. 198.12

9 κατεσκευάσθαι H: *corr. Ald.* προγράψαντα H: *corr. Kühn* 11 ἐπιστημο^νικ~ H: ἐπιστημονικῶς M *Ald.*: *corr. Chart.* 18 τὸν] τὸ *Ald.* 20 καρδίην H: *corr. Kühn* 21 εἰποῦσί] ι[II] *ex* ιν *corr.* H τι *om.* M *Ald.* ἀνεγκεφάλους R² *Ald.* (*cf. supra, p. 194.28 et infra, lin. 28*) 24 μὴ] μήτε *Müller* 28 ἄνδρας H: *corr. Kühn*: ἀνάνδρας *Corn.* 31 μέλλει *Müller* κεκοσμῆσθαι] η *ex* ει *corr.* H 37 θυμητικωτάτην H: *corr. Chart.*

that this is the garrulity of an old woman, or perhaps of a schoolmaster who wishes to list as many verses as possible under the same thought." Well said, Chrysippus! You would have done even better if you had 17 not merely said it, but had avoided this old woman's prating altogether. For indeed what could be more anile, more tedious, more like 18 a schoolmaster, or further removed from the demonstration that a philosopher ought to use, than to mention right at the start the Platonic view and then disregard it and reject it completely, not mentioning how it was supported by his followers, and to neglect also to answer the arguments set forth by these men, or present a refutation, in which he should have confirmed his own doctrine with scientific demonstrations, but instead to quote poets and to call in a multitude of non-experts as witnesses and to record the expressions used by women, and to have no success even with the very witnesses he invokes?

For all the poets are against him in most of what they say, and 19 the ordinary men are also. What poet has not written that many animals experience desire and anger more intensely than man? What 20 ordinary person does not use the terms as Plato's teaching prescribes? He uses 'heartless' as equivalent to cowardly, timid, unmanly, and he says 'take heart' when he is urging his neighbor to a brave deed; he ridicules those who talk nonsense by calling them 'empty-brained' and 'stupid', while he praises others for their intelligence by calling them 'present-minded' and 'full of mind'; and he applies the term 'having no internal organ' to those who pity no one, love no one, and pay no attention whatever to persons who praise, blame, injure, or help (them), but are as insensible as stones. For when they wish to mock 21 people for utter lack of feeling, they say that they lack an internal organ, just as they call cowards heartless and fools brainless. And since there 22 is a third internal organ, the liver, where the desiderative part of the soul resides, and the motions peculiar to it must also be in proper measure if a man's soul is to be perfectly ordered, then with respect to this (part) also, as well as the other two, it would be correct to say of the person who is insensitive and has a faulty disposition that he lacks an organ. His opposite is called 'large-organed'; so Euripides 23 presents Medea as truly 'large-organed', in whom all the powers and movements of the three organs are strong. For he represents the woman as having the most intense desires and the most violent passion, and also as clever at reasoning. Sufficient indications of the 24

284 γνωρίσματα τοῦ μὲν ἐπιθυμητικοῦ τῆς ψυχῆς εἰς / ὅσον ἀμέτρου κινήσεως
ἀφῖκται, τὰ περὶ τὸν ἔρωτα τοῦ Ἰάσονος, ὑφ' οὗ νικηθεῖσα προὔδωκεν
ἅμα καὶ κατέλιπε τοὺς οἰκείους, ἐπηκολούθησε δὲ καὶ τελέως ἐπίστευσεν
ἑαυτὴν ἀνθρώπῳ ξένῳ· τοῦ δὲ θυμικοῦ τῆς σφοδρότητος οἷα περ⟨ὶ⟩ τοὺς
25 παῖδας ἐμήνισεν, οὐ σμικρὰ γνωρίσματα· τοῦ δὲ λογιστικοῦ τῆς συνέσεως,
ὑποτίθεται γὰρ κἀν τούτοις αὐτὴν ὁ Εὐριπίδης οὐ τὴν τυχοῦσαν, |
318 οὐ σμικρὰ σημεῖα ⟨τὰ⟩ πρὸς τὸ τιμωρήσασθαι τοὺς ἐχθροὺς ἐπινοη-
θέντα καὶ ὅσα πρὸς ἑαυτὴν διεξέρχεται καταστέλλουσα καὶ πείθουσα
26 τὸν θυμὸν ἀποχωρεῖν ἔργων ἀνοσίων. ὥστ' εὐλόγως ἐπ' αὐτῆς ὁ Εὐρι-
πίδης εἶπε·

«τί ποτ' ἐργάσεται
μεγαλόσπλαγχνος, δυσκατάπαυστος
ψυχὴ δηχθεῖσα κακοῖσι;»

27 αὕτη μὲν οὖν μεγαλόσπλαγχνος· ἄσπλαγχνος δὲ καὶ μικρόσπλαγχνος ᾧ
φαῦλα καὶ μικρὰ καὶ βραδυκίνητα καὶ δυσκίνητα τὰ τρία τῆς ψυχῆς
μόρια.

285 28 Μεταξὺ δέ μοι τῶν λόγων / ὧν διεξέρχομαι τὸ παραστὰν οὐκ ὀκνήσω
φράσαι· λέλεκται δὲ ὑπὸ τῶν παλαιῶν φιλοσόφων ὡς οὐκ ἐνδέχεταί τινα
διαλεγόμενον ἀδολέσχοις ἀνθρώποις ἀποσχέσθαι τελέως ἁπάσης ἀδο-
29 λεσχίας. ἔγωγ' οὖν ἠναγκάσθην ὑπὸ τῆς Χρυσίππου προαχθεὶς
ἀδολεσχίας ἐξηγεῖσθαι τάς τε τῶν ἰδιωτῶν καὶ τὰς Εὐριπίδου φωνάς,
ὃ μήποτ' ἂν ἑκὼν ἐτόλμησα πρᾶξαι περὶ τηλικούτου δόγματος ἀποδείξεις
319 30 γράφων. οὐχ ὅπως γὰρ Εὐριπίδης ἢ Τυρταῖος ἤ τις ἄλλος ποιη|τὴς
ἢ καὶ παντάπασιν ἰδιώτης ἱκανὸς πιστεύεσθαι περὶ δόγματος ἁπάσης
ἀποδείξεως χωρίς, ἀλλ' οὐδ' αὐτὸς ὁ πάντων ἰατρῶν ὁμολογουμένως ἄρι-
στος Ἱπποκράτης, ὥσπερ οὐδὲ ὁ πρῶτος ἁπάντων φιλοσόφων Πλά-
31 των. οὐδὲ γὰρ ἂν ῥαγῶσιν ὑπὸ φθόνου σύμπαντες οἱ μετ' αὐτὸν οὐδ'
ἂν ὑπὸ φιλονεικίας ἀναίσχυντα σοφίζωνται, καθάπερ οἱ περὶ τὸν Χρύσιπ-
πον, ἢ τὴν δόξαν ὑπερβαλέσθαι ποτὲ δυνήσονται τὴν Πλάτωνος
ἢ τὸν τῶν ἀποδείξεων μιμήσασθαι κόσμον· ἀλλ' ὅμως οὐδὲ τούτοις /
286 τοῖς ἀνδράσι τοσοῦτον ὑπὲρ τοὺς ἄλλους ἐπιστήμῃ τὴν ψυχὴν κεκο-
σμημένοις οὐδεὶς νοῦν ἔχων ἁπλῶς εἰποῦσιν ἀξιοῖ πιστεύειν ἀλλ'
32 ἀναμένει τὴν ἀπόδειξιν. ὁ δέ γε Χρύσιππος ὧν μὲν οὗτοι λέγουσιν
ἀποδείξεων ὑπὲρ τοῦ προκειμένου δόγματος οὔτε ἐμνημόνευσεν οὐδεμιᾶς
οὔτ' ἐξελέγχειν ἐπεχείρησεν, οὐκ αἰδεῖται δὲ Τυρταῖόν τε καὶ Στησί-
χορον ἐπικαλούμενος μάρτυρας οὓς εἰ καὶ ζῶντας ἤρετό τις εἰ τῆς περὶ
τούτων τῶν δογμάτων ἐπιστήμης ἀμφισβητοῦσιν, ἐξωμολογήσαντο ἂν
320 εὖ οἶδ' ὅτι μηδενὸς ἐπαΐειν αὐτῶν, | αὐτοὶ δὲ μᾶλλον ἂν οἶμαι παρὰ
33 Χρυσίππου τι μαθεῖν ἢ παρ' αὐτῶν ἀποδεικνύειν ἠξίωσαν. εἶτα δη-

11–13] Eur. Medea 108–110   20–23] SVF II, p. 256

3 *ante* ἅμα *addiderit* μὲν *Einarson*   4 οἱάπερ H: *corr. Müller*   7 τὰ *add. Ald.*   11 ποτε H: *corr. Kühn*   18 *post* ὑπὸ *add.* τινων *Schöne*   20 ἐγὼ γοῦν R   τῆς *scripsi*: τοῦ H: τῆς *aut* τῆς τοῦ *Petersen*   24 ἱκανῶς H: *corr.* F   25 *post* ὁ *add. et del.* χρύσιππος H   ὁμολογουμένων H: *corr. in textu*, ος *supra lin. add.* F   27 ῥαγεῖεν H: *corr.* F   30 τῶν *ex* τὸν *corr.* H   ἀποδείξεων *ex* ἀδείξεων *corr.* H   36 περὶ τῆς *Müller*   38 μηδὲν M *Ald.*   39 αὐτῶν H: *corr. Müller*

magnitude attained by the immoderate movement in the desiderative
part of her soul are the things she did because of her love for Jason:
overpowered by this love she both betrayed her family and abandoned
them, and she followed a stranger to whom she entrusted herself
completely. No small sign of the violence of the passionate part (of her
soul) is the way that she vented her anger on her children; no small 25
signs of her reasoning power – for here too Euripides portrays her
as no ordinary person – are the schemes she devised for taking ven-
geance on her enemies and all that she said to herself as she tried to
calm her anger and persuade it to refrain from impious deeds. Thus 26
with good reason Euripides said of her:

> "What will this soul,
> large-organed, restless,
> stung by evils, do?"

She, therefore, was large-organed; but a person is lacking organs, and 27
small-organed, if the three parts of his soul are weak and small, and
move slowly and with difficulty.

Interrupting the present discussion, I shall not hesitate to de- 28
scribe my predicament. It was said by the ancient philosophers that
when you converse with babblers you cannot entirely avoid all bab-
bling. So being led on by Chrysippus' chatter, I was compelled to give 29
an account of the words of ordinary men and of Euripides, a thing
that I would never have ventured to do voluntarily while writing the
proofs of such an important doctrine. For not merely is Euripides 30
or Tyrtaeus or any other poet, or any non-expert at all, insufficient
authority for a doctrine in the absence of all proof, but even Hippo-
crates himself, admittedly the best of all physicians, or Plato, the
first of all philosophers, is not sufficient authority. And Plato's 31
successors, even if they all burst with envy or contentiously contrive
shameless sophisms, as Chrysippus and his school did, will never be
able to surpass his reputation or match the beauty of his proofs. And
yet no intelligent person thinks he should accept the mere statement
even of those men whose souls are graced with knowledge so far above
the rest; rather, he waits for the proof. Chrysippus, however, did 32
not mention a single one of the proofs which those men gave in support
of the doctrine now before us, and he made no attempt to answer
(them); but he was not ashamed to call as witnesses Tyrtaeus and
Stesichorus, men who, if asked in their lifetime whether they laid
claim to knowledge about these doctrines, would assuredly have con-
fessed that they were not aware of any of them, and, I fancy, would
have rather expected to receive some instruction from Chrysippus
than to provide any proof themselves. Then Chrysippus, of course, 33

λαδὴ Χρύσιππος ἂν ἐπὶ τοὺς ἰδιώτας ἦγεν αὐτούς, ὁ σοφὸς ἐπὶ τοὺς
ἀμαθεῖς, ὁ σώφρων ἐπὶ τοὺς μαινομένους, ὁ λόγων ἀκολουθίαν εἰδὼς ἐπὶ
τοὺς διαφερομένους πρὸς ἀλλήλους τε καὶ ἑαυτοὺς κατὰ πάντα καιρὸν ἐν
34 λόγοις τε ἅμα καὶ πράξεσιν. ἀλλ' εἰ καὶ μαίνονται τὰ πάντα καὶ δια-
287 φέρονται πρὸς ἀλλήλους τε καὶ ἑαυτοὺς / ἅπαντες οἱ ἰδιῶται, τοῦτο
γοῦν οἶμαι σῶφρον ἔχουσι, τὸ μὴ καλεῖν ἐφ' ἃ λέγουσι τοὺς κατα-
35 μαρτυρήσοντας ἑαυτῶν. ἡ δὲ Χρυσίππου σοφία καὶ τῆς τῶν ἰδιωτῶν
ἀμαθίας ἐπέκεινα προελήλυθεν· ἐπικαλεῖται γοῦν μάρτυρας ὑφ' ὧν κατα-
κρίνεται. τούτου χάριν ἠναγκάσθην κἀγὼ νῦν ἀδολεσχεῖν, ἵν' ἐπι-
36 δείξω τὸν Χρύσιππον ἐν ἅπασι μέγιστα σφαλλόμενον. οὔτε γὰρ ἐ-
μνημόνευσεν οὐδεμιᾶς τῶν ὑπὸ Πλάτωνός τε καὶ Ἱπποκράτους
εἰρημένων ἀποδείξεων οὔτε ἀντεῖπεν οὔτ' αὐτός τινα εἶπεν ἑτέραν ἀπό-
37 δειξιν οὔτε οἶδεν οὓς χρὴ καλεῖν μάρτυρας. ἐπεδείξαμεν οὖν ἤδη καὶ διὰ
821 τοῦ πρώτου βιβλίου περὶ τῆς πρὸς ἑαυτὸν ἐναντιολογίας | τοῦ Χρυ-
σίππου· πρόδηλος δὲ καὶ νῦν ἐστιν ἡ ἀναισθησία τἀνδρός, ἃ χρῆν ἀπο-
κρύπτειν ἐναργῶς καταβάλλοντα τὸν λόγον αὐτοῦ, ταῦτ' οὐ μόνον
⟨οὐκ⟩ ἀποκρύπτοντος, ἀλλὰ καὶ μαρτυρεῖν ὑπολαμβάνοντος.
5. Ἀποχωρήσαντες οὖν ἤδη τῶν τοιούτων ἴδωμεν ἑξῆς ἅπαντας
288 οὓς ἐρωτᾷ λόγους ἐπὶ τὴν ἀρχὴν αὖθις ἀνελθόντες / ἅπαντος τοῦ λόγου
πρὸς τὸ μηδὲν παρελθεῖν. παραθήσομαι δὲ τὴν ῥῆσιν ἅπασαν, εἰ καὶ
2 μακροτέρα πώς ἐστιν, ἔχουσαν ὧδε· «τῆς μὲν οὖν ὀργῆς γιγνομένης
ἐνταῦθα, εὔλογον καὶ τὰς λοιπὰς ἐπιθυμίας ἐνταῦθ' εἶναι καὶ νὴ Δία ⟨καὶ⟩
τὰ λοιπὰ πάθη καὶ τοὺς διαλογισμοὺς καὶ ὅσα τούτοις ἐστὶ παρα-
3 πλήσια. σαινόμενοι δὲ φήμῃ οἱ πολλοὶ τούτων πολλὰ κατὰ τὴν ἀλή-
θειαν ἐπιλέγουσι τοιαῦτα ἐχόμενοι τῆς ῥηθείσης φορᾶς. πρῶτον μὲν
γὰρ πάντες, ἵνα ἐντεῦθεν ἄρξωμαι, κατὰ τοῦτό φασιν ἀναβαίνειν τινῶν
τὸν θυμὸν καὶ καταπίνειν τὴν χολήν τινας ἀξιοῦσι, λέγοντές τε κατα-
πίνεσθαί τινα αὐτοῖς σπαράγματα καὶ μὴ καταπίνεσθαι κατὰ τὴν τοι-
822 4 αύτην φορὰν λέγομεν. οὕτω δὲ λέγεσθαι | καὶ μηδὲν αὐτοῖς τούτων κατα-
βαίνειν καὶ ὅτι 'καταπιὼν τὸ ῥηθὲν ἀπῆλθεν', ὅ τε Ζήνων πρὸς τοὺς
ἐπιλαμβανομένους ὅτι 'πάντα τὰ ζητούμενα εἰς τὸ στόμα φέρεις', ἔφησεν,
'ἀλλ' οὐ πάντα καταπίνεται', οὔτε τῆς καταπόσεως ἄλλως ἂν οἰκει-
289 ότερον λεγομένης / οὔτε τῆς καταβάσεως τῶν ῥηθέντων εἰ μὴ περὶ
5 τὸν θώρακα τὸ ἡγεμονικὸν ἡμῶν ἦν εἰς ὃ ταῦτα πάντα φέρεται. ἐν γοῦν
τῇ κεφαλῇ ὄντος αὐτοῦ γελοίως ῥηθήσεται καὶ ἀλλοτρίως καταβαίνειν,
ἀναβαίνειν [δ'] ἂν οἶμαι οἰκειότερον αὐτῶν λεγομένων καὶ οὐ καταβαίνειν

13–15] libri primi test., *v. supra*, p. 70.10–11 18–202.3] SVF II, p. 242 21–24] *cf. supra*, p. 176.14–16 25 φορᾶς] *cf. supra*, p. 172.15–16 27 καταπίνειν] *cf. infra*, p. 226.27–28 30–32] Zenon. fr. 282: SVF I, p. 64

8 γοῦν] γὰρ *Ald.* 13 οἶδεν] ᾔδειν *coniecerit Einarson* 15 ἐχρῆν p 17 οὐκ *add.* p *Ricci* (non modo non *Andernacus*) 22 νὴ Δία καὶ] ἤδη H: *corr. Müller* (*cf. supra, p. 176.15*) 26 πάντες ἵνα *dubitanter v. Arnim* (omnes, ut *Andernacus*): ἵνα πάντες H: ἵνα πάντως R² *Corn.* 29 λέγεσθαι καὶ] καὶ λέγεται *Müller*: λέγεται καὶ *v. Arnim* 31 φέρειν H: *corr. Corn.*: φέρει *Müller* 36 δ' *del. Müller* οὐκ ἀντιβαίνειν H: *corr. Ald.*

would have taken them to non-experts, the sage to the ignorant, the
sane to the insane, the master of logical consistency to men who
disagree on every occasion with each other and with themselves in
both words and actions. But even if all ordinary men are mad in all 34
respects and disagree with each other and themselves, they have, I
believe, at least this much sense, that they do not summon in behalf
of their views witnesses who will testify against them. But the wisdom 35
of Chrysippus transcends the ignorance of ordinary men; thus he
summons witnesses by whom he is condemned. For this reason I too
was compelled for the present to babble on, that I might exhibit
Chrysippus committing the greatest blunders at every point. For he 36
mentioned not one of the proofs offered by Plato and Hippocrates;
he made no reply to them; he himself did not offer any other proof;
and he does not know what witnesses he ought to call. Already in the 37
first book we showed how Chrysippus contradicted himself, and now
again the man's obtuseness is manifest: he not only failed to conceal
the things he should have concealed, since they clearly refute his
argument, but he even supposed that they corroborate his position.

5. Let us now leave such matters and look next at all the argu-
ments he formulates, returning to the beginning of the whole account
so that nothing may be overlooked. I shall quote the entire passage,
even though it is quite long. It is as follows: "Since anger arises here, 2
it is reasonable that the other desires are here too, and indeed the
remaining affections, and deliberations, and all that resembles these
things. The multitude of men, cajoled by common usage, and holding 3
close to the tendency mentioned above, truthfully apply such terms
to many of these (things). For first, to begin from this point, all people
conform to this when they say that inflamed anger 'rises' in some
persons, and when they demand that some should 'swallow' their
wrath; and again, when we say that certain lacerations are swallowed
or not swallowed by them, we are speaking in conformity with a ten-
dency of this kind. In the same way people say that none of these goes 4
down for them, and 'He swallowed the remark and went away'; and
in reply to the accusation, 'You carry all inquiries to your mouth',
Zeno answered, 'But not all are swallowed'. In no other circum-
stances would it be more appropriate to speak of swallowing remarks,
and of their going down, if our governing part, to which all these
(things) are carried, were not in the region of the chest. Thus if our 5
governing part were in the head, it would be ridiculous and inappro-
priate to say that words go down; I fancy that they would more
properly be said to go up, not down in the manner described earlier.

τὸν προειρημένον τρόπον· τῆς ⟨γὰρ⟩ κατὰ τὴν ἀκοὴν αἰσθήσεως κατα-
φερομένης περὶ τὴν διάνοιαν, ἐὰν ᾖ περὶ τὸν θώρακα, οἰκείως κατά-
6 βασις ῥηθήσεται, ἐὰν δὲ περὶ τὴν κεφαλήν, ἀλλοτριώτερον.» ἐν τού-
τοις πάλιν ὁ Χρύσιππος οὐκ αἰσθάνεται τοὺς ἰδιώτας ἐφ' ἑαυτὸν
καλῶν· τὸ γὰρ ἀναβαίνειν τὸν θυμὸν ἢ καταβαίνειν τὴν χολὴν ὅσα
τ' ἄλλα τοιαῦτα λέγεται μαρτυρεῖ τοῖς τὸν θυμόν τε καὶ ὅλως τὰ πάθη
κάτω που τετάχθαι νομίζουσιν, ὥσπερ ἐν τῇ κεφαλῇ τὸν λογισμόν.
323 7 τηνικαῦτα γὰρ οἶδα καὶ τὸ μὴ | καταβαίνειν ἑαυτοῖς τὰ εἰρημένα λέ-
γοντας τοὺς πολλοὺς οὐκ ἐπειδὰν μὴ παρακολουθῶσι μηδὲ μανθάνωσι
290 τῶν λεγομένων, ⟨ἀλλ'⟩ ἐπειδὰν λέγηται μέν τινα ὡς ὀργὴν ἢ λύ/πην
ἢ θυμὸν ἤ τι τοιοῦτον πάθος ἐκκαλεσόμενα, μὴ φροντίζῃ δὲ αὐτῶν ὁ
ἀκούων μηδὲ κινῆται κατὰ πάθος. αὕτη μὲν οὖν ἡ ἀδολεσχία τοῦτο τὸ
πέρας ἐχέτω.
8 Μετὰ ταῦτα δ' ὁ Χρύσιππος τοιᾶσδ' ἑτέρας μέμνηται· «αἱ δὲ
γυναῖκες καὶ μᾶλλόν τι τούτων ἐμφαίνουσιν. εἰ γὰρ μὴ καταβαίνει αὐ-
ταῖς τὰ λεγόμενα, πολλάκις τὸν δάκτυλον κατάγουσιν ἕως τοῦ κατὰ
9 τὴν καρδίαν τόπου, οὐ φάσκουσαι καταβαίνειν ὧδε τὰ εἰρημένα.» τοῦτο
τὸ ἐπιχείρημα τοῖς ἔμπροσθεν ὁμογενές ἐστι δύο ἕτερα προσειληφὸς
ἐπιχειρήματα πάνσοφα, τό τε γυναῖκας εἶναι τὰς λεγούσας αὐτὰ καὶ μὴ
ὥσπερ τὰ πρόσθεν τοὺς ἄνδρας, τό τε καὶ τῇ δείξει δηλοῦν ὥσπερ
ὀρχουμένας ἅπερ ὁ λόγος ἐπὶ τῶν ἀνδρῶν ἐδήλου. ἀλλά τοι κἀνταῦθα,
γενναιότατε Χρύσιππε, κατὰ σαυτοῦ καλεῖς τὰς γυναῖκας μάρτυρας.
324 10 οὐδὲ γὰρ αὗται λέγουσιν οὕτως οὐδ' | ὀρχοῦνται ταῖς χερσὶν ὡς εἴρηκας,
ἐπειδὰν ἀρνῶνται συνιέναι τῶν λεγομένων, ἀλλ' ὅταν ὑπὸ λοιδορίας ἢ
291 ἀπειλῆς ἤ τινος / τοιούτου μήτε ὀργίζεσθαι φάσκωσι μήτε θυμοῦσθαι
μήθ' ὅλως ἀγανακτεῖν· ὅπερ οὐδ' αὐτὸν οἶμαι λανθάνει τὸν Χρύσιππον.
11 ἀντιφθεγγόμενος γοῦν κἀνταῦθα ἑαυτῷ μετ' ὀλίγον ὡδί πως γράφει·
«ἀφ' ἧς τε φορᾶς λέγομεν μὴ καταβαίνειν τὰ λεγόμενα, εἴτε ἀπειλὰς εἴτε
λοιδορίας, ὥστε καθικέσθαι καὶ ἅπτεσθαι αὐτῶν καὶ οὕτως κινεῖσθαι τὴν
διάνοιαν, ἀπὸ τῆς φορᾶς ταύτης καὶ βαθεῖς τινάς φαμεν εἶναι διὰ τὸ
12 μηδὲν τῶν τοιούτων ἐφικνεῖσθαι καταβὰν αὐτῶν.» ὅτι μὲν οὖν ἐπὶ τῶν
ἀπειλούντων ἢ λοιδορούντων λέγεται τὸ μὴ καταβαίνειν εἰς τὸ στῆθος
13 τὰ εἰρημένα, καὶ αὐτὸς ὁ Χρύσιππος μαρτυρεῖ. προσέρριψε δὲ τῷ λόγῳ
τὸ τῆς διανοίας ὄνομα, δέον εἰπεῖν θυμοῦ· τὸ μὲν γὰρ λογίζεσθαί τε καὶ
νοεῖν τὰ λεγόμενα καὶ τὸ μαχόμενον ἢ ἀκόλουθον ἐπίστασθαι τῆς λογι-
στικῆς δυνάμεως ἔργον· τὸ δὲ ἐπὶ λοιδορίαις ἢ ἀπειλαῖς μήτ' ὀργισθῆναι
325 *292* μήτε | θυμωθῆναι τῆς θυμοει/δοῦς ἴδιον.

8–17] SVF II, p. 243 23–31] SVF II, p. 243 35] *cf. infra*, PHP 732.11 Müller

1 *post* τὸν *dubitanter add.* δὲ *v. Arnim* γὰρ *addidi* 2 *ante* ἐὰν *add.* ἢ *Müller* 5 καλῶν *ex* καλὸς *(?) corr.* H 10 ἀλλ' *add. Corn.*, δὲ *post* ἐπειδὰν *Einarson* 12 κινεῖται H: *corr. Kühn* 17 φάσκουσαι] φ *ex* τ *(?) corr.* H 21 ἀν-δρῶν] ἐδρῶν H: *corr. Ricci* 25 φάσκουσι H: *corr. Kühn* 30 βαθείας H: *corr. Corn. (cf. infra, p. 204.5–6)* 31 ἐφικνεῖσθαι καταβῆναι H: *corr. Einarson*: καταβῆναι καὶ ἐφικνεῖσθαι *Müller*: ἐφικνεῖσθαι *Petersen*

For since auditory sense-perception is carried down to the region of
the mind, if the mind is in the chest, then 'descent' will be the proper
term; but if it is in the head, that expression will be rather inappro-
priate." Here again Chrysippus does not perceive that he is summon- 6
ing the non-experts to his own disadvantage. For the expressions
'anger rises' and 'wrath goes down' and all other such phrases bear
witness for those who believe that anger and the affections generally
are situated somewhere below, just as (they believe that) reason (is
situated) in the head. I know further that the occasion when the many 7
speak of remarks as not 'going down' with them is not when they fail
to follow or understand what is said, but when remarks are made
with the purpose of eliciting anger or distress or inflamed anger or
some such affection, but the person addressed ignores them and is not
emotionally aroused. Let us therefore put an end to this piece of idle
chatter here.

But then Chrysippus brings up another piece of idle chatter: 8
"Women indicate this to a somewhat greater degree than the cases
just mentioned. For if a remark does not go down with them, they
often move their finger to the region of the heart and say that it does
not go down there." This piece of reasoning is of the same class with 9
the earlier ones, to which it adds two other very wise proofs: it is
women who say these things and not men as before; and the women
express by gesture, dancing, as it were, what was expressed verbally
by the men. But even here, most worthy Chrysippus, the women
you summon are witnesses against you. For they speak this way, and 10
they 'dance with their hands', as you called it, not when they deny
that they understand what is said, but when they deny that they are
angered or enraged or at all disturbed by an insult or a threat or
anything of that kind. This fact, I believe, does not escape Chrysip-
pus himself. Thus he contradicts himself here again when he writes a 11
little further on: "And the tendency that leads us to say that remarks,
whether threats or insults, do not go down far enough to reach and
touch the persons so that their minds are set in motion, also leads us
to say that some persons are 'deep', because nothing of that kind
reaches them in its descent." Thus Chrysippus himself also testifies 12
that the reference is to threats and insults when men say that a remark
does not go down to the chest. But he tossed the term 'mind' into the 13
statement, when he should have said 'anger', for reasoning, and
comprehending what is said, and understanding incompatibility and
entailment are the work of the rational power; but not to be angry or
enraged at insults or threats is the concern of the spirited power.

14 'Αλλὰ ταῦτα μὲν ἐν τοῖς ἐφεξῆς ὁ Χρύσιππος λέγει· μεταξὺ δὲ
ταύτης τῆς τε νῦν γεγραμμένης ῥήσεως καὶ ἧς ὀλίγον ἔμπροσθεν ἔγραψα
περὶ τῶν γυναικῶν, ἑτέρα ῥῆσίς ἐστιν ἣν ἤδη παραγράψω πρὸς τὸ
15 μηδὲν ὅλως ὑπερβαίνειν δοκεῖν. ἔχει δὲ ὧδε· «τούτοις δ' ἀκολούθως
ἀνεμεῖν τέ τινάς φαμεν τὰ φανέντα αὐτοῖς καὶ ἔτι τὸν βαθύν, λεγομένων
πολλῶν τοιούτων συμφώνως τοῖς εἰρημένοις· καταπιόντες γάρ, ὅμοιον
εἰπεῖν, ὅτι ἡμέρα ἐστί, καὶ ἐναποθέμενοι τοῦτο εἰς τὴν διάνοιαν καὶ πάλιν
ἐκεῖνο λέγοντες, ὅτι οὐκ ἔστιν ἡμέρα, μενόντων τῶν πραγμάτων, οὐκ
16 ἀλλοτρίως οὐδ' ἀνοικείως ἀνεμεῖν λέγονται.» τοῦτο τὸ ἀνεμεῖν ἐγὼ μὲν
οὐδὲ ἤκουσά τινος λέγοντος, ἀλλὰ μᾶλλον ἀποπτύσαι καὶ ἐκπτύσαι καὶ
ἐκβαλεῖν καὶ ἀπορρῖψαι καὶ ἀποθέσθαι λέγουσιν, ἐπειδὰν λέγωσί τινα
17 δοξῶν ἀποστῆναι μοχθηρῶν. εἰ δ' ἄρα καὶ τὸ ἐξεμέσαι λέγοιτο πρός
τινων, εἴη ἂν ταὐτὸν τῷ ἀποπτύσαι καὶ ἀπορρῖψαι καὶ τοῖς ἄλλοις
293 18 τοῖς ἐκ μεταφορᾶς λεγομένοις ὁμοίως / ἔχον. ὅτι δ' οὐ μόνον ἀνδρὶ
326 φιλοσοφοῦντι τῶν | τοιούτων ἐπιχειρημάτων οὐδέν ἐστι μεταχειριστέον,
ἀλλ' οὐδὲ ῥητορικῷ, δέδεικται μὲν ἤδη μοι καὶ διὰ τῶν ἔμπροσθεν, οὐ
μὴν ἀλλὰ καὶ νῦν ἔνεστιν ἐνδείξασθαι διὰ βραχέων ἀναμνήσαντα τῶν
ῥητορικῶν τεχνῶν ἃς ἐκεῖνοι γράφουσι διδάσκοντες ἡμᾶς τόπους ἐπιχει-
19 ρημάτων εἰς ἑκάστην ὑπόθεσιν. οὐδενὸς γὰρ τοιούτων μνημονεύουσιν
20 οἵων ὁ Χρύσιππος ἐνέπλησε τὰ ἑαυτοῦ συγγράμματα. ἀλλὰ γὰρ
εἴπερ πᾶσαν ῥῆσιν ἀκριβολογεῖσθαι βουληθείην, ὡς μηδὲν τῶν ἁμαρτη-
μάτων ἀνέλεγκτον παραλιπεῖν, εἰς ἄπειρον ἄν τι μῆκος ἐκταθείη τὸ
21 βιβλίον. ἀφέμενος οὖν ἤδη τῶν προγεγραμμένων ἐπὶ τὰ ἐφεξῆς τρέψομαι,
δι' ὧν ὁ Χρύσιππος ἀπάρχεται παρατίθεσθαι τὰς τῶν ποιητῶν
μαρτυρίας μεταξὺ παρεντιθεὶς αὐτῶν ὀλίγους λόγους ἑαυτοῦ, πολλάκις
μὲν ὥσπερ ἐξήγησιν ὧν ἡ ῥῆσις βούλεται, πολλάκις δ' ὥ⟨σ⟩περ ἐπιτομήν
22 τινα καὶ οἷον καθόλου τι κεφάλαιον. ἀρξάμενος οὖν ἀπό τινος Ἐμπεδο-
294 κλείου ῥήσεως ἐξηγεῖταί τε αὐτὴν καί τινων κατὰ τὴν ἐξή/γησιν
327 ἀξιολογ[γ]ωτέρων ἄρχεται | λόγων, ἐν οἷς ἐστι καὶ ὁ περὶ τῆς φωνῆς,
οὗ κατὰ τὸ δεύτερον ἐμνημόνευσα τῶνδε τῶν ὑπομνημάτων, ἐν ᾧ βιβλίῳ
πάντας ἔδοξέ μοι κάλλιον εἶναι παραθέσθαι τοὺς λόγους οἳ τὸ πιθανὸν
ἔχουσι καὶ οὐχὶ ἀπόβλητοι τελέως εἰσὶν οὐδὲ γυναῖκας οὐδὲ ἰδιώτας
οὐδὲ ἐτυμολογίας ἢ φορὰς χειρῶν ἢ ἐπινεύσεις ἢ ἀνανεύσεις κεφαλῆς ἢ
ποιητὰς ἐπικαλοῦνται μάρτυρας· ἐφ' ὧν καὶ μόνων ἐγνώκειν καταμεῖναι
23 μὴ προσθεὶς αὐτοῖς ταυτὶ τὰ νῦν μοι γραφόμενα. δόξαν δὲ τοῖς ἑταίροις
ἄμεινον εἶναι μηδ' ὅσα παντάπασιν ἠδολέσχηται τῷ Χρυσίππῳ, μηδὲ
ταῦθ' ὑπερβῆναι παντελῶς, ἀλλ' ἐπισημήνασθαί τε τὴν ἀτοπίαν αὐτῶν
ἐπιδεῖξαί τε πρὸς τῷ μηδὲν πλέον ἀνύειν αὐτὰ κατὰ τῶν Στωϊκῶν

1–12] SVF II, p. 243   1] *cf. infra*, lin. 23   12 ἐξεμέσαι] *cf.* Arr. Epict. iii. 21.1, 2   23–30] SVF II, p. 237   29–30] *cf. supra*, pp. 130.24–132.2   35–206.11] SVF II, p. 237

5 λέγομεν H: *corr. Kalbfleisch v. Arnim*   14 ἔχον *defendit Kalbfleisch, 1892, pp. 3–4*: ἔχοι *Müller*   24 ἄρχεται *Kühn*   25 ἑαυτοῦ] -οῦ *ex* -ῶν *corr.* H   26 ὥπερ H: *corr. Ald.*   29 ἀξιολογγωτέρων H: *corr. Ald.*   30 ἐν ᾧ *deperdita in* H   31 τοὺς] τ... H   32 οὐδὲ[1]] ου.. H   33 ἐπινεύσεις] ...νεύσεις H   34 μ. .τυρας H   38 τῷ] τὸ H: *corr. Müller*

Chrysippus speaks of these matters in the very next passage; 14
but between the words just quoted and those quoted a short time ago
concerning women, there is another passage that I shall now transcribe
without delay, so that I may not be thought to pass over anything at
all. It is as follows: "In keeping with this we say that some people 15
vomit up their impressions, and further we call a person 'deep', many
expressions of this sort being used in a way that accords with our
previous discussion. Thus when people have swallowed the statement
(let us say) that it is day, and have stored this up in their minds,
and then make that other assertion, that it is not day – the cir-
cumstances remaining the same –, it is not absurd or inappropriate
to say that they vomit up." I have never heard anyone use 'vomit up' 16
in this way; rather, they say 'spit up', 'spit out', 'throw out', 'cast
away', 'put aside', when they speak of relinquishing mistaken opinions.
But if in fact some people should also say 'vomit out', it would be 17
equivalent to 'spit up' and 'cast away', and analogous to the other
metaphorical expressions. I have already shown in an earlier passage 18
that such arguments should not be employed not only by philosophers
but not even by rhetoricians; and here again I can briefly indicate this
by recalling the handbooks written by rhetoricians in which they give
us the places in which to find arguments for each specific case. They 19
make no mention of arguments such as those with which Chrysippus
has filled his volumes. But if I were to examine every passage in detail, 20
so as to leave no error unrefuted, this book would stretch out to endless
length. It is therefore time for me to lay aside the passages quoted 21
earlier and turn to what follows. Here Chrysippus begins with the
evidence of the poets, interlarding the quotations with a few remarks
of his own, often as an explanation of the meaning of the passage,
often as a kind of abridgement and general statement of the main
point. Beginning, then, with a passage from Empedocles, he explains 22
its meaning; and in the course of the explanation he embarks on some
rather important arguments, among them the argument about speech,
which I mentioned in the second book of this work. It seemed better
to me to present in that book all the arguments that have plausibility
and are not completely worthless and do not invoke the testimony of
women, non-experts, etymologies, motions of the hands, upward or
downward movement of the head, or poets. I had decided to limit
myself to these only, and not to add to them the matters that I am
now discussing. But since my friends thought it would be better not 23
even to pass over Chrysippus' utterly foolish talk in complete
silence, but to note its absurdity and point out that the things (he
says) not only fail to advance the argument but even conflict with

δογμάτων παρειλημμένα, διὰ τοῦτο προσέθηκα πάντα ταῦτα κατὰ τόδε
τὸ βιβλίον.
24 Περὶ μὲν δὴ τῆς φωνῆς οὐδὲν ἔτι δέομαι λέγειν ἐν τῷδε σύμπαντα τὸν
τ[ρ]όπον ἱκανῶς ἐξειργασμένος ἐν τῷ πρὸ τούτου βιβλίῳ, ὅσα δὲ ἐφεξῆς
295 ἐστι τοῦ περὶ ταύτης λόγου κατὰ τὸ τοῦ Χρυσίππου βιβλίον / εἰρημένα
828 25 τούτων ἤδη μνημονεύσω. ἔστι δὲ | τά τε κατὰ τὰς φορὰς τῶν χειρῶν,
ὅταν ἐφαπτώμεθα τῶν στέρνων ἡμᾶς αὐτοὺς δεικνύντες, ἔτι τε τὰ κατὰ
τὴν ἐγὼ φωνήν, ἃ δὴ κἀν τοῖς Ἐτυμολογικοῖς εἶπεν, ἔχειν [τε] τι φάσκων
αὐτὴν δεικτικὸν ἐκ τοῦ φαινομένου διὰ τὸ κατὰ τὴν πρώτην ἐν αὐτῇ
συλλαβὴν ὡς ἐπὶ τὸ στῆθος ἀπάγεσθαι τήν τε κάτω γένυν καὶ τὸ
26 χεῖλος. εἴρηταί μοι καὶ περὶ τούτων ἤδη κατὰ τὸ δεύτερον τῶνδε τῶν
27 ὑπομνημάτων κἀν τοῖς Περὶ ὀνομάτων ὀρθότητος. ὅμοια δὲ τοῖς τοιούτοις
ἐπιχειρήμασι καὶ τὰ κατὰ τὴν ἐτυμολογίαν εἰσὶ τοῦ τῆς καρδίας ὀνόματος
ἑξῆς τῶν προειρημένων ὑπὸ τοῦ Χρυσίππου γεγραμμένα κατὰ τὸ
28 πρῶτον Περὶ ψυχῆς ὧδέ πως ἔχοντα· «τούτοις πᾶσι συμφώνως καὶ
τοὔνομα τοῦτ' ἔσχηκεν ἡ καρδία κατά τινα κράτησιν καὶ κυρείαν ἀπὸ
τοῦ ἐν αὐτῇ εἶναι τὸ κυριεῦον καὶ κρατοῦν τῆς ψυχῆς μέρος, ὡς ἂν
29 κρατία λεγομένη.» τὸ μὲν ὡς πρὸς τὴν ζωὴν ἡμῶν κυριώτατον εἶναι τὸ
296 σπλάγχνον / οὐδ' ἡμεῖς ἀμφισβητοῦμεν, ὦ γενναιότατε Χρύσιππε, οὐ
829 30 μὴν ἁπλῶς γε κυριώτατον εἶναι συγχωροῦ|μεν. οὐ γὰρ ἄρχειν αὐτῷ καὶ
δεσπόζειν τῶν ἄλλων ἡ φύσις ἔνειμεν, ὅταν γε προσηκόντως διοικῆται
τὰ κατὰ τὸν ἄνθρωπον, ἀλλ' ἐγκεφάλῳ μὲν ἄρχειν, ὑπακούειν δὲ τῇ
καρδίᾳ, καθάπερ ἡμεῖς ἀποδείκνυμεν.
31 Ἐφεξῆς δὲ τοῖς εἰρημένοις ὁ Χρύσιππος τάδε γράφει· «ὁρμῶμεν
κατὰ τοῦτο τὸ μέρος καὶ συγκατατιθέμεθα τούτῳ καὶ εἰς τοῦτο συντείνει
32 τὰ αἰσθητήρια πάντα.» ταῦτα τὰ κεφάλαια μόνα τῶν ἐπιστημονικῶν
ἐστι καὶ εἴπερ ἀπέδειξεν ὁ Χρύσιππος αὐτά, τότ' ἂν ἐπῃνοῦμέν τε τὸν
33 ἄνδρα καὶ τοῖς δόγμασιν ἐπειθόμεθα τῶν Στωϊκῶν. ἐπεὶ δ' ἀποδεῖξαι
μὲν οὐκ ἐπεχείρησεν, ἀπεφήνατο δὲ μόνον, ἡμεῖς δὲ πρόσθεν μὲν ἤδη περὶ
τῶν αὐτῶν ἀπεδείξαμεν ὡς οὔτε κατὰ τὴν καρδίαν γίγνεται καὶ πάντων
αὐτῶν ἐγκέφαλός ἐστιν ἀρχή, καὶ διὰ τῶν ἐφεξῆς δὲ οὐδὲν ἧττον ἀποδεί-
ξομεν, οὐκέτ' ἂν οἶμαι δίκαιον εἶναι τοῖς Χρυσίππου πιστεύειν δόγμα-
297 34 σιν, / ἀλλὰ τοῖς Ἱπποκράτους καὶ Πλάτωνος. ταυτὶ μὲν οὖν τὰ
κεφάλαια τὸ σύμπαν κῦρος ἐν αὐτοῖς ἔχοντα περὶ τῶν προκειμένων ἡμῖν
830 δογμάτων οὕτως ταχέως ὁ Χρύσιππος παρέδραμεν | ὡς ἐπιμνησθῆναι
μόνον· ἐν οἷς δὲ οὐ χρή, μηκύνει περιττῶς.

8] *cf.* SVF II, p. 9 = Diog. Laert. vii. 200 11–12] *cf. supra*, pp. 104.17–22, 27–106.6 12–18] SVF II, p. 245 12–15] SVF II, pp. 237–238 24–26] SVF II, pp. 245–246 *cf.* SVF II, p. 238 33–36] SVF II, p. 246

4 τρόπον H: *corr. Kühn*: λόγον *Müller* πρὸ] π.. H 5 ἐστι] ἔτι H: *correxi* τὸ *deperditum in* H 6 δὲ *deperditum in* H 7 ἡμ.. H 8 τε *del. Ald.* 9 αὐτὴν] αὐτὰ H: *corr. Corn.* 12 κἀν *in* καὶ *mut.* H³ ὅμοια] ο *e ras.* H 18 *post* μὲν *add.* οὖν M 20 αὐτὸ H R (*e corr.*): *corr. Kalbfleisch* 21 . . . .όζειν H διοικῆσαι H: *corr. Corn.*: μέλλῃ διοικῆσαι *Müller* 22 ἄν. . .πον H 23 ἡμεῖς] . . ῖς H 24 δὲ] δ *e corr.* H ὁρ.ῶμεν H 28 ἐπειθώμεθα H: *corr. Chart.* 29 μὲν^II *om.* M 34 ἐν *deperditum in* H αὐτοῖς H: *corr. Kühn* 35 . .ρέδραμεν H

Stoic doctrines, for that reason I have added all these things in this
book.

I need say nothing further here about speech, as I worked through 24
the whole passage adequately in the preceding book. I therefore pass
now to the things that follow the discussion of speech in Chrysippus'
treatise: the arguments from the movements of the hands when we 25
point to ourselves by touching our chests, and from the word *egō* (I),
points that he also mentioned in his work On Etymologies, claiming
that the word possesses a certain deictic character from our appearance
when we say it, because as we pronounce its first syllable our lower
jaw and lip are drawn away, as though to the chest. But I have already 26
discussed these (things) also in the second book of this work and in my
treatise On the Correctness of Names. In the same class with these 27
arguments is that from the etymology of the word *kardia* (heart),
which comes next in Chrysippus' first book On the Soul. It is as
follows: "Concordant with all this, the heart got its name by virtue 28
of a certain power and sovereignty, from the fact that the sovereign
and ruling part of the soul is in it; it is called, as it were, *kratia* (power)."
We do not deny, noble Chrysippus, that so far as our life is concerned 29
it is the sovereign organ, but we do not agree that it is sovereign in
every way. For nature did not assign to it the government and rule 30
of the rest, at least when a man's affairs are well ordered; rather, it
assigned rule to the brain and obedience to the heart, as we are demonstrating.

Next after this Chrysippus writes: "Our conation is in this part, 31
we assent with this (part), and all the organs of sense extend to this
(part)." These summary statements are the only ones that belong to 32
the class of scientific premises, and if Chrysippus had proved them
we would praise the man and accept the Stoic teaching. But since he 33
did not attempt to prove them, but merely asserted them, and since in
an earlier passage we have already demonstrated, in regard to these
same matters, that they do not take place in the heart, and that the
brain is source of all of them, and since we shall prove this no less in
what follows, it would no longer be right, I think, to accept the teachings of Chrysippus, but (rather) those of Hippocrates and Plato.
These summary statements, then, which have in themselves the full 34
power to decide the issue before us, Chrysippus passed over so
quickly that he only mentioned them; but in matters that he should
not mention he is unnecessarily prolix.

35 Ἑξῆς δὲ περί τε φωνῆς μνημονεύει καὶ νεύρων ἀρχῆς, ὑπὲρ ὧν
36 ἀμφοτέρων εἴρηταί μοι κατὰ τὰ πρόσθεν ὑπομνήματα. καὶ μετὰ ταῦτα
τὴν ἀκάρδιος ἐξηγεῖται προσηγορίαν, ὑπὲρ ἧς ἔμπροσθεν ἤδη μοι
λέλεκται, τοσοῦτον δὲ ἐπισημανοῦμαι καὶ νῦν ἀπ' αὐτῆς τῆς λέξεως τοῦ
37 Χρυσίππου μαρτυρούσης οἷς προεῖπον. ἔχει δὲ ὧδε· «κατὰ τοῦτο καὶ
εὐκάρδιοι λέγονταί ποι εἶναί τινες καθάπερ εὔψυχοι, καὶ καρδίαν ἀλγεῖν
οἱ κηδόμενοί τινων, ὡς ἂν κατὰ τὴν καρδίαν τῆς κατὰ τὴν λύπην
38 ἀλγηδόνος γιγνομένης.» ἐν ταύτῃ γὰρ τῇ ῥήσει σαφῶς ὁ Χρύσιππος
ἐμαρτύρησεν ἡμῖν ὡς οὐδέποτε τὸ λογιζόμενον τῆς ψυχῆς οὐδεὶς τῶν
ἰδιωτῶν ἐν καρδίᾳ νενόμικεν ὑπάρχειν, οὐδ' ὁ ἀκάρδιος τὸν ἄψυχον, ὡς
298 39 οἴεται ὁ Χρύσιππος, ἀλλὰ τὸν ἄτολμον δηλοῖ παρ' αὐτοῖς. / οὕτω δὲ
καὶ τὴν καρδίαν ἀλγεῖν τὸ λυπεῖσθαι λέγουσιν, ὡς καὶ τοῦτ' αὐτὸς
μαρτυρεῖ διὰ τῆς αὐτῆς ταύτης ῥήσεως τῆς νυνὶ γεγραμμένης, ἐν ᾗ φησιν
«ὡς ἂν κατὰ τὴν καρδίαν τῆς κατὰ τὴν λύπην ἀλγηδόνος γιγνομένης».
331 40 οὕτως ἐν | ἅπασι τοῖς λόγοις ὁ Χρύσιππος οὐκ αἰσθάνεται τὰ πάθη
τῆς ψυχῆς ἐν τοῖς κάτω τῆς κεφαλῆς μέρεσιν ὑπάρχειν κατασκευάζων,
οὐ τὸ λογιζόμενον ἢ ἐπιστήμην δεχόμενον ἢ ἀλήθειαν σπουδάζον.
41 οὕτω δὲ κἀπειδὰν ἐπιφέρων εἴπῃ «τὸ γὰρ ὅλον καθάπερ ἐν ἀρχῇ εἶπον
εὖ μάλ' ἐμφαίνουσιν οἵ τε φόβοι καὶ αἱ λῦπαι κατὰ τοῦτο τὸ μέρος
γιγνόμεναι», μαρτυρεῖ κἀνταῦθα τῷ τοῦ Πλάτωνος λόγῳ.
42 Καὶ διὰ τῶν ἑξῆς δὲ κατὰ τὸν παραπλήσιον τρόπον οὐκ αἰσθάνεται
43 κατασκευάζων ὡς ἐν τῇ καρδίᾳ τὸ θυμοειδὲς ἵδρυται τῆς ψυχῆς· «ἥ τε γὰρ
ἐν τοῖς φόβοις πάλσις τῆς καρδίας ἐκφανής ἐστι καὶ ἡ εἰς τοῦτο τῆς ὅλης
ψυχῆς συνδρομὴ οὐκ ἄλλως ἐπιγεν⟨ν⟩ηματικῶς γιγνομένων αὐτῶν,
299 καθάπερ ἄλλοις ἄλλου συμπάσχειν πεφυκότος, / καθὸ καὶ συνιζάνουσιν
εἰς αὐτοὺς συναγόμενοι πρὸς τοῦτο ὡς ἂν τὸ ἡγεμονικὸν καὶ κατ' αὐτὴν
44 ὡς ἂν αὐτῶν τούτου φυλακτικήν. καὶ τὰ τῆς λύπης πάθη ἐνταυθοῖ που
εὐφυῶς γίγνεται οὐδενὸς ἄλλου συμπάσχοντος οὐδὲ συναλγοῦντος
τόπου. ἀλγηδόνων γάρ τινων κατὰ ταῦτα γιγνομένων σφοδρῶν ἕτερος
332 μὲν οὐδεὶς | ἐμφαίνει τόπος τὰ πάθη ταῦτα, ὁ δὲ περὶ τὴν καρδίαν μάλι-
45 στα.» ταῦτα πάντα φήσομεν ἀληθῶς ὑπὸ τοῦ Χρυσίππου λέγεσθαι καὶ
παρακαλέσομέν γε τοὺς ἀπ' αὐτοῦ μεμνῆσθαί τε αὐτῶν καὶ μηκέτι παρ'
ἡμῶν ἑτέραν ἐπιζητεῖν ἀπόδειξιν ὑπὲρ τοῦ τοὺς φόβους καὶ τὰς λύπας
46 καὶ πάνθ' ὅσα τοιαῦτα πάθη κατὰ τὴν καρδίαν συνίστασθαι. ἀλλὰ
τοῦτο μὲν καὶ παρ' αὐτῶν ὁμολογούμενον λαμβάνεται τῶν Στωϊκῶν·

1] SVF II, p. 238 2–8] SVF II, p. 247 *cf.* SVF II, p. 238 2–4] *cf. supra*, pp. 192.7–25; 194.11–16; 196.17–28 18–31] SVF II, pp. 247–248 22–27] *cf.* Nemes. De nat. hom. 20: p. 232.6–9 Matth. 22–23] *cf. supra*, p. 160.19–20 32–210.2] SVF I, p. 51 34–210.2] SVF II, p. 248

6 ποι] τοι *Bas.*: που *Müller* 18 ἐπιφέρον H: *corr. Ald.* 19 ἐμφαίνου. . H
20 . . .τυρεῖ H 21 δὲ *deperditum in* H παραπλήσιον *ex* ἐτήσιον *corr.* H[3]
22 τῇ *deperditum in* H 23 π..σις H 24 ἐπιγενηματικῶς H: *corr. Bas.*
26 κατ' αὐτὴν *scripsi*: κατὰ τὴν H: κατὰ αὐτὴν *Müller*: κατὰ τὴν καρδίαν *v. Arnim*
27 αὐτῶν *del. Müller*: αὐτοῦ *Corn.* 28 εὐφυῶς] "*fortasse* ἐκφανῶς" *v. Arnim*
31 ταῦτα] . . .τα H 32 . . . .καλέσομέν H 35 παρ'] πρὸς *Müller*

Next he takes up speech and the source of the nerves, both of 35
which I discussed in the preceding books. Then he explains the word 36
'heartless', about which I spoke earlier; here I shall note only this
much, taken from Chrysippus' own words, which confirm my earlier
statement. He says: "And in accord with this some people are said to 37
be 'well-hearted', just as (they are called) 'well-souled', and those who
are concerned for someone are said to have pain in their hearts, the
assumption being that the pain of distress arises in the heart." In this 38
passage Chrysippus clearly supports us by testifying that among
ordinary people the rational part of the soul has never been thought
to be in the heart, and that 'heartless' to them does not mean 'soulless',
as Chrysippus supposes, but 'cowardly'. And similarly the ordinary 39
person means by distress a pain in the heart, as Chrysippus himself
testifies in the very passage just quoted, when he says, "the assump-
tion being that the pain of distress arises in the heart". Thus Chry- 40
sippus fails to perceive that in all his arguments he is supporting the
view that the affections of the soul are in the members below the head,
but not the part that reasons or receives knowledge or pursues the
truth. And when in conclusion he says, "For to sum up, as I said in the 41
beginning, fear and distress are very clearly revealed as arising in this
part", here too he supports Plato's account.

Similarly in the next passage he does not perceive that he is 42
supporting the view that the spirited part of the soul is located in the
heart: "For the palpitation of the heart in fear is manifest, and the 43
concourse of the whole soul to that place, these (effects) following not
as a mere aftereffect, as when one part has a natural sympathy with
the others, inasmuch as people shrink into themselves, drawing
themselves together toward this place as being the governing part,
and at the heart as being in them the protector of the governing part.
And the affections of distress arise somewhere there naturally, no 44
other place experiencing sympathy or sharing the affection. For when
certain pains associated with the affections of distress become intense,
no other place exhibits these physical effects, but the region of the
heart does so to a great degree." We shall grant that Chrysippus is 45
correct in all of this, and we shall urge his followers to remember what
he said and no longer demand from us further proof that fear and
distress and all affections of that sort arise in the region of the heart.
This point can be taken as granted by the Stoics themselves, for not 46

οὐ μόνον γὰρ Χρύσιππος, ἀλλὰ καὶ Κλεάνθης καὶ Ζήνων ἑτοίμως
αὐτὰ τιθέασιν· ἐκεῖνο δ' ἐπισκέπτεσθαι χρὴ μόνον ἐν ᾧ τὴν πᾶσαν
ἀμφισβήτησιν εἶναι συμβέβηκεν, εἰ καὶ τὸ λογιζόμενόν ἐστιν ἐνταῦθα.
300 47 εἰ γὰρ ὥσπερ τὸ θυ/μοειδὲς ἐναργῶς ἐπιδείκνυται δι' ὧν ὁ Χρύσιππος
ἤδη πολλάκις εἴρηκε λόγων περιεχόμενον ἐν τῇ καρδίᾳ, ἡμεῖς δὲ καὶ
περὶ τοῦ λογιζομένου παραπλησίας ταύτα⟨ι⟩ς ἢ καὶ σφοδροτέρας ἔτι
προσθείημεν ἀποδείξεις ὑπὲρ τοῦ κατὰ τὴν κεφαλήν τε καὶ τὸν ἐγκέφαλον
333 ὑπάρχειν αὐτό, τί ἄλλο ἢ τὸ Πλάτωνός τε καὶ | Ἱπποκράτους
ἀποδειχθήσεται δόγμα τὰς ἀποδείξεις ἀμφοτέρας ἡμῶν συνθέντων;
6. Ἴσως οὖν ἄμεινον, ἐπειδὴ κατὰ τοῦτο τοῦ λόγου γεγόναμεν,
ἀναμνῆσαι τῶν ἐπιστημονικῶν ἀποδείξεων ὑπὲρ ὧν ἐπὶ πλέον ἐν
τῷ πρὸ τούτου διελέχθην ὑπομνήματι, τὰ λήμματα δεικνὺς ἐξ ὧν ἄν τις
2 ἀποδείξειε τὸ προκείμενον. ἦν δ' αὐτὸ τὸ κεφάλαιον ἐκ τῶν ὑπαρχόντων
καὶ συμβεβηκότων ἑκατέρῳ τῶν σπλάγχνων κατὰ τὴν οὐσίαν τοῦ
ζητουμένου πράγματος ἄρχεσθαι χρῆναι· καὶ δὴ τὰ ὑπάρχοντά τε καὶ
3 συμβαίνοντα καθ' ἑκάτερον ἰδίᾳ πάντα διήλθομεν ἔμπροσθεν. ἦν δὲ καὶ
τούτων κεφάλαια ταυτί· πρῶτον μὲν ὡς τῶν αἴσθησίν τε καὶ κίνησιν τὴν
301 κατὰ προαίρεσιν ἅπασι τοῖς τοῦ / ζῴου [γε] μέλεσι παραγόντων ὀργά-
νων, ἅπερ ὀνομάζεται νεῦρα, τὸν ἐγκέφαλον ἀρχὴν ὑπάρχειν συμβέβη-
4 κεν, ὥσπερ τῶν ἀρτηριῶν τὴν καρδίαν· ἔπειτα δ' ὅτι θλιβεισῶν μὲν ἢ
τρωθεισῶν τῶν κατὰ τὸν ἐγκέφαλον κοιλιῶν ὅλον τὸ ζῷον αὐτίκα
γίνεται καρῶδες, οὐ μὴν ἀπόλλυταί γε οὔτε ἡ κατὰ τὰς ἀρτηρίας οὔτε ἡ
334 κατὰ τὴν | καρδίαν κίνησις, ὥσπερ γε κἀπειδὰν ὁμοίως τὴν καρδίαν
διαθῶμεν, αἱ μὲν κατὰ τὰς ἀρτηρίας κινήσεις παραβλάπτονται, τὸ δ'
ὅλον ζῷον οὔτε εἰς αἴσθησιν οὐδεμίαν οὔτε κίνησιν οὐδὲν φαίνεται
5 βλαπτόμενον. ἐπεδείξαμεν δὲ καὶ ὡς οὐδέτερον οὐδετέρῳ χορηγεῖ τῶν
εἰρημένων δυνάμεων, οὔθ' ἡ καρδία τῷ ἐγκεφάλῳ τῆς αἰσθητικῆς τε καὶ
κατὰ προαίρεσιν κινητικῆς οὔθ' ὁ ἐγκέφαλος τῇ καρδίᾳ τῆς σφυγμικῆς,
ἀλλ' ἔστιν ἑκάτερον τῶν μορίων ἑκατέρας δυνάμεως οἷον πηγή τις.
6 ἐνδείκνυται δ' ὁ λόγος ἤδη καὶ τὴν ἀπὸ τῶν νοσημάτων μαρτυρίαν,
ὑπὲρ ἧς ἐν τοῖς ἑξῆς ἐπὶ πλέον ἐροῦμεν. ἐγκεφάλου μὲν γὰρ πάσχοντος
302 ἕτοιμον παραφρονῆσαί τε καὶ ἀκίνητον καὶ ἀναίσθητον / γενέσθαι τὸ
ζῷον, καρδίας δὲ συγκοπῆναι μὲν καὶ ἀπολέσθαι, τῶν προειρημένων δ'
7 οὐδὲ ἓν παθεῖν. εἴπερ οὖν οὕτως ταῦτ' ἔχει, καθάπερ ἔχει, καὶ οἱ λέγοντες
ἐκ καρδίας πεφυκέναι τὰ νεῦρα λέγειν μὲν δύνανται τοῦτο καὶ γράφειν,
ὥσπερ καὶ ἄλλα πολλὰ λέγουσί τε καὶ γράφουσιν, οὐ μὴν ἐπί γε τῶν
335 8 ζῴων ἐναργῶς δεικνύναι. | τὴν μὲν γὰρ λογιζομένην ἀρχήν, ἀφ' ἧς τὰ
νεῦρα πέφυκεν, ἐγκέφαλον ἀναγκαῖον ὑπάρχειν· ὅσα δ' ὁ Χρύσιππος

1–2] SVF I, p. 130 13–15] *cf. supra*, pp. 108.26–28; 156.31–34 20–26] *cf. supra*, p. 126.11–17

2 αὐτὸ *Müller* 5 δὲ *del. Müller* 6 ταύτας H: *corr. Kühn* 12 . . .λέχθην H 13 ἀποδείξη H: *corr. Kühn* τὸ προκείμενον] . . . . .κείμενον H αὐτὸ] *fort. scribendum est* αὐτῶν 14 συμβεβη. .των H 15 .ρχεσθαι H 16 ἴδια H: *corr. Ald.* 18 γε *om.* M: *delevit Kühn* 20 θλιβεισῶν *ex* λιφθεισῶν *corr.* H²: θλιφθεισῶν R *Ald.* 23 τὴν καρδίαν *sscr.* H² 29 ἑκατέρας] ἑτέρας *Müller* 30 τῇ . . . μαρτυρίᾳ *Corn.* 34 καὶ *del. Müller*

only Chrysippus but also Cleanthes and Zeno readily accept it;
and the only point that must be examined is that in which the whole
controversy happens to lie, whether the rational part is also there.
For if the spirited part is clearly shown to be in the heart by the argu- 47
ments that Chrysippus has already repeated many times over, and
if we should add to these similar or even stronger proofs that the ratio-
nal part is in the head and brain, then when we combine both sets of
proofs, what else will result but the proof of the doctrine of Plato
and Hippocrates?

6. Now perhaps it is better, since we have reached this part of
the discussion, to recall the scientific demonstrations of which I spoke
at length in the preceding book, when I was pointing out the premises
from which a person could prove what we set out to prove. The main 2
point was that one must begin from the properties and attributes of
the two internal organs as they pertain to the essence of the matter
under investigation; and indeed we examined earlier all the properties
and attributes, taking each of the organs separately. And of these pro- 3
perties and attributes the main heads were first, that the brain is the
source of the organs, which we call nerves, that transmit sensation
and voluntary motion to all the limbs of the animal, just as the heart
(is the source) of the arteries; and second, that when the ventricles of 4
the brain have been pressed or wounded, the whole animal immedi-
ately becomes stupefied, but neither the motion in the arteries nor that
in the heart is destroyed; and when we subject the heart to the same
treatment, the movements in the arteries are damaged along
with it, but the animal as a whole is observed to suffer no impairment
either of sensation or of motion. We also showed that neither supplies 5
these powers to the other: the heart (does) not (supply) to the brain
the power of perception and voluntary motion, and the brain (does)
not (supply) to the heart the power to pulsate, but each of the two
parts is as it were the fountain of its own power. And here the argu- 6
ment points to the evidence of diseases, about which we shall speak
more fully in what follows. For if the brain suffers injury the animal
readily becomes delirious and loses motion and sensation; but if the
heart is damaged the animal collapses and dies but suffers none of the
things just mentioned. Now if this is so, and it is so, then those who 7
say that the nerves come from the heart can indeed say and write it,
just as they say and write much else; but they cannot give a clear
demonstration of it in animals. For the seat of reason, from which the 8
nerves come, must be the brain; and all the things that Chrysippus

ἐπὶ πλεῖστον μηκύνων ἐπὶ τῆς καρδίας διεξῆλθεν, οὐ τὸ λογίζεσθαι δείκνυσι τὸ σπλάγχνον, ἀλλὰ τὸ θυμοῦσθαι καὶ τὸ φοβεῖσθαι καὶ τὸ λυπεῖσθαι καὶ πάνθ' ὅσα τοῦ θυμοειδοῦς τῆς ψυχῆς ἐστιν ἔργα τε καὶ πάθη.

7. Ὅπερ οὖν εἶπον ἤδη πρόσθεν ἐν τῷδε τῷ γράμματι, τοῦτο καὶ νῦν ἀναγκαῖον ἀναμνῆσαι, ὅτι ὁ Χρύσιππος ἐν τῇ μετὰ τὰς προγεγραμμένας ῥήσεις λέξει προχείρως πάλιν ἐξ ἑνὸς ἄρχεσθαι μορίου τὰς δυνάμεις ἀμφοτέρας λαμβάνει μηδεμίαν ἀπόδειξιν ἢ παραμυθίαν ἢ πιθανότητα
303 τῷ λόγῳ / προστιθείς, ὡς ἐξ αὐτῆς φανερὸν ἔσται τῆς λέξεως αὐτοῦ
2 τόνδε τὸν τρόπον ἐχούσης· «ἀτόπως οὖν αὐ⟨τοῖς⟩ τὸ κατὰ ταῦτα ἐξαχθησόμενον, ἐάν τε μὴ φῶσι τὴν λύπην καὶ τὴν ἀγωνίαν ⟨καὶ τὴν ὀδύνην⟩ ἀλγηδόνας εἶναι, ἐάν τε ἀλγηδόνας ⟨αἳ⟩ ἐν ἄλλῳ γίνονται τόπῳ
3 ἢ τῷ ἡγεμονικῷ. τὰ δὲ αὐτὰ καὶ ἐπὶ τῆς χαρᾶς καὶ ἐπὶ τοῦ θάρσους
4 ἐροῦμεν, ἅπερ ἐμφαίνει περὶ τὴν καρδίαν γινόμενα. ὃν τρόπον γὰρ ὅταν
336 τὸν | πόδα πονῶμεν ἢ τὴν κεφαλήν, περὶ τούτους τοὺς τόπους ὁ πόνος γίνεται, οὕτως συναισθανόμεθα καὶ τῆς κατὰ τὴν λύπην ἀλγηδόνος περὶ τὸν θώρακα γινομένης, οὔτε τῆς λύπης οὐκ οὔσης ἀλγηδόνος οὔτε ἐν ἑτέρῳ τινὶ τόπῳ ἢ τῷ ἡγεμονικῷ αὐτῆς γινομένης.»

5 Πρὸς ταύτην τὴν ῥῆσιν δίκαιον ἀποκρίνασθαι τῷ Χρυσίππῳ καθ' ἕκαστον ὧν ἐρωτᾷ κεφαλαίων εὐθέως ἀπὸ τῆς ἀρχῆς τὸ πρῶτον ἀναλαβόντας, ἔνθα φησὶ τὴν λύπην καὶ τὴν ἀγωνίαν καὶ τὴν ὀδύνην
6 ἀλγηδόνας ὑπάρχειν. εἴτε γὰρ ἐρωτῶν ἡμᾶς οὕτως εἴποι τις, ὡς Χρύ-/
304 σιππος εἴρηκεν, εἴτε ἀποφαινόμενος, ἐπαινέσομεν αὐτοῦ τὸν λόγον καὶ φήσομεν ἀγωνίαν καὶ λύπην καὶ ὀδύνην ἀλγηδόνας εἶναι τῷ γένει, μᾶλλον δ' εἰ χρὴ τοῖς ὀνόμασι κατὰ τὴν τῶν Ἑλλήνων χρήσασθαι συνήθειαν, ὀδύνας μὲν καὶ ἀλγηδόνας οὐδέτερον ἀλλήλων διαφέρει⟨ν⟩, ὥσπερ οὐδὲ κίονα καὶ στῦλον οὐδ' ὦπας καὶ ὀφθαλμούς· ἀγωνίας μέντοι
7 καὶ λύπης οἷον γένος εἶναί τι τὴν ἀλγηδόνα. τὸ δ' ἐν τῷ ἡγεμονικῷ τόπῳ τὰς ἀλγηδόνας γίνεσθαι, τοῦτ' οὐκέτι τῷ Χρυσίππῳ συγχωρή-
337 σομεν [αὐτῷ τὴν ἀλγηδόνα κατά τε τὸ | ἡγεμονικὸν συνίστασθαι]. δίκαιος οὖν ἐστιν ἐπιδεῖξαι καθ' ἓν ⟨καὶ⟩ ταὐτὸν σπλάγχνον ἀμφοτέρας ᾠκισμένας τὰς δυνάμεις.

8 Καίτοι τί λέγω καὶ καθ' ἓν καὶ ταὐτόν; οὐ γὰρ πρὸς Χρύσιππον οὕτω χρὴ ποιεῖσθαι τὸν λόγον, ἀλλὰ πρὸς Ἀριστοτέλην συγχωροῦντα μὲν εἶναι πλείους δυνάμεις ἡμῶν ἐν τῇ ψυχῇ τῷ γένει διαφερούσας, οὐ μὴν ἐν ἄλλῳ γε καὶ ἄλλῳ σπλάγχνῳ καθιδρῦσθαι· πάντων γὰρ ἀρχὴν

5] *cf. supra*, pp. 176.11–178.6 6–18] SVF II, p. 248 27] *cf.* Gal. De alim. fac. i. 28: CMG V 4.2, pp. 255–256 In Hipp. De artic. comm. i. 20: XVIII A 342 K. 34–214.1] *cf. infra*, p. 222.6–9

7 μορίου] μ. . . H: μόνου *Ald.* 8 ἢ παραμυθίαν] . . . .θίαν H 9 τῆς *deperditum in* H 10 ἀτόπως – 11 ἐξαχθησόμενον] "*fortasse* ἄτοπον οὖν τὸ κ. τ. λεχθησόμενον" *v. Arnim* αὐτοῖς τὸ] αὐτὸ H: *supplevi* 11 . . .χθησόμενον H 11–12 καὶ τὴν ὀδύνην *add. Corn. (cf. infra, lin. 21)* 12 αἳ *add. Einarson* γίνεσθαι *Chart.* 13 αὐ. H 20 ἐρω̄ H: ἐρωτῶ M *Ald.*: *corr. Corn.* 26 μὲν *scripsi*: δὲ H: τε *Corn.*: *del. Müller* διαφέρει H: *corr. Ald.* 27 καὶ[I] *coni. Diels*: οὐδὲ H 30 αὐτῷ – συνίστασθαι *del. Corn.* τε] γε *Kühn* 31 καὶ *add. Corn.*: *ante* καθ' *et post* ἓν *addiderit* καὶ *Einarson (cf. infra, lin. 33)* 33 καὶ[I] *om. Ald.*

recounted at the greatest length about the heart do not prove that that organ exercises reason, but (rather) that it experiences anger and fear and distress and all the activities and affections of the spirited part of the soul.

7. I must now repeat a statement that I made earlier in this book, that in what he says after the passages quoted, Chrysippus again assumes without hesitation that both powers originate from a single member, without adding a single proof or supporting argument or probability, as will be clear from his own words, which are as follows: "Therefore whatever they would reject in this leads to absurdity, 2
whether they say that distress and anxiety and suffering are not pains or are pains that arise in some region other than the governing part (of the soul). We shall say the same also about joy and good cheer, 3
which reveal their origin in the area of the heart. For as when our foot 4
hurts us or our head, the hurting occurs in our foot or head, just so we are conscious of the pain in distress as occurring in the chest; and it is not the case that distress is not a pain, or that it occurs in some place other than the governing part of the soul."

In reply to this passage I must answer Chrysippus on each of 5
his main points, beginning with the first, where he says that distress and anxiety and suffering are pains. For whether a person says this 6
while reasoning with us, as Chrysippus did, or as an assertion, we shall praise his discourse and say that anxiety and distress and suffering belong to the genus pain, or rather, if we must use words in accordance with Greek usage, that there is no difference between suffering and pain, just as there is none between a column and a pillar, or between eyes and organs of sight; but pain is, as it were, the genus of anxiety and distress. But that the pains arise in the place where the 7
governing part is, this we shall no longer concede to Chrysippus. He ought to show, then, that both powers reside in one and the same internal organ.

Yet why do I say "in one and the same"? This is not the way to 8
argue with Chrysippus, but with Aristotle, who agrees that we have in our souls a plurality of powers differing in kind, but (does) not (agree) that they reside in different organs; he wants the heart to be

305 9 εἶναι βούλεται τὴν καρδίαν. / ὁ δὲ Χρύσιππος οὐδὲ τὰς δυνάμεις αὐτὰς
διαλ⟨λ⟩άττειν ἀλλήλων ὁμολογεῖ, οὐδ' ἑτέρᾳ μέν τινι δυνάμει θυμοῦσθαι τὸ
10 ζῷον, ἑτέρᾳ δ' ἐπιθυμεῖν, ἑτέρᾳ δὲ λογίζεσθαι. οὔκουν οὐδ' ἡμᾶς οὕτω χρὴ
προβάλλειν αὐτό, καθάπερ ὀλίγον ἔμπροσθεν εἴπομεν, ἐπιδεῖξαι παρακαλοῦντας ὡς ἐν ταὐτῷ τόπῳ τοῦ ζῴου καὶ τὸ θυμοειδές ἐστι καὶ τὸ
11 λογιστικὸν καὶ τὸ ἐπιθυμητικόν. τὸ τοίνυν πρότερόν τε τούτου καὶ
γενικώτερον ζήτημα τοῦτο παρακαλέσομεν ἢ Χρύσιππον ἤ τινα τῶν
ἀπ' αὐτοῦ καταστήσασθαί τε καὶ ἀποδεῖξαι· τοῦτο δ' ἐστὶ τὸ τῆς
αὐτῆς εἶναι δυνάμεως ἔργα τό τε λογίζεσθαι καὶ τὸ θυμοῦσθαι καὶ τὸ
338 12 βρωμάτων τε | καὶ πομάτων καὶ ἀφροδισίων ἐπιθυμεῖν. ἡμεῖς μὲν
γὰρ ἐπί τε τῶν ἀλόγων ζῴων ἐναργῶς ἐπιδείκνυμεν αὐτὰ κεχωρισμένα
καὶ προσέτι τῶν παίδων, οἳ λογισμῷ μὲν ἥκιστα χρῶνται, θυμοῖς δὲ καὶ
13 ἐπιθυμίαις ἰσχυροτάταις ὥσπερ τὰ θηρία δουλεύουσι. καὶ ἡμῶν γ'
αὐτῶν ὁ μὲν τῷ λογισμῷ μάλιστα χρώμενος ἥκιστ' ἐπιθυμητικός τ' ἐστὶ
306 καὶ θυμικός, ὁ δ' ὑπό τινος τῶν ἀλόγων τῆς ψυχῆς / μορίων ἀρχόμενος
14 ἥκιστα χρῆται λογισμῷ. καὶ τῆς Μηδείας δ' ἀναμνηστέον ἐν τούτῳ
τῆς Εὐριπίδου καὶ τοῦ Ὁμηρικοῦ Ὀδυσσέως, ἐν οἷς ἐστασίασε
μὲν ἑκάτερα πρὸς ἄλληλα τῆς ψυχῆς τὰ μόρια δηλοῦντα σαφῶς ὡς οὐχ
ἕν ἐστιν, ἐνίκησε δὲ ἐπὶ τοῦ σοφωτέρου τὸ βέλτιον, ἐπὶ δὲ τῆς ἀπαιδεύτου
15 τε καὶ βαρβάρου τὸ χεῖρον. καὶ ἐπὶ πολλῶν ἀνθρώπων τοιαῦτ' ἐστὶ
γινόμενα κατὰ τὴν ψυχήν, τοῦ λογισμοῦ ποτὲ μὲν τῷ θυμοειδεῖ μαχομένου
16 ποτὲ δὲ τῷ ἐπιθυμητικῷ. ὁ δὲ Χρύσιππος ἅμα τοῖς ἄλλοις Στωϊκοῖς
ἐπὶ μὲν τῶν ἀλόγων ζῴων ὁμόσε χωρεῖ πρὸς τὸ δόγμα μηδ' ἐπιθυμεῖν
339 φάσκων· καί μοι περὶ τῆς ἀναισχυντίας τοῦ λόγου πρόσθεν | εἴρηται· ἐπὶ
δὲ τῶν παίδων ἄνω καὶ κάτω περιπλέκουσιν, οὐχ ὡσαύτως μὲν ἅπαντες,
ἀναισχυντοῦντες δὲ καὶ παρὰ τὸ φαινόμενον ἀποφαινόμενοι πάντες.
17 εἰρήσεται δέ μοι καὶ περὶ τούτων ἐπὶ πλέον ἐν τοῖς ἐφεξῆς. ὡσαύτως δὲ
καὶ περὶ τῶν κατὰ τὴν ψυχὴν παθῶν τῆς διαφορᾶς οὐδὲν ὁμολογούμενον οὔτε τοῖς ἐναργέσιν οὔτ' ἀλλήλοις λέγουσιν οὐθ' ἕκαστος ἑαυτῷ. /
307 18 περὶ ὧν ἁπάντων ἔγνωκα κατὰ τὸν ἑξῆς λόγον τὸν δ' διελθεῖν· οὑτοσὶ
γὰρ ὁ τρίτος οὐκ οἶδ' ὅπως παρενέπεσε διὰ τὰς τῶν ἑταίρων δεήσεις
ἀξιούντων μη⟨δ'⟩ ὅσα τῶν ὑπὸ Χρυσίππου γεγραμμένων ⟨ἄτοπα
19 παρελθεῖν⟩, ἀλλὰ πρὸς ἅπαντα τὴν ἀντιλογίαν ποιεῖσθαι. ἐγὼ δ' ὧν
μὲν καὶ αὐτὸς ὁ Χρύσιππος ᾔσθετο περιττῶς εἰρημένων ὑφ' ἑαυτοῦ
καὶ τάχ' ἄν τῳ δοξάντων, ὡς αὐτός φησιν, ὑπὸ γραμματιστοῦ τινος

1–3] SVF II, p. 248 16–17] *cf. supra*, pp. 184.14–190.15 22–24] libri primi test., *v. supra*, p. 70.3–5 *cf. supra*, p. 102.22–25 24–27] *cf. infra*, pp. 294.19–20; 316.21–320.13; 340.18–23 33–216.2] *cf. supra*, p. 196.1–3

2 διαλάττειν H M *(e corr.)*: *corr.* F R 3 λογίζεσθαι] λυπεῖσθαι H: λογίσθαι *Ald.*: *corr. Bas. Corn.* 4 προβάλλειν] . . . .λειν H: προβάλειν *Ald.* παρα. . . . .τας H 5 καὶ τὸ[II] *deperdita in* H 7 γε. . .ῶ' (τρ supra) H τοῦτο *ex* τουτου *corr.* H 8 αὐ. . H 9 λογίζεσθαι *coni. Ald.*: λυπεῖσθαι H 21 τῷ *ex* τοῦ *corr.* H 31 ἑταίρων δεήσεις *scripsi*: στωϊκῶν ἔρεις H 32 ἀξιοῦν (τ supra) H: ἀξιοῦνται M: *corr. Ald.* μὴ ὅσα H: *correxi (cf. supra, p. 204.36)*: μὴ πρός τινα *Müller*: μηδὲν παρεῖναι *vel sim. coniecerit Einarson* 32–33 ἄτοπα παρελθεῖν *addidi exempli gratia (cf. infra, p. 216.21; PHP 654.9 Müller)*

the source of all. But Chrysippus does not admit even that the powers 9
themselves differ, or that by one power the animal is angry, by another
desiderative, and by another rational. We should not, then, pose the 10
problem as we did just now, when we called on him to prove that the
spirited, rational, and desiderative parts of the animal are in the same
place. We shall therefore challenge Chrysippus or some follower of 11
his to establish and prove this prior and more general proposition:
that reasoning and being angry and desiring food, drink and sexual
intercourse are activities of the same power. For in the case of irrational 12
animals we can show clearly that they are distinct, and also in children,
who make very little use of reason but, like wild animals, are enslaved
to anger and to very strong desires. And among ourselves the person 13
who uses reason most is least subject to desire and anger, while he who
is ruled by one of the irrational parts of the soul uses reason least.
Here you should recall Euripides' Medea and Homer's Odysseus, 14
in whom two parts of the soul were at war with each other, thus clearly
demonstrating that they are not one; and the better part prevailed in
the wiser (of the two), but the worse in the one who was uneducated
and uncivilized. Such conflicts arise in the souls of many persons, 15
reason conflicting sometimes with the spirited part, sometimes with
the desiderative. But in the case of the irrational animals Chrysippus 16
and the other Stoics boldly attack this view, claiming that the
animals do not even experience desire; I mentioned earlier the shame-
lessness of this statement. And when they speak of children they twist
their arguments up and down. Not all give the same account, but all
are shameless and make statements contrary to the obvious facts.
I shall speak of this later at greater length. And similarly in their 17
accounts of the differences in the affections of the soul they say nothing
consistent with the evident facts or with each other or each with
himself. I have decided to discuss all these matters in the next book, 18
the fourth; for this third book has somehow intruded itself because of
the requests of my friends, who asked me not to omit even the ab-
surdities in Chrysippus' work, but to refute all of it. For my part, 19
I thought it better not to mention at all those statements of Chrysip-
pus which he himself perceived to be absurd and which he says you
might take to be the words of a schoolmaster or a prating old woman.

ἢ γραὸς ἀδολεσχούσης εἰρῆσθαι, βέλτιον ᾤμην εἶναι μηδ' ὅλως μνημο-
νεύειν· τὰ δ' ἄλλα σύμπαντα δίχα τεμὼν ἐν μὲν τῷ πρὸ τούτου διῆλθον
ἅπερ ἦν ἁπάντων ἰσχυρότατα, τοῖς δὲ περὶ τῶν τῆς ψυχῆς παθῶν
ζητουμένοις ἐγνώκειν ἀναθεῖναι [κατὰ] τόδε τὸ γ' τῶν ὑπομνημάτων.|
340 20 τοῦτο μὲν οὖν ἐὰν θεὸς ἡμᾶς σῴζῃ πάντως πράξομεν.
Ἐπεὶ δ' ἐν τῷ νῦν ἐνεστῶτι λόγῳ μνημονεῦσαι πάντων διέγνωμεν ὧν
εἶπεν ὁ Χρύσιππος ἐν τῷ προτέρῳ Περὶ ψυχῆς ⟨ὑπὲρ⟩ ἡγεμονικοῦ
διαλεγόμενος, ἑξῆς ἂν εἴη καιρὸς ἤδη συνάπτειν τοῖς εἰρημένοις τὰ λοι-
308 21 πά. / συνεχὴς οὖν τῇ προγεγραμμένῃ ῥήσει τοῦ Χρυσίππου τοιάδε
τίς ἐστι· «καθ' ἣν ἔτι φορὰν καὶ τὰ τοιαῦτα λέγεται πάντα· 'ἠψάμην
σου τῆς καρδίας' ὥσπερ τῆς ψυχῆς, καὶ 'ἅπτομαι τῆς καρδίας' λέγομεν,
οὐχ ὡς ἂν εἰ παρέλθοιέν τινες ἡμᾶς ἐπὶ τοῦ ἐγκεφάλου καὶ τῶν σπλάγ-
χνων λέγοντες καὶ τοῦ ἥπατος, ἀλλὰ τοῖς προειρημένοις παραπλη-
22 σίως. ἐκεῖνα γάρ μοι δοκεῖ λέγεσθαι ὡς ἄν τις ἔφη 'τῶν ἐντός σου ἅπτομαι',
διϊκνουμένης τῆς κακοποιΐας ἐπὶ τοσοῦτον· τῇ δὲ καρδίᾳ καθάπερ ἂν
23 τῇ ψυχῇ χρώμεθα. καὶ τούτων ἔσται ἔμφασις ἐφιστᾶσι μᾶλλον.» ὅτι
καὶ ταῦτα πρὸς τῷ μηδὲν ἀποδεικνύειν ἀλλ' ἰδιώτας ἐπικαλεῖσθαι μάρ-
τυρας οὐδὲ περαίνει τι τῶν προκειμένων, ἀλλὰ τὸ παθητικόν τε καὶ
ἄλογον τῆς ψυχῆς, οὐ τὸ λογιζόμενον ἐνδείκνυται κατὰ τὴν καρδίαν
341 ὑπάρχειν, ἄντικρυς δῆλον· | ὅθεν οὐδ' ἐπὶ πλέον ἐν αὐτοῖς χρὴ διατρί-
309 βειν ὁμοίαν ἔχουσιν ἀτοπίαν οἷς ἤδη πολλάκις / ἔδειξα.
24 Μετὰ δὲ τὴν προγεγραμμένην ῥῆσιν ἑτέρα τις ἐφεξῆς ἐστιν, ἐν
ᾗ τοὺς ἀσπλάγχνους τε καὶ τοὺς οὐκ ἔχοντας ἐγκέφαλον ἐξηγεῖται πῶς
25 λέγονται, περὶ ἧς αὐτάρκως ἔμπροσθεν εἴρηται. μετὰ δὲ ταῦτα τοιάνδε
τινὰ γράφει[ν] ῥῆσιν· «κατὰ τοιαύτην δέ μοι δοκοῦσι μάλιστα φορὰν καὶ
οἱ τιμωρητικώτερον πρός τινας φερόμενοι ὁρμᾶν ἐπὶ τὸ ταύτην ἐκσπάσαι,
καθ' ἣν φορὰν ἐπιτείνοντες καὶ πρὸς τὰ λοιπὰ τῶν σπλάγχνων ὁμοει-
26 δῶς φέρονται.» ἐνταῦθα πάλιν ὁ Χρύσιππος οὐκ οἶδ' ὅπως ἀγνοεῖ
κατασκευάζων ἕτερόν τι τοῦ προκειμένου σκέμματος. οἱ γὰρ ἀπειλοῦν-
τές τισιν ὥσπερ ἐκκόψαι τοὺς ὀφθαλμοὺς αὐτῶν ἐνίοτε λέγουσιν ἢ
κατάξαι τὴν κεφαλὴν ἢ συντρῖψαι τὰ σκέλη, κατὰ τὸν αὐτὸν τρόπον
27 ἔστιν ὅτε καὶ τὴν καρδίαν ἐκσπάσαι φασὶν ἐν ἴσῳ τῷ ἀποκτεῖναι. ἀλλὰ
τί τοῦτο πρὸς τὰ παρόντα; τὸ γὰρ ἀποτεμεῖν ἐνίοτε τὰ ὦτα καὶ
342 τὴν ῥῖνα καὶ διασπάσαι πολλάκις ἀλλήλους | ἀπειλοῦσιν οἱ ἄνθρω-
310 ποι, καί πού τις εὐχομένη παρὰ τῷ ποιητῇ γυνὴ / τάδε λέγει·

«τοῦ ἐγὼ μέσον ἧπαρ ἔχοιμι
ἐσθέμεναι προσφῦσα.»

6–16] SVF II, pp. 248–249 22–28] SVF II, p. 250 22–24] SVF II, p. 238 24] *cf. supra*, pp. 192.18–198.16 36–37] Hom. Il. xxiv. 212–213.

3 ἰσχυρότατα, τοῖς] ἰσχυ. . . . . H 4 ἀναθεῖναι κατὰ] ει *ex* η *corr.* M²: ἀναθεῖν. . . . . . H: κατὰ *del. Müller* 5 πάντως] π. . . . H 7 ὑπὲρ *add. Müller (cf. supra, pp. 104.28; 170.6–7, 28–29)* 12 ἂν εἰ παρέλθοιέν] ἀντιπαρέλθοιεν H: *corr. Einarson*: ἂν παρέλθοιεν *Corn.*: ἄν τι περιέλθοιέν *Diels* ἡμᾶς] ἡμῖν *Müller* 25 γράφειν H: *corr. Ald.* 26 τιμωρητικώτερον *ex* τιμωρεῖται *corr.* H 33 ἐνίοτε *deperditum in* H 34 ἀλλήλοις *Müller* ἀπει. . . . . H 36 . .σον H 37 αἰσθέμεναι H: *corr. Corn.*

All that remained I divided into two parts: the points that were strongest of all I discussed in the preceding book, and I had decided to devote this third book to questions about the affections of the soul. This I shall certainly do, if god preserves me. 20

But since I decided to mention in the present book all that Chrysippus said in the discussion of the governing part in his first book On the Soul, it is now time to add the remainder to what has already been said. The continuation of the passage quoted earlier 21
from Chrysippus is as follows: "The following expressions, also, are in keeping with this tendency. We say 'I touched your heart', meaning 'your soul', and (we say) 'I touch your heart', not as if people entered into us, as when we speak of touching the brain or internal organs or liver, but in a way similar to the expressions mentioned earlier. For 22
those other expressions, it seems to me, are used as if a person said 'I am touching your inner parts', when the injury penetrates that far, but we use the word 'heart' as we would 'soul'. These matters will become evident as we give more attention to them." It is immediately 23
obvious that these (remarks) too, besides proving nothing and appealing instead to the testimony of non-experts, do not even lead to any of the conclusions that he intends; they indicate rather that the affective and irrational part of the soul, not the rational part, is in the heart. Therefore I need spend no more time on them, as their absurdity is of a kind that I have already exposed on many occasions.

After the passage quoted above there next comes another in which 24
he explains the meaning of 'having no internal organ' and 'having no brain', about which I have said enough already. After that, he writes 25
these words: "It is especially in keeping with a tendency of this kind, I think, that those who are rather strongly moved to punish certain people have an urge to 'tear it out'; and when they are strengthened in this tendency they are moved in the same way toward the rest of the internal organs." Here again Chrysippus somehow fails to 26
perceive that he is making a case for something other than what he wants to prove. For just as in threats men sometimes say that they will knock out a person's eyes or break his head or crush his legs, in the same way they sometimes say that they will tear his heart out, meaning that they will kill him. But what does this have to do with the present 27
problem? People sometimes threaten to cut off ears and nose, and often to tear each other apart, and in a passage in Homer a woman utters this prayer:

> "Would that I might hold the liver in his middle
> and attach myself to it and eat it."

28 τί οὖν οὐ καὶ τὸ ἧπαρ ἀρχὴν τῆς ψυχῆς ἀποφαινόμεθα, φίλτατε Χρύσιππε, καὶ ταῦθ' Ὅμηρον ἔχοντες μαρτυροῦντα, τηλικοῦτον ποιητήν, ᾧ μᾶλλον ἦν σε πιστεύειν δίκαιον ἢ τοῖς ἰδιώταις; οὗτος μέν γε πρὸς τοῖς ἄλλοις ἔτι καὶ ταῦθ' ὑπὲρ ἥπατος ἔγραψε·

29 «καὶ Τιτυὸν εἶδον, γ[ρ]αίης ἐρικυδέος υἱόν,
κείμενον ἐν δαπέδῳ, ὁ δ' ἐπ' ἐννέα κεῖτο πέλεθρα·
γῦπε δέ μιν ἑκάτερθε παρημένω ἧπαρ ἔκειρον
δέρτρον ἔσω δύνοντες, ὁ δ' οὐκ ἀπαμύνετο χερσί.
Λητὼ γὰρ εἵλκυσε Διὸς κυδρὴν παράκοιτιν
Πυθώδ' ἐρχομένην διὰ καλλιχόρου Πανοπῆος.»

30 Ἐν τούτοις ὁ ποιητὴς ἐναργῶς ἐνδείκνυται τὸ τῆς ψυχῆς ἐπι-
311 843 θυμητικὸν μέρος ὑπάρχειν ἐν ἥπατι. διότι γάρ, φησίν, /| ἐπεθύμησεν ὁ Τιτυὸς ὑβρίσαι τὴν Λητώ, διὰ τοῦτο γῦπες αὐτοῦ κείρουσι τὸ ἧπαρ, ὡς εἰς αὐτὸ μάλιστα τιμωρούμενοι τὸ κατάρξαν τῆς ὕβρεως.

31 Ἀλλ' ἐνταῦθα μὲν ἐπαινῶ τὸν Χρύσιππον ἑκόντα σιωπήσαντα τὸ
32 καταβάλλον αὐτοῦ τὴν δόξαν. ἐν οἷς δ' ἤτοι περαίνει μηδὲν ἢ καθ' ἑαυτοῦ καλεῖ τοὺς μαρτυρήσοντας, ἐνταῦθα νομίζω μὴ συνιέναι τῶν ἀκολουθούντων τε καὶ μαχομένων ἀλλήλοις πραγμάτων, ὥσπερ γε κἀν τοῖς ἑξῆς τῶν προγεγραμμένων, ἐν οἷς φησι· «καὶ τὰ τῶν ὀργιζομένων δὲ πάθη περὶ τὸν θώρακα φαίνεται γινόμενα καὶ τὰ τῶν ἐρώντων, ὥστε καὶ τὴν ἐπιθυ-
33 μίαν μάλιστα γίνεσθαι περὶ τούτους τοὺς τόπους.» ἐφ' ἑκάστῃ τῶν τοιούτων ῥήσεων ἐπιφθέγγεσθαι προσήκει, «τί οὖν, ὦ Χρύσιππε, τοῦτο πρὸς τὸ λογιστικόν, ὑπὲρ οὗ ζητοῦμεν;» οὐ γὰρ δὴ περὶ τῶν ὀργιζομένων ἢ ἐπιθυμούντων ἡ ἀμφισβήτησις ἦν, εἰ κατὰ τὸν θώρακά τε καὶ περὶ τὸν θώρακα τοῖς οὕτως ἔχουσι κινεῖται τὰ πάθη, ἀλλ' εἰ καὶ
312 τὸ λογιζόμενον ἐνταῦθά / ἐστιν.

34 Ἐφεξῆς δὲ τούτων τάδε γράφει· «εὖ μάλα δὲ παριστᾶσι τὸ λεγό-
344 μενον, ὡς ἔφην, καὶ αἱ ἐν | αὑτοῖς γινόμεναι μελέται καὶ ῥήσεων καὶ τῶν παραπλησίων. ἐν ᾧ γὰρ ταῦτα πάντα συντελεῖται, πάντως εὔλογον ἐν ἐκείνῳ καὶ τὴν τοῦ λόγου διέξοδον γίνεσθαι καὶ λέγειν ἡμᾶς καὶ δια-
35 νοεῖσθαι κατ' ἐκεῖνο.» ἀληθῆ ταῦτα γράφεις, ὦ Χρύσιππε. καθ' ὃ γὰρ ἐν ἑαυτοῖς μελετῶμεν ἢ καὶ μετὰ σιγῆς διεξερχόμεθα διανοούμενοι, τοῦτό ἐστι
36 τὸ λογιζόμενον. ἀλλὰ πότερον ἐγκέφαλος ἢ καρδία τὸ διανοούμενόν ἐστιν, ὃ ἀπ' ἀρχῆς ἐζητοῦμεν, ἐχρῆν ἀποδεῖξαί σε καὶ μὴ τὸ πρῶτον λῆμμα λαβόντα πρὸς ἁπάντων ὁμολογούμενον ἡγεῖσθαί τι παρ' αὐτοῦ
37 πλέον ἕξειν εἰς τὴν τῶν ζητουμένων εὕρεσιν. οὐδεὶς γοῦν ἐστιν ὃς οὐχ

5–10] Hom. Od. xi. 576–581 *cf. infra*, PHP 578–579 Müller 11–14] *cf.* Gal. De loc. aff. iii. 5: VIII 160 K. 17–18] *cf. infra*, PHP 732.10–12 Müller 18–21] SVF II, p. 250 19–20] *cf. supra*, p. 154.6–8 27–31] SVF II, p. 250

1 ψυχῆς *deperditum in* H 5 γραίης H: *corr. Corn. (cf. infra, PHP 578.16 Müller)* 9 κρύβδην H: *corr. Chart. (cf. infra, PHP 579.4 Müller)* 10 καλλιχώρου H: *corr. Chart. (cf. infra, PHP 579.5 Müller)* 14 εἰς *del. Müller* 17 μαρτυρήσαντας H: *corr. Müller* 20 φαίνεται *ante* περὶ *(lin. 19) trsp. Müller (cf. supra, p. 154.7)* ἐρώντων] ν[1] *inser.* H 23 λογιστικόν] κ *ex* στ *corr.* H 29 παραπλησίων] ω *in* ο *mut., ut vid.*, H 31 καθὸ H: *corr.* R *Ald.* 34 ἀρχῆς ἐζητοῦμεν] ἀ. . . . . τοῦμεν H 35 λαβόντα πρὸς] λαβ. . . . . . H 36 ἕξειν εἰς τὴν] ἕξει. . . . H

Why then, my dear Chrysippus, don't we say that the liver too is 28
the source of the soul, especially as we have Homer as our witness,
a poet of such eminence that you should surely believe him in prefer-
ence to ordinary folk? Furthermore, in addition to his other passages
on the liver, the poet also wrote the following lines:

> "And I saw Tityos, son of glorious earth, 29
> lying on the ground; he covered nine acres.
> Two vultures, sitting on either side, were tearing his liver,
> putting their heads inside his bowels, and he did not
> defend himself with his hands.
> For he had assaulted Leto, glorious wife of Zeus
> as she went to Pytho through Panopeus, a land of
> fair dancing grounds."

In these (lines) the poet clearly indicates that the desiderative 30
part of the soul is in the liver. For, he says, because Tityos desired
to assault Leto, therefore vultures tear his liver, obviously punishing
him most in the very member that initiated the lawless act.

Here I commend Chrysippus for deliberately suppressing a 31
passage that refutes his doctrine. But in the places where either his 32
argument is inconclusive or he calls witnesses against himself, there, in
my opinion, he does not understand entailment and mutual incompati-
bility, as also in the next passage, where he says: "It is evident that
the affections of angry men arise in the region of the chest, and also
those of lovers; therefore desire also arises especially in these regions."
To every such passage the proper response is, "But what, Chrysippus, 33
does this have to do with the rational part, which is the subject of our
inquiry?" For the dispute was not whether persons experiencing anger
or desire have their affections aroused in the chest and the region
around the chest, but whether the rational part is there also.

Next after this he writes: "As I said, our rehearsing speeches and 34
the like in ourselves establishes this point very well. For it is altogether
reasonable that the part in which all these (things) take place is the
part in which the act of going through a discourse is performed, and
that we speak and think there." This statement of yours is true, 35
Chrysippus. That part with which we practice a speech in ourselves
or even silently go through a thing as we think about it is the rational
part. But whether it is the brain or the heart that thinks – which is 36
the question we have been asking from the start –, this you should
have proved. You should not have supposed that by taking as your
first premise a fact agreed to by all, you were thereby in a better
position to find the solution. Surely no one will deny that the govern- 37

ὁμολογήσει καθ' ὃ σκεπτόμεθα καὶ διαλεγόμεθα κατὰ τοῦτο τὸ μόριον
38 εἶναι τὸ τῆς ψυχῆς ἡγεμονικόν. ἀλλ' οὐ τοῦτ' ἦν τὸ ζητούμενον, ἀλλ'
εἰ καρδία τοῦθ' ὑπάρχει τὸ μόριον, ὅπερ οὐκ ἀπέδειξας, εἰ μή τινας ἄρα
313 39 φῇς αἰσθάνεσθαι κατὰ τὴν καρδίαν λογιζομένους. ἀλλ' / ἐν ἀρχῇ γε τοῦ
λόγου παντὸς ἔφησθα κατὰ λέξιν ὧδε· «οὕτω φαίνεται διαφεύγειν ὁ
345 τόπος ἡμᾶς οὔτε αἰσθήσεως ἐκφανοῦς γινομένης, ὅπερ ἐπὶ τῶν | λοιπῶν
συντέτευχεν, οὔτε τῶν τεκμηρίων δι' ὧν ἄν τις συλλογίσαιτο τοῦτο·
οὐδὲ γὰρ ἂν ἐπὶ τοσοῦτον ἡ ἀντιλογία προῆλθε καὶ ἐν ἰατροῖς καὶ ἐν
40 φιλοσόφοις.» ὁ ταῦτ' εἰπὼν Χρύσιππος εἰ πάλιν ἐν ταὐτῷ βιβλίῳ φάσκοι
τῶν διαλογισμῶν ἡμᾶς αἰσθάνεσθαι κατὰ τὴν καρδίαν γινομένων, οὔθ'
41 ἑαυτοῦ δόξει μεμνῆσθαι καὶ καταψεύδεσθαι τῶν ἐναργῶν. οὐ μὴν τοι-
οῦτός γ' ὁ ἀνήρ, ὥστ' οὐκ ἂν εἴποι δι' αἰσθήσεώς τινας ἐπιγινώσκειν
ἐν τῇ καρδίᾳ τῶν προειρημένων ἕκαστον γινόμενον. καὶ μὴν εἰ μὴ δι'
αἰσθήσεως, ἀλλὰ δι' ἀποδείξεώς τινος, ἡδέως ἂν ἀκούσαιμεν αὐτῆς.
42 ἐμοὶ μὲν δὴ δοκεῖ τῷ περὶ τῆς φωνῆς λόγῳ καὶ νῦν προσχρῆσθαι. τεκ-
μαίρομαι δὲ καὶ ἐκ τῶν ἐπιφερομένων· «ἀπὸ γὰρ τῆς διανοίας», φησί,
314 «δεῖ λέγειν καὶ ἐν ἑαυτῷ λέγειν [ἢ φωνὴν διεξιέναι] καὶ / διανοεῖσθαι καὶ
43 ἐν ἑαυτοῖς φωνὴν διεξιέναι καὶ ἐκτὸς ἐκπέμπειν.» ὁμολογούμενον γάρ τι
λαμβάνων ὡς τοῦ αὐτοῦ μορίου τὸ λέγειν εἴη καὶ τὸ ἐν ἑαυτῷ λέγειν,
εἶτα προσλαμβάνων αὐτῷ τῆς καρδίας ἔργον εἶναι τὸ λέγειν, ἐξ ἀμφοῖν
346 44 ἔχει περαινόμενον ἐν τῇ καρδίᾳ | γίνεσθαι τὸ ἐν ἑαυτῷ λέγειν. ἀλλ' ἡμεῖς
γε κατὰ τὸ πρὸ τούτου γράμμα τὸν ὑπὸ τοῦ Ζήνωνος ἐρωτηθέντα
λόγον ὑπὲρ τοῦ τὴν φωνὴν ἀπὸ τῆς καρδίας ἐκπέμπεσθαι μοχθηρὸν
ἐπεδείξαμεν, ὥστε καὶ ὁ νῦν ἐρωτώμενος ὑπὸ τοῦ Χρυσίππου λόγος
ἅμα ἐκείνῳ συνανῄρηται.

45 Ἐπισκεψώμεθα οὖν ἤδη τὸν ἑξῆς· «οἰκείως δὲ τούτῳ καὶ οἱ στεναγ-
μοὶ ἐντεῦθεν προΐενται.» καὶ τοὺς στεναγμούς, ὦ Χρύσιππε, καὶ τὰς
φωνὰς ἐκ τοῦ θώρακος μὲν φήσομεν ἐκπέμπεσθαι καὶ τοῦ πνεύμονος, οὐ
46 μὴν [οὐδ'] ἐκ τῆς καρδίας, ὥσπερ οὐδὲ τὰς φωνάς. ἀποδέδεικται γὰρ
ἡμῖν ὑπὲρ ἑκάστου τούτων ἐν ἑτέροις οὐχ ἁπλῶς οὐδ' ὥσπερ ὑπὸ σοῦ
νῦν οὐδεμίαν ἀπόδειξιν προσθέντος.

315 47 Ἐφεξῆς δὲ / τοῖσδε πλῆθος ἐπῶν ὁ Χρύσιππος γράφει τῶν πλείστων
48 ἑαυτῷ μαχομένων, ὡς ἔμπροσθεν ἔδειξα. τὰ δὲ μεταξὺ τῶν ἐπῶν ἐστι μὲν
ὀλίγιστα, περιέχεται δέ τις ⟨καὶ⟩ κατὰ ταῦτ' ἐναντιολογία τοῦ Χρυσίπ-

5–9] SVF II, pp. 239.10–16; 240.19–23 *cf. supra*, pp. 152.23–27; 170.23–27 15–21] SVF II, p. 250 22–23] *cf. supra*, p. 130.3–5 26–27] SVF II, pp. 250–251 32–222.2] SVF II, p. 238 33–222.1] SVF II, p. 251 33–34] *cf. supra*, p. 204.24–27

1 καθὸ H: *corr.* R *Ald.* ...πτόμεθα H 2 ἡ...νικὸν H 3 τινας *scr. Einarson*: πω H: πως *Petersen* 4 λογιζομένου *Ald.*: λογιζόμενος *Müller* 11 *post* μὴν *add.* ἀλλὰ *Müller* 12 τινος H: *corr. Einarson* 13 μὴ *add.* H[3] 17 ἢ φωνὴν διεξιέναι *secl. v. Arnim*: καὶ φ. δ. *Müller* καὶ διανοεῖσθαι *ex* καρδίαν νοεῖσθαι *corr.* H[2]: καὶ καρδίας ἐστὶ νοεῖσθαι *Müller* 18 *ante* φωνὴν *add.* λέγειν καὶ *Müller* 20 προσλαμβάνον H: *corr. Ald.* αὐτὸ H: *corr. Kalbfleisch* 23 ἀπὸ *ex* ὑπὸ *corr.* H[3] 27–28 καὶ τὰς φωνὰς *secl. Müller*: φωνὰς *deperditum in* H 28–29 οὐ μὴν *deperdita in* H 29 οὐδ'] οὐ *expunxit* H[3]: *del. Castiglioni* γὰρ *deperditum in* H 30 οὐδ'] οὐχ H: *corr. Chart.* 34 καὶ *addidi*

ing part of the soul is in that part in which we inquire and discuss.
But this was not the question. We were asking whether this part is the 38
heart; and you have given no proof of that, unless you actually say
that some men perceive that they are reasoning in their hearts. But at 39
the beginning of the whole account you wrote these exact words:
"Thus the place seems to elude us, since we have neither a clear
perception of it, as was the case with the others, nor sure signs from
which this matter might be inferred; otherwise the disagreement
among physicians and philosophers would not have grown so great."
After Chrysippus has said this, if he should then say in the same 40
book that we perceive the activities of reason taking place in the heart,
he will be thought to have forgotten himself and to be misrepresenting
the evident facts. But he is not that sort of man; therefore he would 41
not say that some persons recognize through perception the occur-
rence of each of these actions in the heart. And if (he does) not (say
that it is) through perception, but by a proof of some kind, I would
gladly hear the proof. It is my opinion that he is still using the argu- 42
ment about speech. I find further evidence for this in what he says
next: "For", he says, "speaking must be from the mind, and also
speaking within oneself, and thinking, and going through an utterance
in oneself, and sending it out." He takes something that is agreed to 43
(as a premise), namely, that speaking and speaking within oneself are
acts of the same member; then he adds to it the further premise that
speaking is an act of the heart; and from these two (premises) he draws
the conclusion that speaking within oneself takes place in the heart.
But we demonstrated in the preceding book that the argument 44
formulated by Zeno to prove that speech is sent out from the heart
is faulty, and therefore the argument now formulated by Chrysippus
is refuted along with it.

Now let us examine the next statement: "It is in accord with this 45
that groans too are emitted from there." We shall say, Chrysippus,
that groans, and words too, are sent out from the chest and the lungs,
but they are not sent out from the heart, nor are words either. Else- 46
where I have demonstrated each of these points separately, not
throwing them all together and not, as you are now doing, without the
addition of a single proof.

After this Chrysippus quotes a multitude of verses, most of 47
which contradict him, as I have already shown. The comments 48
between the verses are very brief, but in these too there is a self-

που πρὸς ἑαυτόν, ἣν ἐν τῷ μετὰ τοῦτ' ἐπιδείξω βιβλίῳ καθ' ὃ περὶ τῶν τῆς
49 ψυχῆς παθῶν ἔγνωκα ποιήσασθαι τὸν λόγον. ἐν δὲ τῷ παρόντι τῶν ῥή-
847 σεων αὐτῶν ἐπιμνησθήσομαι μόνων | ἐχουσῶν ὧδε· «ὁ δὲ ποιητὴς πλεονά-
ζων ἐν τούτοις διὰ πολλῶν παρίστησιν ὅτι καὶ τὸ λογιστικὸν καὶ τὸ
θυμοειδὲς περὶ τοῦτόν ἐστι τὸν τόπον, συνάγων ὡς ταὐτὸν αὐτά, καθ-
50 άπερ καὶ δεῖ ποιῆσαι.» φανερῶς γὰρ ἐνταῦθα συγχωρεῖ μὲν ἕτερόν τι
παρὰ τὸ λογιστικὸν εἶναι τό τε θυμοειδὲς καὶ τὸ ἐπιθυμητικόν, ἐν δὲ τῇ
καρδίᾳ κατῳκίσθαι φησίν, ὅπερ Ἀριστοτέλους ἐστίν, οὐ τῶν Στωϊ-
51 κῶν δόγμα. καὶ διὰ τῶν ἑξῆς δὲ προειπὼν ἐν οἷς ὁ ποιητὴς ἐν τῇ καρδίᾳ
τὸ λογιζόμενον ὑπάρχειν ἀποφαίνεται, μετὰ ταῦτ' ἐπιφέρει· «ὅτι δὲ καὶ
τὸ ἐπιθυμητικὸν ἐνταῦθα διὰ τούτων ἐμφαίνει· /

316 'οὐ γάρ πώποτέ μ' ὧδε θεᾶς ἔρος οὐδὲ γυναικὸς
θυμὸν ἐνὶ στήθεσ⟨σ⟩ι περιπροχυθεὶς ἐδάμασ⟨σ⟩εν.'»

52 εἶτ' ἐφεξῆς· «ὅτι δὲ τὸ θυμοειδὲς [εἰ] ἐνταῦθά πού ἐστι, τὰ τοιαῦτα ἐμφαίνει
πλείονα ὄντα·

'"Ηρῃ δ' οὐκ ἔχαδε στῆθος χόλον, ἀλλὰ προσηύδα.'

καὶ ⟨ἔτι

'καὶ⟩ χόλος, ὅς τ' ἐφέηκε πολύφρονά περ χαλεπῆναι.'» |

848 53 ἐν τοῖς τοιούτοις ἅπασιν ὁ Χρύσιππος ὁμολογεῖ δυνάμεις τινὰς εἶναι
τῆς ψυχῆς τήν τε θυμοειδῆ καὶ τὴν ἐπιθυμητικὴν ἑτέρας τῆς λογιστικῆς.
ἀλλὰ περὶ μὲν τούτων ὡς ἔφην ἐν τῷ τετάρτῳ διαλέξομαι γράμματι.

54 Τὰ δ' ὑπόλοιπα τῶν κατὰ τὸ Χρυσίππου βιβλίον ἐπιδραμὼν
55 ἐνταῦθά που καὶ αὐτὸς ἤδη καταπαύσω τὸν ἐνεστῶτα λόγον. μετὰ δὴ
τὸ πλῆθος τῶν ἐπῶν ἐφεξῆς ὁ Χρύσιππος περί τε φωνῆς καὶ λόγου
καὶ νεύρων ἀρχῆς ὅσα τε τούτοις συνέζευκται διῆλθεν, ἃ δὴ καὶ μόνα /
317 τῶν κατὰ τὸ βιβλίον ἔπρεπεν ἀνδρὶ φιλοσόφῳ, περὶ ὧν καὶ ἡμεῖς ἐν τῷ
πρὸ τούτου λόγῳ διεληλύθαμεν ὑπερβάντες τὰ περιττῶς ἠδολεσχημένα.

8. Νυνὶ μέντοι κατὰ τοῦτο τὸ βιβλίον, ἐπειδὴ καὶ ταῦτ' ἔδοξε προσ-
θεῖναι τά τ' ἄλλα τὰ προηγούμενα διῆλθον, ἑξῆς [τε] προσθήσω τὸν
2 περὶ τῆς Ἀθηνᾶς λόγον. αἰσθόμενος γὰρ ὁ Χρύσιππος ἐναντιού-
μενον τοῖς ἑαυτοῦ δόγμασι τὸν περὶ τῆς θεοῦ μῦθον ἀπὸ τῆς τοῦ Διὸς

2–6] SVF II, p. 251 *cf. infra*, pp. 234.31–236.1 9–18] SVF II, p. 251 *cf. infra*, p. 236.1–13 12–13] Hom. Il. xiv. 315–316 *cf. infra*, p. 236.7–8, 24–25 16] Hom. Il. iv. 24 *cf. supra*, p. 178.18 *infra*, p. 236.11, 27 18] Hom. Il. xviii. 108 *cf. supra*, p. 178.24 *infra*, p. 236.13 22–27] SVF II, p. 238 28–30] SVF II, p. 238 29–228.12] SVF II, pp. 256–258

1 καθὸ H: *corr.* R 3 μόνον *Bas.* 5 συνάγων] συνάπτων *Müller* ὡς ταὐτὸν αὐτά] εἰς ταυτὸν καὶ τὸ ἐπιθυμητικὸν *Corn.* (*cf. infra, p.* 236.1) 6 δεῖ] ἔδει *Müller* (*cf. infra, p.* 236.1) 8 κατωκεῖσθαι H: *corr. Chart.* 8–9 Στωϊκῶν δόγμα] στ, ῶν, δ *in ras.*, *in mg.* οὕτως ἱκανὸν δόγμα H[2] 12 ἔρως H: *corr. Chart.* 13 στήθεσι H: *corr. Bas.* πέρι προχυθεὶς H: *corr. Chart.* ἐδάμασεν H: *corr. Kühn* 14 εἰ *del. Ald.* 17–18 ἔτι καὶ *add. Müller* (*cf. infra, p.* 236.12) 18 χόλον H: *corr. Müller* (*cf. supra, p.* 178.24) 22 τοῦ χρυσίππου βιβλίων H: *corr. Kühn* 23 δή] δὲ *Ald.* 27 ὑπερβάντες τὰ περιττῶς] υ. . . . . .τῶς H 28 βιβλίον, ἐπειδή] β. . . . . H 29 διῆλθον] δ. . . . . H τε *del. Müller* 30 χ. .σιππος H

contradiction of Chrysippus that I shall point out in the next book,
in which I have decided to discuss the affections of the soul. For the 49
present I shall only remind you of his actual words, which are as fol-
lows: "But the poet, who speaks very frequently of these matters,
presents in many verses the view that both the rational and spirited
parts are in this region, bringing them together to the same place, as
indeed one must." Here he clearly agrees that the spirited and deside- 50
rative parts (of the soul) are something other than the rational, and
he locates them in the heart; but that is the view of Aristotle, not of
the Stoics. In what follows he first cites lines in which the poet 51
declares that the rational part is in the heart, and then he adds: "He
indicates in the following lines that the desiderative is there also:

> 'Never before did love of goddess or woman
> so flood my breast and overpower my spirit.'"

Then after this, "That the spirited part is somewhere there is indicated 52
by verses such as these, which are quite numerous:

> 'But Hera's breast could not contain her bitter anger,
> and she spoke out'

and also,

> 'And bitter anger, that drives even the very wise
> to harshness.'"

In all comments of this kind Chrysippus admits that the soul has 53
certain powers, the spirited and the desiderative, that are other than
the rational. But as I said, I shall speak of these matters in the fourth
book.

I shall quickly review here the remainder of Chrysippus' book 54
and then bring this book of my own to a close. After the spate of 55
hexameters, Chrysippus next took up the source of speech, discourse
and nerves, and matters related thereto. These are the only things in
his book that befit a philosopher; I discussed them, omitting the idle
chatter, in the book that preceded this one.

8. But now, since I have decided to include this too in the present
book, and since I have completed my discussion of the more important
points, I shall next add his treatment of Athena. When Chrysippus 2
perceived that the story of the goddess' supposed birth from the head
of Zeus was in conflict with his own doctrines, he made the following

κεφαλῆς ὑπειλημμένης γεγενῆσθαι τοιάδε λέγει· παραγράψω γὰρ |
349 3 ἅπασαν αὐτοῦ τὴν ῥῆσιν, εἰ καὶ μακροτέρα πώς ἐστιν· «ἀκούω δέ τινας
λέγειν παραμυθουμένους πρὸς τὸ ἐν τῇ κεφαλῇ εἶναι τὸ ἡγεμονικὸν τῆς
4 ψυχῆς μέρος. τὸ γὰρ τὴν Ἀθηνᾶν, μῆτιν οὖσαν καὶ οἷον φρόνησιν,
ἐκ τῆς κεφαλῆς γενέσθαι τοῦ Διὸς σύμβολόν φασιν εἶναι τοῦ ταύτῃ τὸ
ἡγεμονικὸν εἶναι· οὐ γὰρ ἄλλως ἂν ἐν τῇ κεφαλῇ γενέσθαι μῆτιν καὶ
318 φρόνησιν, εἰ μὴ τὸ ἡγεμονικὸν ἐν ταύτῃ ἐστί· πιθανοῦ μέν τινος / ἐχόμενοι,
διαμαρτάνοντες δ' ὡς ἐμοὶ φαίνεται καὶ ἀγνοοῦντες τὰ περὶ τούτων ἱστορούμενα, περὶ ὧν οὐ χεῖρόν ἐστιν ἐπὶ πλέον εἰπεῖν τοῖς ἐνεστῶσι ζητήμασι.
5 φασὶ δ' οἱ μὲν οὕτως ἁπλῶς ἐκ τῆς τοῦ Διὸς κεφαλῆς αὐτὴν γενέσθαι
οὐδὲ προσιστοροῦντες τὸ πῶς ἢ κατὰ τίνα λόγον, [ὁ δὲ Ἡσίοδος ἐπὶ πλέον λέγει ἐν ταῖς θεογονίαις] τινῶν μὲν ἐν ταῖς θεογονίαις γραφόντων τὴν γένεσιν αὐτῆς πρῶτον μὲν Μήτιδι συγγενομένου τοῦ Διός, δεύτερον δὲ Θέμιδι, τινῶν δὲ ἐν ἑτέροις ἄλλως γραφόντων τὴν γένεσιν
6 αὐτῆς· ⟨ὁ δὲ Ἡσίοδος ἐπὶ πλέον λέγει ἐν ταῖς θεογονίαις⟩ ὡς ἄρα γε-
350 νομένης ἔριδος τῷ Διὶ καὶ | τῇ Ἥρᾳ γεννήσειεν ἡ μὲν Ἥρα δι' ἑαυτῆς
τὸν Ἥφαιστον, ὁ δὲ Ζεὺς τὴν Ἀθηνᾶν ἐκ τῆς Μήτιδος καταπο-
7 θείσης ὑπ' αὐτοῦ. ἡ μὲν γὰρ εἰς αὐτὸν κατάποσις τῆς Μήτιδος καὶ
ἔνδον τοῦ Διὸς τῆς Ἀθηνᾶς γένεσις κατ' ἀμφοτέρους τοὺς λόγους ἐστίν·
319 διαφέρουσι δ' / ἐν τῷ πῶς ταῦτα συνετελέσθη, πρὸς τὸν ἐνεστῶτα λόγον
8 οὐθενὸς ὄντος ⟨τοῦ⟩ τοιούτου. τὸ γὰρ κοινὸν ἐν αὐτοῖς ὑπάρχον μόνον
χρήσιμόν ἐστι πρὸς τὰ ἐνεστηκότα. λέγεται δ' ἐν μὲν τῇ Θεογονίᾳ οὕτως·

9 'Ζεὺς δὲ θεῶν βασιλεὺς πρώτην ἄλοχον θέτο Μῆτιν,
πλεῖστα θεῶν εἰδυῖαν ἰδὲ θνητῶν ἀνθρώπων.
ἀλλ' ὅτε δή ῥα ἔμελλε θεὰν γλαυκῶπιδ' Ἀθήνην
τέξεσθαι, τότ' ἔπειτα δόλῳ φρένας ἐξαπατήσας
αἱμυλίοισι λόγοισιν ἑὴν ἐγκάτθετο νηδύν·'
'ὥς οἱ συμφράσ⟨σ⟩αιτο θεὰ ἀγαθόν τε κακόν τε.'

10 εἶτα προελθὼν φησιν οὕτως·

'αὐτὸς δ' ἐκ κεφαλῆς γλαυκώπιδα γείνατ' Ἀθήνην, /
320 δεινήν, ἐγρεκύδοιμον, ἀγέστρατον, ἀτρυτώνην,
πότνιαν, ᾗ κέλαδοί τε ἅδον πόλεμοί τε μάχαι τε.' |

10–226.22] *cf.* Hes. fr. dub. 343 Merkelbach-West 24–29] Hes. Theog. 886–890; 900 31–33] Hes. Theog. 924–926

1 ὑπειλημμένης] ης *ex* ας *corr.* H γεγεννῆσθαι *Müller (cf. infra, p. 228.15)* 2 δέ] δή *Ald.* 5 *ante* ταύτῃ *add.* ἐν *Müller* 9 *post* εἰπεῖν *add.* ἐν *Ald.* 11 ὁ – 12 θεογονίαις^{I} *delevi* 12 ταῖς θεογονίαις^{I}] ταῖς *lac. 6 litt. rel.* H: *suppl.* H^{2}? ταῖς θεογονίαις^{II}] τῇ θεογονίᾳ H: *correxi* 14 θέηδι, *ut vid.*, H: θέμηδι H^{2}: *corr.* R *Ald.* 14–15 τὴν γένεσιν αὐτῆς *secl. Hermann* 15 ὁ – θεογονίαις *addidi ex lin. 11–12* 21 οὐθενὸς] ὅθεν ὡς H: οὐθ' ἑνὸς *add. in mg.* H^{2} τοῦ *add. Einarson* 25 ἰδὲ] ἡ δὲ H: *ex Hes. corr. Ald.* 26 δή ῥα *in* δ' ἦρα *mut.* H^{2} 27 τέξεσθαι *deperditum in* H τότ' *deperditum in* H: τότε M 28 λόγοισιν ἑὴν] λό......... H ..κατέθετο H: *corr. Ald.* 29 συμφράσαιτο H: *corr. Chart.* κακόν] ...όν H 31 κεφαλῆς] κ *ex* φ *corr.* H γλαυκώπιδα] δ *ex* π *corr.* H^{2} 33 τε ἅδον] τ' εὔαδον H: *ex Hes. corr. Müller*

statement – I shall quote the entire passage, even though it is rather
long–: "I hear that some people speak in support of the view that the 3
governing part of the soul is in the head. For, they say, the birth of 4
Athena, who is wisdom and, as it were, thought, from the head of
Zeus signifies that the governing part is there; otherwise wisdom and
thought would not arise in the head, if the ruling part is not in it. Their
argument has a certain plausibility, but they are mistaken, as it seems
to me, and they are unaware of the details of the story. A fuller
account of these matters is not irrelevant to our present inquiries.
Some men simply say in this way that she was born from the head of 5
Zeus, and they do not go on to recite the manner of her birth or the
reason for it. Some write in their theogonies that her birth took place
after Zeus lay first with Metis and second with Themis, and others
write it differently in other works. Hesiod, however, relates at 6
greater length in his theogonies that when a quarrel arose between
Zeus and Hera, Hera by herself gave birth to Hephaestus, and
Zeus (gave birth) to Athena as a result of swallowing Metis. Now 7
the swallowing of Metis and the birth of Athena inside Zeus are in
both accounts. They differ about the manner in which these things
were brought about, but that sort of thing is of no importance for the
present argument. The common element in them alone is useful 8
against the objections that have been raised. We read in the Theogony
as follows:

'Zeus, king of the gods, took as his first wife Metis, 9
the wisest of gods and mortal men.
But when she was about to give birth to a goddess,
bright-eyed Athena, he then deceived her mind with guile
and flattering words and put her in his belly;'
'that the goddess might give him knowledge of good and evil.'

Then after a little he says: 10

'He himself gave birth from his head to bright-eyed Athena,
terrifying, stirring up strife, a leader of armies, untiring,
queen, delighting in the din of war and battle.'

351 στήθεσι γὰρ αὐτοῖς ἔνδον εὔδηλον ὅτι ἀπέθετο τὴν Μῆτιν, καὶ οὕτως
11 φησὶν αὐτὴν γεννῆσαι κατὰ τὴν κεφαλήν. ἐν δὲ τοῖς μετὰ ταῦτα πλείω
διεληλυθότος αὐτοῦ τοιαῦτ' ἐστὶ τὰ λεγόμενα·

'ἐκ ταύτης ἔριδος ἡ μὲν τέκε φαίδιμον υἱὸν
Ἥφαιστον τέχνῃσιν ἄνευ Διὸς αἰγιόχοιο,
ἐκ πάντων παλάμῃσι κεκλημένον οὐρανιώνων.
12 αὐτὰρ ὅ γ' Ὠκεανοῦ καὶ Τηθύος ἠυκόμοιο
κούρην νόσφ' Ἥρης παρεδέξατο καλλιπαρῄου,
ἐξαπαφὼν Μῆτιν, καίπερ πολὺ δινεύουσαν.
συμμάρψας δ' ὅ γε χερσὶν ἑὴν ἐγκάτθετο νηδύν,
δείσας μὴ τέξῃ κρατερώτερον ἄλλο κεραυνοῦ.
13 τοὔνεκά μιν Κρονίδης ὑψίζυγος αἰθέρι ναίων /
321 κάππιεν ἐξαπίνης. ἡ δ' αὐτίκα Παλλάδ' Ἀθήνην
κύσατο· τὴν μὲν ἔτικτε πατὴρ ἀνδρῶν τε θεῶν τε
πὰρ κορυφὴν Τρίτωνος ἐπ' ὄχθῃσι⟨ν⟩ ποταμοῖο.
Μῆτις δ' αὖτε Ζηνὸς ὑπὸ σπλάγχνοις λελαθυῖα
ἧστο, Ἀθηναίης μήτηρ, τέκταινα δικαίων, |
352 πλεῖστα θεῶν εἰδυῖα καταθνητῶν τ' ἀνθρώπων.
14 ἔνθα θεὰ⟨ν⟩ παρέδεκτο Θέμιν· παλάμαις περὶ πάντων
ἀθανάτων ἐκέκασθ' ⟨οἳ⟩ Ὀλύμπια δώματ' ἔχουσιν,
αἰγίδα ποιήσασα φοβέστρατον ἔντος Ἀθήνῃ·
σὺν τῇ ἐγείνατό μιν πολεμήια τεύχε' ἔχουσαν.'»

15 ταῦτα προειπὼν ὁ Χρύσιππος ἑξῆς αὐτοῖς συνάπτων τάδε γράφει· «τὰ
μὲν οὖν περὶ τῆς Ἀθηνᾶς λεγόμενα τοιαῦτά ἐστιν, ἄλλου τινὸς συμβό-
16 λου ποιοῦντ' ἔμφασιν. πρῶτον μὲν γὰρ ἡ Μῆτις λέγεται ὡσανεί τις
322 φρόνησις καὶ περὶ τῶν / κατὰ τὸν βίον τέχνη, ἣ τὰς τέχνας δεῖ κατα-
πίνεσθαι καὶ ἐναποτίθεσθαι, καθ' ὃν λόγον καὶ τὰ λεγόμενά τινας κατα-
πίνειν φαμέν, διὰ δὲ τὴν κατάποσιν συνηκολουθηκότως λέγεται καὶ εἰς
17 τὴν κοιλίαν ἀποτίθεσθαι αὐτά. μετὰ ταῦτα τὴν καταποθεῖσαν τοιαύτην
τέχνην τίκτειν εὔλογον ἐν αὐτοῖς παραπλησίαν τῆς τικτούσης μητρός·
πρός τε τούτοις τὰ ὑπὸ τῶν ἐπιστημῶν τικτόμενα ἐν αὐτοῖς· πῶς δ'
18 ἂν ἐκπορεύοιτο καὶ διὰ τίνος μάλιστα, πάρεστι σκοπεῖν. φανερὸν γὰρ ὅτι

4–22] Hes. fr. dub. 343 Merkelbach-West 6] Hes. Theog. 929 18] *cf.* Hes. Theog. 887 *supra*, p. 224.25 26–27] *cf. supra*, p. 200.30

6 κεκλημένος H: *corr. Chart.*: κεκασμένον *ex Hes. Theog. 929* **Ruhnken** οὐρανιόνων H: *corr. Chart.* 8 κάρην H: *corr.* H3? *Corn.*: κούρῃ **Ruhnken** ἥρας H: *corr. Kühn* παρελέξατο **Ruhnken** καλλιπαρήῳ **Ruhnken** 9 πολὺ δινεύουσαν] πολύιδριν ἐοῦσαν **Ruhnken**: πολυδήνε' ἐοῦσαν *Bergk* 10 ἑὴν ἐγκατέθετο H: *corr. Ald.* 13 ἡ δ' H: *corr. Kühn* 15 ὄχθησι H: *corr. Corn.* 16 λελαθηκυῖα H: *corr. Chart.* 17 τέκτηνα H: *corr.* **Ruhnken** 18 κατὰ θνητῶν H: *corr. Chart.* τε H: *corr. Ald.* 19 θεὰ παρέλεκτο H: *corr. Aly* (παρέδεκτο *iam Hermann*) θέμις H: *correxi (cf. supra, p. 224.13–14)* 20 ἐκέκασθ' οἳ] ἐκέκαστο H: *corr.* **Ruhnken** ἐχόντων *Chart.* 21 βοφέστρατον H: *corr. Chart.* ἐντὸς H: *corr. Boissonade* Ἀθήνης *Bergk* 26 δεῖ] δὴ *v. Arnim* 28 συνηκολουθηκότος H: *corr. Chart.* 29 αὐτά] "*fort.* εἶτα" *v. Arnim* 30 αὐτῷ H: *correxi* 31 τε] δὲ *v. Arnim* ἐν αὐτοῖς] "*fort.* ἐντὸς" *v. Arnim* δ' *del. v. Arnim*

It is quite clear that he put Metis, chest and all, inside himself, and thereupon, the poet says, he gave birth to the goddess by way of his head. Subsequently, after having gone through rather many items, 11
the poet speaks in the following way:

'As a result of this quarrel Hera, without aegis-bearing Zeus,
craftily gave birth to a glorious son, Hephaestus,
acclaimed by all the heavenly gods for his skills.
But Zeus, apart from fair-cheeked Hera, took to himself Metis, 12
daughter of Oceanus and fair-haired Tethys,
deceiving her, even though she twisted much this way and that.
He seized her with his hands and placed her in his belly,
fearing that she might give birth to something more powerful than the thunderbolt.
For this reason the high-throned son of Cronos, who dwells in the aether, 13
swallowed her suddenly. And straightway she was big with Pallas Athena,
to whom the father of men and gods gave birth
through the top of his head on the banks of the river Trito;
but Metis lay hidden in Zeus' inner organs,
she the mother of Athena, doer of just deeds,
wisest of gods and mortal men.
Thereupon he received the goddess Themis; she excelled in skill all 14
the immortals who dwell on Olympus,
having made for Athena the aegis, a weapon that terrifies armies;
with it he brought her forth holding her warlike arms.'"

After these preliminaries Chrysippus goes on to say: "Such are the 15
things told of Athena, things that imply a different allegorical meaning. For first of all, Metis is spoken of as if she were a kind of 16
wisdom and art in practical matters, and in this sense the arts must be swallowed and stored up within us. Accordingly we say that certain people swallow the things that are said, and in keeping with this, because of the swallowing, we say also that they are stored in the belly. After this it is reasonable that such an art, on being swallowed, gives 17
birth in them to a daughter similar to the mother; and there are besides the things brought forth in them by the sciences. It is possible to see how and by what route these would most readily emerge.

853 λόγῳ ἐκφέρεται διὰ τοῦ στόματος κατὰ τὴν | κεφαλήν, ἐξ ἴσου οὕτως τῆς
κεφαλῆς λεγομένης ὃν τρόπον προβάτου κεφαλὴ λέγεται καὶ τὰς κεφαλὰς
ἀφαιροῦσί τινων, καθ' ὃν λόγον παραγινόμενον καὶ ἐκ τῆς κορυφῆς
λέγεται γενέσθαι, τῶν τοιούτων παραλλαγῶν κατὰ σύμβολον γινο-
19 μένων πλειόνων. καὶ χωρὶς δὲ τῆς ἱστορίας ταύτης ἀπ' αὐτοῦ μόνον
τοῦ γενέσθαι ταύτην κατὰ τὴν κεφαλὴν τὰ παραπλήσια ⟨ἂν⟩ τις λέγοι·
323 οὐ γὰρ ἐν τῇ κεφαλῇ φησιν αὐ/τὴν γενέσθαι, εἰ μή τινες διαστρέφοντες ἢ
παραλ⟨λ⟩άττοντες τὸν λόγον ἐξελθεῖν ταύτῃ γινομένην ἄλλως ἔροιντο·
ὥστε μᾶλλον καὶ τοῦτο σύμβολον πρὸς τὸν ἕτερον εἶναι, ὡς ἔφην.
τὰ γὰρ ἐν αὐτοῖς γινόμενα τεχνικὰ κατὰ τὴν κεφαλὴν ἐξιόντα μάλιστα
ἀποσημαίνει τὸν προειρημένον λόγον.»

20 Αὕτη μὲν ἡ τοῦ Χρυσίππου ῥῆσις. ἐπεὶ δ' ἐστὶ πάνυ μακρὰ καὶ
διὰ τοῦτ' ἴσως τινὲς οὐκ ἀκριβῶς αὐτῆς ἅπαντα τὸν νοῦν καταμαν-
21 θάνουσιν, ἐγὼ πειράσομαι διὰ βραχέων εἰπεῖν ἃ βούλεται δηλοῦν. οὐ
μάχεταί μοι, φησίν, ὁ μῦθος λέγων ἐκ τῆς τοῦ Διὸς κεφαλῆς γεγεν⟨ν⟩ῆσθαι
22 τὴν Ἀθηνᾶν φρόνησιν ὑπάρχουσαν. οὐ γὰρ αὐτὸ τοῦτο μόνον εἴρηται
854 κατ' αὐτόν, ἀλλ' ὅτι καταπιὼν τὴν Μῆτιν | ὁ Ζεὺς καὶ ὥσπερ ἐγκύμων
ἐξ αὐτῆς γενόμενος τὴν γεννηθεῖσαν ἐν αὐτῷ κόρην ἀπεκύησε διὰ τῆς
23 κεφαλῆς. εἰρῆσθαι δ' οὕτω φησὶ τὰ κατὰ τὸν μῦθον, ἐπειδὴ τὰς τέχνας
324 ἁπάσας ἐν τῇ καρδίᾳ συνι/σταμένας διὰ τὸν λόγον εἰς τὸ φανερὸν
24 ἐκφερόμενοί τινες λόγοι διὰ τῆς κεφαλῆς ἐξιᾶσιν. ἔστι γὰρ καὶ τὸ στόμα
τῆς κεφαλῆς μόριον. οὐ γὰρ τὸ τετριχωμένον μόνον ἀλλὰ καὶ τὸ μετὰ
τὸν τράχηλον ἄνωθεν ἅπαν ὀνομάζεσθαι κεφαλήν, καθ' ὃ σημαινόμενον
25 ἀποτμηθῆναί τινος λέγομεν τὴν κεφαλήν. εἰ δὲ μὴ διὰ τοῦ στόματος τοῦ
Διός, ἀλλ' ἐκ τῆς κορυφῆς ἐμυθολόγησεν ἐξεληλυθέναι τὴν Ἀθηνᾶν,
οὐδὲν ἄτοπον εἶναί φησι τοιούτων παραλλαγῶν κατὰ σύμβολον γι-
νομένων πλειόνων.

26 Ἐν τούτοις τοῖς λόγοις ὁ Χρύσιππος τὰ μὲν ἄλλα πιθανῶς τε
ἅμα καὶ εὐμηχάνως ἐξηγεῖται τοῦ μύθου προσαρμόττων αὐτὸν τῷ
Στωϊκῷ δόγματι· τὸ δὲ συνέχον τε καὶ κυριώτατον τοῦ λόγου παντός,
ὑπὲρ οὗ δίκαιον ἦν ἀγωνίσασθαι, μάλιστα διὰ ταχέων παρέδραμεν ὡς
κἂν τοῖς πρόσθεν ἐποίησεν ἐξηγούμενος ὅπως οἱ πολλοὶ λέγουσι τοὺς |
855 27 μὲν οὐκ ἔχειν, τοὺς δ' ἔχειν ἐγκέφαλον. ὡς γὰρ ἐν ἐκείνοις αὐτὸ τὸ ζητού-
325 μενον τάχιστα παρῆλθεν ἐν τοῖς / ἔξωθεν αὐτοῦ μηκύνας ἐπὶ πλεῖστον,

3–4] *cf. supra*, p. 226.15   31–33] *cf. supra*, pp. 192.19–25; 194.5–6, 22–24

1 τὴν κεφαλήν, ἐξ ἴσου οὕτως] τ. . . . . .τως H   2 κεφαλὴ λέγεται καὶ τὰς] κεφ. . . . . H   3 τῆς κορυφῆς] τ. . . . . H   4 γινο. . . . H   6 γενέσθ. . H   ἂν *add. Müller*   7 φησιν] φ. H: *om.* M: "*malim* φασιν" *v. Arnim*   8 παραλάττοντες H: *corr.* M *Ald.*   *post* λόγον *inserendum putat* ἀλλ' *v. Arnim*   ἀλλ' ὡς H: *corr. Corn.*   ἔροιντο H: *corr. Kühn*: ἔροιεν *Diels*   10 ἐν αὐτοῖς] "*fort.* ἐντὸς" *v. Arnim*   15 γεγενῆσθαι H: *corr. Bas.*   18 αὐτῷ] αὐτῶ H: *corr. Kühn*   20 τῶν λόγων *in textu*, τὸν λόγον *sscr.* H   23 καθὸ H: *corr. Ald.*   25 ἐμυθολόγησαν *Müller*   26 φασὶ H: *corr. Kühn*   33 οὐκ ἔχειν, τοὺς δ' ἔχειν] . . . . .ν H   34 τάχιστα παρῆλθεν] τάχι. . . . . H

Clearly they are carried out by speech through the mouth by way 18
of the head, the word 'head' comprising as much here as it does when we speak of a sheep's head, or of removing the heads of certain persons; and when a thing comes to light in this way it is said also to have been born from the 'crown', such shifts being rather frequent
in allegory. And quite apart from this story, from the mere circum- 19
stance of her being born by way of his head a person could give a similar explanation. For the poet does not say that she came into being in his head, unless some people, by distorting and altering the account, give the erroneous formulation that while she was coming into being she emerged by that route; so that this too is a better allegory, as compared with the other account, as I said. For the fact that things pertaining to the arts and sciences come into being inside these men and come out by way of the head is the best evidence for the account given above."

This is the passage from Chrysippus. Since it is very long 20
and for this reason some may not understand in detail the whole meaning of it, I shall attempt to state briefly the points he wishes to make.
The myth, he says, does not contradict me when it says that Athena, 21
that is, wisdom, was born from the head of Zeus. For this was not 22
the only thing told in the story; it also said that Zeus, after swallowing Metis and becoming pregnant, as it were, from her, delivered through his head the daughter that had been engendered within him.
The mythical account was told in this way, he says, because all the 23
arts and sciences established by reason in the heart are brought to
light by certain utterances which go out by way of the head. For the 24
mouth is also a part of the head. Not only the part covered with hair but all that is above the neck (he says) is called the head, in the
sense in which we say that a person's head has been cut off. And if 25
the poet stated in the myth that Athena emerged, not through the mouth of Zeus, but from his crown, this, Chrysippus says, is not surprising, such shifts being rather frequent in allegory.

In these words, as Chrysippus brings the myth into harmony 26
with Stoic teaching, he gives an explanation that is persuasive and ingenious in other respects; but the essential and crucial point of the whole discussion, on which he should have put forth his best effort, he passed over hastily, just as he did earlier when he was explaining how it is that in ordinary speech we say that some people have a brain
and some do not. For just as in that instance he passed very 27
quickly over the actual question under investigation but spoke at length on matters external to it, so here too he swiftly passed over

οὕτω κἀνταῦθα τὸ συνέχον αὐτὸ τοῦ λόγου διὰ ταχέων παρέδραμεν
ἀρκεσθεὶς εἰπεῖν διὰ τοῦτ' ἐκ τῆς κορυφῆς γεγεν⟨ν⟩ῆσθαι τὴν Ἀθηνᾶν,
οὐκ ἐκ τοῦ στόματος, «τοιούτων παραλλαγῶν κατὰ σύμβολον γινο-
28 μένων πλειόνων». ἐχρῆν γὰρ αὐτὸν ἢ μηδ' ὅλως ἧφθαι τοῦ μύθου μηδέν
γ' ἀναγκαῖον ἔχοντος ἀνδρὶ φιλοσόφῳ πρὸς ἀπόδειξιν δόγματος, ἢ
ἁπτόμενον, ὅπερ ἦν μάλιστα τὴν ἀντιλογίαν συνέχον, ἀκριβῶς ἅπαν
διεξελθεῖν, εἰ καὶ πλειόνων ἔχρῃζε λόγων, οὐκ ὀκνήσαντα τοὺς πολλοὺς
προσγράψαι.
29 Βουλόμενος δ' ἄν τις οἶμαι καὶ τοὺς τοιούτους ἑτέρως ἐξηγεῖσθαι πολ-
λὰς ἐπιχειρημάτων ἀφορμὰς ἐκ τῶν κατὰ τὰς ἀνατομὰς φαινομένων
δύναιτο λαμβάνειν, ὑπὲρ ὧν ἐπὶ πλέον μὲν ἐν τοῖς ἑξῆς ἀναγκαῖον ἔσται
διελθεῖν ἐπειδὰν περὶ τοῦ ψυχικοῦ πνεύματος ὁ λόγος ἡμῖν γίγνηται, διὰ
βραχέων δ' ἂν καὶ νῦν αὐτὰ μόνον εἴποιμι τὰ κεφάλαια τῶν μελλόντων
356 30 ἀποδειχθήσεσθαι. ὥσπερ γὰρ αὐτὸ τὸ | σῶμα τῆς καρδίας ἐξ ἑαυτοῦ
διαστελλόμενόν τε καὶ συστελλόμενον ἐν μέρει τὰς ὕλας τε ἕλκει καὶ αὖθις
326 ἐκπέμπει, κατὰ / τὸν αὐτὸν τρόπον ὁ ἐγκέφαλος ἐπειδὰν προέληται τοῦ
περιεχομένου κατὰ τὰς ἑαυτοῦ κοιλίας πνεύματος, ὃ δὴ καὶ ψυχικὸν
ὀνομάζομεν, ἐπιπέμψαι τινὶ μορίῳ, τὴν εἰς τοῦτ' ἐπιτήδειον κίνησιν
31 κινηθεὶς οὕτως ἐπιπέμπει. γένεσις δὲ τῷ πνεύματι τῷδε τῷ κατὰ τὰς κοιλίας
αὐτοῦ τάχα μέν τις ὀλίγη καὶ ἐκ τῶν εἰς αὐτὰς περαιουμένων γίγνεται
φλεβῶν, τὴν πλείστην δὲ καὶ κυριωτάτην αἱ κατὰ τὸ δικτυοειδὲς πλέγμα
τὸ κατὰ τὴν τοῦ ἐγκεφάλου βάσιν ἀρτηρίαι χορηγοῦσιν, αἵτινες ἀπὸ τῆς
32 καρδίας ἀναφέρονται. ὥστ' εἴ τις βούλοιτο τοῖς ἀληθέσι συνάπτειν τὸν
μῦθον, ἐν τοῖς κάτω μέρεσι κυηθεῖσαν τὴν φρόνησιν, τουτέστι τὸ πνεῦμα
τὸ ψυχικόν, ἐν τῇ κεφαλῇ φήσει τελειοῦσθαι καὶ μάλιστά γε κατὰ τὴν
κορυφήν, ὅτι κατὰ ταύτην ἐστὶν ἡ μέση καὶ κυριωτάτη τῶν ἐγκεφάλου
κοιλιῶν.
33 Ἐγὼ μὲν οὖν, ὥσπερ ὁ Πλάτων αὐτὸς εἶπε, «τὰ τοιαῦτα» πάντα
μυθολογήματα «ἄλλως μὲν χαρίεντα ἡγοῦμαι, λίαν δὲ δεινοῦ καὶ ἐπι-
357 327 πόνου | καὶ οὐ πάνυ εὐτυχοῦς / ἀνδρός, κατ' ἄλλο μὲν οὐδέν, ὅτι δ' αὐτῷ
ἀνάγκη μετὰ τοῦτο τὸ τῶν Ἱπποκενταύρων εἶδος ἐπανορθοῦσθαι
καὶ αὖθις τὸ τῆς Χιμαίρας, καὶ ἐπιρρεῖ δ' ὄχλος τοιούτων Γοργόνων
καὶ Πηγάσων καὶ ἄλλων ἀμηχάνων πλήθη τε καὶ ἀτοπίαι τερατο-
λόγων τινῶν φύσεων, αἷς εἴ τις ἀπιστῶν προσβιβᾷ κατὰ τὸ εἰκὸς ἕκαστον,
34 ἅτε ἀγροίκῳ τινὶ σοφίᾳ χρώμενος, πολλῆς αὐτῷ σχολῆς δεήσει.» ταύτην
τὴν ῥῆσιν ἐχρῆν ἀνεγνωκότα τὸν Χρύσιππον ἀποκεχωρηκέναι τῶν
μύθων καὶ μὴ κατατρίβειν τὸν χρόνον ἐξηγούμενον αὐτῶν τὰς ὑπο-

3–4] *cf. supra*, p. 228.4–5 21] *cf. supra*, p. 88.5–6 *infra*, PHP 603.16; 605.16–606.1 Müller 29–35] Plat. Phaedr. 229 d 3 – e 4

1 κάν. . . . . H *post* ταχέων *add.* αὐτὸ H, *del.* H3? 2 . .κεσθεὶς H γεγενῆσθαι H: *corr. Ald.* 6–7 ἅπασαν ἐξελθεῖν H: *corr. Müller* 7 καὶ εἰ *Chart.* 10 τῶν *ex* τῆς *corr.* H 12 γίγνεται H: *corr. Chart.* 15 ἕλκει τε *Müller* τε[II] *om.* p 28 τὰ – 29 μὲν] ἄλλως μὲν τὰ τοιαῦτα *Plat.* 29 ἡγοῦμαι *add.* H3? 30 εὐτυχοῦς ἀνδρός, κατ'] ε. . . . . .τ' H 31 τὸ τῶν Ἱπποκενταύρων] τ. . . . . .ρων H 32 καὶ ἐπιρρεῖ] κ. . . . . . . H γοργονῶν H: *corr. Ald.* 33 πηγασῶν H: *corr. Kühn* ἀμηχάν. . H ἀτοπώτερα λόγων H: *ex Plat. corr. Müller*

the essential point of the argument, thinking it enough to give as the
reason why Athena was born from Zeus' crown, not from his mouth,
that "such shifts are rather frequent in allegory". Either he should 28
not have used the story at all, as it does not contain anything ne-
cessary to a philosopher for the proof of doctrine; or in using it he
should have dealt carefully and exhaustively with the point that was
the crux of the contradiction, and even if it required a rather full
discussion, he should not have hesitated to add it.

Anyone, I think, who wanted to explain differently even such 29
stories as these could find many points of departure for his arguments
in the observations made in dissections. It will be necessary to discuss
these observations more fully in the following (books), when our account
reaches the psychic pneuma; but here also I might briefly mention the
main points of the proofs that will be given. Just as the body of the 30
heart, as it alternately dilates and contracts of itself, draws matter
in and sends it out again, in the same way the brain, when it chooses
to send to some member a portion of the pneuma contained in its own
ventricles, which we call psychic (pneuma), executes the motion suitable
to this end and thus sends the pneuma. Perhaps in some small part 31
this pneuma in its ventricles is generated from the veins that end in
the ventricles; but the major and principal production (of pneuma) is
supplied by the arteries in the rete mirabile at the base of the brain, and
these (arteries) come up from the heart. Therefore if a person wishes to fit 32
the myth to the facts, he will say that wisdom, that is, psychic pneuma,
after being conceived in the lower parts, reaches full development
in the head, especially the top of the head, because that is the location
of the brain's middle and most important ventricle.

For my part, in the words of Plato himself, I "regard" all 33
"such" interpretations of myth "as otherwise charming, but as the
work of a man who is excessively ingenious and laborious and
not entirely enviable, for no other reason than that after this he
must straighten out the form of the hippocentaurs and then the
Chimera; and a multitude of such shapes comes flooding in, gor-
gons and pegasuses and an absurd crowd of other impossible and
fabulous natures; and if a doubter is going to reduce every one of
them to probability, using a primitive kind of skill, he will need much
leisure time." Chrysippus should have read this passage and then 34
abandoned myths, and he should not have wasted his time explaining

νοίας. ἂν γὰρ ἅπαξ εἰς τοῦτ' ἀφίκηταί τις, ἀνάριϑμον πλῆϑος ἐπιρρεῖ
μυϑολογημάτων, ὥσϑ' ὅλον ἀπολέσει τὸν βίον εἴ τις ἐπεξέρχοιτο
35 πάντα. ἄμεινον δ' ἦν οἶμαι τὸν ἀληϑείας ὄντως ἐφιέμενον ἄνδρα μὴ
τί λέγουσιν οἱ ποιηταὶ σκοπεῖν, ἀλλὰ τῶν ἐπιστημονικῶν λημμάτων
ὑπὲρ ὧν ἐν τῷ δευτέρῳ γράμματι διῆλϑον ἐκμαϑόντα τὴν τῆς εὑρέσεως
328 ὁδὸν ἐφεξῆς μὲν ἀσκῆσαί τε καὶ γυμνάσασϑαι κατὰ ταύτην, / ὅταν δ'
ἱκανῶς ἤδη τὰ κατὰ τὴν ἄσκησιν αὐτῷ προήκῃ τηνικαῦτα ἀφικόμενον |
358 ἐφ' ἕκαστον τῶν προβλημάτων ἐπισκέπτεσϑαι περὶ τῶν εἰς τὰς ἀπο-
δείξεις αὐτοῦ λημμάτων, τίνα μὲν ἐξ αἰσϑήσεως ἁπλῆς, τίνα δ' ἐξ ἐμ-
πειρίας ἤτοι τῆς κατὰ τὸν βίον ἢ τῆς κατὰ τὰς τέχνας, τίνα δὲ ἐκ τῶν
πρὸς νόησιν ἐναργῶν χρὴ λαβόντα περαίνειν ἐξ αὐτῶν ἤδη τὸ προ-
36 κείμενον. εἰ ταύτην τὴν ὁδὸν ὁ Χρύσιππος ἐτράπετο παρελϑὼν τὴν
κατὰ τοὺς μύϑους τε καὶ τὰς ἐτυμολογίας ἀνανεύσεις τε καὶ κατανεύσεις
κεφαλῆς καὶ χειρῶν κινήσεις καὶ χειλῶν σχήματα καὶ ποιητῶν μαρτυ-
ρίας ἅμα γυναιξὶ καὶ τοῖς ἄλλοις ἰδιώταις, αὐτὸς ἂν εὕρισκε τἀληϑὲς
ἡμῶν τε τὸν χρόνον οὐκ ἂν ἀπώλλυεν ἐπιδεικνύντων αὐτῷ μηδὲ ἐν
37 οἷς ἐπικαλεῖται μάρτυσι μηδὲ ἐν τούτοις τι πλέον ἔχοντι. καὶ γὰρ οἱ
ποιηταὶ τὰ πλείω κατὰ τῶν δογμάτων αὐτοῦ λέγουσι καὶ οἱ μῦϑοι καὶ
οἱ ἰδιῶται καὶ τῶν ἄλλων ἕκαστος, οὓς ὡς ἑαυτῷ μαρτυροῦντας ἐν τῷ
προτέρῳ Περὶ ψυχῆς ἔγραψε.

38 Ταῦτ' ἐστὶν ἃ παραλελοίπειν ἐγὼ κατὰ τὸ πρὸ τούτου βιβλίον
329 ὧν / εἰρήκει Χρύσιππος ἐν τῷ περὶ τοῦ τῆς ψυχῆς ἡγεμονικοῦ λόγῳ,
359 νομίζων εἰ κἀκεῖνος οὐκ ᾐδέσϑη πλεονάζειν ἐν αὐτοῖς, | ἐμοὶ γοῦν προσ-
39 ήκειν ἀποχωρῆσαι τῆς τοιαύτης ἀδολεσχίας. ἐπεὶ δ', ὡς ἔφην, ἔδοξε
τῶν ἑταίρων τισί⟨ν⟩ ὑπὸ φιλοτιμίας κινηϑεῖσιν ἐπιμνησϑῆναί με καὶ τῶν
τοιούτων λόγων, ἐκείνοις χαριζόμενος ἔγραψα καὶ τουτὶ τὸ βιβλίον,
ὅσον οἷόν τ' ἦν ἐμοί, μετὰ τοῦ διὰ ταχέων παρέρχεσϑαι τὰ περιττῶς
ὑπὸ τοῦ Χρυσίππου γεγραμμένα, καὶ τῶν χρησίμων τῇ προκειμένῃ
πραγματείᾳ προ⟨σ⟩τιϑεὶς οὐκ ὀλίγα. /|

17–20] *cf. supra*, p. 220.32–33 22] *cf. supra*, pp. 170.30–32; 190.19 24–29] *cf. supra*, pp. 168.26–170.2

7 προήκειν H: *corr.* R *Müller* 15 εὑρίσκετ' ἀληϑὲς H: *corr. Kühn* 16–17 αὐτῷ . . . ἔχοντι] αὐτὸν . . . ἔχοντα *Müller* 21 παρελελοίπειν *Chart.* 23 πλεονάζειν ἐν αὐτοῖς] . . . . .τοῖς H ἔμοιγ' οὖν H: *corr.* R *Bas.* 24 τοιαύτης ἀδολεσχίας] τοι. . . . . .ς H 25 τισὶ H: *corr. Müller* φι. . . . .ας H 26 ἐ. .νοις H 29 προτιϑεὶς H: *corr. Müller* γαληνοῦ περὶ τῶν ἱπποκράτους καὶ πλάτωνος δογμάτων, γ' *subscr.* H

their hidden meanings. For if a person once gets involved in this, a
countless number of mythical narratives 'comes flooding in', so that
anyone who examines them all will spend his whole life at it. It would 35
be better, I think, for the man who really seeks the truth not to ask what
the poets say; rather, he should first learn the method of finding the
scientific premises that I discussed in the second book; then he should
train and exercise himself in this method; and when his training is
sufficiently advanced, then, as he approaches each particular problem,
he should inquire into the premises needed for proving it, which pre-
mises he should take from simple sense-perception, which from experi-
ence, whether drawn from life or from the arts, which from the truths
clearly apprehended by the mind, in order to draw from them the
desired conclusion. If Chrysippus had followed this course and had 36
disregarded the way of myths and etymologies, noddings of the head
up and down, movements of the hands, positions of the lips, and the
testimony of poets, women, and other non-experts, he would himself
have found the truth and would not have caused us to waste our
time pointing out to him that he gains nothing either from the
witnesses he calls or from these other things. For the poets and the 37
myths and the non-experts, and all the others whom he quoted as
friendly witnesses in his first book On the Soul, speak for the most
part against his doctrines.

These are the passages from Chrysippus' account of the gov- 38
erning part of the soul that I had passed over in the preceding book;
I thought that even if he was not ashamed to write at excessive length
about these things, I, at least, might properly refrain from such idle
chatter. But as I said, since some of my friends, moved by a spirit of 39
contention, wanted me to take up the arguments of this kind also,
I yielded to their request and wrote this book; and to the best of my
ability, as I quickly reviewed the superfluous portions of Chrysip-
pus' account, I also added not a few items of use for the present trea-
tise.

ΓΑΛΗΝΟΥ

ΠΕΡΙ ΤΩΝ ΙΠΠΟΚΡΑΤΟΥΣ ΚΑΙ ΠΛΑΤΩΝΟΣ ΔΟΓΜΑΤΩΝ

ΒΙΒΛΙΟΝ ΤΕΤΑΡΤΟΝ

330 360 1. Τῶν μὲν λόγων τοῦ μήκους οὐχ ἡμᾶς αἰτιατέον, ἀλλὰ τοὺς
ἐμπλήσαντας ἃ συνέγραψαν βιβλία μοχθηρῶν ἐπιχειρημάτων, ἅπερ
εἰ μέν τις ἅπαντα παρέρχοιτο, τάχ' ἂν ὑποπτευθείη τῷ μὴ δύνασθαι λύειν
αὐτὰ μᾶλλον, οὐ τῷ καταφρονεῖν αἱρεῖσθαι τὴν βραχυλογίαν· εἰ δ'
ἀκολουθῶν ἐξελέγχοι πάντα, κίνδυνος εἰς τοσαύτην ἐμπεσεῖν μακρο-
361 2 λογίαν ὡς μηδέποτε κεφαλὴν ἐπιθεῖναι | τῇδε τῇ πραγματείᾳ. ταῦτά
τοι κἀγὼ βουληθεὶς ἑκάτερον τῶν ἐγκλημάτων ἐκφυγεῖν εὑρηκέναι μοι
δοκῶ μέσην τινὰ καὶ σύμμετρον ὁδὸν ἴσον ἀφεστῶσαν ἐλλιποῦς τε βρα-
3 χυλογίας καὶ περιττῆς μακρολογίας. ἐάσας γὰρ ἅπαντας τοὺς ἄλλους
331 Στωϊκούς, ὅσα Χρύσιππος / ἔγραψεν εἰς τὸ περὶ τῶν διοικουσῶν
ἡμᾶς δυνάμεων δόγμα, ταῦτ' ἔγνων χρῆναι προχειρισάμενος μόνα παρα-
βάλλειν αὐτὰ τοῖς ὑφ' Ἱπποκράτους τε καὶ Πλάτωνος εἰρημένοις.
4 παμπόλλων δ' ἐπιχειρημάτων γεγραμμένων αὐτῷ περὶ τοῦ τὰ πάθη
τῆς ψυχῆς ἐν τοῖς κατὰ τὸν θώρακα τόποις συνίστασθαι, περὶ δὲ τοῦ
τὸ λογιζόμενον ἐνταῦθ' ὑπάρχειν, οὐδεμιᾶς ἀποδείξεως εἰρημένης, ἀλλ'
ἑτοίμως ἀεὶ λαμβάνοντος τἀνδρός, ἔνθα τὰ πάθη τῆς ψυχῆς συνίσταται,
ἐνταῦθα καὶ τὴν διάνοιαν ὑπάρχειν, εἴρηται μὲν ἤδη μοι πρὸς αὐτὸν
οὐκ ὀλίγα καὶ διὰ τῶν ἔμπροσθεν, εἰρήσεται δὲ καὶ νῦν ὅσον ὑπόλοιπον.
5 Εἰ μὲν οὖν ἀεὶ τὰ αὐτὰ περὶ τῶν αὐτῶν ὁ Χρύσιππος ἔγραφε καὶ
μὴ διεφέρετο πρὸς αὑτὸν ἐν τοῖς πλείστοις δόγμασιν ἐπαμφοτερίζων, οὐδ'
362 ἂν ἐμοὶ μακρὸς ὁ τῆς ἀντιλογίας ἐγίνετο | λόγος. ἐπεὶ δ' ἄλλοτε ἄλλα
περὶ τῶν αὐτῶν εὑρίσκεται γράφων, οὐκέτι ῥᾴδιον οὔτε τὴν γνώμην ἑρμη-
6 νεῦσαι τἀνδρὸς οὔθ' ὅπῃ σφάλλεται δεικνύναι. περὶ γοῦν τῶν διοικουσῶν
332 ἡμᾶς δυνάμεων ἐν τῷ προτέρῳ Περὶ τῆς / ψυχῆς εἰπών, ὡς ὁ Πλάτων
ὑπελάμβανε, τὸ μὲν λογιστικὸν ἐν τῇ κεφαλῇ τετάχθαι, τὸ δὲ θυμοειδὲς
ἐν τῇ καρδίᾳ, τὸ δὲ ἐπιθυμητικὸν περὶ τὸν ὀμφαλόν, ἐν τοῖς ἑξῆς αὐτὸς
7 εἰς τὴν καρδίαν πειρᾶται τὰ τρία συνάγειν. ἔχουσι δὲ αἱ ῥήσεις ὧδε·
«ὁ δὲ ποιητὴς πλεονάζων ἐν τούτοις διὰ πολλῶν παρίστησιν ὅτι καὶ
τὸ λογιστικὸν καὶ τὸ θυμοειδὲς περὶ τοῦτόν ἐστι τὸν τόπον, συνάπτων

4–9] *cf. infra*, PHP 581.1–7 Müller 12–15] *cf. infra*, p. 334.18–20 18–20] *cf. supra*, pp. 156.3–5; 176.24–25 *infra*, PHP 652.5–6 Müller 22–236.15] SVF II, pp. 251–252 24–25] *cf.* Plat. Gorg. 482 a 7–b 1 28–29] *cf. supra*, p. 170.21–23 31–236.1] *cf. supra*, p. 222.3–6

1–3 ἀρχὴ τοῦ τετάρτου H 8 ἐκπεσεῖν *Schöne* 16 παμπόλων H: *corr. Ald.* 17 περὶ δὲ] περί τε *add.* H *in mg.*: καὶ περὶ *coni. Corn.* 18 οὐδεμιᾶς – 238.20 πειρώμενος *om.* H 23 αὐτὸν M *Ald.*: *corr. Chart.*

GALEN

ON THE DOCTRINES OF HIPPOCRATES AND PLATO

BOOK IV

1. We must not be blamed for the length of this discussion; they are rather to blame who filled their books with faulty arguments. If a person were to leave all these arguments unanswered, he might be suspected of choosing brevity from inability to refute them rather than from a scorn for them; but if he were to follow and refute them all, he would run the risk of entering on a discussion of such length that he would never bring this project to an end. For this reason I, 2
too, wishing to escape both charges, believe that I have found a middle and moderate course equally distant from inadequate brevity and excessive prolixity. Dismissing all the other Stoics, I have taken 3
up the things that Chrysippus wrote about the doctrine of the powers that govern us and have decided that they alone should be compared with the words of Hippocrates and Plato. Now he wrote 4
down a great many arguments designed to prove that the affections of the soul arise in the region of the thorax, yet he gave not a single scientific proof that the rational part is there, but always readily assumed that 'Where the affections of the soul arise, there the mind is also'. I have already replied to him at some length in earlier passages, and I shall now say all that remains (to be said).

If Chrysippus always said the same thing about the same 5
subject and did not contradict himself in the majority of his teachings by taking both sides, my refutation too would not be long. But since he is discovered writing different things at different times about the same matters, it is no longer easy to interpret the man's meaning or to point out where he errs. So with reference to the powers that govern 6
us, in his first book On the Soul he takes the Platonic position, that the reasoning part has been assigned to the head, the spirited to the heart, and the desiderative to the region of the navel; but subsequently, going his own way, he tries to gather the three (parts) together into the heart. The passages are as follows: "But the poet, who says more 7
than enough about these (things), presents in many verses the view that both the rational and the spirited parts are in this region, and he

8 εἰς ταὐτὸν καὶ τὸ ἐπιθυμητικόν, καθάπερ καὶ ἔδει ποιῆσαι.» εἶτα ἐπιφέρων φησίν, «ὅτι μὲν γὰρ τὸ λογιστικόν ἐστιν ἐνταῦθα, διὰ τούτων ἐμφαίνεται·

'ἄλλο δ' ἐνὶ στήθεσσι νόος καὶ μῆτις ἀμύμων.'
'ἀλλ' ἐμὸν οὔποτε θυμὸν ἐνὶ στήθεσσιν ἔπειθεν.'» |

363 9 εἶτ' ἐφεξῆς ἔπη παραθέμενος πλείω μετὰ ταῦτά φησιν, «ὅτι δὲ καὶ τὸ ἐπιθυμητικὸν ἐνταῦθα, ἐκ τούτων ἐμφαίνει·

'οὐ γάρ πώποτέ μ' ὧδε θεᾶς ἔρος οὐδὲ γυναικὸς
θυμὸν ἐνὶ στήθεσσι περιπροχυθεὶς ἐδάμασ⟨σ⟩ε.'» /

333 10 καὶ μετ' ὀλίγα πάλιν, «ὅτι δὲ καὶ τὸ θυμοειδὲς ἐνταῦθα αὐτῷ ἐστι, τὰ τοιαῦτα ἐμφαίνει πλείονα ὄντα·

'Ἥρῃ δ' οὐκ ἔχαδε στῆθος χόλον, ἀλλὰ προσηύδα.'

καὶ ἔτι

'καὶ χόλος ὅς τ' ἐφέηκε πολύφρονά περ χαλεπῆναι·
ὅς τε πολὺ γλυκίων μέλιτος καταλειβομένοιο
ἀνδρῶν ἐν στήθεσσιν ἀέξεται ἠύτε καπνός,'»

11 ἐναργέστατα καὶ σαφέστατα διὰ τῶν τοιούτων ἐνδεικνύμενος ὡς ὑπολαμβάνει καὶ αὐτὸς ὁμοίως Ἱπποκράτει καὶ Πλάτωνι δυνάμεις τῆς ψυχῆς ὑπάρχειν ἑτέρας παρὰ τὸν λογισμόν, τήν τε ἐπιθυμητικὴν καὶ τὴν θυμοειδῆ, καὶ καθ' ἕν γε μόνον τοῦτο διαφερόμενος αὐτοῖς, καθ' ὅσον ἐν τῇ καρδίᾳ πάσας εἶναί φησιν, ὡς Ἀριστοτέλης ὑπελάμβανεν, οὐκ ἐν τοῖς τρισὶ σπλάγχνοις, ἐγκεφάλῳ καὶ ἥπατι καὶ καρδίᾳ. |

364 334 12 ἀλλὰ / καὶ τὰ τῶν δυνάμεων ἔργα τε καὶ πάθη διὰ τῶν ἐπῶν ὧν ἔγραψεν αὐτάρκως ἐνεδείξατο, διὰ μὲν τοῦ φάναι·

«οὐ γάρ πώποτέ μ' ὧδε θεᾶς ἔρος οὐδὲ γυναικὸς
θυμὸν ἐνὶ στήθεσσι περιπροχυθεὶς ἐδάμασ⟨σ⟩εν»,

ὡς ὁ ἔρως πάθος εἴη τῆς ἐπιθυμητικῆς δυνάμεως· ἐν δὲ τῷ λέγειν·

«Ἥρῃ δ' οὐκ ἔχαδε στῆθος χόλον, ἀλλὰ προσηύδα»,

13 ὡς ὁ χόλος τῆς θυμοειδοῦς. διαφερέτω δ' ἓν γε τῷ παρόντι μηδέν, εἴτε ἔργα τῶν δυνάμεων εἴτε πάθη τὰ τοιαῦτα πάντα λέγοιμεν, ὕστερον γὰρ ὑπὲρ αὐτῶν ἀκριβῶς ἐπισκεψόμεθα.

3] versus heroici, XIV, ed. Allen 4] Hom. Od. vii. 258 5–8] *cf. supra*, p. 222.10–13 7–8] Hom. Il. xiv. 315–316 *cf. supra*, p. 222.12–13 *infra*, lin. 24–25 9–13] *cf. supra*, p. 222.14–18 11] Hom. Il. iv. 24 *cf. supra*, pp. 178.18; 222.16 *infra*, lin. 27 13–15] Hom. Il. xviii. 108–110 *cf. supra*, p. 178.24–26 13] *cf. supra*, p. 222.18 14–15] *cf. supra*, p. 176.1–2 20–21] *cf. supra*, p. 222.6–9 24–25] *cf. supra*, lin. 7–8 27] *cf. supra*, lin. 11 29–30] *cf. infra*, PHP 491.10–492.6 Müller

2 φησὶ *Ald.* ἐμφαίνει *Müller* 3 δὲ M στήθεσι M 4 στήθεσιν M 7 π ώποτ' ἔμ' *Ald.* ἔρως M *Ald.*: *corr. Chart.* 8 στήθεσι M ἐδάμασε M *Ald.*: *corr. Chart.* 10 ἐκφαίνει M 13 χόλον M *Ald.*: *corr. Müller (cf. supra, p. 178.24)* ὅς τ'] ὥστ' M *Ald.*: *corr. Corn.* 14 ὅς τε] ὥστε M *Ald.*: *corr. Corn.* καταλιβομένοιο M *Ald.*: *corr. Bas.* 15 στήθεσιν M 18 τ' *Ald.* 19 καθ' ἕν γε] καθήγε M: καθ' ἕτερον *Ald.*: καθ' ἓν F: *corr. Müller* 20 πᾶσ' M: πᾶσαν *Ald.*: *corr.* F 21 σπλάγνοις M 22 *ante* πάθη *add.* τὰ *Ald.* ὧν] ὡς M *Ald.*: *corr. Müller* 24 πώποτ' ἐμ' *(sic) Ald.* ἔρως M *Ald.*: *corr. Chart.* 25 στήθεσι M ἐδάμασεν M *Ald.*: *corr. Chart.*

joins the desiderative with them in the same place, as indeed he should." Then he adds: "For the following lines indicate that the rational part is here: 8

'The mind and faultless wisdom in his breast gave other counsel.'
'But she could never persuade my spirit in my breast.'"

Then after citing more lines of verse he says, "He indicates in the following lines that the desiderative is there also: 9

'Never before did love of goddess or woman
so flood my breast and overpower my spirit;'"

and again after a little, "That the spirited part is also here for him is indicated by verses such as these, which are quite numerous: 10

'But Hera's breast could not contain her bitter anger, and she spoke out;'

and also

'And bitter anger, that drives even the very wise to harshness;
far sweeter than dripping honey
it rises up like smoke in men's breasts,'"

indicating most clearly and plainly by such verses that he too, like Hippocrates and Plato, supposes that the soul has other powers besides reason, namely, the desiderative and spirited (powers), and that he differs from them in this one respect only, in his saying that all (the powers) are in the heart, as Aristotle supposed, and not in the three internal organs, brain, liver, and heart. And by the verses he quoted he also indicated adequately the actions and affections of the powers. By saying 11 12

"Never before did love of goddess or woman
so flood my breast and overpower my spirit"

he indicates that love is an affection of the desiderative power; and in stating

"But Hera's breast could not contain her bitter anger, and she spoke out"

he indicates that bitter anger is an affection of the spirited (power). For the moment let us grant that it makes no difference whether we call all such things actions or affections of the powers; for we shall make a detailed examination of them at a later time. 13

14 Κατὰ μὲν ⟨οὖν⟩ τὸ πρότερον Περὶ ψυχῆς βιβλίον ὁ Χρύσιππος
οὐχ ὅπως ἀντιλέγει μηδεμίαν εἶναι τῆς ψυχῆς δύναμιν ἢ ἐπιθυμητικὴν ἢ
θυμοειδῆ, ἀλλὰ καὶ τὰ παθήματ' αὐτῶν ἐκδιδάσκει καὶ τόπον ἀπονέμει
τοῦ σώματος ἕνα· κατὰ δὲ τὰ Περὶ τῶν παθῶν ἅπαντα, τά τε τρία δι'
ὧν ἐπισκέπτεται τὰ λογικὰ περὶ αὐτῶν ζητήματα καὶ προσέτι τὸ Θερα-
335 365 πευτικόν, / ὃ δὴ καὶ Ἠθικὸν ἐπιγράφουσί | τινες, οὐκέθ' ὁμοίως εὑρίσκε-
ται γινώσκων, ἀλλὰ τὰ μὲν ὡς ἐπαμφοτερίζων γράφει, τὰ δὲ ὡς μηδεμίαν
ἡγούμενος εἶναι δύναμιν τῆς ψυχῆς μήτε ἐπιθυμητικὴν μήτε θυμοειδῆ.
15 κατὰ μὲν γὰρ τὴν ἐξήγησιν τῶν ὁρισμῶν τοῦ πάθους ἐμφαίνει τινὰ
δύναμιν ἄλογον ἐν τῇ ψυχῇ τῶν παθῶν αἰτίαν ὑπάρχειν, ὡς ὀλίγον
ὕστερον ἐπιδείξω τὴν ῥῆσιν ἐξηγησάμενος αὐτοῦ· ἐν δὲ τοῖς ἐφεξῆς, ἔνθα
ζητεῖ πότερα κρίσεσιν ἐπιγίγνεται τὰ πάθη, προφανῶς ἀποχωρεῖ τῆς
Πλάτωνος δόξης, ὅς γ' οὐδὲ τὴν ἀρχὴν ἐν τῇ διαιρέσει τοῦ προβλήματος
16 ἠξίωσε καὶ ταύτης ἐπιμνησθῆναι. καίτοι τοῦτο πρῶτον εὐθὺς ἐγκαλέσειεν
ἄν τις αὐτῷ παρὰ τὸ τῆς διαιρέσεως ἐλλιπὲς ἐσφαλμένῳ. τὸ γάρ τοι πά-
θος οἷον ὁ ἔρως ἤτοι κρίσις τίς ἐστιν ἢ κρίσεσιν ἐπιγιγνόμενον ἢ κίνησις
ἔκφορος τῆς ἐπιθυμητικῆς δυνάμεως. οὕτω δὲ καὶ ὁ χόλος ἤτοι κρίσις
ἢ ἑπόμενόν τι ταύτῃ πάθος ἄλογον ἢ κίνησις σφοδρὰ τῆς θυμοειδοῦς
336 17 δυνάμεως. ὁ δέ / γ' οὐδ' οὕτως ἐγχωροῦν εἰς τρία τέμνεσθαι τὸ πρόβλημα
366 μεταχειρί|ζεται τὸν λόγον ἐπιδεικνύναι πειρώμενος ὡς ἄμεινον εἴη κρί-
σεις ὑπολαμβάνειν αὐτὰ καὶ οὐκ ἐπιγινόμενά τινα ταῖς κρίσεσιν, ἐπιλαθό-
μενος ὧν αὐτὸς ἐν τῷ προτέρῳ τῷ⟨ν⟩ Περὶ ψυχῆς ἔγραψε, τὸν μὲν ἔρωτα
τῆς ἐπιθυμητικῆς εἶναι δυνάμεως, τὸν δὲ χόλον τῆς θυμοειδοῦς.

2. Ὥσπερ δ' ἐν τούτοις ἐπελάθετό τε ἅμα τῶν ἑαυτῷ γεγραμμένων
οὐκ ἠξίωσέ τε πρὸς τὸ τῶν παλαιῶν ἀντειπεῖν δόγμα, κατὰ τὸν αὐτὸν
τρόπον ἐν τοῖς ὁρισμοῖς τῶν γενικῶν παθῶν οὓς πρώτους ἐξέθετο, τε-
λέως ἀποχωρεῖ τῆς γνώμης αὐτῶν, τὴν λύπην ὁριζόμενος δόξαν πρό-
σφατον κακοῦ παρουσίας, τὸν δὲ φόβον προσδοκίαν κακοῦ, τὴν δ' ἡδονὴν
2 δόξαν πρόσφατον ἀγαθοῦ παρουσίας. ἄντικρυς γὰρ ἐν τούτοις τοῦ λο-
γιστικοῦ τῆς ψυχῆς μόνου μέμνηται παραλείπων τό τ' ἐπιθυμητικὸν καὶ
τὸ θυμοειδές· καὶ γὰρ τὴν δόξαν καὶ τὴν προσδοκίαν ἐν τῷ λογιστικῷ
337 3 μόνῳ συνίστασθαι νομίζει. / κατὰ μέντοι τὸν τῆς ἐπιθυμίας ὅρον, ἣν
367 ὄρεξιν ἄλογον εἶναί φησιν, | ἐφάπτεται μέν πως ὅσον ἐπὶ τῇ λέξει τῆς
ἀλόγου κατὰ τὴν ψυχὴν δυνάμεως, ἀποχωρεῖ δὲ κἀνταῦθα κατὰ τὴν
ἐξήγησιν αὐτῆς, εἴγε καὶ ἡ ὄρεξις ἣν κατὰ τὸν ὁρισμὸν παρέλαβε τῆς
4 λογικῆς ἐστι δυνάμεως. ὁρίζεται γοῦν αὐτὴν ὁρμὴν λογικὴν ἐπί τι⟨νος⟩
ὅσον χρὴ ἥδον⟨τος⟩.

1–23] SVF III, p. 112 25] *cf. infra*, PHP 652.14–16 Müller 25–240.10] SVF III, pp. 115–116 36–37] *cf. infra*, pp. 250.8–9, 11–12; 342.29–30

1 οὖν *add. Müller* 5 ἐπισκέπτεται *ex* ἐπισκέπτεσθαι *corr.* M 7 γράφειν M 12 *ante* κρίσεσιν *add.* κρίσεις ἐστὶν ἢ *Müller* 15 αὐτῷ] ῶ *ex* ὸ *corr.* M παρὰ] κατὰ *Müller* τὸ τῆς] τῶ M: τῷ τῆς *Ald.*: *corr. Chart.* 16 ἐστὶ *Ald.* κρίσεσιν] κρίσει *Müller* 17 δὲ *om.* M 20 πειρώμενος *ex* -μενον *corr.* M 22 τῶν] τῶ H: *correxi*: *del. Müller* 36–37 τι ὅσον χρὴ ἥδον H: *supplevi (cf. infra, pp. 250.9; 342.30)*

Thus in the first of the two books of his work On the Soul Chrysippus not merely does not reject the view that there is no desiderative or spirited power of the soul but even explains in detail their affections and assigns to them a single locality in the body. But in his entire treatise On the Affections, the three books in which he investigates theoretical questions about them and also the book on their cure, which is also entitled Ethics by some, he is found to hold this same view no longer; at times he writes as if he were on both sides, and at times as if he thought that the soul has neither a desiderative 14
nor a spirited power. For in his explanation of the definitions of affection he implies that some irrational power in the soul is the cause of the affections, as I shall presently show when I comment on his words; but later, when he asks whether the affections supervene on judgments, he clearly departs from Plato's view. Indeed in his division of the problem he did not even consider Plato's view worth mentioning. 15
And yet this is the first charge that one might bring against him, that he was misled by the incompleteness of his division. For an affection such as love either is a judgment or supervenes on judgments or is a runaway movement of the desiderative power. Similarly, bitter anger also is either a judgment or some irrational affection following on this 16
(judgment) or a violent motion of the spirited power. But although the question admits of being divided three ways, he does not handle the argument thus. He tries to show that it is better to suppose that the affections are judgments and are not something supervening on judgments, thus forgetting what he himself wrote in the first book of his work On the Soul, that love is an affection of the desiderative power, and bitter anger of the spirited. 17

2. Just as he here forgot what he himself had written and did not see fit to reply to the teaching of the ancients, similarly in the first definitions that he gives of the generic affections he abandons their opinions completely, defining distress as a fresh belief that evil is present, fear as the expectation of evil, pleasure as a fresh belief that
good is present. In these (definitions) it is obvious that he mentions only the rational part of the soul, omitting the desiderative and the spirited; for he thinks that belief and expectation arise only in the 2
rational part. Nevertheless in his definition of desire, which he calls irrational appetition, he touches in a way, verbally at least, on the irrational power in the soul; but here too he departs from it in his explanation, since even the appetition that he includes in the definition 3
belongs to the rational power. Thus he defines appetition as 'rational conation for something that gives pleasure to the extent that it should'. 4

Ἐν μέντοι δὴ τούτοις τοῖς ὅροις ὁρμὰς καὶ δόξας καὶ κρίσεις ὑπάρ-
χειν οἴεται τὰ πάθη, κατὰ δέ τινας τῶν ἐφεξῆς Ἐπικούρῳ καὶ Ζήνωνι
5 μᾶλλον ἢ τοῖς ἑαυτοῦ δόγμασιν ἀκόλουθα γράφει. τήν τε γὰρ λύπην
ὁριζόμενος μείωσιν εἶναί φησιν ἐπὶ φευκτῷ δοκοῦντι ὑπάρχειν τήν θ'
6 ἡδονὴν ἔπαρσιν ἐφ' αἱρετῷ δοκοῦντι ὑπάρχειν. καὶ γὰρ αἱ μειώσεις καὶ
αἱ ἐπάρσεις καὶ αἱ συστολαὶ καὶ αἱ διαχύσεις – καὶ γὰρ τούτων ἐνίοτε
μέμνηται – τῆς ἀλόγου δυνάμεώς ἐστι παθήματα ταῖς δόξαις ἐπιγιγνό-
μενα. τοιαύτην δέ τινα τὴν οὐσίαν τῶν παθῶν Ἐπίκουρος καὶ Ζήνων,
338 7 οὐκ αὐτὸς ὑπολαμβάνει. ὃ καὶ θαυμάζειν ἐπέρχεταί / μοι τἀνδρὸς ἐν ἐπαγ-
γελίᾳ λογικῆς τε ἅμα καὶ ἀκριβοῦς διδασκαλίας οὐκ ἀκριβοῦντος.
8 Καὶ γὰρ οὐ κατὰ ταῦτα μόνον αὐτὸς ἑαυτῷ διαφέρεται φανερῶς, |
368 ἀλλὰ κἀπειδὰν ὑπὲρ τῶν κατὰ τὸ πάθος ὁρισμῶν γράφων ἄλογόν τε καὶ
παρὰ φύσιν κίνησιν ψυχῆς αὐτὸ φάσκῃ καὶ πλεονάζουσαν ὁρμήν, εἶτα
τὸ μὲν ἄλογον ἐξηγούμενος τὸ χωρὶς λόγου τε καὶ κρίσεως εἰρῆσθαι
φάσκῃ, τῆς δὲ πλεοναζούσης ὁρμῆς παράδειγμα τοὺς τρέχοντας σφο-
δρῶς παραλαμβάνῃ· ταυτὶ γὰρ ἀμφότερα μάχεται τῷ κρίσεις εἶναι τὰ
9 πάθη. εἰσόμεθα δ' ἐναργέστερον αὐτὰς τὰς ῥήσεις αὐτοῦ παραγρά-
10 ψαντες· ἔχει δ' ἡ μὲν ἑτέρα τόνδε τὸν τρόπον· «δεῖ δὲ πρῶτον ἐντεθυ-
μῆσθαι ὅτι τὸ λογικὸν ζῷον ἀκολουθητικὸν φύσει ἐστὶ τῷ λόγῳ καὶ κατὰ
11 τὸν λόγον ὡς ἂν ἡγεμόνα πρακτικόν. πολλάκις μέντοι καὶ ἄλλως φέρεται
ἐπί τινα καὶ ἀπό τινων ἀπειθῶς τῷ λόγῳ ὠθούμενον ἐπὶ πλεῖον, καθ'
ἣν φορὰν ἀμφότεροι ἔχουσιν οἱ ὅροι, τῆς παρὰ φύσιν κινήσεως ἀλόγως /
339 12 οὕτως γινομένης καὶ τοῦ ἐν ταῖς ὁρμαῖς πλεονασμοῦ. τὸ γὰρ ἄλογον τουτὶ
ληπτέον ἀπειθὲς λόγῳ καὶ ἀπεστραμμένον τὸν λόγον, καθ' ἣν φορὰν
369 καὶ ἐν τῷ ἔθει τινάς φαμεν ὠθεῖσθαι καὶ ἀλόγως | φέρεσθαι ἄνευ λόγου
⟨καὶ⟩ κρίσεως· ⟨οὐ γὰρ⟩ ὡς εἰ διημαρτημένως φέρεται καὶ παριδών τι
κατὰ τὸν λόγον, ταῦτ' ἐπισημαινόμεθα, ἀλλὰ μάλιστα καθ' ἣν ὑπο-
γράφει φοράν, οὐ πεφυκότος τοῦ λογικοῦ ζῴου κινεῖσθαι οὕτως κατὰ τὴν
ψυχήν, ἀλλὰ κατὰ τὸν λόγον.»
13 Ἡ μὲν οὖν ἑτέρα τῶν τοῦ Χρυσίππου ῥήσεων ἐξηγουμένη τὸν
πρότερον τῶν ὅρων τοῦ πάθους ἐνταυθοῖ τελευτᾷ. τὴν δ' ὑπόλοιπον
ἐν ᾗ τὸν ἕτερον ὅρον ἐξηγεῖται γεγραμμένην ἐφεξῆς τῇδε κατὰ τὸ πρῶ-
14 τον σύγγραμμα Περὶ παθῶν ἤδη σοι παραθήσομαι· «κατὰ τοῦτο δὲ καὶ ὁ
340 πλεονασμὸς τῆς ὁρμῆς εἴρηται, διὰ τὸ τὴν / καθ' αὑτοὺς καὶ φυσικὴν τῶν
15 ὁρμῶν συμμετρίαν ὑπερβαίνειν. γένοιτο δ' ἂν τὸ λεγόμενον διὰ τούτων
γνωριμώτερον, οἷον ἐπὶ τοῦ πορεύεσθαι καθ' ὁρμὴν οὐ πλεονάζει ἡ τῶν

1–9] Usener, Epicurea, fr. 410 5–9] *cf. infra*, pp. 246.38–248.3; 292.18–20 11–242.11] SVF III, pp. 113–114 23–27] *cf. infra*, p. 242.29–32 23–26] *cf. infra*, p. 242.18–19 26–27] *cf. infra*, pp. 256.1–2; 316.6–7

1 μέντοι] μὲν *Müller* 2 ἑξῆς *v. Arnim* 4 θ'] δ' H: *corr. Müller* 11 οὐ κατὰ] οὐκ αὐτὰ H: *corr. Corn.*: οὐ κατὰ αὐτὰ *Müller* 15 φάσκει H: *corr. Müller* 16 παραλαμβάνει H: *corr. Müller* 25 τινά *Müller* 26 καὶ[I] *add. Petersen* οὐ – εἰ] ὡς εἰ H: *supplevi*: οὐχὶ εἰ *Ricci Corn. Al. Just.*: καὶ οὐχὶ εἰ *Müller*: καὶ γὰρ οὐχὶ εἰ *Pohlenz* 27 *post* λόγον *add.* ἀλλὰ ἀπεστραμμένως τε καὶ ἀπειθῶς αὐτῷ *Müller* ἐπισημαινόμενοι *v. Arnim* ἀλλὰ] ἄλογα *Diels*: *del. Müller* ὑπογράφομεν *Müller*

In these definitions he indeed fancies that the affections are
conations and opinions and judgments; yet in some of the very next
definitions he says things that follow from the views of Epicurus and
Zeno rather than from his own. For in defining distress he says that 5
it is a shrinking before what is thought to be a thing to avoid, and
pleasure he defines as a rising up at what is thought to be a thing to
pursue. But shrinking and rising up, and contraction and expansion – 6
for sometimes he mentions these – are affections of the irrational
power which supervenes on opinions. Epicurus and Zeno suppose
that the affections have such a nature as this, but Chrysippus does
not. And it strikes me as surprising that the man who professes to be 7
giving both logical and precise instruction is not precise.

These are not the only definitions in which he clearly contradicts 8
himself. He does so also in his account of the definitions of affection,
when he says that affection is an irrational and unnatural movement
of the soul and an excessive conation, then says, in explaining 'irratio-
nal', that it means 'without reason and judgment' and takes as a model
of excessive conation persons who are running hard. These are both
in conflict with the statement that affections are judgments. We shall 9
see this more clearly when we have quoted his own words. The first
passage is as follows: "First one must keep in mind that the rational 10
animal is by nature such as to follow reason and to act with reason as
his guide. But often he moves in another way toward some things and 11
away from some things in disobedience to reason when he is pushed
too much. Both definitions refer to this movement; the unnatural
motion arises irrationally in this way, and also the excess in the
conations. For this irrationality must be understood as disobedient to 12
reason and rejecting it; and with reference to this motion we say in
ordinary usage that some persons are pushed and moved irrationally,
without reason and judgment. For when we use these expressions it is
not as if a person is carried away by error and from a misapprehension
of something that is in accord with reason; we use them most of all
with reference to the movement that he describes, since it is not the
nature of a rational animal to move thus in his soul, but in accordance
with reason."

The first passage from Chrysippus, expounding the first of the 13
definitions of affection, ends here. The remaining passage, in which
he expounds the second definition, comes next after this in the first
book On the Affections; I shall now place it before you. "In this con- 14
text we have spoken also of excess of conation, because their conations
exceed the measure that accords with themselves and with nature.
My meaning would be made clearer by the following examples. When 15
a man walks in accordance with a conation, the motion of his legs is

σκελῶν κίνησις ἀλλὰ συναπαρτίζει τι τῇ ὁρμῇ ὥστε καὶ στῆναι, ὅταν ἐθέλῃ,
16 καὶ μεταβάλλειν. ἐπὶ δὲ τῶν τρεχόντων καθ' ὁρμὴν οὐκέτι τοιοῦτον γί-
νεται, ἀλλὰ πλεονάζει παρὰ τὴν ὁρμὴν ἡ τῶν σκελῶν κίνησις ὥστε
17 ἐκφέρεσθαι καὶ μὴ μεταβάλλειν εὐπειθῶς οὕτως εὐθὺς ἐναρξαμένων. αἷς
870 οἶμαί τι παραπλήσιον καὶ ἐπὶ τῶν ὁρμῶν γίνεσθαι διὰ τὸ τὴν | κατὰ
λόγον ὑπερβαίνειν συμμετρίαν, ὥσθ' ὅταν ὁρμᾷ μὴ εὐπειθῶς ἔχειν πρὸς
αὐτόν, ἐπὶ μὲν τοῦ δρόμου τοῦ πλεονασμοῦ λεγομένου παρὰ τὴν ὁρμήν,
18 ἐπὶ δὲ τῆς ὁρμῆς παρὰ τὸν λόγον. συμμετρία γάρ ἐστι φυσικῆς ὁρμῆς
ἡ κατὰ τὸν λόγον καὶ ἕως τοσούτου, [καὶ] ἕως αὐτὸς ἀξιοῖ. διὸ δὴ καὶ
341 τῆς ὑπερβάσεως κατὰ τοῦτο καὶ οὕτως γινομένης / πλεονάζουσά τε
ὁρμὴ λέγεται εἶναι καὶ παρὰ φύσιν καὶ ἄλογος κίνησις ψυχῆς.»
19 Αἱ μὲν τοῦ Χρυσίππου ῥήσεις αὗται. σκεψώμεθα δ' ἀκριβέστερον
ὑπὲρ ἑκατέρας αὐτῶν ἀπὸ τῆς προτέρας ἀπαρξάμενοι, καθ' ἣν ἐξηγεῖται
20 πῶς εἴρηται τὸ πάθος ἄλογος καὶ παρὰ φύσιν κίνησις ψυχῆς. ἐπειδὴ γὰρ
ἠπίστατο δύο σημαινόμενα πρὸς τῆς ἄλογος φωνῆς ὧν τὸ ἕτερον βού-
λεται μόνον δηλοῦσθαι κατὰ τὸν ὅρον, τὸ χωρὶς κρίσεως, ὀρθῶς ἐποίησε
μηδεμίαν ὑπολιπόμενος ἀμφιβολίαν ἀλλ' αὐτὸς δηλώσας ὅτι τὴν κατὰ
τὸ πάθος ὁρμὴν ἄλογον εἶναί φησι καθ' ὅσον ἀπέστραπται τὸν λόγον
21 καὶ ἀπειθεῖ τῷ λόγῳ καὶ χωρὶς κρίσεως γίνεται. διὰ μὲν οὖν τοῦ ἀπε-
871 στράφθαι φάναι τὸν λόγον ἐχώρισε | τὴν κατὰ τὸ πάθος ἄλογον κίνησιν τῶν
22 ἀψύχων τε καὶ τῶν ἀλόγων ζῴων. κινεῖται μὲν γὰρ καὶ λίθος καὶ ξύλον ἐνίοτε
καὶ τῶν ἄλλων ἕκαστον τῶν ἀψύχων, ἀλλ' οὐχ ὡς ἀπεστραμμένον τὸν
342 λόγον οὐδ' ὡς ἀπειθοῦν. ᾧ γὰρ τὴν ἀρχὴν μὴ μέτεστι / τοῦ πείθεσθαί τε
καὶ ἕπεσθαι τῷ λόγῳ, τοῦτο πῶς ἂν ἢ ἀπειθεῖν ἢ ἀπεστράφθαι ποτὲ
23 δύναιτο τὸν λόγον; ἀλλ' ὅλως μὴ χρῆσθαι λέγοιτο ἂν εἰκότως. ἀπε-
στράφθαι δὲ καὶ ἀπειθεῖν λεχθήσεται τὸ φύσιν μὲν ἔχον ἕπεσθαί τε καὶ
πείθεσθαι, παρὰ φύσιν δέ ποθ' ἑτέρως φερόμενον. ἐκ μὲν δὴ τῶν τοιούτων
δείκνυται τὸ μήτ' ἀψύχῳ τινὶ μήτ' ἀλόγῳ ζῴῳ πάθος ἐγγίνεσθαι
24 ψυχικόν. ἐπειδὰν δὲ γράφῃ χωρὶς λόγου καὶ κρίσεως γίγνεσθαι τὴν
κατὰ πάθος κίνησιν, εἶτα συνάπτων ἐφεξῆς λέγῃ «οὐχὶ εἰ διημαρτημένως
φέρεται καὶ παριδών τι κατὰ τὸν λόγον, καὶ ἀπεστραμμένως τε καὶ
ἀπειθῶς αὐτῷ», διορίζει τῶν ἁμαρτημάτων τὰ πάθη καὶ πάνυ δεόντως.
25 τὰ μὲν γὰρ ἁμαρτήματα μοχθηραὶ κρίσεις εἰσὶ καὶ ὁ λόγος ἐψευσμένος |
872 τῆς ἀληθείας καὶ διημαρτημένος· τὸ δὲ πάθος ἔμπαλιν οὐδὲν μὲν ἡμαρτη-
μένον οὐδὲ παρορώμενον κατὰ τὸν λογισμόν, ἀπειθὴς δέ ἐστι τῷ λόγῳ
26 κίνησις ψυχῆς. ὁ μὲν γὰρ ὑπὲρ τοῦ σῶσαι τὴν πατρίδα τῆς ζωῆς τῶν
343 τέκνων καταφρονήσας / καὶ ἤτοι παραδοὺς ἑτέροις ἀποσφάττειν ἢ αὐτὸς

14–21] SVF III, p. 114 27–36] *cf.* SVF III, p. 114 29–32] *cf. supra*, p. 240.23–27 33–244.9] *cf.* Reinhardt, 1921, pp. 305–306 33–36] *cf.* Gal. De affect. dignot. 1: CMG V 4.1.1, pp. 3–4

1 τῆς ὁρμῆς H: *corr. Müller* 4 ἐναρξαμένων *ex* -μένως *corr.* H οἷς *Müller* 9 καὶ[II] *del. Müller* 13 ἀρξάμενοι *Schöne* 19 *ante* κρίσεως *add.* λόγου *Müller*, λόγου καὶ *Wilamowitz* 20 *post* κίνησιν *add.* τῆς *Müller* 26 ἀπειθεῖν *ex* ἀπειθοῦν *corr.* H 27 ποθ'] θ *ex* τ *corr.* H 29 καὶ *om. Müller* 30 *ante* πάθος *add.* τὸ *Ald.* λέγειν H: λέγει *Ald.* (*cf. supra, p. 240.13–16*): *corr. Kühn* 31 καὶ[II]] ἀλλὰ *Müller* 33 ὁ *del. Müller*

not excessive but is in some way commensurate with the conation, so that he may stop when he wishes, or change his pace. But when 16 persons run in accordance with a conation, this sort of thing no longer happens. The movement of the legs exceeds the conation, so that they are carried away and do not obediently change their pace, (as they did before,) the moment they set out to do so. I think that something 17 similar to these (movements of the legs) happens also in conations because of an excess beyond the rational measure, so that when a man exercises the conation he is not obedient to reason; and whereas the excess in running is termed contrary to the conation, the excess in conation is termed contrary to reason. For the proper measure of 18 natural conation is that which is conformable to reason and which goes only so far as reason thinks right. Therefore when excess arises in this respect and under these conditions, it is said to be an excessive conation and an unnatural and irrational movement of the soul."

These are the passages from Chrysippus. Let us examine them 19 both rather carefully, beginning with the earlier one, in which he explains what he meant when he said that affection is an irrational and unnatural movement of the soul. Since he understood that the 20 word 'irrational' has two meanings and intended it to have only one of these meanings in the definition, the meaning 'without judgment', he was right not to leave any ambiguity but to make his meaning clear, that an affective conation is irrational insofar as it rejects and disobeys reason and occurs without judgment. Now by saying that it 21 rejects reason he removed the irrational movement of affection from inanimate objects and irrational animals. Stone and wood move some- 22 times, and every other inanimate object; but not as something that has rejected reason or is disobedient to it. For when a thing has nothing at all to do with obeying and following reason, how could it ever disobey or reject it? One might reasonably say that it makes no use of reason at all. But rejection and disobedience will be ascribed to 23 something that by nature follows and obeys yet sometimes, contrary to its nature, moves the other way. By such considerations as this it is shown that no affection of the soul arises in an inanimate object or an irrational animal. And when he writes that affective movement 24 arises apart from reason and judgment, then joins to this the following statement, "It is not the case that if a person is carried away by error and from a misapprehension of something that is in accord with reason, he is also acting in a way that rejects and disobeys reason", he very properly distinguishes affections from errors. For errors are 25 faulty judgments and reason that has been mistaken about the truth and has erred. But affection, on the contrary, is not something that has erred or makes a mistake in its reasoning; it is a motion of the soul disobedient to reason. A man who scorns his children's life in order to 26 save his country, whether surrendering them to others to slay, or

ὑπομείνας σφάξαι τῇ γε τοῦ καλοῦ φαντασίᾳ τοῦτο δρᾷ καὶ λογισμῷ
27 τινι χρησάμενος· ἡ Μήδεια δ' ἔμπαλιν οὐ μόνον ὑπ' οὐδενὸς ἐπείσθη
λογισμοῦ κτείνειν τοὺς παῖδας, ἀλλὰ καὶ τοὐναντίον ἅπαν, ὅσον ἐπὶ τῷ
λογισμῷ μανθάνειν φησὶν οἷα δρᾶν μέλλει κακά, τὸν θυμὸν δὲ εἶναι κρείτ-
τονα τῶν βουλευμάτων, τουτέστιν οὐχ ὑποτετάχθαι καὶ πείθεσθαι καὶ
ἕπεσθαι καθάπερ τινὶ δεσπότῃ τῷ λόγῳ τὸ πάθος ἀλλ' ἀφηνιάζειν καὶ
ἀποχωρεῖν καὶ ἀπειθεῖν τῷ προστάγματι, ὡς ἑτέρας τινὸς ἔργον ἢ
πάθημα δυνάμεως ὑπάρχον, οὐ τῆς λογιστικῆς. πῶς γὰρ ἂν ἢ ἀπειθεῖν
ἑαυτῷ τι δύναιτο ἢ ἀποστρέφεσθαι ἑαυτὸ ἢ μὴ ἕπεσθαι ἑαυτῷ;
28 Ταυτὶ μὲν οὖν ἅπαντα πρὸς τῷ μηδὲν ἔχειν μεμπτὸν ἔτι καὶ ἀληθῶς
τε καὶ διωρισμένως καὶ κατὰ τὴν Πλάτωνος εἴρηται γνώμην, παραπλη-
873 σίως δὲ καὶ | τὰ κατὰ τὴν ἐξήγησιν τοῦ δευτέρου τῶν ὅρων ὑπ' αὐτοῦ
γεγραμμένα, δι' ἧς ἐμνημόνευσε καὶ τῶν τρεχόντων ὠκέως, οἳ μηδ' εἰ
344 29 στῆναι βούλοιντο παραχρῆμα δύναιντο πράττειν / αὐτό. σαφῶς γὰρ
κἀνταῦθα ἔνδειξις γίγνεται δυνάμεως ἑτέρας παρὰ τὸν λόγον, ὑφ' ἧς ἀπο-
τελεῖται τὰ παθήματα. γνοίημεν δ' ἂν ἐναργέστερον εἰ τὴν αἰτίαν ἐξεύ-
ροιμεν ὑφ' ἧς συμβαίνει μὴ δύνασθαι στῆναι παραχρῆμα πολλοὺς τῶν
30 θεόντων. ἡ δ' εὕρεσις ἐξ αὐτοῦ γένοιτ' ἂν ἡμῖν τοῦ μὴ πᾶσιν οὕτως
συμβαίνειν ἀλλ' ὅσοι δι' ὁμαλοῦς τινος ἢ κατάντους φέρονται. τῶν μὲν
γὰρ ἀνάντη χωρία διαθεόντων οὐκ ἔστιν ὅτῳ τοῦτο συμπίπτει· παρα-
χρῆμα γοῦν ἵστανται βουληθέντες, ὡς ἂν τῆς ῥοπῆς τοῦ σώματος μὴ φε-
31 ρούσης αὐτοὺς βιαίως [κάτω] καθάπερ ἐκείνους ἔφερε. σύνθετος γὰρ αὐτῶν
ἔνεστιν ἡ τῆς φορᾶς αἰτία, ἡ μέν τις ὡς ζῴων ὑφ' ὁρμῆς κινουμένων ἡ δ' ὡς
ἀψύχων σωμάτων τῷ βάρει ῥεπόντων. οὕτω γοῦν καὶ λίθοι πολλάκις
874 ὀρῶν καταφέρονται στῆναι μεταξὺ μὴ δυνάμενοι πρὶν ἐξικέσθαι | πρός τι
32 χωρίον ὁμαλὸν ἢ κοῖλον. ὥστε καὶ κατὰ τοῦτο τὸ παράδειγμα δυνάμεώς
ἐστιν ἔνδειξις ἑτέρας παρὰ τὸν λογισμόν, ἀλόγου τὴν φύσιν οἷά πέρ ἐστιν
345 33 ἐν τοῖς τῶν ζῴων σώμασι τὸ βάρος. ὅτι δ' οὐ δύνανται / διὰ τοῦτο στῆναι
βουληθέντες, οὐ μόνον ἐκ τῆς τῶν ἀναντῶν τε καὶ καταντῶν χωρίων
διαφορᾶς ἔνεστι μαθεῖν, ἀλλὰ καὶ ἐκ τῆς ἐν αὐτοῖς τοῖς ὁμαλέσι διαφόρου
34 κινήσεως. ὁ μὲν γὰρ εἰς τοὐπίσω τὴν ῥοπὴν τοῦ σώματος ποιησάμενος
ἐν τῷ τρέχειν αὐτοκράτωρ ἐστὶ τοῦ στῆναι, ὁ δ' εἰς τὸ ἔμπροσθεν ὑπ'
35 ἐκείνης κωλύεται. καὶ δι' αὐτό γε τοῦτο οὕτω θέουσιν ἅπαντες ὑπ' αὐτῆς
τοῦ πράγματος τῆς φύσεως διδασκόμενοι συντελεῖν τὴν εἰς τὸ πρόσω
36 ῥοπὴν τῷ τάχει τῆς κινήσεως. ὥσπερ οὖν ἐπὶ τοῦ παραδείγματος, ὦ
γενναιότατε Χρύσιππε, τοῖς μὲν μηδὲν ὑπὸ τοῦ κατὰ τὸ σῶμα
βάρους εἰς τάχος κινήσεως ὠφελουμένοις ἕτοιμον τὸ στῆναι, τοῖς δ'
ἐκ διττῆς αἰτίας τὸ τάχος γεννῶσιν οὐκέθ' ἡ βούλησις ἱκανή, κατὰ
τὸν αὐτὸν τρόπον ἐπὶ τῶν τῆς ψυχῆς ὁρμῶν, ὅταν μὲν ὁ λογισμὸς μόνος
875 ἔχῃ τὴν αἰτίαν, ἐπ' αὐτῷ παῦσαι τὴν ὁρμήν· | ὅταν δ' ἤτοι θυμὸς ἢ

2–5] Eur. Medea 1078–1079 *cf. supra*, p. 188.27–28 *infra*, p. 274.13–14
11–13] *cf. supra*, p. 242.2–4 24–26] *cf.* Hom. Il. xiii. 136–142

3 λογισμῷ H: *corr. Chart.* 7 ἀπωθεῖν H: *corr. Kühn* 16 μαθήματα H: *corr. Ald.* 22 κάτω *delevi* ἔφερον H: *corr. Ald.* 27 οἷαπερ H: *corr. Kühn*
29 ἀνάντων ... κατάντων H: *corr. Chart.* 37 ὠφελουμένοις] ου *ex* ω *corr.* H
39 ὁρμῶν *in* ὅρμον *mut.* H

taking on himself the burden of the deed, acts as he does because it
seems to him noble to do so, and he engages in a certain reasoning.
Medea, on the other hand, was not persuaded by any reasoning to 27
kill her children; quite the contrary, so far as reasoning goes, she says
that she understands how evil the acts are that she is about to perform,
but her anger is stronger than her deliberations; that is, her affection
has not been made to submit and does not obey and follow reason as
it would a master, but throws off the reins and departs and disobeys
the command, the implication being that it is the action or affection
of some power other than the rational. For how could anything disobey
itself or reject itself or fail to follow itself?

All these statements are not only irreproachable; they are also 28
true, they make the proper distinctions, and they are in accord with
Plato's view. And so it is with the things he wrote in his explanation
of the second definition, in which he also mentioned the swift runners
who could not stop instantly even if they wished to do so. Here again 29
there is a clear indication of a power other than reason which causes
the affections. We could further clarify our knowledge of this if we
should discover why it is that many runners cannot stop instantly.
We could make the discovery from the very fact that this is not the 30
case with all runners, but only with those who are moving on a level
or downhill course. Persons who are running uphill do not experience
this; they come to a halt immediately when they wish to, the impli-
cation being that the impetus of the body does not carry them along
forcibly, as it did the others. For the cause of motion in them is com- 31
pound: they move on the one hand as living things moved by conation,
and on the other as inanimate bodies carried along by their weight.
Thus stones also are often carried down a mountainside, unable to
stop on the way until they reach some level or hollow ground. So this 32
example also indicates that there is a power other than reason, irra-
tional by nature, of the same description as the weight in the bodies of
animals. That this power makes them incapable of stopping when they 33
wish can be learned not only from the difference between uphill and
downhill courses, but also from the difference in motion even on level
ground. For the person who draws the weight of his body backward 34
as he runs has full control over stopping, but the person who draws it
forward is prevented by it from stopping. This is the reason why 35
everyone runs in this latter way, taught by the very nature of the
thing to use the forward imbalance to increase the speed of the motion.
Therefore, most worthy Chrysippus, as in the example those who 36
derive no advantage from their body's weight for the speed of their mo-
tion can stop at will, but for those who generate speed from both causes
the will to stop is no longer enough, so it is with conations of the soul.
When reason alone is responsible, it is in the power of reason to stop
the conation, but when some anger or desire – irrational powers, similar

ἐπιθυμία τις αὐτῷ προσέλθῃ – δυνάμεις ἄλογοί τε καὶ παραπλήσιαι τῷ
κατὰ τὸ σῶμα βάρει –, παραχρῆμα μὲν οὐχ οἷόν τε στῆναι, χρόνῳ δ' ἂν
346 37 ἴσως γένοιτο / καὶ τοῦτο καθάπερ ἐπὶ τῶν θεόντων. τὸ δ' ἴσως τῷ λόγῳ
προσέθηκα διὰ τὴν τῶν κατὰ μέρος αἰτίων ὅσα γε κινεῖ τὴν ὁρμὴν ἄνισον
δύναμιν. ἐπειδὴ γὰρ καὶ λογισμὸς αὐτὴν κινεῖ καὶ ἐπιθυμία καὶ θυμός,
ἡ μὲν ὑφ' ἑνὸς αὐτῶν συστᾶσα τῶν ἄλλων ἡσυχαζόντων ὑπ' ἐκείνου
38 μόνου δεσπόζεται. ὥστ' εἰ μὲν ὑπὸ τοῦ λογισμοῦ γένοιτο, καὶ καταπαύ-
[σ]ειν αὐτὴν καὶ αὖθις ἐπεγείρειν οἷόν τε διὰ μόνου τοῦ βουληθῆναι, εἰ δ'
ὑπὸ θυμοῦ τινος ἢ ἐπιθυμίας, ὅταν ἐκεῖνα λωφήσῃ· εἰ δ' ὑφ' ἑκατέρων
ἐνεργούντων γίγνοιτο, λογισμοῦ θ' ἅμα καί τινος ἀλόγου δυνάμεως,
εἰ μὲν οὖν ἀντισπῶντος τοῦ λογισμοῦ, κρατήσει τὸ ἰσχυρότερον, εἰ δὲ
συνεκθέοντος, οὐδέποτε παύσεται.
39 Λέγω δὲ συνεκθεῖν τῷ πάθει τὸν λογισμὸν ὅταν ἅπερ ἐκεῖνο προσ-
τάττει καὶ ὁ λογισμὸς δοξάζῃ, ὥσπερ ἐπὶ τῶν ἀκολάστων. δοξάζουσι
876 γὰρ ἀγαθὸν εἶναι μέγιστον οὗτοι τὴν ἀπόλαυσιν τῶν ἡδίστων | ἑκου-
40 σίως ἑπομένου κατὰ τὴν ψυχὴν αὐτῶν τοῦ λογισμοῦ τῇ ἐπιθυμίᾳ. ἀντι-
347 τείνειν δέ φημι τὸν / λογισμὸν τῷ πάθει μὴ δοξάζοντος μὲν τἀνθρώπου
καλὸν ἢ ἀγαθὸν εἶναι τὴν ἀπόλαυσιν τῆς προκειμένης ἡδονῆς, ἑλκο-
μένου δέ πως ἐπ' αὐτὴν διὰ τὴν τῆς ἐπιθυμητικῆς δυνάμεως ἰσχυρὰν
41 κίνησιν. ἀλλ' εἰ μὲν ὁ λογισμὸς κρατήσειεν, ἐγκρατὴς ἑαυτοῦ τε καὶ τῶν
ἑαυτοῦ παθῶν ὁ τοιοῦτος ἄνθρωπός ἐστί τε καὶ λέγεται, εἰ δ' ἐπιθυμία,
42 τοὐναντίον τῷδε πρόσρημα λαβὼν ἀκρατὴς ὀνομάζεται. ὅταν δ' ὑπὸ
τοῦ λογισμοῦ μόνου πρὸς τὴν τῶν ἡδέων ἄγηται χρῆσιν, ὁ τοιοῦτος
σώφρων καλεῖται, σκοπὸν τῆς αἱρέσεως αὐτῶν οὐ τὴν ἀπόλαυσιν ἀλλὰ
τὴν ὠφέλειαν πεποιημένος, ὥσπερ γε καὶ ἀκόλαστος ὁ πρὸς τῆς ἐπιθυ-
μίας μόνης ἀγόμενος, ἀκολουθοῦντος αὐτῇ τοῦ λόγου καθάπερ τινὸς
43 οἰκέτου. τῇ τοιαύτῃ συμπλοκῇ τῶν τὰς ὁρμὰς κινούντων αἰτίων μαρ-
τυρεῖ καὶ τὸ τοῦ Χρυσίππου παράδειγμα. τῶν μὲν γὰρ πρὸς ἄναντες
θεόντων ἡ λογικὴ μόνη δύναμις ἡγεῖται, τῶν δ' ἀκουσίως κατὰ κρημνοῦ
877 φερομένων ἡ ἄλογος, ἥνπερ δὴ τὸ βάρος τοῦ σώματος ἔφαμεν | ὑπάρ-
44 χειν, τῶν δ' ἐς τὸ κάταντες θεόντων ἀμφότεραι. οὕτω δὲ καὶ τῶν ἐφ'
348 ὁμαλοῦς εἰ πρόσω ῥέποιεν· ὡς εἴγε ἀνα/νεύοιεν ὀπίσω, θέοιε⟨ν⟩ μὲν
ἂν οὕτω γε τῶν ἑτέρων ἧττον, ἵσταιντο δ' ἂν ὁπότε βουληθεῖεν. ὥστε
οὐδὲν ἄχρι γε τῆς τῶν ὅρων ἐξηγήσεως ὁ Χρύσιππος ἐναντίον ἀπ-
εφήνατο τοῖς παλαιοῖς.
3. Ὁπόταν δ' ἐφεξῆς ἐπισκέπτηται πότερα κρίσεις τινά⟨ς⟩ ἢ κρί-
σεσιν ἑπόμενα χρὴ νομίζειν εἶναι τὰ πάθη, καθ' ἑκάτερα μὲν ἀποχωρεῖ
2 τῶν παλαιῶν, πολὺ δὲ μᾶλλον ἐν τῷ τὸ φαυλότερον ἡγεῖσθαι. καὶ γὰρ
Ζήνωνι κατά γε τοῦτο καὶ ἑαυτῷ καὶ πολλοῖς ἄλλοις μάχεται τῶν

36–248.32] Posid. fr. 34 Edelstein-Kidd **36–37]** *cf. supra*, p. 238.20–21
38–248.3] SVF I, p. 51 *cf. supra*, p. 240.5–9 *infra*, p. 292.18–20

4 γε] τὲ H: *correxi*: *del. Müller* 7 γίνοιτο *Müller* καταπαύσειν H: *corr. Kühn* 11 οὖν *inser.* M: *del. Müller, sed cf. J. D. Denniston, The Greek Particles, ed. 2, Oxford, 1954, p. 473* 12 συνεκθέοντες H: *corr. Ald.* 13 προστάττῃ H (η *in* ει *mut.*) M²: πράττῃ *Ald.*: πράττει *Kühn* 24 σκοπῶν H: *corr. Ald.* 29 ἐπὶ κρημνοῦ H: *corr. Einarson*: ἐπὶ κρημνὸν *Kühn* 32 θέοιε H: *corr. Corn.* 36 πό-τερον R *Ald.* τινὰ H: *corr. Ald.*

to weight in the body – is added to reason, it is not possible to stop instantly, although this too could perhaps be done after an interval, as with runners. I added 'perhaps' to the statement because of the 37
unequal power of the causes that move conation in particular cases. For since reason moves it, and desire and anger also (move it), the conation that arises through the agency of one of these, while the others are inactive, is controlled by that one alone. Thus if it is caused by 38
reason, it can be stopped and aroused again by a mere act of will; and if it comes from some anger or desire, it ceases when they subside. But if it is the product of the combined action of reason and some irrational power, then if reason resists, the stronger will prevail; but if reason joins forces with the irrational power, the conation will never stop.

I speak of reason joining forces with an affection when reason 39
makes its opinions conform to the demands of the affection, as is the case with the self-indulgent. These persons hold the opinion that the greatest good is the enjoyment of the pleasantest (objects), for in them the soul's reason willingly follows its desire. I speak of reason resisting 40
an affection when a person does not hold the opinion that the enjoyment of the pleasure at hand is noble and good but is somehow pulled toward the pleasure through the strong motion of the desiderative power. If reason prevails, such a man is, and is said to be, in control 41
of himself and his affections; if desire (prevails), he is described in the opposite way and is said to be incontinent. But when a person is led 42
by reason alone to the experience of pleasant things, such a person is called temperate, for he has made his aim in choosing them not the enjoyment but the benefit; and in the same way, the man who is led by desire alone is self-indulgent, his reason following his desire like a servant. Chrysippus' example also testifies to such a pairing of the 43
causes that arouse conation. When the runner runs uphill, the reasoning power alone is guiding him; when he is carried against his will down a precipice, the irrational power prevails, that is, the weight of his body, as we said; and when he runs downhill, both causes are at work. This 44
is true also of those who throw their weight forward while running on level ground; for if they leaned backward they would not run so fast as the others but they would stop when they wished. So far, then, up to and including his explanation of the definitions, Chrysippus has said nothing contrary to the ancients.

3. But when he turns next to the question whether the affections should be regarded as judgments of some kind or as following on judgments, he departs from the ancients on both points; and he departs even further by accepting the worse (of the two alternatives). In doing 2
this he contradicts Zeno and himself and many other Stoics, who

Στωϊκῶν, οἳ οὐ τὰς κρίσεις αὐτὰς τῆς ψυχῆς ἀλλὰ καὶ τὰς ἐπὶ ταύταις
ἀλόγους συστολὰς καὶ ταπεινώσεις καὶ δήξεις ἐπάρσεις τε καὶ διαχύσεις
3 ὑπολαμβάνουσιν εἶναι τὰ τῆς ψυχῆς πάθη. Ποσειδώνιος μέν γε τελέως
ἀπεχώρησεν ἀμφοτέρων τῶν δοξῶν· οὔτε γὰρ κρίσεις οὔτε ἐπιγιγνόμενα
κρίσεσιν, ἀλλ' ὑπὸ τῆς θυμοειδοῦς τε καὶ ἐπιθυμητικῆς δυνάμεως ἡγεῖται
4 γίγνεσθαι τὰ πάθη κατὰ πᾶν ἀκολουθήσας τῷ παλαιῷ λόγῳ. καὶ
878 πυνθάνεταί γε τῶν περὶ | τὸν Χρύσιππον οὐκ ὀλιγάκις ἐν τῇ Περὶ
349 παθῶν / ἑαυτοῦ πραγματείᾳ, τίς ἡ τῆς πλεοναζούσης ὁρμῆς ἐστιν αἰτία.
ὁ μὲν γὰρ λόγος οὐκ ἂν δύναιτό γε πλεονάζειν παρὰ τὰ ἑαυτοῦ πράγ-
5 ματά τε καὶ μέτρα. πρόδηλον οὖν ὡς ἑτέρα τις ἄλογός ἐστι δύναμις αἰτία
τοῦ πλεονάζεσθαι τὴν ὁρμὴν ὑπὲρ τὰ μέτρα τοῦ λόγου, καθάπερ τοῦ
πλεονάζεσθαι τὸν δρόμον ὑπὲρ τὰ μέτρα τῆς προαιρέσεως ἄλογος ἡ
αἰτία, τὸ βάρος τοῦ σώματος.
6 Ἀλλ' οὐ τοῦτο θαυμαστὸν εἰ πολλοῖς ἐναντία λέγει Χρύσιππος,
ὥσπερ οὐδ' ὅτι τῆς ἀληθείας ἀπέσφαλται – συγγνώμη γὰρ ἀνθρώπῳ
γε ὄντι καὶ ἁμαρτάνοντι –, ἀλλ' ὅτι μήτε ἐπεχείρησεν ὅλως τὰ πρὸς τῶν
παλαιῶν εἰρημένα διαλύσασθαι καὶ πρὸς αὐτὸν διαφέρεται νυνὶ μὲν
γίνεσθαι νομίζων τὰ πάθη ἄνευ λόγου καὶ κρίσεως, νυνὶ δ' οὐ μόνον
7 κρίσεσιν ἕπεσθαι φάσκων, ἀλλ' αὐτὸ δὴ τοῦτο κρίσ⟨ε⟩ις εἶναι. τὸ γὰρ
μηδ' ὅλως ἐφάπτεσθαι κρίσεως ἐναντιώτατον δήπου τῷ κρίσιν εἶναι τὸ
879 πάθος, εἰ μὴ νὴ Δία βοηθῶν τις αὐτῷ φαίη πλείω ση|μαίνειν τὸ τῆς
350 κρίσεως / ὄνομα καὶ κατὰ μὲν τὴν ἐξήγησιν τοῦ ὅρου τὴν οἷον περίσκεψιν
εἰρῆσθαι κρίσιν, ὡς εἶναι τὸ ἄνευ κρίσεως ἴσον ⟨τῷ⟩ ἄνευ περισκέψεως,
ἔνθα δὲ κρίσεις εἶναί φησι τὰ πάθη, τὰς ὁρμάς τε καὶ τὰς συγκαταθέσεις
8 ὀνομάζεσθαι κρίσεις. ἀλλ' εἴπερ τοῦτό τις δέξαιτο, πλεονάζουσα συγκα-
τάθεσις ἔσται τὸ πάθος, καὶ πάλιν ὁ Ποσειδώνιος ἐρήσεται τὴν αἰτίαν
ὑφ' ἧς πλεονάζεται, πρὸς τῷ καὶ μέγιστον ἁμάρτημα κατὰ τὴν διδασκα-
9 λίαν ἡμαρτῆσθαι τῷ Χρυσίππῳ. εἰ γὰρ ἐν αὐτῷ δὴ τούτῳ τὸ κῦρος
τοῦ δόγματός ἐστιν, ἐν τῷ διαστείλασθαι τὴν ὁμωνυμίαν καὶ δεῖξαι κατὰ
τί μὲν σημαινόμενον ἄνευ κρίσεως γίνεται τὰ πάθη, κατὰ τί δὲ κρίσεις
εἰσίν, ὁ δ' οὐδὲ καθ' ἓν τῶν τεττάρων βιβλίων ἃ Περὶ τῶν παθῶν
10 ἔγραψεν ἐποίησεν αὐτό, πῶς οὐκ ἄν τις αὐτὸν δικαίως μέμψαιτο; τάχα
μὲν γὰρ οὐδὲ βραχυλογίαν τις ἄκραν ἐζηλωκὼς ὀρθῶς ἂν ὑπερβαίνοι[το]
351 τὰ οὕτως ἀναγκαῖα, πολὺ δ' οὖν μᾶλλον / ὅταν ἐπὶ μήκιστον ἐκτείνῃ

4–6] *cf. infra*, pp. 286.8; 292.20–25 6] Posid. test. 102 Edelstein-Kidd
16–32] *cf.* SVF III, p. 115 25–27] *cf.* Reinhardt, 1921, p. 298

1 καὶ *del. Corn.* 5 *post* κρίσεσιν *add.* εἶναι *Müller* 7 τῶν] τοὺς H: *corr. Kidd* 10 *post* ἄλογός *iter. et del.* πρόδηλον – ἄλογος H 16 ἁμαρτάνειν *coniecerit Einarson* 18 καὶ *del. Müller* 19 αὐτὰ δὴ ταῦτα *Müller* κρίσις H: *corr. Ald.*: κρίσεως M 22 τὴν[II] *supra lin. inser.* C *aut* C[2] 23 ἴσον] ἢ C τῷ *add. Bake* 24 τὰ πάθη *om., ut vid.,* C ὁρμάς] δόξας *Bake* 28 ἐν αὐτῷ] . . .ὐ.ῶ C 30 κρίσεως] κρ΄. C τὰ πάθη *om., spat. 4 litt. rel.,* C 31 ὅ δ' H: *corr. Bake*: οἳ δ' C οὐδὲ *ex* οὐδὲν, *ut vid., corr.* H 32 αὐτό] α.΄. .΄ C αὐτὸν δικαίως] δικαίως α.τῶ C 33 ὑπερβαίνοιτο H C: *corr. Kühn*

do not suppose that the judgments of the soul themselves, but the
irrational contraction, abasement and affliction, and the rising up and
expansion, that attend on judgments are the affections of the soul.
Posidonius, however, completely rejected both views. He does not 3
regard the affections as judgments or as supervening on judgments,
but he holds that they are caused by the spirited and desiderative
power, thus following the ancient account in every respect. And on no 4
few occasions in his work On the Affections he asks Chrysippus,
what is the cause of excessive conation? For reason could not exceed
its own acts and measures. Thus it is evident that some other irrational 5
power causes conation to exceed the measures set by reason, just as
the cause that makes the running exceed the measures set by choice is
irrational, the weight of the body.

The surprising thing is not that Chrysippus contradicts many 6
others, or even that he has missed the truth – we pardon him for that,
as he is human and fallible –, but that he made no attempt at all to
refute the statements of the ancients, and that he contradicts himself,
holding at one time that the affections arise without reason and judg-
ment, and at another saying not only that they supervene on judg-
ments but that they actually are judgments. To state that an affec- 7
tion has nothing to do with judgment is surely the exact opposite of
stating that it is a judgment, unless indeed one might say in his defense
that the word judgment has more than one meaning, and that in his
explanation of the definition he used the word in the sense of circum-
spection, so that 'without judgment' equals 'without circumspection',
but when he says that the affections are judgments, he is using
judgment as a name for conation and assent. But if you accept this, 8
then affection will be an excessive assent, and Posidonius will again
ask what causes the excess. Chrysippus, moreover, will have made
a very great mistake in his manner of teaching. For if the crucial point 9
of the doctrine lies precisely here, in removing the ambiguity and
pointing out by which meaning (of 'judgment') affections arise without
judgment, and by which meaning they are judgments, and if Chry-
sippus did not make this point in any one of the four books he wrote
On the Affections, how would it be unjust to censure him? Perhaps 10
even a writer who aimed at extreme brevity would be wrong to omit
such necessary things; surely, then, the omission is much more culpable

τοὺς λόγους, ὥσπερ ὁ Χρύσιππος. ἀλλὰ περὶ μὲν τούτου καὶ μικρὸν
ὕστερον ἐπισκεψόμεθα. |
380 4. Περὶ δὲ τοῦ μὴ φροντίζειν τῆς πρὸς ἑαυτὸν ἐναντιολογίας αὐτὸν
ἔχων ἔτι μυρία λέγειν, ἃ τάχ' ἂν καὶ ὕστερον εἰ μακροτέρας ἐπιλαβοίμην
σχολῆς εἰς μίαν ἀθροίσαιμι πραγματείαν, ἅπαντα παραλιπὼν τἆλλα
2 μόνων τῶν οἰκείων τοῖς νῦν προκειμένοις μνημονεύσω. τὴν τοίνυν
ἐπιθυμίαν ἐν τῷ πρώτῳ Περὶ παθῶν ὁρισάμενος ὄρεξιν ἄλογον, αὐτὴν
πάλιν τὴν ὄρεξιν ἐν ἕκτῳ τῶν κατὰ γένος ὅρων ὁρμὴν λογικὴν εἶναί φησιν
ἐπί τι⟨νος⟩ ὅσον χρὴ ἥδοντος [αὐτῷ], οὕτω δὲ αὐτὴν ὁρίζεται κἀν τοῖς
Περὶ τῆς ὁρμῆς, ὥστε τὸν τῆς ἐπιθυμίας ὅρον ἀναπτυσσόμενον γίγνεσθαι
τοιοῦτον· ἐπιθυμία ἐστὶν ὁρμὴ λογικὴ ἐπί τι⟨νος⟩ ὅσον χρὴ ἥδοντος
3 [αὐτῷ], ἄλογος. ἀλλὰ τὸ μὲν ἐν διαφέρουσιν ἤτοι βιβλίοις ἢ χωρίοις βι-
βλίων ἀναισθήτως ἔχειν τῆς ἐναντιολογίας ἧττον δεινόν· ὅταν δ' ἐν
352 αὐτοῖς οἷς φθέγγεταί τις ἐναντία τε καὶ / παντοίως μαχόμενα συμπλέξῃ,
συγχεῖ καὶ ταράσσει τὴν διδασκαλίαν ἐν τῷδε καὶ πολλὴν ἀπορίαν
881 παρέχει τοῖς ἐξελέγχειν αὐτὰ πειρωμένοις, ὥσπερ ἂν εἰ καὶ | οὕτω τις
εἴποι γε, καταβὰς ἄνω καὶ διαλεχθεὶς τῷ λίθῳ καὶ πλεύσας διὰ μέσης τῆς
4 πέτρας ἀνελθεῖν εἰς τὸν βυθὸν τῆς λίμνης. ἄν τε γὰρ ὡς οὐ καταβάντα
διελέγχῃς φάσκων αὐτὸν ἄνω μεμενηκέναι [καταβάντα], τοῦτ' αὐτὸ
δήπου φήσει καὶ αὐτὸς εἰρηκέναι κατὰ τὸν λόγον ἐν τῷ προσθεῖ-
ναι τὸ ἄνω, ἄν θ' ὡς οὐδενὶ διαλεχθέντα, καὶ τοῦτ' εἰρῆσθαι φήσει,
ταὐτὸ γὰρ εἶναι τὸ λίθῳ διαλέγεσθαι τῷ μηδὲ λίθῳ, τῷ λίθῳ γὰρ
οὐδεὶς διαλέγεται, καὶ τἆλλα οὕτως ἅπαντα σοφιστικῶς ἐπανορθοῦσθαι
δυνήσεταί τις· ὥστε κατ' ἀρχὰς εὐθὺς δεῖν ἀποδρᾶναι λόγων εἶδος
τοιούτων ἐν ᾧ χρὴ τοὺς ἀκούοντας οὐχ ἃ σημαίνεται συνήθως ὑφ' ἑκά-
στου τῶν ὀνομάτων μανθάνειν, ἀλλ' ἕτερ' ἄττα.
5 Τοιοῦτον γάρ τι καὶ ὁ Χρύσιππος ἀξιώσει, ἐπειδὰν μὲν ἄνευ /
353 κρίσεως λέγῃ [τις] γίνεσθαι τὰ πάθη τῆς ψυχῆς, ἀκούειν ἡμᾶς ἀξιῶν ὅτι
μετὰ κρίσεώς τε γίνεται καὶ κρίσεις εἰσίν· ἐπειδὰν δ' ἄνευ λόγου καὶ ἄλογα,
τὸ μήτ' ἄλογα μήτ' ἐν ἀλόγῳ τινὶ δυνάμει τῆς ψυχῆς ἀλλ' ἐν τῇ λογι-
882 6 ζομένῃ καὶ λογικά, | τὸ γὰρ κρίνειν ταύτης ἔργον ὑπάρχειν· ἐπειδὰν

1–2 μικρὸν ὕστερον] *v. infra*, lin. 27–29 *cf. infra*, p. 262.29–30 3–10] *cf.* SVF III, p. 116 4–5] *cf. infra*, p. 280.18–19; PHP 596.4–6; 662.10–13 Müller 7–9] *cf. supra*, p. 238.32–33 *infra*, p. 344.1–2 8–11] *cf. supra*, p. 238.36–37 *infra*, lin. 11–12; p. 342.29–30 31–252.5] *cf.* SVF III, p. 115

1 τουˀ C: τούτων *Ald.* 3 δὲ] τε C ἀντιλοˠ' C αὐτῶν C 4 μικροτέ-
προκειμένης
ρας H 6 τοῖς νῦν προκειμένοις] τῆς νῦν πραγματείας C 9 τι H C: *correxi* ὅσον] ὡς ὧν C ἧδον H: ἤδη ὄντος C: *ex p. 342.30 correxi* αὐτῷ *del. Einarson* 10 ὥστε] ἕως τε C 11 ὁρμὴ *ex* ὁρμὴν *corr.* H τι H C: *correxi* ὅσον] ὡς ὧν C ἧδον H: ⁚.η ὀντ. . C: *ex p. 342.30 correxi* 12 αὐτῷ *del. Einarson* ἄλογος *om.* C χωρίοις] χωρὶς H βίβλων H 14 αὐτοῖς οἷς φθέγγεταί] *vestigia tantum in* C 17 εἴποι] ἤτοι C 18 ἀνελθεῖν] ἀ. . . .ει C 19 διηλέγχθης C αὐτὸν] αὐτῶ C μεμνηκέναι H: βεβηκέναι *Müller* καταβάντα H: τὰ πάντα C: *del. recens. anon.* 21 τὸ *ex* τὰ *corr.* C[2] διελέχθη H: διαλεχθῇ C: *correxi* 22 ταυτὸν C εἶναι τὸ] εἴτε τῶ C μηδὲ λίθῳ] μηδενὶ *Castiglioni* 26 μανθάνειν *om.* C ἕτερ' ἄττα] *vestigia tantum in* C 28 τις *del. Müller* 29 ἐπειδὰν] ἐπεί C 31 ἔργον ταύτης C

in a person who prolongs his account to the greatest length, as Chry-
sippus does. But we shall look into this (matter) again a little later.

4. Although I could still say thousands of things about his un-
concern at his own self-contradictions – perhaps I shall some day
collect them into a single treatise if I should get an extended period of
leisure time –, I shall now put all the rest aside and mention only what
is relevant to our present purpose. After defining desire in his first 2
book On the Affections as irrational appetition, he defines appetition
itself in the sixth of his generic definitions as 'rational conation
toward something that gives pleasure to the extent that it should';
and he defines it this way also in his work On Conation. Therefore the
definition of desire, when expanded, is this: 'Desire is an irrational
rational conation toward something that gives pleasure to the extent
that it should.' To fail to notice contradictions in different books or 3
parts of books is less serious; but when a person combines in the very
statements he is making things that are contrary and utterly incompat-
ible, he thereby confounds and disrupts the presentation and causes
great difficulty for those who try to test his statements. It is as if a
person should say "descending up", or "talking with a stone", or
"after sailing through the middle of the rock I rose to the bottom of the
lake". If you challenge him on the grounds that the man did not 4
descend, asserting that he remained up, your adversary will of course
reply that he too said exactly this by adding the word 'up' to his
statement. And if you challenge him on the grounds that the man
talked with no one, he will reply that he said this too, since talking
with a stone is the same as not talking with even a stone, for no one
talks with a stone. And a person could justify all the rest by this kind
of sophistry. Right from the start, therefore, you should avoid the
kind of statement that makes it necessary for the hearer to give to
each word a meaning other than the usual one.

Chrysippus will be making a demand of this kind when he says 5
that the affections of the soul arise without judgment but demands
that we take this to mean that they arise along with judgment and
that they are judgments; when he says that they arise without reason and
are irrational but demands that we take this to mean that they are
not irrational and do not arise in some irrational power of the soul but
arise in the reasoning power and are rational, since judgment is an
operation of the reasoning power; and when he says that they arise in 6

δ' ἀπειϑῶς τε καὶ ἀπεστραμμένως τοῦ λόγου, τὸ μηδεμίαν ἐπιζητεῖν
ἑτέραν ἐν τῇ ψυχῇ δύναμιν ἧς κινουμένης ἀπειϑῶς τῷ λόγῳ γίγνεσϑαι
τὰ πάϑη· μηδὲ γὰρ εἶναί τινα τοιαύτην, ὡς ἔνιοι τῶν φιλοσόφων ὑπο-
λαμβάνουσιν ἐπιϑυμητικήν τε καὶ ϑυμοειδῆ προσαγορεύοντες, τὸ ὅλον
7 γὰρ εἶναι τὸ τῶν ἀνϑρώπων ἡγεμονικὸν λογικόν. εἰ μὲν γὰρ εἰς πρόβλημά
τις ἀπὸ στόματος ἐπὶ καιροῦ λέγοι, κάλλιον μὲν καὶ τούτῳ διωρισμένως
τε χρῆσϑαι καὶ σαφῶς τοῖς ὀνόμασιν, ἕξει δ' οὖν ὅμως συγγνώμην
αὐτοῦ τὰ σφάλματα· τὸ δ' ἐπιστημονικὴν καὶ λογικὴν πραγματείαν
ἐπαγγειλάμενον γράφειν ἀπειϑῆ μὲν τῷ λόγῳ τινὰ κίνησιν ὀνομάζειν,
354 ἀξιοῦν δ' ἡμᾶς ἀκούειν / αὐτὴν λογικὴν ἢ ἀπεστράφϑαι μὲν τὸν λόγον,
εἶναι δ' οὐδὲν ἄλλο ἢ λόγον τε καὶ κρίσιν αὐτήν, οὐκ οἶδ' εἰ μὴ
8 τῆς μεγίστης μέμψεως ἄξιον ὑπάρχει· [ἄνϑρωπος] μὴ συγχωρῶν ἐπὶ
ταὐτοῦ λέγειν αἰσχύνεσϑαι καὶ αἰδεῖσϑαι μηδ' ἥδεσϑαι καὶ χαίρειν, ἀλλ'
383 ἀκριβοῦν ἅπαντα καὶ μέχρι | τῶν ὀνομάτων ἀξιῶν αὐτὸν ἐν τοῖς συγ-
γράμμασιν, ὃ μικρὸν ἔμπροσϑεν οὐκ ἐκ λόγου καὶ κρίσεως ἔφησε γίγνε-
σϑαι, προελϑὼν ἐν λόγῳ καὶ κρίσει συνίστασϑαί φησιν, ἑνὸν ἐκφυγεῖν μὲν
ἁπάσας τὰς οὕτως ἀκαίρους τε ἅμα καὶ παρὰ τὸ τῶν Ἑλλήνων ἔϑος
ἀναπεπλασμένας ὁμωνυμίας, ἀκριβῶσαι δὲ καὶ διαρϑρῶσαι τὸν λόγον
Ἑλληνικοῖς τε καὶ σαφέσιν ὀνόμασιν.

9 Τὸ γοῦν ἄλογον ὡσαύτως ἀφώνῳ τε καὶ ἀτραχήλῳ διχῶς ἅπαντες
ἄνϑρωποι λέγουσι καὶ τρίτον οὐδέν ἐστιν ἐπ' αὐτῶν σημαινόμενον
εὑρεῖν οὔτε παρὰ τοῖς νῦν Ἕλλησιν οὔτε παρὰ τοῖς παλαιοῖς, εἴ τι χρὴ
355 10 τεκμαίρεσϑαι τοῖς βιβλίοις αὐτῶν. ἄφω/νον δὲ δὴ πῶς λέγουσι καὶ ἀτράχη-
λον; – ἀναγκάζει γὰρ ἡμᾶς [τὰ ῥήματα] ἡ Χρυσίππειος ἑρμηνεία καὶ
ταῦτ' ἐξηγεῖσϑαι. – τὸ μὲν οἶμαι στερήσει φωνῆς ἢ τραχήλου, τὸ δὲ
11 κακώσει. εἰ μὲν γάρ τις φάσκοι τοὺς ἰχϑῦς ἀφώνους ὑπάρχειν ἢ τὰ φυτά,
τῷ μηδ' ὅλως ἔχειν φωνὴν οὕτως αὐτὰ προσαγορεύει· εἰ δέ τις ἄφωνον
εἶναι λέγοι τὸν κιϑαρῳδὸν ἢ τὸν κήρυκα, κάκωσίν τινα ἐνδείκνυται τῆς
384 φωνῆς τἀνϑρώπου· ἢ γὰρ μικρόφωνον | ἢ τραχύφωνον ἢ μελάμφωνον ἤ
τι τοιοῦτον ἕτερον εἶναί φησιν αὐτόν, οὐ μὴν παντελῶς γ' ἐστερῆσϑαι
12 φωνῆς. οὕτω δὲ καὶ ἀτραχήλους τινὰς ὀνομάζουσιν ἀνϑρώπους, οὐ μὰ
Δί' ὥσπερ τοὺς ἰχϑῦς ἀτραχήλους ἄν τις εἴποι, διότι μηδ' ὅλως αὐτοῖς
ὑπάρχει τράχηλος – οὐδεὶς γὰρ ἂν οὕτως γε ἄνϑρωπος ἀτράχηλος εἴη,
ὡς ἐστερῆσϑαι τὸ πάμπαν τραχήλου –, ἀλλὰ τῷ μικρὸν ἔχειν τὸν τράχη-
λον ὀνομάζονταί τινες οὕτως καὶ μένει κἀνταῦϑα τὰ παραπλήσια δύο

1] *cf. supra*, p. 242.18–19 12–15] SVF III, p. 107.33–35 *cf.* ibid. 20–22

1 τὸν λόγον *Diels* 2 τῇ *om.* C 3 μὴδὲν H 6 στόματος] *vestigia tantum in* C ἐπικαίρου H C: *correxi* λέγει C τούτῳ *ex* τοῦτο *corr.* H 9 ὀνο-μάζει C 10 τὸν] τῶ C 11 δ' *om.* C 12 ἄξιος *Ald.* ἄνϑρωπος *delevi*: ἄνϑρωπος ὃς *Müller*: ἄλλους γὰρ *Wilamowitz* 13 αἰσχύνεσϑαι καὶ *om.* C μήϑ' C 14 αὐτὸν (αὑ *ex* αὐ *mut.*) H C: αὐτὸς *Müller* 15 οὐκ *om.* C 16 προελϑόν C ἑνὸν ἐκφυγεῖν] ἢ :μφύειν C 18 ἀναπιμπλαμένας H: ἀναπιμπλάνειν C: *corr. Müller* 21 ἐπ' – 22 εὑρεῖν] εὑρεῖν :. ἀ. .ῶν . . .αινόμενον C 23 δή πως H C: *corr. Müller* 24 τὰ ῥήματα *del. Wilamowitz* ἡ Χρυσίππειος ἑρμηνεία] χρύσιππος ἑρμηνεῦσαι C 25 φωνῆς ἢ τραχήλου] *vestigia tantum in* C 27 προσαγορεύειν C 29 μελάμφωνον] μεγάφωνον *Corn.* 31 μὰ] .ὰ C

disobedience to reason and in rejection of it but demands that we seek no other power in the soul whose movements in disobedience to reason give rise to the affections, since there is no power of the kind posited by some philosophers when they speak of the desiderative and the spirited, inasmuch as the ruling power in men is all of it rational. Now 7
if a person speaks to a problem from memory on the spur of the moment, the better course even for him is to give clear and distinct meanings to the words he uses; his errors, however, will be pardoned. But to announce that one is writing a scientific and theoretical treatise and then to call a certain motion disobedient to reason yet demand that we take the motion to be rational, or to speak of it as rejecting reason yet demand that we take it to be nothing other than reason and judgment – I am inclined to think that such behavior deserves the severest censure: he does not allow men to use the expression 'being 8
ashamed' synonymously with 'having respect', or 'experiencing pleasure' with 'taking delight', and he demands of himself complete precision in his writings, even to the use of words; nevertheless, after saying of a thing a short time before that it does not arise from reason and judgment, he says later on that it comes to exist in reason and judgment. He could have avoided all these ambiguities, fabricated so ineptly and so contrary to Greek usage, and made his argument exact and articulate by using words correctly and clearly.

Now all men use the word *alogon* (irrational or reasonless) in two 9
senses, as they do 'voiceless' and 'neckless'. There is no third meaning to be found in addition to these among Greeks of today or of earlier times, if we are to make any inference from their books. And how do 10
they use 'voiceless' and 'neckless'? – Chrysippus' language compels us to explain these words also. – They refer, I believe, either to the absence of voice and neck, or to their impairment. If a person says that 11
fishes or plants are voiceless, he gives them this name because they have no voice at all. But if he says that a singer to the cithara or a herald is voiceless, he is indicating some impairment of the person's voice; he is saying that the person is weak-voiced or harsh-voiced or has an indistinct voice or something else of that kind, but not that he is completely without a voice. And in the same way people call some 12
men neckless, obviously not as you might call fishes neckless because they have no neck at all – no man would be neckless in the sense that he lacked a neck completely –, but some men are given this name because they have a small neck. Here too, then, the two meanings

13 σημαινόμενα καθάπερ ἐπὶ τῆς ἄφωνος προσηγορίας. οὕτω δὲ καὶ ἄπους
356 καὶ ἀσκελὴς καὶ ἀκοίλιος καὶ ἄπλευρος καὶ ἄχειρ καὶ / πάνθ' ὅσα τοιαῦτα,
ποτὲ μὲν ἀναιρούσης τῆς ᾱ φωνῆς τὸ σημαινόμενον ἑκάστου τῶν ὀνομά-
14 των οὗ προτάττεται, ποτὲ δ' οὐκ ἀναιρούσης. οὕτως εὑρίσκω καὶ τὸ
ἄλογον ὄνομα παρά τε τοῖς παλαιοῖς ἅπασιν εἰρημένον ὑπό τε τῶν νῦν
ἀνθρώπων λεγόμενον. ἐπειδὰν μὲν γὰρ ἢ τὸν ἰχθῦν τις ἢ τὸν καρκίνον
ἄλογον εἶναι φάσκῃ, παντάπασιν ἀναιρεῖ τὸ σημαινόμενον ἐκ τῆς λόγος
15 φωνῆς. ἐπειδὰν δὲ τόδε τι τὸ ὑπὸ τοῦδε λεγόμενον ἐπιμεμφόμενοι φάσκω-
385 σιν | ἄλογον, οὐχ ὡς οὐδένα λόγον ἔχον ἀλλ' ὡς μεμπτέον καὶ μοχθηρῶς
ἔχον οὕτως ὀνομάζουσιν. ἄλλο δὲ τρίτον ἢ καὶ νὴ Δία τέταρτον, ὡς
οὗτοι βιάζονται, σημαινόμενον οὐκ ἔστιν ἐν ἔθει τοῖς Ἕλλησιν, ὧν
ἐξηγεῖσθαι τὴν φωνὴν ἐπαγγέλλονται.
16 Δηλοῖ δὲ τοῦτο καὶ αὐτὸς ὁ Χρύσιππος ἐν τῇδε τῇ ῥήσει· «διὸ καὶ
οὐκ ἀπὸ τρόπου λέγεται ὑπό τινων τὸ τῆς ψυχῆς πάθος εἶναι κίνησις
17 παρὰ φύσιν, ὡς ἐπὶ φόβου ἔχει καὶ ἐπιθυμίας καὶ τῶν ὁμοίων. πᾶσαι γὰρ
357 αἱ τοιαῦται κινή/σεις τε καὶ καταστάσεις ἀπειθεῖς τε τῷ λόγῳ εἰσὶ καὶ
ἀπεστραμμέναι· καθὸ καὶ ἀλόγως φαμὲν φέρεσθαι τοὺς τοιούτους οὐχ
οἷον κακῶς ἐν τῷ διαλογίζεσθαι, ὡς ἄν τις εἴποι κατὰ τὸ ἔχειν ἐναν-
18 τίως πρὸς τὸ εὐλόγως, ἀλλὰ κατὰ τὴν τοῦ λόγου ἀποστροφήν.» ἐναργῶς
ἐν τούτοις ὁ Χρύσιππος ἐνδείκνυται τὰ δύο σημαινόμενα τῆς ἄλογον
φωνῆς, ἅπερ καὶ ὄντως ἐστὶ παρὰ τοῖς Ἕλλησι, τὸ μὲν ἕτερον ᾧ τὸ
19 εὔλογον ἐναντίον ἐστί, τὸ δ' ἕτερον ᾧ μηδὲν μέτεστι λόγου. τὸ μὲν οὖν
ἀντικείμενον τῷ εὐλόγῳ ἁμάρτημά ἐστι καὶ κρίσις μοχθηρά· τὸ δ' ἕτερον,
386 20 ὃ χωρὶς | λόγου γίγνεται παντός, ἡ κατὰ τὸ πάθος ὁρμὴ καὶ κίνησις. εἰ
δέ γε ἦν πλείω τὰ σημαινόμενα τοῦ ἄλογον ὀνόματος, οὐκ ἂν ὤκνησεν
οὐδὲ περὶ ἐκείνων εἰπεῖν ἐπιδεικνὺς ὡς οὐδὲ καθ' ἓν αὐτῶν ἄλογον
εἴρηται τὸ τῆς ψυχῆς πάθος, ἀλλὰ κατὰ μόνον ὅπερ αὐτὸς ὠνόμασε τὸ
358 21 κατὰ τὴν ἀποστροφὴν τοῦ λόγου γινόμενον. / ὅσα μὲν γάρ τις ἔκρινε
κακῶς, οὐκ ἀπέστραπται τὸν λόγον, ἀλλ' ἔσφαλται κατ' αὐτόν· ὅσαι δ'
ὁρμαὶ κατὰ θυμὸν ἢ ἐπιθυμίαν ἀποτελοῦνται μὴ προσχρώμεναι λόγῳ,
ταύτας ἀλόγους ὀνομάζει κατὰ τὸ ἕτερον τῶν σημαινομένων, ἐν ᾧ τὴν ᾱ
φωνὴν ἀποφάσκειν τε καὶ ἀναιρεῖν ἐλέγομεν τὸ σημαινόμενον τῆς μετ'
22 αὐτὸ τεταγμένης. ἡ γὰρ ἀπειθὴς λόγῳ κίνησις ψυχῆς ἄλογός ἐστι κατὰ
23 τοῦτο τὸ σημαινόμενον ἐν ᾧ τὸ μηδὲ ὅλως χρῆσθαι λόγῳ περιέχεται. ὡς
εἴγε χρώμεθα λόγῳ καὶ κατ' αὐτήν, οὐκ ὀρθῶς ὁ Χρύσιππος εἶπεν ἐν

10–19] *cf.* SVF III, p. 126 16–17] *cf. supra*, pp. 240.24; 242.18–19, 31–32 34–256.5] SVF III, pp. 126–127

3 τῆς ᾱ *om.* C 4 οὗ] οὐ C 5 ἄλογος *Müller* τοῖς *om.* C 7 λόγος] ἄλογος H 8 δὲ *om.* C 9 μοχθηρῶς] πονηρῶς H 11 ὧν] ὃ H 16 αἱ – τε[I]] *vestigia tantum in* C 17 καθ' ὃ C τοὺς *inser.* C 18 εἴποι (ε supra lin.) C 20 δύο] . . . C ἀλόγου H: ἀλό(γ)' C: *corr. Kühn*: ἄλογος *Müller* 22 *ante* λόγου *add.* τοῦ C

24 παντός] πάντως ὡς C 24–25 εἰ δέ γε] εἰ . ε δὲ C 25 ἀλό(γ) C: ἄλογος *Müller* 26 ὡς *om.* C 27 εἰρῆσθαι H C: *correxi* πάθος] ὀνό(μ) C 31 ᾱ *om.* C 33 αὐτὸ *in textu*, αὐτοῦ *supra lin.* H: αὐ(τ)' C 34 περιέχεται] ει *e corr.* H ὡς] ὥστε *Müller*

remain, similar to those of 'voiceless'. It is the same with footless, 13
legless, stomachless, ribless, handless, and all such expressions: some-
times the *a* negates the meaning of the word to which it is prefixed,
and sometimes it does not. And I find the word *alogon* (irrational) used 14
in this way by all the ancients and by men of today. When a person
says that a fish or a crab is *alogos* (irrational), he completely negates
the meaning of the word *logos* (reason); but when men criticise a partic- 15
ular statement of a particular person by saying that it is *alogon*
(irrational), they do not give it this name because it has no *logos*
(reason), but because it is blameworthy and faulty. There is no third
meaning, and indeed no fourth meaning either, as they try forcibly to
impose, in current use among the Greeks, whose speech they claim
to be expounding.

Chrysippus himself makes this clear in the following passage: 16
"Therefore some people say not inappropriately that an affection of
the soul is a movement contrary to nature, as in fear and desire and
the like. For all such movements and states are disobedient to reason 17
and reject it; accordingly we say that such persons are moved irration-
ally, not in the sense of reasoning poorly, as one might speak of a
person who reasons the opposite of well, but in the sense of rejecting
reason." Here Chrysippus clearly indicates the two meanings of 18
alogon (irrational) that actually exist in Greek usage, one the opposite
of well-reasoned, the other the complete absence of *logos* (reason). Now 19
that which is opposed to what is well reasoned is error and faulty
judgment; but the other, which takes place apart from all *logos* (reason),
is the conation and motion attendant on affection. If there were even 20
more meanings of the word *alogon* (irrational), he would not have
hesitated to speak of them also, demonstrating that no one of them is
meant when the affection of the soul is called *alogon* (irrational), but
only the meaning that he named, the irrationality that follows from
the rejection of reason. For a person's faulty judgments are not a 21
rejection of reason but a mistaken use of it; but the conations that
result from anger or desire without resort to reason he calls irrational
in the other of its meanings, that in which, as we said, the *a* denies and
negates the meaning of the word to which it is prefixed. When the 22
soul's movement disobeys reason it is *alogos* (irrational) in this latter
meaning, which includes not using reason at all. For if we use reason 23
in this movement also, Chrysippus was mistaken when he said in

τε τῷ πρώτῳ Περὶ παθῶν οὐχὶ «διημαρτημένως φέρεται καὶ παριδών τι
κατὰ τὸν λόγον», ἀλλ' «ἀπεστραμμένως τε καὶ ἀπειθῶς αὐτῷ» καὶ πάλιν
387 ἐν τῷ Θεραπευτικῷ τῶν παθῶν | αὐτὰ δὴ ταῦτα τὰ μικρῷ πρόσθεν μοι
παραγεγραμμένα διὰ τῆς ῥήσεως ἐν ᾗ τὸ μὲν ἐναντίως τῷ εὐλόγως λεγόμε-
νον ἄλογον οὐκ ἔφασκεν ἐν τῷ τοῦ πάθους ὁρισμῷ σημαίνεσθαι, θάτερον
24 δὲ τὸ ἀπειθές τε καὶ ἀπεστραμμένον τὸν λόγον. ἐπιφέρων γοῦν φησιν·
359 «οἷαι καὶ ἀκρατεῖς αἱ τοιαῦται κατα/στάσεις εἰσίν, ὡς ἂν οὐ κρατούντων
ἑαυτῶν, ἀλλ' ἐκφερομένων καθάπερ οἱ τῷ τόνῳ τρέχοντες προσεκφέ-
25 ρονται οὐ κρατοῦντες τῆς τοιαύτης κινήσεως. οἱ δὲ κατὰ τὸν λόγον
κινούμενοι ὡς ἂν ἡγεμόνα καὶ τούτῳ οἰακίζοντες, κἂν ὁποιοσοῦν ᾖ,
κρατοῦσιν ἤτοι ἀπαθεῖς εἰσι τῆς τοιαύτης κινήσεως καὶ τῶν κατ' αὐτὴν
26 ὁρμῶν.» ἐνταῦθα γὰρ πάλιν τὸ «κἂν ὁποιοσοῦν ᾖ» προσκείμενον ἐπὶ τοῦ
λόγου σαφῶς ἐνδείκνυται τὸν ἀπὸ τῶν ἁμαρτημάτων διορισμὸν τοῦ
27 πάθους. εἴτε γὰρ ὑγιὴς εἴη καὶ ἀληθὴς ὁ λόγος εἴτε μοχθηρός τε καὶ
28 ψευδής, ὁ κινούμενος κατ' αὐτὸν οὐκ ἄν ποτε γένοιτ' ἐν πάθει. κατὰ μὲν
γὰρ τὸν ἀληθῆ προσηκόντως τε καὶ κατωρθωμένως κινεῖται, κατὰ δὲ τὸν
ψευδῆ μοχθηρῶς τε καὶ διημαρτημένως. ἵνα γὰρ ὁ λόγος ἡγεμών ἐστιν,
388 29 ἡ ἀρετὴ | ἕπεται ἢ ἁμάρτημα, πάθος δ' οὐδέποτε. τὸ γοῦν οἰηθῆναι τὴν
360 ἡδονὴν ἀγαθὸν εἶναι, καθάπερ ὁ Ἐπίκουρος, ἡμαρτημένος τε / λόγος
ἐστὶ καὶ ψευδής, ἁπάσας τε τὰς ἐνεργείας καὶ κατὰ μέρος κινήσεις [ἐκ] τῆς
ψυχῆς ὅσαι τῆς ἡδονῆς ὡς τέλους στοχάζονται μοχθηρῶς, μοχθηρὰς
μὲν ἐξ ἀνάγκης ἔχει καὶ διημαρτημένας, οὐ μὴν ἤδη γέ πω καὶ πάθη· τὸ
γὰρ ἴδιον τοῦ πάθους αὐτὸ δὴ τοῦτ' ἔστι, τὸ χωρὶς λόγου κινεῖσθαι τὴν
30 ψυχήν. ὅθεν καὶ δεόντως ὁ Χρύσιππος ἔγραψεν «οἱ δὲ κατὰ λόγον
κινούμενοι ὡς ἂν ἡγεμόνα καὶ τούτῳ οἰακίζοντες» τὰς κατὰ μέρος δηλονότι
κινήσεις τῆς ψυχῆς «κρατοῦσι τῶν κατ' αὐτὰς ὁρμῶν ἀνάλογον τοῖς
περιπατοῦσιν ἀλλ' οὐχ ὑπ' αὐτῶν ἐκφέρονται βιαίως, ὥσπερ οἱ κατὰ
31 πρανοῦς θέοντες». συνάπτων γοῦν τῇ προγεγραμμένῃ ῥήσει καὶ ταυτὶ
προσγράφει· «οἱ δέ γε κατὰ λόγον κινούμενοι ὡς ἂν ἡγεμόνα καὶ τούτῳ
οἰακίζοντες καὶ ἐὰν ὁποιοσοῦν ᾖ, κρατοῦσι τῶν κινήσεων καὶ τῶν κατ'
αὐτὰς ὁρμῶν, ὥστε πεισθῆναι ἐάνπερ ἐνδεικνύηται αὐτός, παραπλησίως
389 32 τοῖς περιπατοῦσιν.» οὐκ ἀρκεσθεὶς δὲ τούτοις ἐπιφέρει· «διὸ καὶ | αἱ οὕτως
361 ἄλογοι / κινήσεις πάθη τε λέγονται καὶ παρὰ φύσιν εἶναι ἅτ' ἐκβαίνουσαι

1–2 αὐτῷ] *cf. infra*, p. 316.6–8 1–2 λόγον] *cf. supra*, p. 240.26–27 2] *cf. supra*, pp. 240.24; 242.18–19, 30–32 3–4] *cf. supra*, p. 254.17–19 7–12] SVF III, p. 127 7–9] *cf. supra*, pp. 238.16–17; 242.3–4; 244.13 *infra*, p. 276.35 9–12] *cf. infra*, lin. 24–27, 29–31 18–20] Usener, Epicurea, fr. 404 24–32] *cf. supra*, p. 242.2–4 30–258.1] SVF III, p. 127

1 *post* οὐχὶ *add.* εἰ *Müller (cf. supra, p. 242.30)* τι] τὲ H: *lect. incert.* C: *corr. Chart.* 4 παραγεγραμμένα] *vestigia tantum in* C εὐλόγω C 5 ἔφασκεν] ἔπασχεν C 6 τῶν λόγων C 7 οἷαι] ὅθεν *vel* διὸ *coni. Müller* 8 ἐκφερομένων] ομ *e corr.* H 9 τὸν *om.* C 10 τοῦ$^{\tau}$ C 11 κρατοῦσι C ἤτοι ἀπαθεῖς εἰσι *om.* C *(cf. infra, lin. 29–30)* τοιαύτης *om.* C 12 . . .κείμενον C 14 τε] γε C 15 πάθει *e ras.* C 16 κατωρθω. ! .ως C: κατορθωμένως H 18 ἡ ἀρετὴ ἕπεται *om.* C τὸ *om.* C 19 ἀγαθὸν εἶναι, καθάπερ] *vestigia tantum in C, qui his verbis des.* 20 ἐκ *del. Müller* 24 *ante* λόγον *add.* τὸν *Müller (cf. supra, lin. 9)* 29 *ante* λόγον *add.* τὸν M *Ald.* 31 ἐνδείκνυται H: *corr. Müller*

his first book On the Affections that a person is not "carried away by
error and from a misapprehension of something that is in accord with
reason", but "in a way that rejects and disobeys reason"; and again in
his book on the Cure of the Affections he was mistaken when he made
those very remarks that I quoted a short time ago from the passage in
which he said that in the definition of affection *alogon* (irrational) does
not mean the opposite of well-reasoned but has its other meaning,
that of disobeying and rejecting reason. Indeed he adds the words: 24
"Such states as these are the sort that are out of control, as if the men
had no power over themselves but were carried away, just as those
who run hard are carried along and have no control over that sort of
movement. But those who move with reason as their guide and steer 25
their course by it, no matter what the nature of the reasoning, have
control over, or are not subject to, that kind of movement and its
conations." Here again the added words "no matter what the nature 26
of the reasoning" clearly indicate the distinction made between error
and passion. Whether the reasoning be valid and true, or faulty and 27
false, the person who moves in accordance with it would never be in a
state of affection. If he is guided by true reason, his motions are 28
fitting and right; if by false, they are faulty and mistaken. For where
reason leads, virtue or error follows, but never affection. To believe, 29
like Epicurus, that pleasure is a good thing is erroneous and false
reasoning; and the actions and particular movements of his soul that
mistakenly aim at pleasure as the end are all necessarily faulty and
erroneous; but one could not go so far as to call them affections. For
the distinguishing mark of affection is precisely this, that the soul
moves without reasoning. Therefore Chrysippus wrote as he ought 30
when he said, "Those who move with reason as their guide and steer
by it" the particular movements of the soul, obviously, "have control
over the conations accompanying the movements, as walkers do, and
are not carried away forcibly by them, like those who run downhill."
Thus he appended the following words to the passage just quoted: 31
"Those who move with reason as their guide and steer their course by
it, no matter what the nature of the reasoning, have control over their
movements and the conations pertaining to them, so that they obey,
like walkers, if reason shows itself." But not content with this, he adds: 32
"Therefore the motions that are irrational in this sense are also said
to be affections and contrary to nature because they go beyond a

33 τὴν λογικὴν σύστασιν.» πῶς «οὕτως»; ἢ δηλονότι χωρὶς λόγου παντὸς
καὶ ἀπεστραμμέναι τὸν λόγον, ὃν ἡγεμόνα ἔδωκεν ἡμῖν ἡ φύσις ἁπασῶν
τῶν κατὰ μέρος ἐνεργειῶν; οὐχ ἡγεῖται δ' ἐν τοῖς πάθεσιν· ὅθεν ἐκβεβη-
κέναι φησὶ τὴν λογικὴν σύστασιν ἁπάσας τὰς κατὰ πάθος κινήσεις,
34 ὀρθότατα λέγων. εἰ γὰρ ἡ μὲν λογικὴ τοῦ ζῴου σύστασις ἡγεμόνα κέκτη-
ται τὸν λόγον, οὐ κρατεῖ δ' οὗτος οὐδ' ἡγεῖται τῶν κατὰ πάθος κινήσεων,
ἐκβέβηκε τὴν λογικὴν φύσιν ὁ κατὰ πάθος κινούμενος.
Καὶ μὴν εἴπερ οὐ λόγος ὁρμῆς ἡγεῖται, ἀποκρινάσθωσαν ἡμῖν οἱ
35 περὶ τὸν Χρύσιππον ὅ τί ποτέ ἐστι τὸ ἡγούμενον. οὐ γὰρ δὴ ἀποχρήσει
γε αὐτοῖς εἰπεῖν ὡς οὔτε λόγος οὔτε ἄλλη δύναμις οὐδεμία. συγχωροῦσι
γὰρ οὕτως ἀναίτιόν τινα κίνησιν ὃ παντὸς μᾶλλον φυλάττεσθαι παραι-
νοῦσι καὶ μέμφονταί γε τὸν Ἐπίκουρον ἐπειδάν τινα τοιαύτην ὑποτιθῆ-
36 ται. εἴπερ οὖν μηδὲν ἀναιτίως γίγνεται καὶ τοῦτ' ἔστιν ἁπάντων σχεδόν
362 390 τι τῶν / φιλοσόφων | ὁμολόγημα κοινόν, οὐ Χρυσίππου μόνον ἢ
Ἀριστοτέλους ἢ Πλάτωνος, ἀποκρινάσθωσαν ἡμῖν, ἥτις ποτ' ἐστὶν
37 αἰτία τῆς κατὰ πάθη κινήσεως. οὐ γὰρ δὴ ὁ λόγος γε νῦν ἡγεμὼν οὐδ'
αἴτιος αὐτοῖς ὑπάρχει, καθάπερ ἔν τε τοῖς ἁμαρτήμασι καὶ κατορθώμα-
σιν.
38 Ὁ μὲν οὖν Ποσειδώνιος, ὡς ἂν οἶμαι τεθραμμένος ἐν γεωμετρίᾳ
καὶ μᾶλλον τῶν ἄλλων Στωϊκῶν ἀποδείξεσιν ἕπεσθαι συνειθισμένος,
ᾐδέσθη τήν τε πρὸς τὰ σαφῶς φαινόμενα μάχην καὶ τὴν αὑτοῦ πρὸς
αὑτὸν ἐναντιολογίαν τοῦ Χρυσίππου καὶ πειρᾶται μὴ μόνον ἑαυτὸν
τοῖς Πλατωνικοῖς, ἀλλὰ καὶ τὸν Κιττιέα Ζήνωνα προσάγειν· οἱ
δ' ἄλλοι Στωϊκοὶ σχεδὸν ἅπαντες οὐκ οἶδ' ὅπως ἕπεσθαι μᾶλλον οἷς
ἐσφάλη Χρύσιππος ὑπομένουσιν ἢ τἀληθὲς αἱρεῖσθαι.
5. Καὶ οἵ γε νῦν αὐτῶν ἐνδοξότατοι πυνθανομένων ἡμῶν ἑκάστοτε
τίνα ποτὲ χρὴ τίθεσθαι τὴν αἰτίαν τῆς κατὰ τὰ πάθη κινήσεως, ἄνω μὲν
καὶ κάτω τοὺς λόγους ἑλίττουσιν, ἀποσαφοῦσι δ' οὐδέν, ἀλλ' ἐνίοτε μὲν
363 391 τὸν ἡμαρτημένον / λόγον φασὶ καὶ τὴν δόξαν τὴν ψευδῆ τῶν | κατὰ τὰ
πάθη κινήσεων αἴτιον ὑπάρχειν, δυσωπούμενοι δ' αὖθις ὑπὸ τῶν
Χρυσίππου ῥήσεων ὑποχωροῦσί τε τούτων καὶ κινήσεις τινὰς ἀναι-
τίους ὑποτίθενται καὶ μένουσιν οὐδέποτ' ἐπὶ τῶν αὐτῶν ἀποκρίσεων,
ἀλλ' Εὐρίπου δίκην ἑκάστοτε μεταρρέουσιν ἀπὸ μὲν τοῦ τὸν λόγον τε
καὶ τὴν δόξαν αἰτιᾶσθαι τῶν παθῶν ἐπὶ τὸ χωρὶς αἰτίας οὑτωσί πως
κινουμένην τὴν ψυχὴν ἐμπίπτειν τοῖς πάθεσιν, ἀπὸ δ' αὖ τῆς εἰκαίας τε
2 καὶ ἀναιτίου κινήσεως ἐπὶ τὸ λογικὰς εἶναι τὰς κινήσεις τῶν παθῶν. ὁ
γὰρ ἔλεγχος ἑκατέρων τῶν ἀποκρίσεων ἐκ προχείρου παρακείμενος οὐκ
ἐᾷ καταμένειν ἐπ' οὐδετέρας αὐτῶν ἐν μὲν τῷ τὰς κατὰ τὰ πάθη κινήσεις

19–22] Posid. test. 83 Edelstein-Kidd 22–23] Posid. test. 99 Edelstein-Kidd 23–25] Posid. test. 59 Edelstein-Kidd 27–28] *cf. supra*, p. 192.36–37 33] *v.* Gal. Meth. med. i. 4: X 35 K. UP vi. 10: III 454 K. Plat. Phaedo 90 c 5 Chalcid. In Tim. comm., p. 51.17 Waszink Müller, Beweis, p. 32

1 δηλονότι] ηλο *e corr.* H 5 ὀρθότητα H: *corr. Ald.* 6 *ante* πάθος *add.* τὸ *Ald.* 9–10 δὴ γε ἀποχρήσει αὐτοῖς H: *corr. Müller* 14 μόνου H: *corr. Ald.* 21 αὐτὴν H: *corr. Müller* 22 αὐτὸν *ex* αὐτῷ *corr.* H 27 ἄνω – 266.10 ἐμπίπτουσι *om.* H 33 εὐρίππου M

rational constitution." What does he mean by "in this sense"? Is it 33
not obviously 'apart from all reason and rejecting reason', which nature
gave us as guide of all particular actions? Reason is not the guide in
the affections; therefore he says that all the movements of affection
have gone beyond a rational constitution, and he is entirely right to
say so. For if the rational constitution of the animal possesses reason as 34
its guide, but reason does not control or guide the movements of affec-
tion, then the person moved by affection has gone beyond his rational
nature.

But if reason does not guide conation, let Chrysippus and his
followers tell us what does guide it. It will not do for them to answer 35
that neither reason nor any other power guides it, for that answer is an
admission that there is an uncaused motion, a doctrine that they
advise us to avoid at all costs; indeed they censure Epicurus for
making such an assumption. If then nothing happens without a cause, 36
and this is a point of common agreement among just about all philo-
sophers, not merely Chrysippus, Aristotle and Plato, let them
tell us what is the cause of the movement attendant on the affections.
For reason is not the guide or cause for them now, as it was in errors 37
and right actions.

Now Posidonius, a man reared in geometry, as I believe, and 38
trained beyond the other Stoics to follow demonstrative proofs, was
ashamed of Chrysippus' conflict with evident facts and of his self-contradictions; and Posidonius tries to bring not only himself but also Zeno of Citium into the company of the Platonists. Just about all the other Stoics, however, somehow consent to follow Chrysippus' errors rather than to choose the truth.

5. And the most celebrated of the Stoics of today, whenever we ask them what cause we should assign to the motion attendant on the affections, twist the arguments up and down and make nothing clear; sometimes they say that mistaken reasoning and false opinion cause the motions attendant on the affections, but at another time, put to shame by Chrysippus' words, they retreat from this position and posit certain uncaused motions. They never remain with the same answers but on every occasion they ebb and flow like the Euripus. After making reason and opinion the cause of the affections, they change to the position that when the soul moves in a certain way without a cause it falls into the affections; and again from this random and uncaused motion they return to the view that the movements
of the affections are rational. For the refutation of either answer is at 2
hand, and it allows them to persist in neither: when they claim that

ὑπὸ τοῦ λόγου γίγνεσθαι φάσκειν οὐκ ἐχόντων αὐτῶν ἁμάρτημα δια-
κρῖναι πάθους, ἐν δὲ [καὶ] τῷ καὶ τοῦτον ἀφελεῖν εἰς ἀναίτιόν τινα κίνησιν
ἐμπιπτόντων, ἐνὸν αὐτοῖς ἐξ ἑτοίμου φυγεῖν ἀμφοτέρας τὰς ἀτοπίας,
τὴν μὲν τοῦ μὴ δύνασθαι διορίσαι πάθους ἁμάρτημα χωρίζοντας τοῦ
364 λόγου τὰ πάθη, τὴν δὲ τοῦ γίνεσθαί τι χωρὶς αἰτίας / ὁμολογήσαντας
892 ἀλόγους τινὰς εἶναι δυνάμεις ἐν τῇ ψυχῇ | τῶν κατ' αὐτὴν παθῶν
αἰτίας.
3 Οὐ μόνον τοίνυν οἱ ἄλλοι, ἀλλὰ καὶ ὁ Χρύσιππος αὐτὸς ἐν τοῖς
Περὶ παθῶν συγγράμμασιν ἐπ' οὐδεμιᾶς ὁρ⟨μ⟩ίζει βεβαίως δόξης, ἀλλ'
4 ἀεὶ σαλεύει καθάπερ ἐν κλύδωνι. καὶ γὰρ καὶ χωρὶς λόγου παντὸς
γίγνεσθαί φησιν τὰ πάθη καὶ αὖθις τῆς λογικῆς εἶναι δυνάμεως μόνης,
ὥστε διὰ τοῦτο μηδὲ ἐν τοῖς ἀλόγοις ζῴοις συνίστασθαι, καὶ χωρὶς
5 κρίσεως γίνεσθαι καὶ αὖθις κρίσεις εἶναι. ἐμπίπτει δέ ποτε καὶ εἰς τὸ
φάσκειν εἰκῇ γίνεσθαι τὰς κατὰ τὰ πάθη κινήσεις, ὅπερ οὐδὲν ἄλλο
6 ἐστὶν ἢ ἀναιτίως, εἴ τις ἀκριβῶς ἐξετάζοι τὸ ῥῆμα. αἷς γοῦν ὀλίγον
ἔμπροσθεν γέγραφα ῥήσεσιν ἐφεξῆς φησιν «οἰκείως δὲ τῷ τῶν παθῶν
γένει ἀποδίδοται καὶ ἡ πτοία κατὰ τὸ ἐνσεσοβημένον τοῦτο καὶ φερόμενον
7 εἰκῇ.» ἀλλ' εἰ μὲν τὸ ἀναιτίως ⟨τὸ⟩ εἰκῇ λέγεις, ὦ Χρύσιππε, καὶ σεαυτῷ
μάχῃ καὶ Ἀριστοτέλει καὶ Πλάτωνι καὶ ταῖς ἁπάντων ἀνθρώπων
365 ἐννοίαις καὶ πολὺ / πρότερον αὐτῇ τῶν πραγμάτων τῇ φύσει μηδενὸς
ἀναιτίως γίνεσθαι δυναμένου· εἰ δὲ τὸ χωρὶς λόγου σημαίνει σοι τὸ εἰκῇ,
893 τὸ μὲν ἄλογον οὕτω | γε μετειλημμένον ἂν εἴη, τὸ δ' ἐξ ἀρχῆς ζητούμενον
8 ἔτι μένει· τὴν παράλογον ταύτην κίνησιν, τὴν ὑπὸ λόγου μὲν μὴ γινο-
μένην, ὑπ' αἰτίας δέ τινος γινομένην, ἐρωτῶμέν σε, τίς ἐδημιούργησεν
αἰτία; ἡμεῖς μὲν γάρ φαμεν ἐνίοτε μὲν τὴν θυμοειδῆ δύναμιν, ἐνίοτε δὲ τὴν
9 ἐπιθυμητικήν· σὺ δὲ οὔτε ταῦτα ὁμολογεῖς οὔτε τὴν λογικὴν εἰπεῖν
τολμᾷς, ἀλλ' εἰκῇ γίνεσθαι φήσας ἀπηλλάχθαι νομίζεις τοῦ ζητήματος,
οὐκ εἰδὼς ὅτι πᾶν ὅ τί περ ἂν εἰκῇ καὶ ἀπὸ ταὐτομάτου γίνεσθαι λέγηται
κατὰ τὴν ὡς πρὸς ἡμᾶς γνῶσιν οὕτω προσαγορεύεται, ταῖς δ' ἀληθείαις
οὐδὲν αὐτῶν οὕτω γίγνεται, καθάπερ καὶ ὁ θειότατος Ἱπποκράτης
10 εἶπεν· «ἡμῖν μὲν αὐτόματον, αἰτίᾳ δ' οὐκ αὐτόματον.» οὕτω δὲ καὶ τὸ
πλεονάζουσαν ὁρμὴν εἶναι τὸ πάθος ἐξηγούμενος ὁ Χρύσιππος ἔν τε
366 τῷ Περὶ παθῶν Ἠθικῷ κἀν τῷ πρώτῳ τῶν / λογικῶν ὑπὲρ τὴν τοῦ λόγου
συμμετρίαν γίνεσθαί φησιν τὴν ὑπερβολὴν τῆς κινήσεως, οὐ μὴν τήν γ'
11 αἰτίαν αὐτῆς προστίθησιν. ἐχρῆν δέ γε κἀνταῦθα μὴ περιπλέκειν καὶ
894 ταράττειν τὸν λόγον εἰς περιττὸν ἐκτείνοντα μῆκος, ἀλλὰ τοῦ | πλεονά-

8–18] SVF III, p. 127 12] *cf. supra*, p. 102.23–24 15–16] *cf. supra*, pp. 256.32–258.1 31] Hipp. De alim. 14: CMG I 1, p. 80.9–10 = p. 141.21–22 Joly 32–34] *cf. supra*, pp. 240.33–242.11

2 καὶ *om. Ald.* 4 χωρίζοντος M *Ald.*: *corr. Corn.* 9 ὁρίζει M *Ald.*: *corr. Müller* 12 *ante* διὰ *spat. 3 litt. in* M 16 γέγραφε M *Ald.*: *corr. Müller* εἰκείως *Ald.* 18 ἀλλ' – εἰκῇ *om.* M ἀναιτίως] ἐναντίας *Ald.*: *corr. Corn.* τὸ II *add. Kühn* 20 ἐννοίαις *ex* ἐνοίας *corr.* M 23 παράλογον] γὰρ ἄλογον *Petersen* τὴν II – μὲν] ὑπὸ λόγου μὲν τὴν M: ὑπὸ λόγου μὲν *Ald.*: *corr. Einarson* 24 ὑπ' – γινομένην *om.* M 25 αἰτία *ex* αἰτίαν *corr.* M 31 αὐτόματοι ... αὐτόματοι *Müller* αἰτίῃ *Müller*: ἐτεῇ *Bywater* 33 κἂν *Ald.*

the movements of the affections are produced by reason, they cannot distinguish error from affection; and when they remove reason as the cause, they are driven to the view that some motion is uncaused. Yet the way was open to them to escape both absurdities, the absurdity of being unable to distinguish error from affection by separating affections from reason, and the absurdity of saying that something happens without a cause by admitting that certain irrational powers in the soul are the causes of its affections.

Not only the others, but Chrysippus himself in his treatise On 3
the Affections also fails to anchor firmly to any one doctrine; he tosses
continually as on a stormy sea. He says that the affections arise apart 4
from all reason, and again that they pertain to the rational power
only, and that is why they do not occur in irrational animals. He says
that they arise apart from judgment, and again that they are judg-
ments. And sometimes he falls into the assertion that the movements 5
of the affections happen 'at random', which is not different from 'un-
caused', if one give the expression its exact meaning. Thus, directly 6
after the passages that I quoted a short time ago, he says: "'Flutter-
ing' too has been appropriately used to characterize the affections as a
class in respect of this 'being ruffled' and 'moving at random'." If 7
by 'random', Chrysippus, you mean 'uncaused', you are in
conflict with yourself and Aristotle and Plato and the notions of
all men, and long before that you are in conflict with the very nature
of things, since nothing can happen without a cause. But if by 'ran-
dom' you mean 'apart from reason', irrationality would thereby be
given a place alongside rationality, and the original question remains
unanswered: this strange motion, which does not arise through the 8
agency of reason yet has some cause – what cause, we ask you, pro-
duced it? Our answer is that the cause is sometimes the spirited power,
sometimes the desiderative. But you neither agree to this nor make 9
bold to assert that its cause is the rational power, but you say that it
occurs at random and think you have got rid of the question. You do
not know that whatever is said to happen at random or spontaneously
is so described with reference to the knowledge that we have of it; in
reality none of these things happens in this way, as the most divine
Hippocrates said: "Spontaneous with reference to us, but with
reference to cause, not spontaneous." Thus when Chrysippus in his 10
Ethics of the Affections and in the first of his theoretical books ex-
plains the definition of affection as excessive conation, he says that
the excess of motion goes beyond the measure that accords with
reason, but he does not add the cause of this excess. And here again 11
he should not have complicated and confused the account by extending
it to excessive length; he should have put an end to it by stating the

12 ζεσθαι τὴν ὁρμὴν εἰπόντα τὴν αἰτίαν ἀπηλλάχθαι. ὡς γὰρ ἐπὶ τῶν εἰς
τὸ κάταντες θεόντων ἅμα τῇ βουλήσει τὸ βάρος τοῦ σώματος αἴτιον
ὑπάρχει τῆς κινήσεως, οὕτως ἐν τοῖς τῆς ψυχῆς πάθεσιν ὅ τί ποτ' ἄλλο
τῇ λογικῇ δυνάμει προσιὸν αἴτιον γίνεται τῆς ἀμέτρου καὶ ὡς αὐτὸς
13 εἴωθεν ὀνομάζειν ἐκφόρου κινήσεως, ἐχρῆν αὐτὸν διελθεῖν. ἡ δ' οὖν
ῥῆσις ἡ κατὰ τὸ Θεραπευτικὸν τῶν παθῶν βιβλίον ὧδ' ἔχει· «οἰκείως
δὲ καὶ ὁρμὴ πλεονάζουσα λέγεται εἶναι τὸ πάθος, ὡς ἄν τις ἐπὶ τῶν
ἐκφερομένων κινήσεων πλεονάζουσαν κίνησιν εἴποι, τοῦ πλεονασμοῦ ἐν
αὐτῇ γινομένου κατὰ τὴν τοῦ λόγου ἀποστροφήν, καὶ τὸ ἄνευ τοῦ
14 πλεονασμοῦ τούτου σωστικόν. ὑπερβαίνουσα γὰρ τὸν λόγον ἡ ὁρμὴ καὶ
367 παρὰ / τοῦτον ἀθρόως φερομένη οἰκείως τ' ἂν πλεονάζειν ῥηθείη καὶ κατὰ
τοῦτο παρὰ φύσιν γίγνεσθαι καὶ εἶναι ἄλογος, ὡς ὑπογράφομεν.»
15 «ὑπερβαίνουσα», φησί, «τὸν λόγον ἡ ὁρμὴ καὶ παρὰ τοῦτον ἀθρόως φερο-
μένη» τὴν κατὰ τὸ πάθος ἔκφορον ἀπεργάζεται κίνησιν. οὔκουν ὁ λόγος
395 16 αἴτιος ὦ Χρύσιππε τῆς ἐκφόρου τε καὶ | ἀμέτρου κινήσεως. αὐτὸς γὰρ
ὁμολογεῖς αὐτὴν γίνεσθαι παρὰ τὸν λόγον· οὐκ ἐγχωρεῖ δ' ἅμα τε παρὰ
τὸν λόγον γίνεσθαί τι καὶ ὑπὸ τοῦ λόγου· πάντως δ' ὑπό τινος αἰτίας·
οὐκ ἔστι δ' ἐκείνη λογική· ἄλογος ἄρα τις ἡ τὸ πάθος ἐργαζομένη δύναμις.
17 καὶ «τάδ' οὐχ ὑπ' ἄλλων, ἀλλὰ τοῖς αὐτῶν πτεροῖς ἁλισκόμε⟨σ⟩θα»,
καίτοι γ' ἐνὸν ἡμῖν λέγειν, ὦ γενναιότατε Χρύσιππε, δυοῖν θάτερον,
ἢ ὡς οὐδὲν διαφέρει πάθος ἁμαρτήματος ἢ ὡς ἐπιγίνεται τοῖς ἁμαρτήμασι
τὰ πάθη· τούτων γὰρ ὁποτερονοῦν εἰπόντες οὐκ ἂν ἠναγκαζόμεθα τὴν
18 αἰτίαν ἀποκρίνεσθαι τῆς παρὰ τὸν λόγον ἀμέτρου κινήσεως. ἀλλὰ τού-/
368 των μὲν οὐδέτερον ὑπέμεινας εἰπεῖν αἰδούμενος ἐναντία λέγειν τοῖς ἐναρ-
γῶς φαινομένοις, αὐτὸς δὲ πρὸς αὑτὸν ἐναντιολογούμενος οὐκ αἰσθάνῃ
παρὰ τὸν λόγον γίνεσθαι φάσκων τινὰς κινήσεις καὶ ἀπεστράφθαι τὸν
λόγον καὶ ἀφηνιάζειν αὐτὸν κἄπειτα μικρὸν ὕστερον τὰς αὐτὰς ταύτας
ὑπὸ λογικῆς γίνεσθαι δυνάμεως φάσκων.
19 Ἡ δ' αὐτὴ μάχη κἀν [ἐν] τῷ κρίσεις τε φάσκειν εἶναι τὰ πάθη τῆς
396 20 ψυχῆς καὶ χωρὶς κρίσεως | γίνεσθαι. τὴν μὲν οὖν ἐκ τοῦ πρώτου Περὶ
παθῶν ῥῆσιν, ἔνθα φησὶ χωρὶς κρίσεως γίνεσθαι τὰ πάθη, παρεθέμην
ἔμπροσθεν. ὅτι δὲ καὶ κατὰ τὸ Θεραπευτικὸν αὐτοῦ βιβλίον, ὃ δὴ καὶ
Ἠθικὸν ἐπιγράφεται, τῆς αὐτῆς δόξης ἔχεται, μαθεῖν ἔνεστιν ἐκ τῆσδε
21 τῆς ῥήσεως· «οὐ γὰρ ἐν τῷ κρίνειν ἀγαθὰ ἕκαστα τούτων λέγεται ἀρ-
ρωστήματα ταῦτα, ἀλλὰ καὶ κατὰ τὸ ἐπὶ πλέον ἐκπεπτωκέναι πρὸς

1–3] *cf. supra*, p. 244.22–24, 36–38 4–12] SVF III, p. 130 4–5] *cf. comm. ad* p. 238.16–17 19] Aesch. Myrmid. fr. 139 Nauck = 231 Mette 20] *cf. supra*, p. 244.35–36 21–22] *cf. supra*, p. 238.20–21 29–30] *cf. supra*, p. 248.19–21 30–264.1] SVF III, p. 130 *cf.* Pohlenz, 1898, p. 545 31–32] *cf. supra*, p. 240.15–16, 25–26 32–33] *cf. supra*, p. 238.4–7

6 χρῆσις M: *corr.* R² *Ald.* 9 *ante* καὶ *add.* ὡς *v. Arnim* 11 παρὰ] περὶ M 19 τάδ'] τάχ' M *Ald.*: *corr. Cobet* αὐτῶν M *Ald.*: *corr. Kühn* πτεροῖς] πικροῖς M *Ald.*: *corr. Kühn* ἁλισκόμεθα M *Ald.*: *corr. Cobet* 20 λέγειν *ex* λέγει *corr.* M² 21 ἢ[I]] ἡ *Ald.* διαφέροι M *Ald.*: *corr. Chart.* ὡς[II]] ὧς *Ald.* 22 ἂν *om. Kühn* ἀναγκαζόμεθα *Ald.* 23 *post* αἰτίαν *add.* οὐκ *Ald.* 25 αὑτὸν] αὐτὸν M 29 κἀν ἐν M *Ald.*: *corr. Müller* 32 αὑτοῦ *Kühn* 33 ἔνεστιν] ἐστιν *Ald.*: ἔστιν *Kühn* 35 καὶ *om. Ald.* τὸ] τὰ *Ald.*

cause that makes the conation excessive. For as when persons run 12
downhill the weight of their bodies together with their volition is the
cause of their motion, so in the affections of the soul he should have
explained what that other thing is which, on being added to the
rational power, becomes the cause of the immoderate and, as he
habitually calls it, runaway motion. At all events, the passage in his 13
Cure of the Affections is as follows: "And affection is also appropri-
ately called excessive conation, as one might say of a runaway motion
that it is an excessive motion, the excess in it arising along with the
rejection of reason, and what is without excess is preservative of
reason. For conation that goes beyond reason and moves in a rush 14
contrary to reason would appropriately be said to be excessive and in
this respect to arise unnaturally and to be irrational, as we indicate."
"Conation", he says, "that goes beyond reason and moves in a rush 15
contrary to reason" produces the runaway motion of affection. There-
fore, Chrysippus, reason is not the cause of the runaway and immod-
erate motion. You yourself agree that it arises contrary to reason; it 16
is not admissible that something arise both contrary to reason and by
the agency of reason; but (it must) by all means (arise) from some
cause; that cause is not rational; therefore it is some irrational power
that produces affection. "Indeed we are caught, not by others, but by 17
our own feathers", even though, most worthy Chrysippus, either
of two statements was open to us: that there is no difference between
affection and error, or that affections supervene on errors; for if we
had made the one statement or the other, we would not be forced to
account for the cause of the motion that is contrary to reason and
immoderate. You could not bring yourself to make either of these 18
statements, for fear of contradicting obvious facts; but you do not
see that you are contradicting yourself when you say that certain
motions arise contrary to reason and that they reject reason and
rebel against it, and then say a little later that these same motions
arise by the agency of a rational power.

There is the same conflict also in his asserting that the affections 19
of the soul are judgments, and that they arise apart from judgment.
I have already quoted the passage from the first book On the Affec- 20
tions in which he says that the affections arise apart from judgment.
That he holds to the same view in his Cure of the Affections, which is
also called the Ethics, can be learned from this passage: "For we do 21
not speak of these infirmities as being in the judgment that each of
these things is good, but in also being drawn to them in excess of what

22 ταῦτα τοῦ κατὰ φύσιν.» ἴσως δ' ἂν τινος «ἐν τῇδε τῇ ῥήσει» λέγοντος
«οὐκ ἀπεστέρηκε μὲν τοῦ κρίσιν εἶναι τὸ ἀρρώστημα, οὐ μὴν ἐν αὐτῇ γε
369 μόνῃ τῇ ψευδεῖ κρίσει τὴν γένεσιν αὐτοῦ τίθεται, / ἀλλὰ προσέρχεσθαί
φησι τὸ ἐπὶ πλέον,» ἐκ τῶν ἐπιφερομένων ἡ γνώμη τοῦ Χρυσίππου
καταφανήσεται «ὅθεν οὐκ ἀλόγως γυναικομανεῖς τινες λέγονται καὶ
23 ὀρνιθομανεῖς». εἰ γὰρ δὴ μὴ μάτην ἐγκείσεται τὸ τῆς μανίας ὄνομα τῷ τοῦ
ἀρρωστήματος προσρήματι, μανία δ' ὑπὸ τῆς ἀλόγου κατὰ τὸ σῶμα
γίνεται δυνάμεως, οὐδὲν ἧττον τῶν ἀρρωστημάτων λογικόν.
397 24 Ἀλλὰ νὴ Δί' ἴσως ἄν τις φήσειε | τὸ μανιῶδες οὐ διὰ τὴν ἄλογον
γίνεσθαι δύναμιν, ἀλλὰ διὰ τὸ ἐπὶ πλέον ἢ προσῆκεν ἐξῆχθαι τήν τε
κρίσιν καὶ τὴν δόξαν, ὡς εἰ καὶ οὕτως ἔλεγεν, ἀρρωστήματα γίνεσθαι
κατὰ τὴν ψυχὴν οὐχ ἁπλῶς τῷ ψευδῶς ὑπειληφέναι περί τινων ὡς
25 ἀγαθῶν ἢ κακῶν, ἀλλὰ τῷ μέγιστα νομίζειν αὐτά· μηδέπω γὰρ ἀρρώστημα τὴν περὶ τῶν χρημάτων εἶναι δόξαν ὡς ἀγαθῶν, ἀλλ' ἐπειδάν τις
αὐτὰ μέγιστον ἀγαθὸν εἶναι νομίζῃ καὶ μηδὲ ζῆν ἄξιον ὑπολαμβάνῃ τῷ
στερηθέντι χρημάτων· ἐν τούτῳ γὰρ συνίστασθαι τήν τε φιλοχρηματίαν
370 26 καὶ τὴν φιλαργυρίαν ἀρρω/στήματα οὔσας. ἀλλὰ τῷ ταῦτα φάσκοντι
Ποσειδώνιος ἀντιλέγων ὧδέ πώς φησι· «τοιούτων δ' ὑπὸ τοῦ Χρυσίππου λεγομένων διαπορήσειεν ἄν τις πρῶτον μὲν πῶς οἱ σοφοὶ μέγιστα
καὶ ἀνυπέρβλητα νομίζοντες εἶναι ἀγαθὰ τὰ καλὰ πάντα οὐκ ἐμπαθῶς
κινοῦνται ὑπ' αὐτῶν ἐπιθυμοῦντές τε ὧν ὀρέγονται καὶ περιχαρεῖς
27 γινόμενοι ἐπὶ τοῖς αὐτοῖς ὅταν τύχωσιν αὐτῶν. εἰ γὰρ τὸ μέγεθος τῶν
398 φαινομένων ἀγαθῶν ἢ κακῶν κινεῖ τὸ νομί|ζειν καθῆκον καὶ κατ' ἀξίαν
εἶναι παρόντων αὐτῶν ἢ παραγινομένων ⟨ἐμπαθῶς κινεῖσθαι⟩ καὶ
μηδένα λόγον προσίεσθαι περὶ τοῦ ἄλλως δεῖν ὑπ' αὐτῶν κινεῖσθαι, τοὺς
ἀνυπέρβλητα νομίζοντας εἶναι τὰ περὶ αὐτοὺς τοῦτ' ἔδει πάσχειν,
28 ὅπερ οὐχ ὁρᾶται γινόμενον. ὁμοίως δὲ καὶ εἰς τοὺς προκόπτοντας καὶ
μεγάλας βλάβας ὑπὸ τῆς κακίας ὑπολαμβάνοντας παρεῖναι· ἔδει δὲ καὶ
ὑποφέρεσθαι φόβοις καὶ λύπαις περιπίπτειν μὴ μετρίαις, ὅπερ οὐδ' αὐτὸ
371 29 συμβαίνει.» τούτοις δ'/ ἐφεξῆς ὁ Ποσειδώνιος καὶ τάδε γράφει· «εἴ τε

4–6] SVF III, p. 130 *cf.* SVF III, p. 167 9–270.8] Posid. fr. 164 Edelstein-Kidd 9–19] SVF III, p. 130 9–16] *cf.* Hirzel, Unters. III, p. 462 n. 14–16] *cf.* Aristoph. Nubes 1074 17–30] *cf.* Hirzel, Unters. III, p. 435 Reinhardt, 1921, pp. 278–279 18–266.21] Pohlenz, 1898, pp. 613–614 *cf.* ibid., pp. 545–547 19–22] *cf.* Philod. De ira, ed. Wilke, p. XXVI Edelstein, 1936, p. 311 22–24] Pohlenz, 1906, p. 333 24–25] Pohlenz, 1906, p. 336 27–30] *cf. infra*, pp. 282.3–5; 332.2–4 Edelstein, 1936, p. 311 30–266.21] *cf.* Reinhardt, 1921, pp. 281–284

1 λέξοντος M *Ald.*: *corr.* R^2 (γ *in ras.*): λέξαντος *Kühn* 3 ψευδῆ M: *corr.* R^2 *Ald.* 6 ἐγγείσεται M 7 προσαρτήματι M *Ald.*: *corr. Schöne* 8 ἧττον] ἧττον ἢ *Ricci*: ἥπται *Müller* τὸ ἀρρώστημα τῶν λογικῶν M *Ald.*: *corr. Einarson* 12 περί τινων] περίτιμον M 14 ἐπεὶ δὴ (η *e corr.*) δάν M 15 νομίζοι (*ex* νομίζειν *supra lin. corr.*) M *Ald.*: *corr. Kühn* ὑπολαμβάνοι M *Ald.*: *corr. Kühn* 18 ποσειδόνιος *ex* ποσειδόνειος *mut.* M 19 μέγιστοι M: μέγιγα *Ald.*: *corr. Bas.* 20 ἐμπαθῶν M 22 γενόμενοι *Hirzel* 24 ἐμπαθῶς κινεῖσθαι *addidi*: ἐν πάθει γίνεσθαι *add. Pohlenz* 26 αὐτούς (-οὺς *Ald.*) M *Ald.*: *corr. Bake* 27 εἰς *del. Müller* καὶ[II] *scr. Einarson*: ἢ M *Ald.*: *del. Müller* 28 ὑπολαμβάνονται R: ὑπολαμβάνοντες *Bake* δὲ *del. Müller*

is natural." If someone should perhaps remark, "In this passage 22
Chrysippus has not denied to infirmity its being a judgment; rather,
he does not place its origin in the false judgment alone but says that
excess is also present", Chrysippus' opinion will become completely
clear in the words that follow: "And therefore it is not unreasonable
that some are called 'woman-mad' and 'bird-mad'." If the inclusion 23
of 'mad' in the name of the infirmity is not to be meaningless, and if
madness arises by the agency of the irrational power in the body,
nothing is less rational than infirmities.

Perhaps someone may protest that the madness does not arise 24
because of the irrational power but because the judgment and the
opinion have gone beyond what is fitting, as if he said that infirmities
arise in the soul not simply from the false supposition about something,
that it is good or evil, but from the supposition that it is the greatest
(good or evil); the opinion about money, that it is good, is not yet an 25
infirmity, but it becomes an infirmity when one holds that money is
the greatest good and even supposes that life is not worth living for
the man who has lost it: this constitutes 'love of money' and 'love of
wealth', which are infirmities. Posidonius answers this objection in 26
the following way: "On this interpretation of Chrysippus' words one
might first raise the question how it is that wise men, who hold that all
honorable things are good to the highest degree and unsurpassed, are
not moved affectively by them, desiring the things they seek and
taking excessive delight in these same things whenever they obtain
them. For if the magnitude of apparent goods or evils moves one to 27
believe that it is proper and in accordance with one's estimate of them
to be moved affectively when they are present or approaching and to
accept no reasoning that says one should be moved by them in another
way, then the persons who think that the good they enjoy is unsurpas-
sed ought to have been thus affected; but we observe that this does
not happen. There is a similar difficulty in the case of those who are 28
making progress and who suppose that their vice brings them great
harm: they ought to have been carried away by fear and to have fallen
victim to immoderate distress, but this too does not happen." After 29
this Posidonius writes as follows: "And if they should say that in

πρὸς τῷ μεγέθει τῶν φαινομένων καὶ τὴν ἀσθένειαν τῆς ψυχῆς αἰτιάσοιντο
καὶ διὰ τοῦτο τοὺς μὲν σοφοὺς τὸ παράπαν ἐροῦσιν ἀπηλλάχθαι τῶν
παθῶν, τοὺς δὲ φαύλους, ὅταν ἀσθενεῖς ὦσι μὴ κατὰ τὴν κοινὴν ἀσθένειαν
ἀλλὰ κατὰ τὴν ἐπὶ πλεῖον ἐρρυηκυῖαν, ⟨οὔ⟩, οὐδ' οὕτως λέλυται τὸ
30 ζητούμενον. ὅτι γὰρ διὰ τὴν νόσον τῆς ψυχῆς ἐν τοῖς πάθεσι γίνονται,
πάντες ὁμολογοῦσι· πῶς μέντοι γε κινηθείσης καὶ πῶς κινούσης ζητεῖται
31 μέν, οὐχ ὑποδείκνυται δέ.» εἶτ' ἐφεξῆς καὶ τάδε γράφει· «οὐ μόνον δ' οἱ
399 ἐπὶ πλέον ἐρρυηκυῖαν ἔχοντες τὴν κακίαν | καὶ ἐν ταῖς εὐεμπτωσίαις
ὄντες ἐμπίπτουσιν εἰς τὰ πάθη ἀλλὰ πάντες οἱ ἄφρονες ἕως ἂν ἔχωσι τὴν
32 κακίαν καὶ εἰς μεγάλα πάθη καὶ εἰς μικρὰ ἐμπίπτουσι.» καὶ τούτων ἑξῆς
τάδε· «τὸ δ' ὑπολαμβάνειν κατ' ἀξίαν [εἶναι] τῶν συμβεβηκότων οὕτως
372 κεκινῆσθαι, ὥστε ἀποστρέφεσθαι τὸν / λόγον μέγα πάθος ἐμφαίνει, οὐ
καλῶς ὑπολαμβάνειν ἐστί· γίνεται δὲ καὶ διὰ σύμμετρον καὶ μικρόν.»
33 ἐχόμενα δὲ τούτων ὁ Ποσειδώνιος καὶ τάδε γράφει· «δυοῖν τε τὴν
αὐτὴν ἀσθένειαν ἐχόντων καὶ τὴν ὁμοίαν λαμβανόντων φαντασίαν
ἀγαθοῦ ἢ κακοῦ ὁ μὲν ἐν πάθει γίνεται, ὁ δὲ οὔ, καὶ ὁ μὲν ἧττον, ὁ δὲ
μᾶλλον, καὶ ἐνίοτε ὁ ἀσθενέστερος μεῖζον ὑπολαμβάνων τὸ προσπεπτω-
κὸς οὐ κινεῖται· καὶ ὁ αὐτὸς ἐπὶ τοῖς αὐτοῖς ὁτὲ μὲν ἐν πάθεσι γίνεται,
34 ἔστιν ὅτε δ' οὔ, καὶ ὁτὲ μὲν μᾶλλον, ὁτὲ δ' ἧττον. οἱ γοῦν ἀήθεις μᾶλλον
πάσχουσιν ἐν φόβοις, ἐν λύπαις, ἐν ἐπιθυμίαις, ἐν ἡδοναῖς, καὶ οἱ κακώτεροι
συναρπάζονται ταχέως ὑπὸ τῶν παθῶν.»

35 Ἐφεξῆς δὲ τούτων ὁ Ποσειδώνιος ῥήσεις τε ποιητικὰς παρα-
τίθεται καὶ ἱστορίας παλαιῶν πράξεων μαρτυρούσας οἷς λέγει. καὶ μετὰ
400 ταῦτα | ἐπιφέρων φησί· «τὸ μὲν ἄρα κακὸν ὑπὸ τοῦ ἀσυνήθους ταχὺ
συναρπάζεται, τὸ δ' ἐναντίως ἡγμένον χρόνῳ μετασυνεθιζόμενον· ἐν
373 οἷς αἱ μὲν ὑπολήψεις ἴσαι πολλάκις / καὶ τὰ τῆς ἀσθενείας, τὰ πάθη δ'
36 οὔτ' ἐπίσης οὔτε ἴσα γίγνεται.» καὶ μὴν καὶ τούτων ἑξῆς τοιάσδε τινὰς
ἐρωτήσεις ἐρωτᾷ· παραγράψω δὲ καὶ ταύτας αὐτοῖς ὀνόμασι, κἂν μα-
κρότεραί πως αἱ ῥήσεις ὦσι· «διὰ τί δέ τινες τῶν μεγάλα νομιζόντων
καίπερ ἀσθενεῖς ὄντες ταῖς γνώμαις βουλεύονταί τε καὶ συμφράδμονας
37 ἄλλους παραλαμβάνουσιν, ὡς ὁ διαγρυπνῶν Ἀγαμέμνων; οὗτος γὰρ

14–19] *cf.* Philod. De ira, ed. Wilke, p. XXVI 22–270.3] Pohlenz, 1898, pp. 614–615 *cf.* ibid., pp. 547; 551 Reinhardt, 1921, pp. 285–286 22–23] Posid. test. 104 Edelstein-Kidd 30 συμφράδμονας] *cf.* Hom. Il. ii. 372 31] Hom. Il. x. 1–4

1 αἰτοιάσοιντο M: αἰτιάσονται *Müller* 3 *post* φαύλους *add.* οὐκ ἀπηλλάχθαι *vel* ἐν τοῖς πάθεσι γίνεσθαι *Müller*, εὐεμπτώτους εἶναι *Pohlenz* ὅτε M *Ald.*: *corr. Pohlenz*: ὅτι R ἀσθενεῖς *e corr.* R: ἀσθενὲς M ὦσι] ζῶσι *Müller* 4 ἐρρυκυῖαν *Ald.* οὐ *add. Einarson* 8 ἐρρυκυῖαν *Ald.* 9 βάθη M 11 εἶναι *delevi* 12 κεκινεῖσθαι H: *corr. Bas.*: γε κινεῖσθαι R *post* μέγα *add.* δὲ *Bake*, μὲν *Wyttenbach* ἐμφαίνειν *Bake* 12–13 οὐ καλῶς] καὶ οὐχ ἁπλῶς *Pohlenz*: οὐ καλῶς δὲ *Wyttenbach*: οὐκ ἄλλως *Reinhardt* 18 πάθει *Bake* 19 ὁτὲ . . . ὁτὲ] ὅτε . . . ὅτε H: *corr. Kühn* οὖν H: *corr. Müller* 20 *ante* καὶ *add.* εἰ *Pohlenz* 24 *ante* ταχὺ *add. et del.* φησὶ H 25 συναρπάζει *maluerit Müller* τὸ δ'] τότ' H: *corr. Bake* ἡγμένον] ἡγημένον *Corn.*: ἢ γενόμενον *Pohlenz* *post* χρόνῳ *add.* ἢ *Pohlenz* *post* μετασυνεθιζόμενον *lac. pos. Wyttenbach* 29 με^γλ' H: μεγάλων M *Ald.*: *corr. Corn.*: μεγάλα κακὰ παρεῖναι *Petersen* νομιζομένων *Bake*

addition to the magnitude of the apparent good or evil, weakness of
soul is also to blame, and for that reason the wise are completely rid
of the affections, but inferior men, when their weakness is not a weak-
ness of the ordinary kind but one that has gone to extremes, are not,
even so the problem is not resolved. For all agree that men fall into 30
affections because of sickness of soul; but the question asked is how
the soul has been moved and what motion it causes, and that question
is not answered." His next words are: "But not only those who have 31
a vice that has gone to extremes and who fall easily into affections,
but all unwise men, so long as they have their vice, fall into affections
both great and small." And he continues, "To suppose that a person 32
has been moved in this way in accordance with his estimate of events,
so that the rejection of reason indicates a great affection, is to suppose
wrongly; for this happens also through a moderate and a small
(affection)." After this Posidonius writes the following: "When two 33
persons have the same weakness and receive a like impression of
good or evil, one is moved affectively, the other not; and one (is
moved) more, the other less. And sometimes the weaker (of two
persons), who supposes that what has befallen him is greater, is not
moved. And the same person is sometimes moved affectively, some-
times not, at the same things, and sometimes more, sometimes less.
Thus those who are unused (to a thing) are more greatly affected in 34
situations of fear, distress, desire and pleasure; and the more vicious
are quickly seized by their affections."

Posidonius next presents quotations from the poets and histor- 35
ical accounts of ancient exploits which testify to his statements. And
after that he adds: "So what is evil is quickly seized by an unaccusto-
med thing, but what is given the opposite evaluation is seized only
when its habituation is changed in the course of time; in these cases
the suppositions held are often equal, and so is the degree of infirmity,
but the affections do not arise equally and are not equal." Thereupon 36
he poses questions such as the following; I shall quote them in his own
words, even though the passages are rather long: "Why is it that some
who believe that what is happening is of great import, even though
they are infirm in judgment, nevertheless deliberate and call on others
to advise them, as sleepless Agamemnon did? Because of the rout 37

διὰ τὴν τροπὴν εὐϑὺς ἅμα τοῖς ἄλλοις ἀριστεῦσιν ἀρρήτῳ τινὶ πένϑει
βέβλητο κατὰ τὸν ποιητήν. λωφήσαντος δὲ τοῦ πάϑους καίπερ τῆς
τῶν συμβεβηκότων ὑπολήψεως ἅμα τῇ τῶν λογισμῶν ἀσϑενείᾳ δια-
μενούσης οὐδαμῶς ἡσυχάζειν ἐδοκίμαζεν·

38 ‘ἥδε δέ οἱ κατὰ ϑυμὸν ἀρίστη φαίνετο βουλή,
Νέστορ' ἐπὶ πρῶτον Νηλήϊον ἐλϑέμεν ἀνδρῶν, /
374 εἴ τινά οἱ σὺν μῆτιν ἀμύμονα τεκτήναιτο,
ἥτις ἀλεξίκακος πᾶσι⟨ν⟩ Δαναοῖσι γένοιτο.’ |

401 39 ἐπεὶ δὲ καὶ αὐτὸς ὁ Νέστωρ ϑεασάμενος διὰ τῆς ὄρφνης πόρρωϑεν
προσιόντα τίς ἐστιν ἐπερωτᾷ, δηλώσας μετά τινος σχετλιασμοῦ φησι·

‘πλάζομαι ὧδ', ἐπεὶ οὔ μοι ἐπ' ὄμμασι νήδυμος ὕπνος
ἱζάνει, ἀλλὰ μέλει πόλεμος καὶ κήδε' Ἀχαιῶν.
αἰνῶς γὰρ Δαναῶν πέρι δείδια οὐδέ μοι ἦτορ
ἔμπεδον, ἀλλ' ἀλ⟨αλ⟩ύκτημαι, κραδίη δέ μοι ἔξω
στηϑέων ἐκϑρώσκει, τρομέει δ' ὑπὸ φαίδιμα γυῖα.’

40 εἰ μὲν δὴ τὴν καρδίαν σαλευόμενος οὕτως ὑπὸ τοῦ φόβου πάρεστι συμβου-
λευόμενος, οἱ ἐν τοῖς πάϑεσιν ὄντες οὐ κατ' ἀξίαν τῶν συμβεβηκότων
καϑήκειν νομίζοντες μηδένα λόγον προσίεσϑαι κινοῦνται κατὰ τὰ πάϑη·
41 εἰ δὲ μηκέτι φοβούμενος, ἀνανεούμενος δὲ τὰ ἐν τῷ φόβῳ ταῦτά φησι,
375 διὰ τί / ποτε τῆς αὐτῆς ὑπολήψεως καὶ ἀσϑενείας ὑποκειμένης οἱ μὲν
ἀποκλίνουσι τὸν λόγον, οἱ δὲ προσίενται, διαπορήσειεν ἄν τις εὐλόγως.
42 τὸ δ' αἴτιον τοῦ πάϑους παντὸς οὐκ εἴρηκεν.» ἑξῆς τούτοις ὁ Ποσει-
δώνιος καὶ τάδε φησί· «τὸ δὲ δὴ μὴ μόνον ἀποστρέφεσϑαι τὸν λόγον ἐν
402 ταῖς ἐπιϑυμίαις, ὥς φησιν, ἀλλὰ καὶ προσυπολαμβάνειν ὅτι εἰ | καὶ μὴ
συμφέρον ἐστί, καὶ οὕτως ἑκτέον, μάχην περιέχει[ν], φέρεσϑαί τε ὡς
ἐπὶ μέγα συμφέρον καὶ διὰ τὸ μέγεϑος αὐτοῦ, εἰ καὶ ἀσύμφορόν ἐστιν,
ἄξιόν ⟨τε⟩ ἡγεῖσϑαι τοῦ μεγέϑους αὐτοῦ, εἰ καὶ μηδὲν ἔχει ὄφελος ἀλλὰ
43 καὶ τοὐναντίον, ὅμως ἀντέχεσϑαι οὕτως αὐτοῦ. ἔστω γὰρ τοὺς λέγοντας
ὅτι οὐκ ἔστι συμφέρον ἀποστρέφεσϑαι καὶ τοὺς ἐπαγγελλομένους δεί-
ξειν ὅτι ἀσύμφορόν ἐστι λήρους ἡγεῖσϑαι καὶ διὰ τὸ μέγα ὄφελος εἶναι τὸ
376 διωκόμενον· ἀλλ' ἐκεῖνό γε / ἀπίϑανον διὰ τὸ μέγα αὐτὸ ἀγαϑὸν ὑπολαμ-
βάνειν οἴεσϑαι δεῖν, κἂν ᾖ μέγιστον κακόν, ὅμως αὐτὸ λαμβάνειν ἐπιφω-
νοῦντας

1–2] Hom. Il. ix. 3, 9 5–8] Hom. Il. x. 17–20 9–10] *cf.* Hom. Il. x. 82–83 11–15] Hom. Il. x. 91–95

3 τῆς ... ἀσϑενείας H: *corr. Müller*: *ante* τῆς *add.* καὶ *Kühn*, τε *Pohlenz* 6 ἐλ-ϑέμεν' (= ἐλϑέμεναι) H: *corr.* M *Ald.* 7 τεκτήνοιτο H: *ex Hom. corr. Bake* 8 πᾶσι H: *ex Hom. corr. Bake* 9 ὄρφνης] ὁρμῆς H: *corr. Müller (cf. Hom. Il. x. 83)* 14 ἀλύκτημαι H: *corr. Bake* 15 ὑποφαιδιμα H: *corr. Corn.* 16 οὗτος H: *corr. Ald.* πάρεισι *Müller* συμβουλευσόμενος *Kühn* 22 δ' αἴτιον] δ' αἴτιον οὖν *Bake*: δὴ αἴτιον *Pohlenz* πάντως *Corn.* 25 περιέχειν H: *corr. Corn.* 27 τε *add. Einarson* τοῦ μεγέϑους αὐτοῦ] ἢ διὰ τὸ συμφέρον αὐτοῦ *Corn.*: τοῦ διώκειν αὐτὸ ἢ διὰ τὸ συμφέρον *Müller*: *del. Wilamowitz* ὄφελος *coni. Pohlenz*: μέγεϑος H 28 *ante* οὕτως *add.* καὶ *Reinhardt* 29 *post* ἀποστρέφεσϑαι *add.* τὸν λόγον *Bake* 30 καὶ *del. Müller* ὄφελος *del. Reinhardt*

he had immediately been struck, as were the other heroes, with an unspeakable grief, as the poet says. But when the affection abated, although his supposition about what had happened remained, along with the weakness of his reasoning, he thought it not at all right to lie quiet:

> 'This plan seemed best to him in his spirit, 38
> to go first among men to Nestor, son of Neleus,
> to see if he might devise with him some faultless plan
> that would drive the evil away from all the Danaans.'

And when Nestor from a distance saw him approaching through the 39 darkness and asked him who he was, he made himself known with a complaint:

> 'I wander thus because sweet sleep does not settle on my eyes;
> I am troubled by the war and by the Achaians' woes.
> For I am in great fear for the Danaans and my heart
> is not steady; I am in anguish, my heart leaps out
> of my chest, and my shining limbs tremble beneath me.'

If he is present taking counsel while his heart is thus shaking with 40
fear, then persons in affective states who do not think it is in accord with their estimate of what has happened to accept no reasoning are being moved affectively. But if he is no longer afraid but is recalling 41
the experience of fear when he says this, one might reasonably ask why it is that when the same supposition and the same weakness underlie (their acts) some persons reject reasoning whereas others accept it. He has not given the cause of the affection in its entirety."
After this Posidonius continues: "But the view that a person not 42
only rejects reason in desires, as he says, but also makes in addition the supposition that he should cleave to the thing even if it is not beneficial, contains a contradiction: being carried to the thing as to a great benefit just because of its greatness, even if it has no benefit, and considering it appropriate to the greatness of the thing that although it brings no profit but even does the opposite, nevertheless one should in such circumstances cling to it. Let us grant that those 43
who say that the thing is of no benefit are rejected, and those who announce that they will prove it unbeneficial are held to be fools, on the grounds that what is pursued is of great profit; but what is unconvincing is that because you suppose it is a great good you think that even if it is the greatest evil you ought nevertheless to take hold of it, exclaiming,

'ἔα μ' ἀπολέσθαι· τοῦτό μοι νῦν συμφέρει.'
44 τούτου γὰρ τὴν αἰτίαν οὐ πιθανόν ἐστιν ἐν τῇ ὑπολήψει κεῖσθαι τοῦ
45 μέγα ἀγαθὸν ὑπάρχειν ἐφ' ὃ ὠθοῦνται· ζητητέον δέ.» ἐγὼ μὲν οὐκ ἔχω
πρὸς ταῦτα οὐδὲν ἀποκρίνασθαι τῷ Ποσειδωνίῳ, νομίζω δὲ μηδ' ἄλλον
τινὰ ἕξειν, εἴ γε χρὴ τεκμαίρεσθαι τῇ τε φύσει τῶν πραγμάτων αὐτῇ
403 46 καὶ τοῖς νῦν οὖσι Στωϊκοῖς. οὐκ ὀλίγων γὰρ οὐδὲ τῶν ἐπιτυχόντων | ἐν
τοῖς καθ' ἡμᾶς χρόνοις γεγονότων οὐδενὸς αὐτῶν οὐδὲν ἤκουσα πιθανὸν
εἰπόντος εἰς τὰς ὑπὸ τοῦ Ποσειδωνίου προβληθείσας ἀπορίας. ἀλλὰ
περὶ μὲν ἐκείνων καὶ αὖθις ἐροῦμεν.

6. Ὅτι δ' ὁ Χρύσιππος οὐχ ἅπαξ ἢ δὶς ἀλλὰ πάνυ πολλάκις
377 αὐτὸς ὁμολογεῖ δύναμίν τινα ἑτέραν εἶναι τῆς λογικῆς / ἐν ταῖς ψυχαῖς
τῶν ἀνθρώπων αἰτίαν τῶν παθῶν, ἔνεστιν ἡμῖν ἐκ τῶν τοιούτων καταμαθεῖν ἐν οἷς αἰτιᾶται τῶν πραττομένων οὐκ ὀρθῶς ἀτονίαν τε καὶ
ἀσθένειαν τῆς ψυχῆς· οὕτω γὰρ αὐτὰς ὀνομάζει, καθάπερ γε καὶ τἀναντία
2 τὸ μὲν εὐτονίαν τὸ δ' ἰσχύν. ὅσα γὰρ οὐκ ὀρθῶς πράττουσιν ἄνθρωποι,
τὰ μὲν εἰς μοχθηρὰν κρίσιν ἀναφέρει, τὰ δ' εἰς ἀτονίαν καὶ ἀσθένειαν
τῆς ψυχῆς, ὥσπερ γε καὶ ὧν κατορθοῦσιν ἡ ὀρθὴ κρίσις ἐξηγεῖται μετὰ
3 τῆς κατὰ τὴν ψυχὴν εὐτονίας. ἀλλὰ τοιούτων ὥσπερ ἡ κρίσις ἔργον
ἐστὶ τῆς λογικῆς δυνάμεως, οὕτως ἡ εὐτονία ῥώμη τε καὶ ἀρετὴ δυνάμεως ἑτέρας παρὰ τὴν λογικήν, ἣν αὐτὸς ὁ Χρύσιππος ὀνομάζει τόνον,
404 ἀφίστασθαί τέ φησιν | ἔστιν ὅτε τῶν ὀρθῶς ἐγνωσμένων ἡμῖν ἐνδόντος
τοῦ τόνου τῆς ψυχῆς καὶ μὴ παραμείναντος ἕως παντὸς μηδ' ἐξυπηρετήσαντος τοῖς τοῦ λόγου προστάγμασιν, ἐναργῶς ἐν τοῖς τοιούτοις ἐνδεικνύ-
4 μενος οἷόν τι τὸ πάθος ἐστίν. ἤδη δὲ καὶ ῥῆσιν αὐτοῦ τινα παραγράψω
378 5 περὶ τούτων ἐκδιδάσκουσαν· ἔστι δ' ἐκ τοῦ Περὶ παθῶν / Ἠθικοῦ· «ἔτι δὲ
καὶ κατὰ τοῦτ' ἴσως ⟨ὡς⟩ οἱ ἐπὶ τοῦ σώματος λέγονται τόνοι ἄτονοι καὶ
εὔτονοι εἶναι κατὰ τὸ νευρῶδες τῷ δύνασθαι ἡμᾶς ἢ ἀδυνατεῖν ἐν τοῖς
διὰ τούτων ἐπιτελουμένοις ἔργοις, καὶ ὁ ἐν τῇ ψυχῇ λέγεται τόνος ὡς
6 εὐτονία καὶ ἀτονία.» καὶ ἐφεξῆς, «ὥσπερ γὰρ ἐν δρόμῳ καὶ ἀνθέξει τινὸς
καὶ τοῖς παραπλησίοις ἤδη, ἃ διὰ τῶν νεύρων ἐνεργεῖται, ἔστι τις ἐπιτελεστικὴ κατάστασις καὶ ἐνδοτική, τῶν νεύρων προεκλελυμένων καὶ
ἀνειμένων, ἀναλόγως καὶ ἐπὶ ψυχῆς ἐστι τοιοῦτον νευρῶδες, καθὸ καὶ
7 κατὰ μεταφορὰν ἀνεύρους τινὰς λέγομεν καὶ νεῦρα ἔχειν.» εἶθ' ἑξῆς ἐξηγούμενος αὐτὸ τοῦτο τάδε γράφει· «ὁ μὲν δειμῶν ἐπιγινομένων ἀφίσταται,
405 ὁ δὲ κέρδους ἢ | ζημίας φερομένης ἐξελύθη καὶ ἐνέδωκεν, ὁ δὲ καθ' ἕτερα
8 τοιαῦτα οὐκ ὀλίγα. ἕκαστον γὰρ τῶν τοιούτων τρέπεταί τε καὶ δου-

1] Com. adesp. fr. 217: III, p. 450 Kock = III A, p. 390 Edmonds 3–8] Posid. test. 60 Edelstein-Kidd 10–272.8] SVF III, pp. 122–124 *cf.* F. L. Ganter, Philologus 53 (1894), pp. 500–501 24–33] *cf.* Philod. De ira, ed. Wilke, p. XXXIX

1 ἔα μ'] ἐᾶν H: *ex Plut. Mor. 446 A corr. Müller (cf. Wyttenbach apud Bake, p. 284)* μοι νῦν] γάρ μοι *ex Plut. Mor. 446 A Müller* 5 εἴ γε] εἴτε H: *corr. Kühn* 18 τοιούτων] τοίνυν *v. Arnim*: τοι τούτων *Einarson* 22 μήτ' H: *corr. Müller* 25 ἔτι *ex* ἔστι *corr.* H 26 ὡς *add. Einarson* 28 τόνος λέγεται *v. Arnim* ὡς *del. Müller* 29 τρόμω H: *corr. Müller* 30 τῶν παραπλησίων H: *corr. Müller* 32 τοιοῦτο M καθ' ὃ R 34 δείμων H: *corr. Kühn*

'Let me be undone; this now is good for me.'

For it is not convincing that the cause in this case lies in the suppo- 44
sition that what one is pushed toward is a great good; but the question
must be asked." I can give Posidonius no answer to his question, 45
and I believe that no one else will be able to do so, if I am to judge by
the actual nature of the facts and by the Stoics of the present. In my 46
time there have been no few (Stoics), and these not undistinguished;
but I have heard none of them say anything convincing in answer to
the question raised by Posidonius. But we shall return to them at
another time.

6. Now Chrysippus himself admits not once or twice but very
many times that some power in men's souls other than the rational is
the cause of the affections. We may see this in such passages as those
wherein he gives 'softness' and 'weakness' of soul as the cause of in-
correct actions. These are the names he gives them, and he calls their
opposites 'firmness' and 'strength'. Some of men's incorrect actions 2
he refers to faulty judgment, others to softness and weakness of soul,
just as right judgment together with firmness of soul guides them to
correct actions. In persons of the latter sort, as the judgment is the 3
work of the rational power, so the firmness is the strength and virtue
of a power other than the rational. This power Chrysippus himself
calls 'tone'; and he says that there are times when we abandon correct
judgments because the tone of the soul yields and does not persist to the
end or carry out fully the commands of reason. Thus he clearly indi-
cates the kind of affection that is found in persons of this sort. I shall 4
now quote a passage in which he gives a full account of these matters;
it is from the Ethics of his work On the Affections. "Furthermore, it is 5
also in accord with this that as 'tones' in the body are called soft and
firm with reference to its sinewy character, insofar as we have power
or lack it in actions performed by their means, so too perhaps the tone
in the soul is called firmness and softness." Then he says, "As in running, 6
holding fast to something, and similar actions that are performed by
means of the sinews, there is a condition that is able to accomplish what
it undertakes, and another that gives in, the sinews becoming limp and
slack too soon, so in the soul there is a sinewy character of this kind,
in terms of which we speak metaphorically of men without sinew, and
of having sinew." He then writes an explanation of this very statement: 7
"One person desists when dangers arise, another became limp and gave
in when a reward or penalty was brought, another on encountering
other such things, which are not few in number. Every such situation 8

λοῦται ἡμᾶς, ὡς ἐνδιδόντας αὐτοῖς καὶ φίλους καὶ πόλεις προδιδόναι καὶ
379 αὐτοὺς εἰς πολλὰς καὶ / ἀσχήμονας πράξεις ἐπιδιδόναι τῆς πρόσθεν
9 φορᾶς ἐκλυθείσης. οἷος εἰσῆκται καὶ τῷ Εὐριπίδῃ ὁ Μενέλαος· σπα-
σάμενος γὰρ τὴν μάχαιραν φέρεται ἐπὶ τὴν Ἑλένην ὡς ἀναιρήσων, ἰδὼν
δὲ καὶ καταπλαγεὶς [εἰς] τὸ κάλλος ἐξέβαλε τὴν μάχαιραν, οὐδὲ ταύτης
ἔτι δυνάμενος κρατεῖν, καθὰ καὶ ἡ ἐπίπληξις αὔτη εἴρηται αὐτῷ·

> 'σὺ δ' ὡς ἐσεῖδες μαστὸν [ἐκείνης] ἐκβαλὼν ξίφος
> φίλημ' ἐδέξω προδότιν αἰκάλ⟨λ⟩ων κύνα·'»

ἃ πάντα εἴρηται ὀρθῶς τῷ Χρυσίππῳ, μάχεται δὲ τῷ κρίσεις εἶναι
10 τὰ πάθη. κρίνας γοῦν ὁ Μενέλαος ἀποκτεῖναι τὴν Ἑλένην καὶ σπασά-
μενος τὸ ξίφος, ἐπειδὴ πλησίον ἧκεν αὐτῆς, ἐκπλαγεὶς τοῦ κάλλους διὰ
τὴν ἀτονίαν καὶ ἀσθένειαν τῆς ψυχῆς – τοῦτο γάρ ἐστιν ὃ κατασκευάζει
παρ' ὅλον τὸν λόγον ὁ Χρύσιππος –, οὐ μόνον ἀπέρριψε τὸ ξίφος
406 ἀλλὰ καὶ καταφιλεῖ τὴν γυναῖκα καὶ | ὥσπερ ἂν εἴποι τις αὐτὸν δοῦ-/
380 λον ἐγχειρίζει οὐ μεταπεισθεὶς ὑπὸ λόγου τινός, ὡς ἑτέραν κτήσασθαι
κρίσιν, ἀλλ' ἀκρίτως τε καὶ ἀλόγως ὁρμήσας ἐπὶ τἀναντία τοῖς ἐξ ἀρχῆς
11 κεκριμ[μ]ένοις. ὅθεν καὶ αὐτὸς ὁ Χρύσιππος ἐπιφέρων ἐρεῖ· «διὸ πάντων
τῶν φαύλων οὕτω πραττόντων ἀποστατικῶς καὶ ἐνδοτικῶς κατὰ πολ-
λὰς αἰτίας, ἀσθενῶς καὶ κακῶς ἕκαστα πράττειν ἂν λέγοιτο.»
12 Τὸ μὲν οὖν ἀποστατικῶς μὲν τοῦ λόγου, τοῖς πάθεσι δ' ἐνδοτικῶς ἁπάν-
των τῶν φαύλων πραττόντων ἀσθένειάν τινα καὶ ἀτονίαν ἐμφαίνεσθαι
κατὰ τὴν ψυχὴν αὐτῶν ἀληθέστατα λέγεται· τὸ δὲ κατὰ πολλὰς αἰτίας,
ὃ δὴ καὶ αὐτὸς προσέθηκεν ἐν τῇ ῥήσει, καλῶς μὲν εἴρηται πρὸς αὐτοῦ,
κάλλιον δ' ἦν εἰ καὶ τὰς πολλὰς ταύτας αἰτίας αἵτινές ποτ' εἰσὶν ἐφεξῆς
13 αὐτὸς διεληλύθει. εἰ γάρ τις προσέχοι τὸν νοῦν, οὐδὲν οὕτως εὑρήσει
συνέχον τὴν Περὶ τῶν παθῶν πραγματείαν καὶ μάλιστα τὴν Θερα-
πευτικήν, ἐν ᾗ ταῦτ' ἔγραφεν, ὡς τὸ πάσας γνῶναι τὰς αἰτίας ὑφ' ὧν
381 ἀποχωροῦσι τῶν ἐξ ἀρχῆς κρίσεων οἱ / κατὰ πάθος τι πράττοντες.
407 14 ὁ δέ γε τοσούτου | δεῖ συμπάσας ἀκριβῶς ἐκδιδάσκειν ὥστ' οὐδ' αὐτὴν
ταύτην ἧς μέμνηται νῦν ἐδήλωσε σαφῶς. οὐ γὰρ δὴ ἀποχρήσει[ς] γ'
ἡμῖν εἰπεῖν ὡς ἡ τῆς ψυχῆς ἐστιν ἀσθένεια· κοινὴ γὰρ αὕτη γε κατὰ
15 πάντα τὰ πάθη καὶ μία. Χρύσιππος δὲ πολλὰς εἶναί φησιν αἰτίας
τὰς ἐξελεγχούσας δηλονότι τὴν ἀσθένειαν τῆς ψυχῆς, ὥσπερ ἐπὶ μὲν
τοῦ Μενέλεω τὸ κάλλος τῆς Ἑλένης, ἐπὶ δὲ τῆς Ἐριφύλης τὸν χρυσόν,
16 ἐπ' ἄλλου δέ τινος ἄλλο. μυρία γάρ ἐστι τὰ κατὰ μέρος ὑφ' ὧν ἐξίστανται
17 τῆς ἀρχαίας κρίσεως οἱ κατὰ πάθος ζῶντες. ἀλλ' οὐ χρὴ τῶν μυρίων
τούτων μνημονεύειν ἀλλ' εἰς ὀλίγα κεφάλαια τὸν λόγον ἄγειν, ὡς ὁ
Πλάτων ἐποίησε βασιλικὸν μέν τι λέγων εἶναι καὶ δεσποτικὸν ἐπιστήμην

7–8] Eur. Andromache 629–630 17–19] SVF III, p. 124 25–30] SVF III, p. 124 25–28] *cf. infra*, p. 284.26–28

1 φίλους] πολλοὺς H: *corr. Corn.* 2 πρόσθεν] πρὸς θέατρα H: *corr. Schöne*: πρὸς θάτερα *Diels* 4 φέρεται *ex* φαίνεται *corr.* H 5 εἰς *del. Porson* 6 αὐτῇ εἴρηκεν H: *corr. Diels* 7 ἐς εἶδες H: *corr. Ald.* ἐκείνης *del. Greenhill* 8 αἰκάλων H: *corr. Chart.* 9 ἃ πάντα] ἅπαντα R 14 αὐτὸν H: *corr. Ald.* 17 κεκριμμένοις H: *corr. Chart.* 19 λέγοιντο *Müller* 25 προύχοι H: *corr. Kühn* 27 ἔγραψεν *Chart.* 30 ἀποχρήσεις H: *corr. Ald.* 38 ἐποίησε] ε[II] *ex* εν *corr.* H

defeats and enslaves us, so that by yielding to it we betray friends and
cities and offer ourselves up to many shameful acts after our former
impetus has gone slack. Euripides has presented Menelaus as this 9
kind of person. He drew his sword and rushed at Helen to kill her,
but on seeing (her) and being struck by her beauty he let the sword
drop, no longer able even to keep his hold on it. He was accordingly
rebuked with these words:

'When you caught sight of her breast you dropped your sword
and took her kiss, fawning on the shameless traitor.'"

In all of this Chrysippus' statements are true; but they are not
consistent with the view that affections are judgments. Menelaus 10
had formed the judgment to kill Helen and had drawn his sword, but
when he drew near he was struck by her beauty and, because of his
soul's softness and weakness – this is the point that Chrysippus is
establishing throughout the discussion – he not only threw away the
sword but also kissed the woman and, one might say, surrendered
himself to her to be her slave; he was not persuaded by any argument
to exchange one judgment for another, but without recourse to judg-
ment or reason he set his course toward the very opposite of the
action he had originally decided on. For that reason Chrysippus 11
himself adds: "Therefore, since all inferior men act in this way,
abandoning their course and yielding for many causes, it might be
said that they act in every case weakly and badly."

Now he spoke very truly when he said that all inferior persons, 12
by acting in a way that abandons reason and yields to the affections,
reveal a certain weakness and softness in their souls. He spoke well
also when he said that it is 'for many causes', the phrase that he
himself added in the passage; but it would have been better if he had
also gone on to explain what these many causes are. For if you attend 13
carefully, you will find that nothing so unifies the treatise On the
Affections, and especially the Cure, where this passage occurs, as (the
aim) to know all the causes through which persons who take some
action because of an affection depart from their initial judgments. But 14
he falls so far short of expounding them all in precise terms that he
did not even give a clear account of the very cause he just now men-
tioned. It will not satisfy us to say that it is the soul's weakness; this
is a cause common to all the affections, and it is but one. But Chry- 15
sippus says that there are many causes – (causes,) he obviously
means, which convict one of weakness of soul, just as Helen's beauty
was the cause for Menelaus, gold for Eriphyle, other things for
other persons. There are tens of thousands of particular items that 16
cause those who live by the affections to abandon their initial judg-
ments. But one must not mention these tens of thousands; one must 17
bring the account to a few main heads, as Plato did when he said
that knowledge is a royal and despotic thing and that no one errs in

καὶ μήποτε ἂν ἁμαρτεῖν μηδένα κατὰ μηδὲν ἐπιστήμης παρούσης, τοὺς
μέντοι μεταπεισθέντας ἢ ἐπιλαθομένους [αὐτῶν] ἢ βιασθέντας ἢ δε-
18 λεασθέντας ἐξαμαρτάνειν, ἄλλον ἐν ἄλλῃ πράξει. ἀλλὰ τὸ μὲν ἐπιλα-
382 θέσθαι καὶ τὸ μεταπεισθῆναι / πάθος οὐδέπω, καθάπερ οὐδὲ τὸ μηδὲ
408 19 ὅλως ἔχειν ἐπιστήμην· ἀμαθία γὰρ τοῦτο καὶ | ἄγνοιά ἐστιν, οὐ πάθος. εἰ
δέ τις ὑπὸ θυμοῦ βιασθεὶς ἢ δελεασθεὶς ὑφ' ἡδονῆς ἀπέστη τῶν ἐξ ἀρχῆς
κεκριμ[μ]ένων, ἀσθενὴς μὲν ἡ ψυχὴ τούτῳ καὶ ἄτονος, ἡ κίνησις δ' αὐτῆς
τὸ πάθος ἐστίν, ὥσπερ που καὶ ἡ τοῦ κατὰ τραγῳδίαν ὑποκειμένου
Μενέλεω ψυχὴ δελεασθεῖσα πρὸς τῆς ἐπιθυμίας ἐξέστη τῶν κεκριμ[μ]έ-
νων, ἡ δέ γε Μηδείας βιασθεῖσα πρὸς τοῦ θυμοῦ, περὶ ἧς καὶ αὐτῆς οὐκ
οἶδ' ὅπως ὁ Χρύσιππος οὐκ αἰσθάνεται καθ' ἑαυτοῦ τῶν Εὐριπίδου
μεμνημένος ἐπῶν

«καὶ μανθάνω μὲν οἷα δρᾶν μέλλω κακά,
θυμὸς δὲ κρείσσων τῶν ἐμῶν βουλευμάτων.»

20 οὐ γὰρ μανθάνειν ἐχρῆν εἰρηκέναι τὸν Εὐριπίδην, εἰ τοῖς τοῦ Χρυσίπ-
που δόγμασιν ἔμελλε μαρτυρήσειν, ἀλλ' αὐτὸ τὸ ἐναντιώτατον, ἀγνο-
21 εῖν τε καὶ μὴ μανθάνειν οἷα δρᾶν μέλλει κακά. τὸ δὲ γινώσκειν μὲν αὐτὸ
νικᾶσθαι δ' ὑπὸ τοῦ θυμοῦ τί ἄλλο ἐστὶν ἢ δύο ἀρχὰς εἰσάγοντος ἀνθρώ-
383 που τῶν / τῆς Μηδείας ὁρμῶν, ἑτέραν μὲν ᾗ γιγνώσκομέν τε τὰ πράγμα-
409 τα καὶ ἐπιστήμην ἔχομεν αὐτῶν, ἥτις ἐστὶν ἡ | λογικὴ δύναμις, ἑτέραν δ'
22 ἄλογον, ἧς ἔργον τὸ θυμοῦσθαι; αὕτη μὲν οὖν Μηδείας ἐβιάσατο τὴν
ψυχήν· ἡ δ' ἑτέρα ἡ ἐπιθυμητικὴ τὴν τοῦ Μενέλεω δελεάσασα κατηνάγ-
23 κασεν ἀκολουθεῖν οἷς αὐτὴ προσέταττε. Χρύσιππος δ' οὔτε τῆς ἐν
τούτοις ἐναντιώσεως αἰσθάνεται καὶ μυρί' ἕτερα γράφει τοιαῦτα, καθ-
άπερ ἐπειδὰν λέγῃ «ἔστι δὲ ὡς οἶμαι κοινότατον ἡ ἄλογος αὕτη φορὰ
καὶ ἀπεστραμμένη τὸν λόγον, καθὸ καὶ θυμῷ φαμέν τινας φέρεσθαι.»
24 καὶ πάλιν «διὸ καὶ ἐπὶ τῶνδε τῶν ἐμπαθῶν ὡς περὶ ἐξεστηκότων ἔχομεν
καὶ ὡς πρὸς παρηλλαχότας ποιούμεθα τὸν λόγον καὶ οὐ παρ' ἑαυτοῖς
25 οὐδ' ἐν αὐτοῖς ὄντας.» καὶ ἐφεξῆς δὲ πάλιν ἐξηγούμενος αὐτὰ ταῦτα,
«ἡ δὲ παραλλαγὴ γίγνεται καὶ ἡ ἐξ αὐτοῦ ἀναχώρησις οὐ κατ' ἄλλο τι
26 ἢ τὴν τοῦ λόγου ἀποστροφήν, ὡς προείπομεν.» τό τε γὰρ «θυμῷ φέ-
384 ρεσθαι» καὶ «ἐξεστηκέναι» καὶ «οὐ παρ' ἑαυτοῖς / οὐδ' ἐν ἑαυτοῖς εἶναι» καὶ
πάνθ' ὅσα τοιαῦτα φανερῶς ⟨κατα⟩μαρτυρεῖ τοῦ κρίσεις εἶναι τὰ πάθη
κἀν τῇ λογικῇ δυνάμει τῆς ψυχῆς συνίστασθαι, καθάπερ καὶ τὰ οὕτως
410 27 ἔχοντα· | «διὸ καὶ τοιαύτας ἔστιν ἀκοῦσαι φωνὰς ἐπί τε τῶν ἐρώντων καὶ
τῶν ἄλλως σφόδρα ἐπιθυμούντων καὶ ἐπὶ τῶν ὀργιζομένων, ὅτι τε τῷ
θυμῷ θέλουσι χαρίζεσθαι καὶ ἐᾶν αὐτούς, εἴτε ἄμεινον εἴτε μή, καὶ μηθὲν
λέγειν αὐτοῖς, καὶ ὡς τοῦτο ἐκ παντός γε τρόπου ποιητέον, καὶ εἰ δια-
μαρτάνουσι καὶ εἰ ἀσύμφορόν ἐστιν αὐτοῖς.»

10–14] SVF III, p. 124 13–14] Eur. Medea 1078–1079 *cf. supra*, pp. 188.27–28; 244.2–5 23–276.1] SVF III, p. 125

2 αὐτῶν *del. Müller* 7 *et* 9 κεκριμμένων H: *corr. Chart.* 10 μήδεια H: *correxi (cf. infra, lin. 21)* 26 καθ' ὃ *Kühn* 27 περιεξεστηκότων H: *corr. Ald.* 28 προσπαρηλλαχότας H: *corr. Ald.* 29 αὐτοῖς H: *correxi*: ἑαυτοῖς *Ald.* 30 ἀποχώρησις *Müller* 31 τό] τῷ H: *corr. Müller* 33 μαρτυρεῖ H: *corr. Kalbfleisch*: ἀντιμαρτυρεῖ *v. Arnim* 38 λέγειν] μέλειν *Diels*

anything when knowledge is present; errors, however, are committed
by those who have been persuaded to change their minds or have for-
gotten or have been forced or deceived, one in one act, one in another.
Forgetting and changing one's mind are not yet affections, nor is it an 18
affection to have no knowledge at all; that is ignorance and stupidity,
not affection. But if a person is forced by anger or beguiled by pleasure 19
to depart from his initial judgment, his soul is weak and soft, and its
motion is the affection; thus the soul of Menelaus, as presented
in the tragedy, abandoned its decision because it was beguiled by
his desire, Medea's soul because it was forced by anger. Somehow
in her case Chrysippus does not perceive that he is testifying against
himself when he quotes Euripides' words:

> "I understand the evils I am going to do,
> but anger prevails over my counsels."

If Euripides was to give evidence in support of the teachings of 20
Chrysippus, he should not have said that she understands but the
very opposite, that she is ignorant and does not understand what evils
she is going to do. But to say that she knows this and yet is overcome 21
by anger – what is that but the act of a man who introduces two
sources for Medea's appetitions, one by which we recognize things
and have knowledge of them, which is the rational power, and another
irrational (power), whose function it is to be angry? This latter 22
(power), then, coerced Medea's soul, while the other (irrational
power), the desiderative, by beguiling Menelaus' soul, compelled him
to follow its commands. But Chrysippus does not notice the contra- 23
diction here, and he makes other statements of this kind by the
thousands, as when he says, "This movement, irrational and rejecting
reason, is, as I think, most widely shared; by reference to it we say
that some are moved by anger." And again, "Therefore we behave 24
toward these persons suffering from affection as we do toward persons
out of their minds, and we talk to them as to persons who have taken
leave of their senses and are not in their right minds or in possession of
their faculties." Then he explains again this last point: "This taking 25
leave and withdrawing from oneself is occasioned by nothing other
than the rejection of reason, as we said before." Here the words 26
"moved by anger", "out of their minds", "not in their right minds or
in possession of their faculties" and all such expressions clearly testify
against the view that the affections are judgments and that they arise
in the rational power of the soul. So also the following: "For that 27
reason we can hear utterances of the following kind both in the case
of lovers and persons with other violent desires, and of angry persons,
that they want to gratify their anger and to let them be, whether it
is better or not, and to say nothing to them, and that this is to be
done by all means, even if they are wrong and if it is not to their
advantage."

28 Καὶ γὰρ καὶ τὰ οὕτως ὑπὸ τοῦ Χρυσίππου λεγόμενα τὴν θυ-
μοειδῆ δύναμιν ἑτέραν τινὰ τῆς λογιζομένης ἐνδείκνυται καὶ τὴν ὁρμὴν
τοῦ ζῴου ποτὲ μὲν ὑπ' ἐκείνης ἄρχεσθαι διδάσκει, ποτὲ δ' ὑπὸ τῆς
ἐπιθυμητικῆς, ὅταν γ' ἐν πάθει καθεστήκῃ, καθάπερ ὅταν ἔξω πάθους ὑπὸ
29 τῆς λογικῆς. ὅμοια δὲ τοῖς προγεγραμμένοις καὶ τὰ οὕτως ὑπὸ τοῦ
Χρυσίππου λεγόμενα, καθάπερ ἔχει καὶ τάδε· «οἵας μάλιστα φορὰς καὶ
385 οἱ ἐρώμενοι ἀξιοῦσι πρὸς ἑαυτοὺς / ἔχειν τοὺς ἐραστάς, ἀπερισκεπτότερον
καὶ ἄνευ ἐπιστροφῆς λογικῆς ἱσταμένους καὶ ἔτι τοῦ παραινοῦντος λόγου
αὐτοῖς ὑπερβατικοὺς ὄντας, μᾶλλον δ' οὐδ' ὅλως ὑπομονητικοὺς ἀκοῦσαί
30 τινος τοιούτου.» καὶ γὰρ καὶ τὰ τοιαῦτα πάντα τῇ παλαιᾷ δόξῃ μαρ-
411 τυρεῖ, | καθάπερ καὶ τὰ ἐφεξῆς αὐτῶν τάδε· «οὕτως τε μακρὰν ἀπέχουσιν
ἀπὸ τοῦ λόγου, ὡς ἂν ἀκοῦσαι ἢ προσέχειν τινὶ τοιούτῳ, ὥστε μηδὲ τὰ
τοιαῦτα ἀπὸ τρόπου ἔχει⟨ν⟩ γ' αὐτοῖς λέγεσθαι·

'Κύπρις γὰρ οὐδὲ νουθετουμένη χαλᾷ·
ἂν γὰρ βιάζῃ, μᾶλλον ἐντείνειν φιλεῖ.
νουθετούμενος δ' Ἔρως
μᾶλλον πιέζει.'»

31 καὶ γὰρ καὶ ταῦτα καὶ τὰ ἐφεξῆς λεγόμενα τῷ παλαιῷ μαρτυρεῖ δόγματι
περὶ τῆς τῶν παθῶν γενέσεως· ἔχει δ' οὕτως· «ἔτι δ' ὥσπερ ἄκαιρον
ἐπιτιμητὴν καὶ οὐκ ἐπιγνώμονα τοῖς γινομένοις ἐν τῷ ἐρᾶν ἀποκλίνουσι
386 τὸν λόγον, καθάπερ ἄνθρωπον ἀκαίρως δοκοῦντα νουθετεῖν, / ἡνίκα
32 δὴ καὶ οἱ θεοὶ δοκοῦσιν αὐτοῖς ἐφιέναι ἐπιορκεῖν.» καὶ ἔτι τὰ τούτων
ἑξῆς ἔτι μᾶλλον· «ἐξείη – φασίν – αὐτοῖς τὸ ἐπιὸν ποιεῖν ἀκολουθοῦσι
τῇ ἐπιθυμίᾳ.» ἐνταῦθα μέν γε ναὶ μὰ τὸν Δία σαφῶς εἶπεν «ἀκολουθοῦσι
33 τῇ ἐπιθυμίᾳ» καθάπερ ἔμπροσθεν ἔφη[ν] «τῷ θυμῷ». λόγῳ δ' οὔτ' ἐν
412 τούτοις οὔτ' ἐν | ἄλλῳ τινὶ τῶν ἑξῆς ἀκολουθεῖν φήσει τοὺς ἐν πάθει
καθεστηκότας, ἀλλ' ἀπεστράφθαι διὰ παντὸς αὐτὸν καὶ φεύγειν καὶ μὴ
34 προσίεσθαι καὶ πάνθ' ὅσα τοιαῦτα. καὶ μὲν δὴ καὶ ὅταν μνημονεύῃ τοῦ
Μενανδρείου ἔπους, ἐν ᾧ φησι

«τὸν νοῦν ἔχων ὑποχείριον
εἰς τὸν πίθον δέδωκα»,

φανερῶς κἀνταῦθα μαρτυροῦσαν ἀπόφασιν τῇ παλαιᾷ δόξῃ παρα-
τίθεται, καθάπερ κἀπειδὰν ἐξηγούμενος τὸ μὴ παρ' ἑαυτοῖς εἶναι μηδ'
35 ἐν ἑαυτοῖς λέγῃ ταυτί· «οἰκείως δὲ καὶ ἐκφέρεσθαι λέγονται οἱ οὕτως
ὀργιζόμενοι τοῖς ἐπὶ τῶν δρόμων προεκφερομένοις παραπλησίως κατὰ
τὸ πλεονάζον τῶν μὲν παρὰ τὴν ἐν τῷ τρέχειν ὁρμήν, τῶν δὲ παρὰ τὸν /
387 ἴδιον λόγον. οὐ γὰρ ἂν οὕτως ⟨ὡς⟩ οἵ γε κρατοῦντες τῆς κινήσεως καθ'

5–24] SVF III, pp. 125–126 14–15] Eur. fr. 340 Nauck, p. 462 16–17] Eur. fr. 665 Nauck, p. 570 19–22] *cf.* Plat. Symp. 183 a–b 28–278.4] SVF III, p. 128 30–31] Menand. fr. 702 Körte-Thierfelder 33–34] *cf. supra*, p. 274.28–29

5 δὲ] δὴ *Kalbfleisch* οὕτως] ἑξῆς *Petersen* 6 φορᾶς H: *corr. Bas.* 10 καὶ[II] *del. v. Arnim* 13 ἔχει H: *corr. Chart.* 19 ἔτι] ὅτι M *Ald.* 23 *ante* ἐξείη *add.* ἂν *Müller* ἐξείη φησὶν H: *corr. Einarson*: ἐξεῖναί φασιν *v. Arnim* αὐτοῖς H: *corr. v. Arnim* 25 ἔφην H: *corr. Müller* 26 φησι *Diels* 30 ὑποχείριον ἔχων H: *trsp. Bergk* 31 δέδυκα *Cobet* 35 δρομέων H: *corr. Diels* 37 ὡς *add. Einarson*, μὴ *post* γε *v. Arnim*

The expressions of this sort that Chrysippus cites indicate that 28
the spirited power is something other than the rational, and they
inform us that a person's conation is sometimes ruled by the spirited,
sometimes by the desiderative power, when, that is, he is in a state of
affection; and when he is free from affection his conation is ruled by
the rational power. These expressions that Chrysippus cites are also 29
similar to those previously quoted, and it is the same with the follow-
ing: "Loved ones especially expect that the conduct of their lovers
toward them should be of this kind, that their attitude should be
rather uncalculated and without concern for reason, and furthermore,
that they should defy the discourse that gives them advice, or rather,
have no patience whatever with any discourse of that kind." All such 30
statements support the ancient view, and his next words do also:
"They keep so far away from admonitory discourse, from listening or
attending to anything of the kind, that it is not out of place to say to
them such things as these:

'Even when censured Cypris does not let go;
if you use force she loves to strive the more.
Eros, when admonished,
presses more heavily.'"

This passage and the next support the ancient view about the origin 31
of the affections. He next says, "Furthermore they reject the dis-
course as an untimely censor, unsympathetic to the affairs of love,
like a man who is held to admonish unseasonably, at a time when
even the gods are thought to permit them to swear false oaths." The 32
words that follow (give) even more (support to the ancient view):
"Permit us – they say – to do what occurs to us and follow our
desire." Here indeed he clearly says "follow our desire", just as he
said earlier, "our anger". Neither here nor anywhere in the subsequent 33
discussion will he say that persons in an affected state follow reason,
but that they reject it entirely, flee from it, do not admit it, and
every expression of that kind. And when he recalls the lines where 34
Menander says,

"I got my mind in hand
and stowed it in a pot",

he again cites a statement that clearly testifies to the ancient view.
He does so also when in his explanation of 'not being in their right
minds or in possession of their faculties', he says, "Persons thus an- 35
gered are also appropriately said to be carried away, like those who
are carried too far onward in races, the similarity being in the excess,
which in the runners goes counter to their conation in running, and
in the persons angered, counter to their own reason. For they could
not be said, like those who are in control of their movement, to be

ἑαυτοὺς ἂν κινεῖσθαι λέγοιντο, ἀλλὰ κατ' ἄλλην τινὰ βίαν ἔξωθεν
36 αὐτῶν.» ὁμολογεῖ κἀνταῦθα βίαν τινὰ τὴν κινοῦσαν εἶναι πᾶσι τοῖς
ἐμπαθέσιν ὁρμάς, ὀρθότατα γιγνώσκων, πλὴν ὅτι τὴν βίαν ἔξωθεν αὐτῶν
ἔφησεν εἶναι, δέον οὐκ ἔξωθεν ἀλλ' ἐν τοῖς ἀνθρώποις ὑπάρχειν εἰπεῖν.
37 οὐ γὰρ διὰ τοῦτο λέγομεν αὐτοὺς ἑαυτῶν ἔξω καθεστηκέναι καὶ μὴ
418 ἐν αὐτοῖς εἶναι, διότι τὸ | βιαζόμενον αὐτοὺς ὁρμᾶν κατὰ τὸ πάθος
ἔξωθέν ἐστιν, ἀλλ' ὅτι παρὰ φύσιν ἔχουσιν, εἴγε τὸ λογικὸν τῆς ψυχῆς
ᾧ κρατεῖν καὶ ἄρχειν τῶν ἄλλων ἦν κατὰ φύσιν, οὐ κρατεῖ νῦν ἀλλὰ
38 κρατεῖται καὶ ἄρχεται πρὸς τῶν ἀλόγων τῆς ψυχῆς δυνάμεων· ὅπερ
οἶμαι καὶ διὰ τῶν τοιούτων παραδειγμάτων ὁ Χρύσιππος κατασκευ-
άζων οὐκ αἰσθάνεται. παρατίθεται γοῦν τὸν Εὐριπίδῃ γεγραμμένον
Ἡρακλέους πρὸς Ἄδμητον διάλογον· ἔχει δ' ὧδε· /
388 «τί δὲ ἂν προκόπτοις, εἰ θέλεις στένειν ἀεί;»
ταυτὶ μὲν Ἡρακλῆς λέγει, ὁ δ' Ἄδμητος ἀποκρίνεται
«ἔγνωκα καὐτός, ἀλλ' ἔρως τις ἐξάγει.»
39 δῆλον γὰρ ὅτι τῆς ἐπιθυμητικῆς δυνάμεως οὐ τῆς λογικῆς ὁ ἔρως πάθος
ὑπάρχων ἐξάγει τὴν ὅλην ψυχὴν καὶ ἄγει τὸν ἄνθρωπον εἰς ἐναντίας
40 πράξεις ὧν ἐξ ἀρχῆς ἐκεκρίκει. παρατίθεται δὲ καὶ τὰ τοῦ Ἀχιλλέως
πρὸς τὸν Πρίαμον εἰρημένα·
«ἄνσχεο μηδ' ἀλίαστον ὀδύρεο σὸν κατὰ θυμόν·
οὐ γάρ τι πρήξεις ἀκα[σ]χήμενος υἷος ἑῆος |
414 οὐδέ μιν ἀνστήσεις· πρὶν καὶ κακὸν ἄλλο πάθησθα.»
41 ταῦτα μέν φησι λέγειν αὐτὸν «παρ' αὑτῷ διαλεγόμενον» — οὕτω γὰρ ἔγρα-
ψεν αὐτοῖς ὀνόμασιν —, ἐξίστασθαι δ' οὐκ ὀλιγάκις ἐκ τῶν αὐτῶν τούτων
κρίσεων ἐν τοῖς συμπίπτουσι καὶ μὴ κρατεῖν ἑαυτοῦ νικώμενον ὑπὸ τῶν
389 42 παθῶν. καὶ γὰρ οὖν / κἀνταῦθα τό τε τῶν κρίσεων ἐξίστασθαι καὶ τὸ μὴ
κρατεῖν ἑαυτοῦ καὶ τὸ ποτὲ μὲν εἶναι παρ' ἑαυτῷ, ποτὲ δ' οὔ, καὶ πάνθ' ὅσα
τοιαῦτα τοῖς τε φαινομένοις ἐναργῶς ὁμολογεῖ καὶ τῇ παλαιᾷ δόξῃ περὶ
43 παθῶν τε καὶ ψυχῆς δυνάμεων, οὐ μὴν οἷς ὑπέθετο Χρύσιππος. ὁμοίως
δ' εἴρηται καὶ τὰ τοιαῦτα κατὰ τὸ Περὶ τῶν παθῶν βιβλίον· «τὸ γὰρ
δὴ σεσοβημένον καὶ παρηλλαχὸς ἐν ἡμῖν καὶ ἀπειθὲς τῷ λόγῳ οὐχ ἧττον
44 ἐπὶ τῆς ἡδονῆς καταγίνεται.» καὶ πάλιν, «οὕτω γὰρ ἐξιστάμεθα καὶ ἔξω
γινόμεθα ἑαυτῶν καὶ τελέως ἀποτυφλούμεθα ἐν τοῖς σφαλλομένοις, ὥστε
ἔστιν ὅτε σπόγγον ἔχοντες ἢ ἔριον ἐν ταῖς χερσὶ τοῦτο[ν] διαράμενοι
βάλλομεν ὡς δή τι περα[ι]νοῦντες δι' αὐτῶν. εἰ δ' ἐτυγχάνομεν μάχαιραν

9–280.15] SVF III, pp. 128–130 13 *et* 15] Eur. Alcestis 1079–1080 20–22] Hom. Il. xxiv. 549–551

2 *post* εἶναι *add.* ἐν *Müller* 3 πάθεσιν H: *corr. Müller* 4 τοῖς *bis scr.* H: *corr.* R² *Ald.* 5 διὰ τοῦτο] δι' αὐτὸ H: *correxi* ἑαυτῶ H: *corr. Müller*: ἑαυτοῖς *Ald.* 11 εὐριπίδου H: *correxi*: ὑπὸ Εὐριπίδου *Müller* 12 ἡρακλεῖ H: *corr. Müller* 13 θέλοις *Kühn* 15 ἔγνωκ' αὐτοὺς H: *ex Eur. corr. Chart.* ἐξάγει] μ' ἐξάγει *Eur.* 18 *ante* τοῦ *add.* ὑπὸ *Müller* 21 ἀκασχή' H: *corr. Chart.* ἑῆος H: *corr. Ald.* 22 οὐδὲ μίαν H: *corr. Ald.* ἂν στήσεις H: *corr. Kühn* 23 αὑτῷ] αὐτῶ H: *corr. Kalbfleisch* 25 νικωμένου H: *corr. Müller* 34 *post* ἔχοντες *add. et del.* ἢ – παραπλησίως *(p. 280.1)* H τοῦτον H: *corr. Müller* 35 περαινοῦντες H: *corr. Chart.* δὲ τυγχάνομεν H: *corr.* M

moving in conformity with themselves, but instead to be moving in
conformity with some force external to themselves." Here again 36
he grants that there is some force that arouses conations in all the
affections, and his understanding is correct, except that he said that
the force was external to them, when he should have said that it is
not external but in the men. It is not because the force that compels 37
their conations to conform to their affections is external, that we say
that they 'have got outside themselves' and are not 'in themselves',
but because they are in an unnatural state, since the rational part
of the soul, which by nature had the government and rule of the
rest, does not now govern but is governed and ruled by the soul's
irrational powers. In my opinion Chrysippus was not aware that 38
with examples like these he is supporting that very position. Thus he
quotes from Euripides the exchange between Heracles and Ad-
metus. It goes like this:

"What would you gain if you let yourself grieve forever?"

This line is spoken by Heracles, and Admetus answers,

"I too know that, but a certain love distracts me."

It is clear that his love, being an affection of the desiderative power, 39
not of the rational, distracts his whole soul and leads the man to acts
contrary to his initial judgment. He also cites Achilles' words to 40
Priam:

"Bear up and do not let the grief in your spirit be inflexible.
You will do nothing by mourning for your son.
You will not bring him back; sooner you will suffer yet
another evil."

He says that Achilles says these things "speaking in his right mind" – 41
these are the very words he wrote – but that Achilles not infre-
quently abandons these same judgments in adverse circumstances
and does not have power over himself when overcome by affections.
Here too 'abandoning one's judgments' and 'not having power over 42
oneself' and being sometimes 'in one's right mind' and sometimes not,
and all such expressions, are in clear agreement with the observed
facts and the ancient view about the affections and the soul's powers,
but (they are) not (in agreement) with the suppositions of Chry-
sippus. Such statements as the following in his book On the Affec- 43
tions are to the same effect: "That in us which is agitated and off
course and disobedient to reason arises no less in the case of pleasure."
And again, "We take such leave of ourselves and get so far outside 44
ourselves and are so completely blinded in our frustrations that some-
times if we have a sponge or (a piece of) wool in our hands we lift
it up and throw it, as if we would thereby accomplish anything. If

415 45 ἔχοντες ἢ ἄλλο τι, τούτῳ ἂν ἐχρησά|μεθα παραπλησίως.» καὶ ἐφεξῆς
«πολλάκις δὲ κατὰ τὴν τοιαύτην τυφλότητα τὰς κλεῖς δάκνομεν καὶ τὰς
390 θύρας τύπτομεν οὐ ταχὺ αὐτῶν / ἀνοιγομένων πρός τε τοὺς λίθους
ἐὰν προσπταίσωμεν, τιμωρητικῶς προσφερόμεθα καταγνύντες καὶ ῥι-
πτοῦντες αὐτοὺς εἴς τινας τόπους καὶ ἐπιλέγοντες καθ' ἕκαστα τούτων
46 ἀτοπώτατα.» ὡσαύτως δὲ κἀν τοῖς ἑξῆς φησιν «ἐννοήσειε δ' ἄν τις ἐκ
τῶν τοιούτων καὶ τὴν ἐν τοῖς πάθεσιν ἀλογιστίαν καὶ ὡς ἐν τοῖς τοιού-
τοις ἀποτυφλούμεθα καιροῖς ὡς ἂν ἕτεροί τινες γεγονότες τῶν προ[σ]-
47 διαλελογισμένων.» ὅλως δ' εἴ τις ἐκλέγοι πάντα καὶ παραγράφοι νῦν
ὅσα κατὰ τὸ Περὶ παθῶν εἴρηται βιβλίον αὐτῷ, μαχόμενα μὲν οἷς αὐτὸς
ὑπέθετο δόγμασιν ὁμολογοῦντα δὲ τοῖς τε φαινομένοις ἐναργῶς καὶ τῇ
48 Πλάτωνος δόξῃ, μῆκος ἂν ἄμετρόν τι γένοιτο τοῦ βιβλίου. μεστὸν
γάρ ἐστιν αὐτῶ⟨ν⟩ τὸ γράμμα, τῶν τε κρίσεων ἐξίστασθαι λέγοντι καὶ
τῶν προδιαλελογισμένων διὰ τὸν θυμὸν ἢ τὴν ἐπιθυμίαν ἢ τὴν ἡδονὴν ἤ
τι τοιοῦτον μανιωδῶς τε κινεῖσθαι καὶ οὐκ ἐν ἑαυτῷ οὐδὲ παρ' ἑαυτῷ
416 391 εἶναι | τετυφλῶσθαί τε τὴν διάνοιαν ἀλογίστως τε φέρεσθαι / καὶ πάνθ'
ὅσα τοιαῦτα.

7. Τὰς μὲν δὴ τοιαύτας ῥήσεις αὐτοῦ τινι κατὰ σχολὴν ἐκλέγειν
ἐπιτρέπω, δεδειγμένου γε ἤδη σαφῶς αὐτῶν τοῦ τύπου. μεταβήσομαι
δ' ἐπί τινα τῶν ὑπὸ τοῦ Ποσειδωνίου πρὸς τὸν Χρύσιππον ἀντ-
2 ειρημένων. «ὁ γοῦν ὅρος οὗτος», φησίν, «ὁ τῆς ἄτης, ὥσπερ οὖν καὶ
ἄλλοι πολλοὶ τῶν παθῶν ὑπό τε Ζήνωνος εἰρημένοι καὶ πρὸς τοῦ
Χρυσίππου γεγραμμένοι, σαφῶς ἐξελέγχουσι τὴν γνώμην αὐτοῦ.
3 δόξαν γὰρ εἶναι πρόσφατον τοῦ κακὸν αὐτῷ παρεῖναί φησι τὴν λύπην.
ἐν ᾧ καὶ συντομώτερον ἐνίοτε λέγοντες ὧδέ πως προ[σ]φέρονται· λύπη
4 ἐστὶ δόξα πρόσφατος κακοῦ παρουσίας.» εἶναι μὲν δὴ τὸ πρόσφατόν
φησι τὸ ὑπόγυον κατὰ τὸν χρόνον, ἀξιοῖ δὲ τὴν αἰτίαν αὐτῷ ῥηθῆναι δι'
ἣν ἡ τοῦ κακοῦ δόξα πρόσφατος μὲν οὖσα συστέλλει τε τὴν ψυχὴν καὶ
392 λύπην ἐργάζεται, χρονισθεῖσα δ' ἢ οὐδ' ὅλως ἢ οὐκ ἔθ' ὁμοίως / συστέλ-
417 5 λει. καίτοι οὐδὲ τὸ πρόσφατον ἐχρῆν ἐγκεῖσθαι κατὰ | τὸν ὅρον, εἴπερ
ἀληθῆ τὰ Χρυσίππου. κατὰ γὰρ τὴν γνώμην αὐτοῦ μᾶλλον ἦν με-
γάλου κακοῦ ἢ ἀνυπομονήτου ἢ ἀκαρτερήτου, καθάπερ αὐτὸς εἴωθεν
ὀνομάζειν, τὴν λύπην εἰρῆσθαι δόξαν, οὐ προσφάτου.

9–10] *cf. supra*, p. 278.30 15] *cf. supra*, pp. 264.5–6; 274.28–29 19–290.22] Posid. fr. 165 Edelstein-Kidd 19–30] *cf.* Reinhardt, 1921, pp. 291–292 21–282.7] SVF III, p. 131 21–26] SVF I, p. 52 Pohlenz, 1898, p. 616 30–282.7] Reinhardt, 1921, p. 292 30–282.3] *cf.* Pohlenz, 1898, pp. 549–550

4 καταγνοῦντες H: *corr. Ai. Just.* 5 ἐπιλέγοντας H: *corr. Chart.* 8 προσδιαλελογισμένων H: *corr. Chart.* 9 παραγράφοι *ex* -ει *corr.* H *supra lin.* 13 αὐτῶ H: *corr. Einarson* γραμμάτων H: *corr. Diels* 16 τετυφλῶσθαι *ex* τυφλῶσθαι *corr.* H 18 αὐτῶ H: *corr. Kühn* 19 γε] δὲ *Ald.* 20 ἐπί] ἐπεί H: *corr.* R² *Ald.* 21 ἄτης] λύπης *Corn.* 24 τοῦ] τὸ H: *corr. Müller* ἑαυτῷ *Bake* 25 ἐν ᾧ] ὃν *vel* ὃ *v. Arnim*: ἔνιοι *Reinhardt* προσφέρονται H: *corr. Ald.* 27 αὐτῶν H: *corr. Einarson*: ὑπὸ αὐτῶν *Müller* 31 ἦν *Wilamowitz apud Pohlenz*: ἐχρῆν *Wilamowitz apud Petersen*: τὴν H: τοῦ *Ald.*: *del. Müller*: τὸ *Einarson* 33 *post* εἰρῆσθαι *add.* ἐχρῆν *Corn.*, ἔδει *Wyttenbach* πρόσφατον *Müller*

we had happened to have a knife or some other object, we should have
used it in the same way." He continues: "Often in this kind of blind- 45
ness we bite the keys and beat against the doors when they are not
quickly opened, and if we stumble on a stone we take punitive meas-
ures, breaking it and throwing it somewhere, and all the while we use
the strangest language." What he says next is in the same vein: "From 46
such actions a person would get a notion of the irrationality in the affec-
tions and would perceive how we are blinded on such occasions, as
though we were no longer the same persons who had earlier engaged in
philosophical conversations." In short, if a person were to collect and 47
now transcribe all the statements made by Chrysippus in his book
On the Affections that contradict his own assumptions but agree with
the evident facts and the Platonic view, this book would extend
to an immoderate length. For his treatise is full of them, as when he 48
speaks of abandoning one's judgments and one's prior discussions
through anger or desire or pleasure or some such thing, and of being
moved like a madman and not being in possession of one's faculties
or in one's right mind, and of being blinded in thought and carried
away irrationally, and everything of that kind.

7. I leave it to someone else to excerpt at his leisure these passages
from Chrysippus' writings, as their character has now been clearly
revealed. I pass to some of Posidonius' answers to Chrysippus:
"This definition of *atē* (baneful blindness)", he says, "and also many 2
other (definitions) of affections that were pronounced by Zeno and re-
corded by Chrysippus clearly refute his view. Indeed he says that 3
distress is a fresh opinion that one is in the presence of evil. Sometimes
they express it even more briefly: distress is a fresh opinion of the
presence of evil." He says that what is fresh is recent in time, and he 4
asks that they tell him why it is that when the opinion of evil is fresh
it contracts the soul and produces distress, but after an interval it
either does not contract (the soul) at all, or no longer to the same
extent. And yet if Chrysippus' teachings were true, the word 'fresh' 5
should not even have been included in the definition. It would have
been more consistent with his view to call distress an opinion of the
presence of a great or intolerable or unbearable evil – this is his usual
term –, rather than a fresh evil.

6 Ἔνθα καὶ διχόθεν ὁ Ποσειδώνιος ἀντιλέγει τῷ Χρυσίππῳ,
κατὰ μὲν τοῦτον τὸν δεύτερον ὁρισμὸν ἀναμιμνήσκων τῶν τε σοφῶν
καὶ τῶν προκοπτόντων, ὡς ἔμπροσθεν εἴρηται· οἱ μὲν γὰρ ἐν μεγίστοις
ἀγαθοῖς, οἱ δ' ἐν μεγίστοις κακοῖς ἑαυτοὺς ὑπολαμβάνοντες εἶναι ὅμως
7 οὐ γίνονται διὰ τοῦτ' ἐν πάθει. κατὰ δὲ τὸν πρῶτον ἐρωτᾷ τὴν αἰτίαν
δι' ἣν οὐχ ἡ τῆς τοῦ κακοῦ παρουσίας δόξα τὴν λύπην, ἀλλ' ἡ πρόσφατος
ἐργάζεται μόνη· καί φησι διὰ τί πᾶν τὸ ἀμελέτητον καὶ ξένον ἀθρόως
προσπῖπτον ἐκπλήττει τε καὶ τῶν παλαιῶν ἐξίστησι κρίσεων, ἀσκηθὲν
δὲ καὶ συνεθισθὲν καὶ χρονίσαν ἢ οὐδ' ὅλως ἐξίστησιν, ὡς κατὰ πάθος κι-
393 νεῖν, ἢ ἐπὶ μικρὸν κομιδῇ· διὸ καὶ / προενδημεῖν φησι τοῖς πράγμασι
8 μήπω τε παροῦσιν οἷον παροῦσι χρῆσθαι. βούλεται δὲ τὸ προενδημεῖν
418 ῥῆμα τῷ Ποσειδωνίῳ τὸ οἷον προανα|πλάττειν τε καὶ προτυποῦν
τὸ πρᾶγμα παρ' ἑαυτῷ τὸ μέλλον γενήσεσθαι καὶ ὡς πρὸς ἤδη γενό-
9 μενον ἐθισμόν τινα ποιεῖσθαι κατὰ βραχύ. διὸ καὶ τὸ τοῦ Ἀναξαγό-
ρου παρείληφεν ἐνταῦθα, ὡς ἄρα τινὸς ἀναγγείλαντος αὐτῷ τεθνάναι
τὸν υἱὸν εὖ μάλα καθεστηκότως εἶπεν «ᾔδειν θνητὸν γεννήσας» καὶ ὡς
τοῦτο λαβὼν Εὐριπίδης τὸ νόημα τὸν Θησέα πεποίηκε λέγοντα

10 «ἐγὼ δὲ παρὰ σοφοῦ τινος μαθὼν
εἰς φροντίδας νοῦν συμφοράς τ' ἐβαλλόμην,
φυγάς τ' ἐμαυτῷ προ⟨σ⟩τιθεὶς πάτρας ἐμῆς
θανάτους τ' ἀώρους καὶ κακὰς ἄλλας ὁδούς,
ὥστ', εἴ τι πάσχοιμ' ὧν ἐδόξαζόν ποτε,
μή μοι νεῶρες προσπεσὸν ψυχὴν δάκοι.»/

394 11 οὕτως δὲ εἰρῆσθαί φησι καὶ τὰ τοιαῦτα·

«εἰ μὲν τόδ' ἦμαρ πρῶτον ἦν κακουμένῳ
καὶ μὴ μακρὰ⟨ν⟩ δὴ διὰ πόνων ἐναυστόλουν,
εἰκὸς σφαδᾴζειν ἦν ἂν ὡς νεόζυγα
πῶλον χαλινὸν ἀρτίως δεδεγμένον· |
419 νῦν δ' ἀμβλύς εἰμι καὶ κατηρτυκὼς κακῶν.»

3] *cf. supra*, p. 264.17–30 5–11] *cf.* Hirzel, Unters. III, p. 428 n. 2 7–284.17] Pohlenz, 1898, pp. 616–618 7–284.2] SVF III, pp. 131–132 7–17] *cf.* Reinhardt, 1921, pp. 292–293 8–10] *cf.* Cic. Tusc. Disp. iii. 26; 52 10–23] Anax. fr. A 33 D.-K. 16] *cf.* Diog. Laert. ii. 13 Cic. Tusc. Disp. iii. 30; 58 18–23] Eur. fr. 964 Nauck, p. 672 25–29] Eur. fr. 821 (Phrixus) *cf.* Nauck, p. 628 Snell, Supplementum, p. 13

7 *ante* καί *lac. statuit Müller* διὰ τί] διότι H: *corr. Pohlenz* 8 ἐκπίπτει τὲ H: *corr. Wyttenbach*: ἐκπτοεῖ τε *Bake*: ἐκπίπτειν τε ποιεῖ *Pohlenz* 10 δι' ὃ *Pohlenz* φησι] δεῖ *Corn.*: δεῖν φησι *Kühn* 11 μήπω τε] μήποτε H: *corr. Müller*: καὶ μήπω *Kühn* χρῆσαι, *ut vid.*, H: *corr.* M *Ald.* 12 Ποσειδωνίῳ] Χρυσίππῳ *Bake*: *ante* Ποσ. *indicem corruptionis inser. Müller* 15 ἀπαγγείλαντος *Kühn* 16 καθεστηκότως] ω *ex* ο *corr.* H 18 *ante* παρὰ *add.* τοῦτο *Musgrave*, ταῦτα *Nauck* 20 φυγάς τ'] φυγάδ' H: *corr. Musgrave*: φυγὰς δ' *Chart.* ἐμαυτὸν H: *ex Plut. Mor. 112 D corr. Chart.* προτιθεὶς H: *ex Plut. Mor. 112 D corr. Chart.* 21 θανάτους τ'] *ν e corr.*, τ' *sscr.* H 22 πάσχοιμι H: *corr. Chart.* 23 νεωραῖς H: *corr. Müller*: νεωρὲς *Musgrave Greenhill*: νεαρὸν *Plut. Mor. 112 D* 25 τόδε ἦμαρ H: *corr. Chart.* 26 μακρὰ H: *corr. Greenhill* 27 ἦν] "μ' ἦν *malim*" *Nauck*

Here Posidonius also gives a double refutation of Chrysippus. 6
In answer to this second definition he mentions the wise and those
progressing toward wisdom, as I said before; the one group suppose
themselves to be in the presence of the greatest goods, the other of
the greatest evils, yet neither is for that reason in an affected state.
With reference to the first definition he asks why it is not the belief 7
that evil is present, but only the fresh belief, that causes distress;
and he asks why all that is unprepared for and strange, falling on a
person in a sudden burst, confounds him and causes him to abandon
his earlier judgments, but if prepared for, made familiar and pro-
longed, either it does not upset him at all, so as to cause an affective
movement, or it does so to a very limited extent. That is the reason
why he says to 'dwell in' things 'in advance' and to behave toward
things not yet present as though they were present. The word *pro-* 8
endēmein (dwell in in advance) means to Posidonius to imagine,
as it were, in advance and to prefigure in one's mind what is going
to happen, and to bring about a gradual habituation to it, as to some-
thing that has happened before. And that is why he cited here the 9
story about Anaxagoras, that when someone brought him the
news that his son was dead, he said with great composure, "I knew
I had begotten a mortal"; and he mentioned also how Euripides
took this idea and portrayed Theseus as saying:

"Taught by a certain sage, I 10
cast my mind into cares and calamities
and added to my lot flight from my native land,
untimely death, and other passages of woe,
so that if ever I suffered any of the things I kept
imagining,
it might not fall on me as new and sting my soul."

The following lines, he says, make the same point: 11

"If this were the first day of my afflictions,
if I were not voyaging far and wide through evils,
I might be expected to rear up like a new-yoked
colt that has just received the bit;
but now I am dulled and tamed to evils."

ἔσθ' ὅτε τὰ τοιαῦτα· [μακρὸς]
«χρόνος μαλάξει, νῦν δ' ἔθ' ἡβάσκει κακόν.»
12 Ὅτι δ' ἐν τῷ χρόνῳ μαλάττεται τὰ πάθη, κἂν αἱ δόξαι μένωσι τοῦ
κακόν τι αὐτοῖς γεγονέναι, καὶ ὁ Χρύσιππος ἐν τῷ δευτέρῳ Περὶ παθῶν
13 μαρτυρεῖ γράφων ὧδε· «ζητήσαι δ' ἄν τις καὶ περὶ τῆς ἀνέσεως τῆς
λύπης, πῶς γίνεται, πότερον δόξης τινὸς μετακινουμένης ἢ πασῶν δια-
14 μενουσῶν, καὶ διὰ τί τοῦτ' ἔσται.» εἶτ' ἐπιφέρων φησί, «δοκεῖ δέ μοι ἡ
395 μὲν τοιαύτη δόξα διαμένειν, ὅτι κακὸν αὐτὸ ὃ δὴ πάρεστιν, / ἐγχρονι-
ζομένης δ' ἀνίεσθαι ἡ συστολὴ καὶ ὡς οἶμαι ἡ ἐπὶ τὴν συστολὴν ὁρμή.
15 τυχὸν δὲ καὶ ταύτης διαμενούσης οὐχ ὑπακούσεται τὰ ἑξῆς, διὰ ποιὰν
16 ἄλλην ἐπιγινομένην διάθεσιν δυσσυλλόγιστον τούτων γινομένων. οὕτω
γὰρ καὶ κλαίοντες παύονται καὶ μὴ βουλόμενοι κλαίειν κλαίουσιν, ὅταν
μὴ ὁμοίας τὰς φαντασίας τὰ ὑποκείμενα ποιῇ καὶ ἐνιστῆταί τι ἢ μηθέν.
420 17 ὃν τρόπον γὰρ ἡ θρήνων παῦσις γίνεται καὶ | κλαυθμοί, τοιαῦτα εὔλογον
καὶ ἐπ' ἐκείνων συντυγχάνειν ἐν ταῖς ἀρχαῖς μᾶλλον τῶν πραγμάτων
κινούντων, καθάπερ ἐπὶ τῶν τὸν γέλωτα κινούντων γίνεσθαι ἔφην, καὶ
τὰ ὅμοια τούτοις.»
18 Ὅτι μὲν οὖν ἐν τῷ χρόνῳ παύεται τὰ πάθη καίτοι τῆς δόξης δια-
μενούσης, αὐτὸς ὁ Χρύσιππος ὁμολογεῖ· διὰ τίνα μέντοι τὴν αἰτίαν
19 τοῦτο γίνεται, δυσλόγιστον εἶναί φησιν. εἶθ' ἑξῆς ἕτερα παραπλησίως
γινόμενα γράφει περὶ ὧν οὐδ' αὐτῶν δηλονότι τὴν αἰτίαν ἐπαγγέλ-
396 λεται γιγνώσκειν. / ἀλλ' οὐ Ποσειδώνιός γε, Χρύσιππε, τὰς αἰτίας τῶν
τοιούτων ἀγνοεῖν φησιν, ἀλλ' ἐπαινεῖ καὶ ἀποδέχεται τὰ ὑπὸ τῶν παλαιῶν
20 εἰρημένα, ἃ ἐφεξῆς ἐρῶ. σὺ δ' οὔτ' ἐκείνων μνημονεύσας οὔτ' ἄλλην αὐτὸς
εἰπὼν οἴει λελύσθαι τὸ ζητούμενον, ἂν ὁμολογήσῃς ἀγνοεῖν τὴν αἰτίαν.
21 καίτοι τό γε συνέχον ὅλην τὴν πραγματείαν τήν τε τῶν λογικῶν ζητημά-
των καὶ τὴν θεραπευτικὴν τῶν παθῶν οὐδὲν ἄλλο ἐστὶν ἢ τὸ τὰς αἰτίας
22 ἐξευρεῖν ὑφ' ὧν γίνεταί τε καὶ παύεται τὰ πάθη. οὕτω γὰρ ἄν τις οἶμαι καὶ
τὴν γένεσιν αὐτῶν κωλύσειε καὶ γενομένας παῦσαι δυνηθείη. συναναι-
421 ρεῖσθαι | γὰρ εὔλογον οἶμαι ταῖς αἰτίαις τάς τε γενέσεις καὶ τὰς ὑπάρ-
23 ξεις τῶν πραγμάτων. ταῦτά τοι καὶ ἀπορεῖς κατὰ τὸ Περὶ τῶν παθῶν
βιβλίον τι καὶ γράψαι τοιοῦτον ἡμῖν, ᾧ προσέχοντες τὸν νοῦν κωλύσομέν
τε τῶν παθῶν ἕκαστον γίνεσθαι καὶ γενόμενον ἰασόμεθα, καίτοι ταῦτα
καὶ τοῦ Πλάτωνος θαυμαστῶς γράψαντος, ὡς καὶ ὁ Ποσειδώνιος

2] Eur. Alcestis 1085 3–22] SVF III, pp. 117–118 10–11] *cf. infra*, p. 288.19–21 11–13] Pohlenz, 1898, p. 590 11–13 ποιῇ] *cf. infra*, p. 288.23–24 15–22] Reinhardt, 1921, p. 306 18–24] Posid. test. 101 Edelstein-Kidd 19–20] *cf. supra*, lin. 11 *infra*, p. 288.12–13 21–22] *cf. infra*, p. 316.14–15 24–33] SVF III, p. 118 26–28] *cf. supra*, p. 272.25–28 31–33] *cf. infra*, p. 314.4–5 33–286.7] Posid. fr. 150a Edelstein-Kidd 33–286.4] Posid. test. 97 Edelstein-Kidd 33–34] *cf. infra*, p. 316.13–14

1 μακρὸς *del. Müller* 2 δέ θ' H: *corr.* R 5 ζητῆσαι H: *corr. Kühn* 11 δισυλλόγιστον H: *corr. Pohlenz*: δυσσιλλόγιστον R²: δυσυλλόγιστον *Ald.*: δυσλόγιστον *Bas.*: ἀσυλλόγιστον *Müller (cf. infra, lin. 20* δυσλόγιστον, *p. 288.12, 32* ἀσυλλόγιστον, *et VIII 882 K.* δυσσυλλόγιστα*)* 13 μὴ *del. Ricci (cf. infra, p. 288.24)* καὶ] καθὸ ἂν *v. Arnim* 14 κλαυθμῶν *Müller* 18 ἐν *del. v. Arnim* γίνεται *in textu*, παύεται *sscr.* H 20 παραπλησίως *ex* -ήσια *corr.* H

Sometimes words such as these (are spoken):

"Time will soften it; now the evil still has the strength of youth."

Chrysippus also testifies in the second book On the Affections 12
that the affections are softened in time, even though the opinion remains that some evil has befallen one. He writes as follows: "A person 13
might inquire about the abatement of distress, how it comes about, whether at the alteration of some opinion, or while all continue (as they were), and why this will occur." Then he continues, "It seems 14
to me that an opinion of this kind remains, that the actual present thing is evil, but as the opinion grows older the contraction is eased and, as I believe, the conation that follows on the contraction. It 15
might also happen that although the conation persists, the things that follow will not conform to it, this being due to another supervening disposition of some sort which is not easily reasoned out. Thus 16
people cease weeping, and people weep against their will, when the underlying circumstances create unlike impressions and something or nothing stands in the way. For in the same way that cessation 17
from laments and outbreaks of weeping occur, so it is reasonable that there should be occurrences of this and similar kinds also in those other cases, since things cause greater motion initially, as I stated with reference to the causes of laughter."

Thus Chrysippus admits that the affections cease in time, 18
even though the opinion persists; but the reason why this happens is, he says, difficult to reason out. He then goes on to write about other 19
things that happen in similar ways, and here again, of course, he does not profess to know the causes. But, Chrysippus, Posidonius does not say that he is ignorant of the causes of such things; he praises and accepts the account of the ancients, which I shall presently relate. But you, without mentioning them or stating another (cause) 20
on your own authority, think the problem has been solved if you admit to ignorance of the cause. And yet the unifying theme in your 21
whole treatise, both on the theory of the affections and on their cure, is none other than the discovery of the causes by which the affections are aroused and allayed. This discovery, I believe, would enable a 22
person to prevent the affections from arising and to put an end to those that have arisen. For it is reasonable, I think, that the genesis and the existence of things are removed along with their causes. This is why you are at a loss in your book On the Affections to write 23
anything for us of such a kind that by attending to it we shall prevent the several affections from arising and heal them when they have arisen. And yet Plato wrote of these matters marvellously well, as Posidonius too points out; for Posidonius admires the

397 ἐπισημαίνεται / θαυμάζων τὸν ἄνδρα καὶ θεῖον ἀποκαλῶν ὡς καὶ πρε-
σβεύων αὐτοῦ τά τε περὶ τῶν παθῶν δόγματα καὶ τὰ περὶ τῶν τῆς ψυχῆς
δυνάμεων ὅσα τε περὶ τοῦ μὴ γίνεσθαι τὴν ἀρχὴν ἢ γενόμενα παύεσθαι
24 τάχιστα τῆς ψυχῆς τὰ πάθη γέγραπται πρὸς αὐτοῦ. συνῆφθαι δὲ καὶ
τὴν περὶ τῶν ἀρετῶν διδασκαλίαν τούτοις φησὶ καὶ τὴν περὶ τοῦ τέλους
καὶ ὅλως πάντα τὰ δόγματα τῆς ἠθικῆς φιλοσοφίας ὥσπερ ἐκ μιᾶς
μηρίνθου δεδέσθαι τῆς γνώσεως τῶν κατὰ τὴν ψυχὴν δυνάμεων, αὐτός
τε δείκνυσιν ὡς ὑπὸ θυμοῦ καὶ ἐπιθυμίας γίγνεται τὰ πάθη καὶ
διὰ τίνα τὴν αἰτίαν ἐν τῷ χρόνῳ καθίσταται, κἂν αἱ δόξαι τε καὶ αἱ
25 κρίσεις ἔτι μένωσι τοῦ κακὸν ὑπάρχειν αὐτοῖς ἢ γεγονέναι. προσχρῆται
422 δ' εἰς τοῦτο μάρτυρι καὶ αὐτῷ τῷ Χρυσίππῳ | κατὰ τὸ δεύτερον Περὶ
26 τῶν παθῶν ὧδέ πως γράφοντι· «ἐπὶ δὲ τῆς λύπης καὶ ὡς ἂν ἐμπλη-
σθέντες τινὲς ὁμοίως φαίνονται ἀφίστασθαι, καθάπερ καὶ ἐπὶ Ἀχιλλέως
ταῦτα λέγει ὁ ποιητὴς πενθοῦντος τὸν Πάτροκλον· /

398 'ἀλλ' ὅτε δὴ κλαίων τε κυλινδόμενός τ' ἐκορέσθη
καί οἱ ἀπὸ πραπίδων ἦλθ' ἵμερος ἠδ' ἀπὸ γυίων,'

ἐπὶ τὸ παρακαλεῖν ὥρμησε τὸν Πρίαμον τὴν τῆς λύπης ἀλογίαν αὐτῷ
27 παριστάς.» εἶτ' ἐφεξῆς ἐπιφέρει καὶ ταῦτα· «καθ' ὃν λόγον οὐκ ἂν ἀπελ-
πίσαι τις οὕτως τῶν πραγμάτων ἐγχρονιζομένων καὶ τῆς παθητικῆς
φλεγμονῆς ἀνιεμένης τὸν λόγον παρεισδυόμενον καὶ οἱονεὶ χώραν λαμ-
28 βάνοντα παριστάναι τὴν τοῦ πάθους ἀλογίαν.» ἐναργῶς γὰρ ἐν τούτοις
ὁ Χρύσιππος ὁμολογεῖ τήν τε παθητικὴν φλεγμονὴν ἀνίεσθαι κατὰ
τὸν χρόνον, ἔτι τῆς ὑπολήψεώς τε καὶ δόξης μενούσης, ἐμπίπλασθαί τε
τῶν παθητικῶν κινήσεων τοὺς ἀνθρώπους καὶ διὰ τοῦτο παῦλάν τινα
λαμβάνοντος τοῦ πάθους καὶ ἡσυχάσαντος τὸν λόγον ἐπικρατέστερον
423 29 γίνε|σθαι. ταῦτα γὰρ ἀληθῆ μέν ἐστιν εἴπερ τινὰ καὶ ἄλλα, μάχεται δὲ
ταῖς ὑποθέσεσιν αὐτοῦ καθάπερ καὶ τὰ ἐπιφερόμενα τόνδε τὸν τρόπον
30 ἔχοντα· «λέγεται δὲ καὶ τοιαῦτα εἰς τὴν μεταβολὴν τῶν παθῶν·/

399 'λαιψηρὸς δὲ κόρος στυγεροῖο γόοιο'

καὶ ἔτι τὰ τοιαῦτα εἰς τὸ κατὰ τὴν λύπην ἀγωγόν·

'τοῖς δὲ δυστυχοῦσί πως
τερπνὸν τὸ κλαῦσαι κἀποδύρασθαι τύχας·'»

31 καὶ ἔτι τούτων ἐφεξῆς,

«ὣς φάτο, τοῖσι δὲ πᾶσιν ὑφ' ἵμερον ὦρσε γόοιο»

6–7] *cf.* Gal. Quod opt. med. sit etiam philos.: I 61 K. 10–288.12] SVF III, pp. 118–119 12–21] Pohlenz, 1898, p. 618 15–16] *cf.* Hom. Od. iv. 541 Il. xxiv. 514 17–18] *cf.* Hom. Il. xxiv. 518–551 24] *cf. infra*, p. 322.13–14 28–288.3] Pohlenz, 1898, pp. 618–619 29] Hom. Od. iv. 103 31–32] *cf.* Eur. fr. 563 Nauck, p. 537 Aesch. Prom. Vinct. 637 Porson, Adversaria, p. 134 34] Hom. Od. iv. 113

1 ἀποκαλεῖ H: *corr.* F ὡς *del. Müller* πρεσβεύειν *Schöne* 3 παύεσθαι *bis scr.* H: *corr.* M *Ald.* 9 διά τινα H: *corr. Ald.* 12 ἐπὶ] περὶ *Ald.*: ἔτι *Kalbfleisch (cf. supra, pp. 270.25; 276.19)* τῆς λύπης καὶ] καὶ τῆς λύπης *Kalbfleisch*: καὶ *del. Müller* 13 ὁμοίως] ὅμως *coni. Bake* 16 ἦδ' H: *corr. Bake* γυιῶν H: *corr. Chart.* 18 ἐπιφέρει *in* -η *mut.* H² 25 ἡσυχάσαντας H: *corr.* R² *Ald.* 26 ἐστιν] εσ *e corr.* H 27 τόνδε *bis scr.* H: *corr.* M *Ald.* 31 πῶς H: *corr. Chart.* 32 καὶ ἀποδύρασθαι H: *corr. Kühn*

man and calls him divine inasmuch as he holds in honor Plato's
teaching about the affections and about the powers of the soul, and
all that he wrote on the subject of the soul's affections not arising at
all, or if they arise, ceasing most quickly. He says that instruction 24
about the virtues and about the end is tied to these teachings, and,
in short, that all the doctrines of ethical philosophy are bound to-
gether by the knowledge of the soul's powers as by a single cord.
And Posidonius himself shows that the affections arise from anger
and desire, and he gives the reason why they subside in time, even
though a person continue in the opinion and judgment that an evil
exists or has arisen for him. In support of this point he even invokes 25
the testimony of Chrysippus himself, who writes as follows in the
second book of his work On the Affections: "In the case of distress 26
also there are some who appear similarly to take leave of it as though
sated. Thus the poet speaks in this way about Achilles grieving
for Patroclus:

'But when he had his fill of weeping and rolling
on the ground,
and the longing for such things had gone from his mind
and limbs'

he undertook to comfort Priam by setting before him the irrationality
of his distress." Then he continues, "By this account a person would 27
not give up hope that with the passage of time, when the inflammation
of the affection has abated, reason will make its way in and find room,
so to speak, and expose the irrationality of the affection." Here Chry- 28
sippus clearly admits that the inflammation of affection subsides
in time, while the supposition and opinion still persist; men get their
fill of the affective motions, and when because of this the affection
has a kind of respite and grows quiet, reason gains the upper hand.
This is the truth, if anything is, but it is in conflict with Chrysippus' 29
assumptions. It is the same with the next passage, which goes as fol-
lows: "Such words as these are spoken also with reference to the 30
alteration of the affections:

'Swift is the satiety of hateful grief;'

and also words like these about the attraction of grief:

'Somehow when ill fortune strikes
it is pleasant to weep and mourn one's lot;'"

and next after these Chrysippus cites 31

"Thus he spoke, and he aroused in them all a longing
for lamentation",

καὶ

«τὸν αὐτὸν ἔγειρε γόον
ἄναγε πολύδακρυν ἀδονάν.»

32 ἔ⟨σ⟩τι δὲ ἀμέλει πάμπολ⟨λ⟩α καὶ ἄλλα τοιαῦτα παρὰ τῶν ποιητῶν
ἀθροῖσαι μαρτύρια τοῦ καὶ λύπης καὶ δακρύων καὶ κλαυθμῶν καὶ θυμοῦ
καὶ νίκης καὶ τιμῆς καὶ πάντων [τε] τῶν τοιούτων ἐμπίπλασθαι τοὺς
ἀνθρώπους, ἐφ' οἷς οὐδὲν χαλεπόν ἐστι συλλογίζεσθαι τὴν αἰτίαν δι'
424 ἣν ἐν τῷ χρόνῳ παύεται μὲν τὰ πάθη, κρατεῖ δὲ τῶν ὁρμῶν | ὁ λόγος.
33 ὡς γὰρ ἐφίεται τὸ παθητικὸν τῆς ψυχῆς οἰκείων τινῶν ὀρεκτ[ικ]ῶν,
400 οὕτως καὶ τυγχάνον αὐτῶν ἐμπίπλαται κἀν τούτῳ τὴν / ἑαυτοῦ κίνησιν
καθίστησιν, ἥτις ἐκράτει τῆς ὁρμῆς τοῦ ζῴου καὶ καθ' ἑαυτὴν ἦγεν ἐφ'
34 ὅ τι παρήγετο. οὔκουν ἀσυλλόγιστοι τῆς παύλης τῶν παθῶν εἰσιν αἱ
αἰτίαι, καθάπερ ὁ Χρύσιππος ἔλεγεν, ἀλλὰ καὶ πάνυ σαφεῖς τῷ γε
35 μὴ βουλομένῳ φιλονεικεῖν τοῖς παλαιοῖς. οὐδὲν γὰρ οὕτως ἐναργές ἐστιν
ὡς τὸ δυνάμεις τινὰς ἐν ταῖς ἡμετέραις εἶναι ψυχαῖς ἐφιεμένας φύσει, τὴν
μὲν ἡδονῆς τὴν δὲ κράτους καὶ νίκης, ἃς ἐναργῶς ὁρᾶσθαί φησι κἀν τοῖς
ἄλλοις ζῴοις ὁ Ποσειδώνιος, ὥσπερ καὶ ἡμεῖς ἐπεδείξαμεν εὐθὺς ἐν
ἀρχῇ τοῦ πρώτου γράμματος.

36 Ἐπιμέμφεται δ' ὀρθῶς τοῦ Χρυσίππου καὶ τὸ φάναι «τυχὸν δὲ
τῆς ὁρμῆς διαμενούσης οὐχ ὑπακούσεται τὰ ἑξῆς διὰ ποιάν ἄλλην ἐπι-
γινομένην διάθεσιν.» ἀμήχανον γὰρ εἶναί φησι παρεῖναι μὲν τὴν ὁρμήν,
37 ὑπ' ἄλλης δέ τινος αἰτίας κωλύεσθαι τὴν κατ' αὐτὴν ἐνέργειαν. ὅθεν κἀ-
425 πειδὰν λέγῃ, «οὕτω γὰρ καὶ | κλαίοντες παύονται καὶ μὴ βουλόμενοι
κλαίειν κλαίουσιν, ὅταν ⟨μὴ⟩ ὁμοίας τὰ ὑποκείμενα φαντασίας ποιῇ»,
401 τὴν / αἰτίαν ἐρωτᾷ κἀνταῦθα ὁ Ποσειδώνιος δι' ἣν καὶ οἱ πολλοὶ μὴ
βουλόμενοι πολλάκις κλαίουσιν ἐπισχεῖν μὴ δυνάμενοι τὰ δάκρυα καὶ
ἄλλοι κλαίειν ἔτι βουλόμενοι φθάνουσι[ν ἔτι] παυόμενοι, ⟨δηλονότι⟩
διὰ τὰς παθητικὰς κινήσεις σφόδρα ἐγκειμένας ὡς μὴ κρατεῖσθαι πρὸ⟨ς⟩
τῆς βουλήσεως, ἢ παντελῶς πεπαυμένας ὡς μηκέτ' ἐπεγείρεσθαι δύνα-
38 σθαι πρὸς αὐτῆς. οὕτω γὰρ ἥ τε τοῦ λόγου μάχη τε καὶ διαφορὰ πρὸς
τὸ πάθος εὑρεθήσεται καὶ τῆς ψυχῆς αἱ δυνάμεις ἐναργῶς σωθήσονται,
οὐ μὰ Δία ὡς Χρύσιππός φησι διά τινας αἰτίας ἀσυλλογίστους τούτων

2–3] Eur. Electra 125–126 9–18] Posid. fr. 158 Edelstein-Kidd 9–12] *cf.* Pohlenz, 1898, pp. 554; 628 13] *cf. supra*, p. 284.19–20 14–18] libri primi test., *v. supra*, p. 66.8–11 15–16] *cf.* Pohlenz, 1898, p. 619 Cic. De off. i. 13 19–21] *cf. supra*, p. 284.10–11 23–24] *cf. supra*, p. 284.11–13 27–30] Pohlenz, 1898, pp. 628–629

1 *post* καὶ *spat. 4 litt. in* H 2 *ante* τὸν *habet* ἴθι *Eur.* ἀνέγειρε H: *corr. Bergk apud Müller* 3 ἀηδόνα H: *ex Eur. corr. Kühn* 4 ἔστι] ἔτι H: *corr. Corn.* πάμπολα H: *corr. Ald.* 5 ῥ θμοῦ H: *corr. Diels Kalbfleisch*: θρήνου *Ald.* 6 τε *del. Müller*: γε *Einarson* 9 ὀρεκτικῶν *(in* ὀρεκῶν *mut.* H[3?]*)* H *Ald.*: *corr.* M 10 τυγχάνον] τυγχανόντων καὶ τυγχανόντων H: *correxi*: τυγχάνον τῶν *Pohlenz* ἑαυτοῦ] ἑαυτῶν H: *corr. Müller* 12 παύλας H: *corr. Müller* 19 τῷ Χρυσίππῳ *Müller* καὶ τὸ] κἀν τῷ *Ald.* 24 μὴ *add. Corn. (cf. supra, p. 284.13)* 25 καὶ οἱ *del. Müller,* οἱ *tantum Kalbfleisch* 27 φθάνουσιν ἔτι H: *corr. Müller* δηλονότι *add. Einarson,* καὶ τοῦτο γίνεσθαι φησὶ *Corn.,* ἤτοι *Bake,* γίνεσθαι δέ φησι *Müller* 28 *ante* σφόδρα *add.* ἢ *Müller* πρὸ H: *corr.* R *Corn.* 30 αὐτῆς *in* αὐτῶν *mut.* H *supra lin.* τε[II] *del. Müller*

and

"Raise up the same lament,
renew the tearful joy."

It is quite easy to collect many other such passages from the poets 32 which testify that men become sated with distress, tears, laments, anger, victory, honor, and all such things; and it is not difficult in these cases to infer the reason why the affections cease after a time and reason gains control of the conations. For as the affective part of 33 the soul strives after certain objects of desire that are proper to it, so when it obtains them it is satiated; and thereupon it puts an end to its own motion, which was controlling the animal's conation and in keeping with its nature was leading (the animal) to this or that misguided end. Therefore the causes of the cessation of the affections 34 are not inaccessible to reason, as Chrysippus said, but they are very clear to anyone who does not wish to compete with the ancients. Nothing is so evident as that there are certain powers in our souls, 35 one of which naturally pursues pleasure, the other mastery and victory. These powers, Posidonius says, are clearly seen also in the lower animals; and we too made this same point at the very beginning of the first book.

Posidonius is right also to find fault with Chrysippus' saying, 36 "It might happen that although the conation persists, the things that follow will not conform to it because of another supervening disposition of some sort." Posidonius says that it is impossible that the conation be present and the activity in accord with it be obstructed by some other cause. Therefore when Chrysippus says, 37 "Thus people cease weeping, and people weep against their will, when the underlying circumstances create unlike impressions", Posidonius again asks the reason why ordinary men often weep when they do not wish to and are unable to check their tears, while in others the tears stop before the wish – obviously because the affective motions press so hard that they cannot be mastered by the will, or are brought to so complete a halt that it can no longer arouse them. In 38 this way the conflict and disagreement between reason and affection will be laid bare and the powers will clearly be saved, since these things happen not indeed as Chrysippus said, because of some causes

39 γινομένων ἀλλὰ διὰ τὰς ὑπὸ τῶν παλαιῶν εἰρημένας. οὐ γὰρ Ἀριστοτέλης μόνον ἢ Πλάτων ἐδόξαζον οὕτως ἀλλ' ἔτι πρόσθεν ἄλλοι τέ τινες καὶ ὁ Πυθαγόρας, ὡς καὶ ὁ Ποσειδώνιός φησιν ἐκείνου πρώτου μὲν εἶναι λέγων τὸ δόγμα, Πλάτωνα δ' ἐξεργάσασθαι καὶ κατασκευάσαι
402 40 τελεώτερον αὐτό. διὰ τοῦτο τοίνυν καὶ τὰ / ἔθη φαίνεται πλεῖστον δυνά-
426 41 μενα καὶ ὅλως ὁ | χρόνος εἰς τὰς παθητικὰς κινήσεις. ἐν μὲν γὰρ τοῖς ἔθεσιν οἰκειοῦται κατὰ βραχὺ τὸ τῆς ψυχῆς ἄλογον οἷς ἂν ἐντρέφηται, κατὰ δὲ τὸν χρόνον ὡς προείρηται παῦλα γίνεται τῶν παθῶν ἐμπιπλαμένων τῶν ἀλόγων τῆς ψυχῆς δυνάμεων ὧν ἐπεθύμουν ἔμπροσθεν.
42 αἱ δὲ λογικαὶ γνώσεις τε καὶ κρίσεις καὶ ὅλως ἐπιστῆμαι πᾶσαι καὶ τέχναι διὰ τὸν χρόνον αὐτὸν μόνον ψιλὸν οὔτε δύσλυτοι φαίνονται γίγνεσθαι καθάπερ οἱ κατὰ πάθος ἐθισμοί, οὔτε μετατίθεσθαί τε καὶ παύεσθαι
43 καθάπερ ἡ λύπη καὶ ἄλλα πάθη. τίς γὰρ τοῦ τὰ δὶς δύο τέσσαρα εἶναι διὰ τὸν χρόνον ἐμπλησθεὶς ἀπέστη καὶ μετεδόξασεν; ἢ τίς τοῦ [μὴ] πάσας
44 ⟨ἴσας⟩ εἶναι τὰς ἐκ τοῦ κέντρου τοῦ κύκλου; καθ' ἕκαστόν τε τῶν ἄλλων θεωρημάτων οὐδείς ἐστιν ὅστις ἐμπλησθεὶς ἀπέθετο τὴν παλαιὰν δόξαν, ὥσπερ ἀποτίθεται τὸ κλαίειν τε καὶ λυπεῖσθαι καὶ στένειν οἰμώζειν /
403 τε καὶ θρηνεῖν ὅσα τε ἄλλα τοιαῦτα, κἂν αἱ περὶ τῶν γεγενημένων ὡς κακῶν ὅμοιαι διαμένωσιν ὑπολήψεις.
427 45 Ἱκανὰ μὲν οὖν ἀμέλει καὶ ταῦτα πρὸς ἔνδειξιν ὧν οὐκ ὀρθῶς | ἔγραψεν ὁ Χρύσιππος ὑπέρ τε τῶν τῆς ψυχῆς παθῶν, καὶ πολὺ πρότερον ἔτι περὶ
46 τῶν ἐργαζομένων αὐτὰ δυνάμεων· οὐ μὴν ἀλλὰ διὰ τοῦ πέμπτου γράμματος ἔγνωκα περὶ τῶν αὐτῶν ἔτι διαλεχθῆναι παραλείπων μὲν τὰ πλεῖστα τῶν οὐκ ὀρθῶς εἰρημένων αὐτῷ, μόνων δὲ ἐκείνων μνημονεύων ἐν οἷς ἐναντιολογεῖται πρὸς ἑαυτὸν ἐναντία τε τολμᾷ φθέγγεσθαι τοῖς ἐναργῶς φαινομένοις· ἐπιμνησθήσομαι δ' ἐν αὐτοῖς ἔτι καὶ τῶν ὑπὸ τοῦ Ποσειδωνίου πρὸς τὸν Χρύσιππον ἀντειρημένων. /|

1–5] Posid. test. 95 Edelstein-Kidd 6–7] Pohlenz, 1898, p. 629 8] *cf. supra*, p. 286.23–25 20–27] Posid. test. 61 Edelstein-Kidd

4 μὲν] τὲ H: *corr.* F 6 ὅλος H: *corr. Pohlenz* 14 διὰ τὸν] διτὸν H: *corr.* R *Ald.* μὴ *del. Müller* 15 ἴσας *add. Müller*, γράμμας *(sic)* ἴσας *post* κύκλου *(lin. 15) Corn.*, εὐθείας ἴσας *Edelstein* κέντρου] μέτρου H: *corr. Ald.* 19 διαμένουσιν H: *corr. Chart.* 27 γα(ληνοῦ) περὶ τῶν ἱπποκράτ(ους) καὶ πλάτωνος δογμάτων τὸ τέταρτον *subscr.* H

inaccessible to reason, but because of the causes stated by the ancients. This was not the opinion of Aristotle or Plato only; it was held 39 even earlier by certain others, among them Pythagoras, who, as Posidonius also says, was the first to hold that view, while Plato worked it out and made it more complete. For this reason, therefore, 40 habits and time in general are seen to have the greatest importance for affective movements. The irrational part of the soul gradually 41 conforms to the habits in which it is nurtured; and in time, as I said earlier, there is a cessation of the affections, when the irrational powers of the soul get their fill of the things they previously desired. But it does not appear that from the mere passage of time rational 42 opinions and judgments, and in general all sciences and arts, become difficult to dislodge, as affective habituations do, or that they shift and cease, like distress and other affections. Who ever because of the 43 passing of time had his fill of 'two times two are four' and so abandoned it and changed his opinion? Or who ever had his fill of the opinion that all the radii of a circle are equal? And so it is with every 44 theorem: there is no one who from satiety has put aside his earlier view, as he put aside weeping, grieving, groaning, wailing, mourning, and all other such things, even when his assumption about what happened, that it was bad, remains the same.

These remarks are quite sufficient to indicate the errors in Chrysippus' statements about the affections of the soul, and still more 45 about the powers that produce them. Nevertheless, I have decided to 46 continue in the fifth book the discussion of these same matters, passing over most of his errors and mentioning only those in which he contradicts himself and ventures to make pronouncements inconsistent with clearly observed facts. And in the course of the discussion I shall also mention Posidonius' criticisms of Chrysippus.

ΓΑΛΗΝΟΥ

ΠΕΡΙ ΤΩΝ ΙΠΠΟΚΡΑΤΟΥΣ ΚΑΙ ΠΛΑΤΩΝΟΣ ΔΟΓΜΑΤΩΝ

ΒΙΒΛΙΟΝ ΠΕΜΠΤΟΝ

404 428 1. Ὁ περὶ τῶν παθῶν τῆς ψυχῆς λόγος ἀναγκαῖος μὲν ἦν ἡμῖν
ἐσκέφθαι καὶ δι' ἑαυτόν, ἀναγκαιότερον δὲ ἐποίησαν αὐτὸν οἱ περὶ τὸν
Χρύσιππον εἰς ἀπόδειξιν τοῦ περιέχοντος τόπου τὸ τῆς ψυχῆς ἡγεμο-
2 νοῦν προσχρησάμενοι. δείξαντες γάρ, ὡς μὲν αὐτοὶ νομίζουσιν, ἅπαντα
τὰ πάθη συνιστάμενα κατὰ τὴν καρδίαν, ὡς δὲ τἀληθὲς ἔχει, τὰ κατὰ
429 μόνον τὸν θυμόν, ἔπειτα προσλα|βόντες ὡς ἔνθα ἂν ᾖ τὰ πάθη τῆς
ψυχῆς, ἐνταῦθ' ἐστὶ καὶ τὸ λογιζόμενον αὐτῆς, οὕτως ἤδη περαίνουσιν
3 ἐν τῇ καρδίᾳ τὸ λογιστικὸν ὑπάρχειν. ἡμεῖς δὲ ὅτι μὲν ἐντεῦθεν ὁρμᾶται
τὰ κατὰ τὸν θυμὸν ἀληθεύειν αὐτούς φαμεν, οὐ μὴν οὐθ' ὅτι καθ' ἕνα
405 τόπον ἀναγκαῖόν / ἐστι τό τε θυμούμενον εἶναι καὶ τὸ λογιζόμενον οὐθ'
ὅτι μιᾶς δυνάμεώς ἐστον ἔργα συγχωροῦμεν, ἀλλ' ἀποδεικνύειν αὐτοὺς
ἀξιοῦμεν, ὥσπερ τἆλλα τὰ κατὰ τὸν λόγον, οὕτω καὶ ὅτι τὴν αὐτὴν
ἀρχὴν ἀναγκαῖόν ἐστιν εἶναι τῶν τε παθῶν καὶ τοῦ λογισμοῦ.
4 Χρύσιππος μὲν οὖν ἐν τῷ πρώτῳ Περὶ παθῶν ἀποδεικνύναι
πειρᾶται κρίσεις τινὰς εἶναι τοῦ λογιστικοῦ τὰ πάθη, Ζήνων δ' οὐ τὰς
κρίσεις αὐτάς, ἀλλὰ τὰς ἐπιγιγνομένας αὐταῖς συστολὰς καὶ χύσεις
5 ἐπάρσεις τε καὶ ταπεινώσεις τῆς ψυχῆς ἐνόμιζεν εἶναι τὰ πάθη. ὁ Πο-
σειδώνιος δ' ἀμφοτέροις διενεχθεὶς ἐπαινεῖ τε ἅμα καὶ προσίεται
τὸ Πλάτωνος δόγμα καὶ ἀντιλέγει τοῖς περὶ τὸν Χρύσιππον οὔτε
κρίσεις εἶναι τὰ πάθη δεικνύων οὔτε ἐπιγιγνόμενα κρίσεσιν, ἀλλὰ κινήσεις
430 τινὰς ἑτέρων | δυνάμεων ἀλόγων ἃς ὁ Πλάτων ὠνόμασεν ἐπιθυμητικήν
6 τε καὶ θυμοειδῆ. πολλῶν δ' εἰρημένων αὐτῷ πρὸς ἀπόδειξιν τοῦ παλαιοῦ
δόγματος, ἃ μέν ἐστιν ἐπίκαιρα, ταῦτ' ἐν τῷ πρὸ τούτου λόγῳ τετάρτῳ
406 τῆς ὅλης ὄντι πραγματείας ἐπειράθην εἰπεῖν διὰ βραχέων / ἐπὶ τῇ
7 τελευτῇ τοῦ γράμματος. ἐν μὲν γὰρ τοῖς ἔμπροσθεν αὐτὸς ἐπ' ἐμαυτοῦ

3–11] SVF II, p. 236 9–10] *cf. supra*, pp. 176.16–17; 234.19–20 *infra*, p. 346.21–22 11–12] *cf. supra*, p. 208.31 17–25] Posid. fr. 152 Edelstein-Kidd 17–20] SVF III, p. 113 17–18] *cf. supra*, p. 238.4–23 *infra*, p. 314.8–10 18–20] SVF I, p. 51 *cf. supra*, pp. 240.5–9; 246.38–248.3 *infra*, p. 334.24–28 20–22] Posid. test. 98 Edelstein-Kidd 22–25] *cf. supra*, p. 248.4–6 25–294.3] Posid. test. 62 Edelstein-Kidd 25–26] Posid. fr. 157 Edelstein-Kidd

1–3 ἀρχὴ τοῦ πέμπτου λόγου H 14 ἔστων H: *corr. Chart. (cf. supra, p. 52)*: αὐτῶν R² *in mg.* 19 χύσεις] λύσεις *Ald.*: διαχύσεις *Müller* 20 ταπεινώσεις] τὰς πτώσεις H: *corr. Petersen*: πτώσεις *Bake* 23 κρίσεσιν] κρίσει H: *corr. Müller*: "*f.* κρίσεσι" *Bake*

GALEN

ON THE DOCTRINES OF HIPPOCRATES AND PLATO

BOOK V

1. The theory of the affections of the soul had to be examined for its own sake, but the inquiry was made even more necessary by Chrysippus and his followers, who used it for proving the location of the soul's governing part. Having shown, as they themselves thought, 2
that all the affections arise in the region of the heart – but in fact that only the affections of the spirited part arise there –, and then having added (as a second premise) that where the affections of the soul are, there its reasoning part is also, they then proceeded to draw the conclusion that reason is in the heart. We grant that 3
they are right when they say that the affections of the spirited part arise here, but we do not grant that the spirited and rational parts must be in one place or that they are the work of one power: and as with the other points of their argument, so here too we ask the Stoics to prove that the affections and reason must have the same source.

Now Chrysippus in the first book of his work On the Affec- 4
tions tries to prove that the affections are certain judgments of the reasoning part. Zeno, however, held that the affections are not the actual judgments but the contractions and expansions, risings and fallings of the soul that supervene on judgments. Posidonius, 5
disagreeing with both, both praises and accepts the Platonic view and refutes Chrysippus. He points out that the affections are not judgments and do not supervene on judgments; they are certain motions of other, irrational powers, which Plato called desiderative and spirited. He said many things in support of the ancient doctrine; 6
and I tried to mention briefly his most important points at the end of the preceding book, the fourth of the entire treatise. In the earlier 7

διῆλθον ὅσα τε μάχεται τῶν ἐναργῶς φαινομένων τῷ Χρυσίππου
δόγματι καὶ ὅσα πρὸς ἑαυτὸν ἐναντιολογούμενος εἴρηκεν οὐκ ἀναμείνας
τὸν ἔξωθεν κατήγορον.
8 Ἱκανὰ μὲν οὖν ἦν καὶ ἐκεῖνα πρὸς ἀπόδειξιν τοῦ πλείους εἶναι
δυνάμεις αἷς ἐπιθυμοῦμέν τε καὶ θυμούμεθα καὶ λογιζόμεθα καὶ μὴ μίαν,
ὡς ὁ Χρύσιππος οἴεται. προσκείσεται δ' οὐκ ὀλίγα καὶ κατὰ τοῦτον
ἔτι τὸν λόγον ὅσα ὁ Χρύσιππος αὐτὸς ἐναντιολογούμενος αὐτῷ
9 μαρτυρεῖ τοῖς τ' ἀληθέσιν ἅμα καὶ τῷ παλαιῷ δόγματι. τὰ μὲν γὰρ ἄλλα
τὰ κακῶς εἰρημένα παρ' αὐτοῦ καίτοι πάμπολ⟨λ⟩α τὸν ἀριθμὸν ὄντα
παρελθεῖν ἔκρινα πολύβιβλόν τε ἅμα τὴν πραγματείαν ἔσεσθαί μοι
431 νομίζων εἰ πάντ' ἐξελέγχοιμι καλῶς, πεπεισμένος τε | ὑπὸ φιλονεικίας τῆς
πρὸς τοὺς παλαιοὺς ἐριστικώτερον ὑπὲρ αὐτῶν ἀντεροῦντάς μοι τοὺς
10 ἐπαινοῦντας τὰ Χρυσίππου δόγματα· ἐν οἷς δὲ αὐτὸς ἑαυτὸν καταβάλ-
λει μετὰ τοῦ καὶ μάχεσθαι τοῖς ἐναργῶς φαινομένοις, ἐν τούτοις ἡγοῦμαι
407 τάχ' / ἂν αἰδεσθῆναί τέ τινα καὶ μεταστῆναι πρὸς τὰ βελτίω καθάπερ
καὶ ὁ Ποσειδώνιος ἐποίησεν αἰδεσθεὶς συναγορεῦσαι ψευδεῖ φανερῶς
δόγματι τῷ τῶν ἄλλων Στωϊκῶν, οἵ γε μέχρι τοσούτου φιλονεικίας
ἥκουσιν ὥστ' ἐπειδὴ τῆς λογικῆς δυνάμεως ἔφασαν εἶναι τὰ πάθη, τοῖς
ἀλόγοις ζῴοις μὴ μετέχειν αὐτῶν συγχωρεῖν, οἱ πλεῖστοι δ' οὐδὲ τοῖς
11 παιδίοις ὅτι δηλαδὴ καὶ ταῦτ' οὐδέπω λογικά. τὸ μὲν οὖν οὕτως
ἀναισχυντεῖν πρὸς τὰ πᾶσιν ἀνθρώποις ἐναργῶς φαινόμενα σοφιστῶν
ἔργον ἐστί, τὸ δὲ μηδὲ ἅπερ ὑπέθεντο δύνασθαι διαφυλάττειν, ἀλλ'
ἐναντία γράφειν αὐτῶν, ἀγυμνάστων περὶ λόγον ἀνθρώπων, οἷόσπερ
καὶ ὁ θαυμασιώτατος Χρύσιππος ἐν παμπόλ⟨λ⟩αις εὑρίσκεται πραγ-
ματείαις. ἀλλὰ περὶ μὲν τῶν ἄλλων ἑτέρωθι. |
432 2. Περὶ δὲ τῶν τῆς ψυχῆς παθῶν ὡς οὐκ ἔστι τῆς λογιστικῆς δυνά-
μεως ἤδη μέν μοι καὶ τὸ πρὸ τούτου πεπλήρωται βιβλίον ὧν αὐτὸς
ἄκων ὁμολογεῖ, πληρωθήσεται δ' οὐδὲν ἧττον καὶ τοῦτο τὴν ἀρχὴν
408 2 ἐνθένδε ποιησαμένῳ. τὸ πάθος / τῆς ψυχῆς κίνησίν τινα παρὰ φύσιν
ἄλογον ὑπάρχειν οὐχ οἱ παλαιοὶ μόνον, ἀλλὰ καὶ Χρύσιππος ὁμολογεῖ.
καὶ μὲν δὴ καὶ ὡς ἡ κίνησις αὕτη ταῖς τῶν ἀστείων οὐκ ἐγγίνεται ψυχαῖς,
3 ὡμολόγηται παρ' ἀμφοῖν. ὁποία δέ τίς ἐστιν ἡ τῶν φαύλων ψυχὴ κατά
τε τὰ πάθη καὶ πρὸ τῶν παθῶν οὐκέθ' ὁμοίως ἐξηγοῦνται. Χρύσιππος
μὲν γὰρ ἀνάλογον ἔχειν αὐτήν φησι τοῖς ἐπιτηδείοις σώμασιν εἰς πυρετοὺς
ἐμπίπτειν ἢ διαρροίας ἤ τι τοιοῦτον ἕτερον ἐπὶ μικρᾷ καὶ τυχούσῃ
4 προφάσει. καὶ μέμφεταί γε ὁ Ποσειδώνιος αὐτοῦ τὴν εἰκόνα· χρῆναι
γάρ φησιν οὐ τούτοις ἀλλὰ τοῖς ἁπλῶς ὑγιαίνουσι σώμασιν εἰκάσαι τὴν
τῶν φαύλων ψυχήν· εἴτε γὰρ ἐπὶ μεγάλοις αἰτίοις εἴτ' ἐπὶ μικροῖς πυρέτ-
433 τοιεν οὐδὲν διαφέρειν ὡς πρὸς τὸ πάσχειν τε αὐτὰ καὶ εἰς πάθος | ἄγεσθαι
καθ' ὁτιοῦν, ἀλλὰ τῷ τὰ μὲν εὐέμπτωτα εἶναι τὰ δὲ δύσπτωτα διαφέρειν

13–20] Posid. fr. 159 Edelstein-Kidd 17–20] SVF III, p. 127 22–25] SVF III, p. 116 29–36] SVF III, p. 116 32–296.36] Posid. fr. 163 Edelstein-Kidd 36–296.1] Pohlenz, 1898, p. 630 Reinhardt, 1921, p. 311

4 ἦν *sscr.* H 8 μαρτυρεῖ *ex* εἴρηκε *corr.* H 9 πάμπολα H: *corr. Ald.* 23 αὐτοῖς *Müller* 24 παμπόλαις H: *corr. Ald.* 26 λογικῆς R *(in* -ιστικῆς *corr.) Bas.* 28 ἀκούων H: *corr. Müller* 32 ὁποῖα H: *corr. Chart.*

books I gave my own account of the evident facts that are in conflict
with Chrysippus' teaching and of the things he said in opposition
to his own views, not waiting for someone else to attack him.

That earlier discussion would have been enough to prove that 8
the powers by which we desire and are angry and reason are more
than one, not one only, as Chrysippus imagines. But again in this
book no few instances will be added where Chrysippus, in contra-
dicting himself, bears witness both to the truth and to the ancient
view. I decided to pass over the rest of his errors, numerous as they 9
are; for I considered that a treatise of many books would be required
if I were to refute all of them properly, and I was convinced that the
champions of Chrysippus' doctrines would answer me rather con-
tentiously on these matters because of their desire to compete with
the ancients. But in the places where he refutes himself and at the 10
same time contradicts obvious facts, I think a person might feel
shame and change to the better view, as Posidonius did; he was
ashamed to defend the doctrine, obviously false, of the other Stoics,
who went to such an extreme of contentiousness that they admitted
that since, as they maintained, the affections belong to the reasoning
power, irrational animals have no share in them; and most (of the
Stoics) admitted that children do not share in them either, because,
obviously, children too are not yet rational. Such shamelessness in 11
the face of facts obvious to all mankind is the work of sophists; but
not to be able to maintain even their own assumptions but to write
things inconsistent with them, that is the mark of persons untrained
in reasoning. Chrysippus, that most remarkable man, is found in
very many of his treatises to be of this description. We shall postpone
the other items.

2. But on the subject of the soul's affections, that they do not
belong to the reasoning power, I have already filled the book before
this one with his own involuntary admissions, and I shall fill the
present (book) no less, taking my start from the following point. That 2
affection is an unnatural and irrational motion of the soul is acknowl-
edged not only by the ancients but also by Chrysippus. Further-
more, both (parties) admit that this motion does not arise in the souls
of the better sort of men. But when they come to describe the soul 3
of inferior men, both during and prior to affections, their accounts
are no longer the same. Chrysippus says that their soul is analogous
to a body which is apt to fall into fever or diarrhoea or something
else of that kind from a small and chance cause. Posidonius is critical 4
of this comparison; he says that the soul of inferior persons should not
be compared to these (bodies) but simply to healthy bodies. For with
respect to their experiencing the affection and being led to suffer
it in any way whatever, it makes no difference whether the cause of
their fever is large or small; the difference between them is that the
one kind (of body) contracts the disease easily, while the other does

5 ἀλλήλων. οὔκουν ὀρθῶς εἰκάζεσθαί φησιν ὑπὸ τοῦ Χρυσίππου τὴν
μὲν ὑγίειαν τῆς ψυχῆς τῇ τοῦ σώματος ὑγιείᾳ, τὴν δὲ νόσον τῇ ῥᾳδίως
409 εἰς νόσημα ἐμπιπτούσῃ καταστάσει / τοῦ σώματος· ἀπαθῆ μὲν γὰρ
γίγνεσθαι ψυχὴν τὴν τοῦ σοφοῦ δηλονότι, σῶμα δ' οὐδὲν ὑπάρχειν
ἀπαθές· ἀλλὰ δικαιότερον εἶναι προσεικάζειν τὰς τῶν φαύλων ψυχὰς
«ἤτοι τῇ σωματικῇ ὑγιείᾳ ἐχούσῃ τὸ εὐέμπτωτον εἰς νόσον» — οὕτω
γὰρ ὠνόμασεν ὁ Ποσειδώνιος — «ἢ αὐτῇ τῇ νόσῳ», εἶναι γὰρ ἤτοι
6 νοσώδη τινὰ ἕξιν ἢ ἤδη νοσοῦσαν. συμφέρεται μέντοι τῷ Χρυσίππῳ
καὶ αὐτὸς ὡς νοσεῖν τε λέγειν τὴν ψυχὴν ἅπαντας τοὺς φαύλους ἐοικέναι
7 τε τὴν νόσον αὐτῶν ταῖς εἰρημέναις τοῦ σώματος καταστάσεσι. λέγει
γοῦν ὧδε κατὰ λέξιν· «διὸ καὶ ἡ νόσος τῆς ψυχῆς ἔοικεν οὐχ ὡς ὁ Χρύ-
σιππος ὑπείληφε τῇ νοσώδει καχεξίᾳ τοῦ σώματος, καθ' ἣν ὑποφέρεται
ῥεμβώδεσιν οὐχὶ περιοδικοῖς οἷά τ' ἐμπίπτειν πυρετοῖς, ἀλλὰ μᾶλλον
434 ἔοικεν ἡ ψυχικὴ νόσος ἤτοι σωματικῇ | ὑγιείᾳ ἐχούσῃ τὸ εὐέμπτωτον
εἰς τὴν νόσον ἢ αὐτῇ τῇ νόσῳ. ἔστι γὰρ ἡ μὲν σωματικὴ νόσος ἕξις ἤδη
410 νοσοῦσα, / ἡ δὲ ὑπὸ τοῦ Χρυσίππου λεγομένη νόσος εὐεμπτωσίᾳ
μᾶλλον ἔοικεν εἰς πυρετούς.»

Ἐν τούτοις τὸν Ποσειδώνιον ἐπαινῶ μὲν ὅτι τοῖς ὑγιαίνουσι
σώμασιν ὁμοίως ἔχειν φησὶ τὰς τῶν φαύλων ψυχὰς ὅταν ἔξω παθῶν
καθεστήκωσιν, οὐκ ἐπαινῶ δὲ νόσον ὀνομάζοντα τὴν τοιαύτην κατάστα-
9 σιν. ἐχρῆν γάρ, εἴπερ ὀρθῶς εἴκαζε, τὰς μὲν τῶν σπουδαίων ψυχὰς ὁμοίως
ἔχειν φάναι τοῖς ἀπαθέσι σώμασιν, εἴτ' οὖν ἐστιν εἴτ' οὐκ ἔστιν τινὰ
τοιαῦτα, περιττὸν γὰρ ὡς πρὸς τὴν προκειμένην εἰκόνα διασκέπτεσθαι
τοῦτο, τὰ⟨ς⟩ δὲ τῶν προκοπτόντων τοῖς εὐεκτικοῖς, τὰς δὲ τῶν μετρίων
ἀνδρῶν τοῖς ὑγιαίνουσι χωρὶς εὐεξίας, τὰς δὲ τῶν πολλῶν τε καὶ φαύλων
τοῖς ἐπὶ σμικρᾷ προφάσει νοσοῦσι, τὰς δὲ τῶν ὀργιζομένων ἢ θυμουμέ-
10 νων ἢ ὅλως ἐν πάθει τινὶ καθεστώτων τοῖς ἤδη νοσοῦσιν. ἀλλὰ γὰρ
εὐλαβηθῆναί μοι δοκεῖ διαφερόμενος ἐν ἅπασι φωραθῆναι Χρυσίππῳ· |
435 τίνα γὰρ ἄν τις ἄλλην αἰτίαν εἴποι τοῦ τὴν νόσον τῆς ψυχῆς ὁμοιοῦν αὐτὸν
411 τῇ καταστάσει / τῶν θ' ὑγιαινόντων σωμάτων τῶν τ' ἤδη νοσούντων;
11 οὐ γὰρ ἀμφοτέροις ἀλλὰ μόνοις τοῖς νοσοῦσι δικαιότερον ἦν παραβεβλῆ-
σθαι τὰς νοσούσας ψυχάς· ἀδύνατον γὰρ ἓν πρᾶγμα τὴν νόσον τῆς ψυχῆς
12 δυσὶν ἐναντίοις ὡμοιῶσθαι πράγμασιν, ὑγ⟨ι⟩είᾳ τε ἅμα καὶ νόσῳ. εἰ γὰρ
δὴ τοῦτο, καὶ τὴν ὑγίειαν ἀναγκαῖον ἔσται τῇ νόσῳ παραπλησίαν ὑπάρ-
χειν, εἴ γε δὴ τῇ τῆς ψυχῆς νόσῳ προσέοικεν ἑκάτερον αὐτῶν· τὰ γὰρ τῷ
αὐτῷ παραπλήσια πάντως που καὶ ἀλλήλοις ἐστὶ παραπλήσια.

3–5] *cf.* Cic. Tusc. disp. iv. 31 Sen. Ep. 72.6 6–7] *cf. infra*, lin. 14–15
11–17] Pohlenz, 1898, p. 630 27–28] Posid. test. 94 Edelstein-Kidd

2 ὑγείαν H: *corr. Chart.* 5 προσεικάζειν] ει *ex* η *corr.* H 13 ῥομβώδεσιν H: *corr. Corn.* οἷά τ' ἐμπίπτειν] οἷς τ' ἐμπίπτει *Ald.*: *del. Müller*: *obelum ante* οἷά *pos. Pohlenz* 14 *post* ἤτοι *add.* τῇ R² *(cf. supra, lin. 6)* 15 τὴν *del. Müller* 20 καθεστήκασιν H: *corr. Kühn* 23 εἰκός H: *corr. Al. Just.* 24 τὰ H: *corr.* R² 31 παραβεβλῆσθαι] $\pi^{\alpha\rho\alpha}$ *ex* π^{ε}, *ut vid.*, *corr.* H 33 ὑγεία H: *corr. Chart.*

so with difficulty. Thus Chrysippus erred, he says, in his comparison 5
of health of soul to health of body, and disease (of soul) to a bodily
state that easily falls into disease, for there is a soul – that of the
wise man, obviously – that becomes immune to affection, whereas no
body is immune to disease; it would be more correct to compare the
souls of inferior persons "either to physical health with a proneness
to disease" – that is Posidonius' phrase – "or to the disease itself";
for there is a constitution that is either sickly or already laboring
from a disease. But he himself agrees with Chrysippus to the ex- 6
tent of saying that all inferior men are diseased in soul and that their
disease is comparable to the above-mentioned states of the body.
His actual words are as follows: "Therefore the disease of the soul 7
does not resemble, as Chrysippus had supposed, the sickly consti-
tution of the body, whereby it is carried off in such a way as to fall
into irregular, non-periodic, fevers; rather, disease of the soul resembles
either physical health with a proneness to disease, or the disease itself.
For disease of the body is a state already diseased, but what Chry-
sippus calls disease resembles rather a proneness to fever."

In this passage I commend Posidonius for stating that the 8
souls of inferior persons, when free from affections, are like healthy
bodies; but I do not approve his calling such a state a disease. If the 9
comparison were properly made, the souls of virtuous men ought to
be compared to bodies immune to disease, whether any such bodies
exist or not – for that inquiry is not germane to the analogy now before
us –; the souls of those progressing in virtue should be compared to
bodies of robust constitution, souls of intermediate persons to bodies
that are healthy without being robust, souls of the multitude of or-
dinary men to bodies that become ill at a slight cause, and souls
of men who are angry or enraged or in any affected state whatever
to bodies that are actually diseased. Still it is my opinion that Po- 10
sidonius was careful not to be caught disagreeing with Chrysippus
at every point. What other reason could be given for his making the
disease of the soul similar to the condition both of healthy bodies
and of (bodies) that are actually diseased? He would have done 11
better not to compare diseased souls to both, but only to diseased bod-
ies; for it is impossible that one thing, disease of the soul, be assim-
ilated to two opposites, health and disease. If that is the case, then 12
health will necessarily be like disease, since each of them resembles
disease of the soul. For surely things that are like the same thing
are also like each other.

13 Χρύσιππος δ' ἀτοπώτερον ἔτι μηδ' ἐν ταῖς περιοδικαῖς τισι
νόσοις καθεστῶσιν, οἱονεὶ τριταίοις ἢ τεταρταίοις πυρετοῖς, ὡμοιῶσθαι
14 συγχωρῶν τὴν νόσον τῆς ψυχῆς. γράφει γοῦν ὧδε· «ὑπονοητέον τοίνυν
τὴν μὲν τῆς ψυχῆς νόσον ὁμοιοτάτην εἶναι τῇ τοῦ σώματος πυ-
ρετώδει καταστάσει καθ' ἣν οὐ περιοδικῶς ἀλλ' ἀτάκτως πυρετοὶ καὶ
φρῖκαι γίνονται καὶ ἄλλως ἀπὸ τῆς διαθέσεως καὶ μικρῶν ἐπιγινομένων
412 436 15 αἰτίων.» οὐκ οἶδα τί ποτε δόξαν αὐτῷ τοὺς μὲν / ἑτοίμως | ἔχοντας πρὸς
τὸ νοσῆσαι νοσεῖν ἤδη φησί, τοὺς δ' ἤδη νοσοῦντας οὐδ' ὅλως νοσεῖν.
16 οἱ γὰρ ἐν τεταρταίαις καὶ τριταίαις περιόδοις ὄντες, ἐπειδὰν μὲν ῥιγῶσί τε
καὶ πυρέττωσιν, ἐν πάθει καθεστήκασι, κινουμένης δ' αὐτῶν τῆς νοσώ-
δους κατασκευῆς ἐπειδὰν μηδὲν τούτων πάσχωσιν ἀλλ' ἐν τοῖς καλου-
17 μένοις διαλείμμασιν ὦσιν, ἔξω τῶν παθῶν εἰσι. τὴν μέντοι νοσώδη
κατάστασιν εἰκάζοι[τό] τις ἄν, οἶμαι, τοῖς ἤτοι πενθοῦσιν ἢ ἐρῶσιν ἢ
18 φθονοῦσιν ἤ τι τοιοῦτον ἕτερον πάσχουσι. καὶ γὰρ οὗτοι, καθ' ὃν μὲν
ἂν χρόνον ἢ ὑπνώττωσιν ἢ πρὸς ἄλλῳ τινὶ τὴν διάνοιαν ἔχωσιν, ἔξω
τῶν παθῶν γίνονται, μετ' ὀλίγον δὲ ἀναμνησθέντες αὐτῶν εἰς παρα-
πλησίαν τινὰ κατάστασιν ἀφικνοῦνται ταῖς καταβολαῖς τῶν πυρετῶν.
ὅσοις μέντοι μήτε πένθος ἐνέστηκε μήτ' ἐπιθυμία τις ὑπόγυος ἢ θυμός,
19 οὗτοι τοῖς ὑγιαίνουσι τὰ σώματα παραπλησίως ἔχουσιν. ἐπεὶ δὲ καὶ
τούτων αὐτῶν ἔνιοι μέν εἰσιν εὐάλωτοι νόσοις, ἔνιοι δ' οὔ, καὶ τῶν τὰς
ψυχὰς ὑγιαινόντων οἱ μὲν τούτοις οἱ δ' ἐκείνοις ὁμοίως ἕξουσιν, οὐ μὴν
413 437 λεχθήσονταί γε νοσεῖν / | τὰς ψυχὰς εἴπερ μηδὲ ἐκεῖνοι τὰ σώματα.
20 Ἀλλὰ νὴ Δία, φήσει τις ἴσως τῶν Στωϊκῶν, ὥσπερ οὖν καὶ
λέγουσιν, οὐ τὴν αὐτὴν ἀναλογίαν εἶναι τῇ ψυχῇ πρὸς τὸ σῶμα κατά τε
21 τὰ πάθη καὶ τὰ νοσήματα καὶ τὴν ὑγίειαν. τί ποτ' οὖν, ὦ βέλτιστοι,
φαίημεν ἂν ἡμεῖς πρὸς αὐτούς, εἰκάζετε τοῖς κατὰ τὸ σῶμα πάθεσί τε καὶ
νοσήμασι τὰ τῆς ψυχῆς πάθη; τί δὲ Χρύσιππος ἐν τῷ Περὶ παθῶν
22 Ἠθικῷ γράφει ταυτί; «οὔτε γὰρ περὶ τὸ νοσοῦν σῶμά ἐστί τις τέχνη ἣν
προσαγορεύομεν ἰατρικήν, οὐχὶ δὲ καὶ περὶ τὴν νοσοῦσαν ψυχήν ἐστί τις
τέχνη οὔτ' ἐν τῇ κατὰ μέρος θεωρίᾳ τε καὶ θεραπείᾳ δεῖ λείπεσθαι
23 ταύτην ἐκείνης. διὸ καὶ καθάπερ τῷ περὶ τὰ σώματα ἰατρῷ καθήκει τῶν
τε συμβαινόντων αὐτοῖς παθῶν ἐντὸς εἶναι, ὡς εἰώθασι τοῦτο λέγειν,
καὶ τῆς ἑκάστῳ οἰκείας θεραπείας, οὕτω καὶ τῷ τῆς ψυχῆς ἰατρῷ ἐπιβάλ-
24 λει ἀμφοτέρων τούτων ἐντὸς εἶναι ὡς ἔνι ἄριστα. καὶ ὅτι οὕτως ἔχει
414 μάθοι ἄν τις τῆς πρὸς ταῦτ' ἀναλογίας παρατε/θείσης ἀπ' ἀρχῆς. ἡ γὰρ
πρὸς ταῦτα ἀντιπαρατείνουσα οἰκειότης παραστήσει, ὡς οἴομαι, καὶ
438 τὴν | τῶν θεραπειῶν ὁμοιότητα καὶ ἔτι τὴν ἀμφοτέρων τῶν ἰατρειῶν
25 πρὸς ἀλλήλας ἀναλογίαν.» ὅτι μὲν οὖν ἀναλογίαν τινὰ βούλονται εἶναι
τῶν ἐν τῇ ψυχῇ τοῖς κατὰ τὸ σῶμα, δῆλον οἶμαι γεγονέναι καὶ οὐ μόνον

1–8] SVF III, pp. 116–117 3–7] Pohlenz, 1898, p. 630 18–20] SVF III, p. 117 23–25] SVF III, p. 120 *cf.* Pohlenz, 1898, p. 556 27–300.12] SVF III, pp. 120–121 27–28] *cf. supra*, p. 238.6

1 ἀτοπώτερος *Kühn* 2 τριταίων ἢ τεταρταίων πυρετῶν H: *corr. Einarson* 7 αἰτιῶν *Müller* 10 νοσω^δ' H: νοσώδου M *Ald.*: *corr. Chart.* 13 εἰκάζοιτό H: *corr. Müller* 18 ὑπόγυιος *Ald.* 34 ἔχοι H: *corr. Kühn* 38 τινὲς H: *corr. Corn.*

Chrysippus even more absurdly does not even grant that 13
disease of the soul is comparable to the state of a person who is suf-
fering from a recurrent fever, tertian or quartan for example. He 14
writes: "We must suppose that the disease of the soul is most sim-
ilar to a feverish physical state in which fevers and chills do not
occur at regular intervals but irregularly and at random from the
constitution (of the man) and at the incidence of small causes." I 15
don't know what he was thinking when he said that persons prone
to disease are already diseased, and persons already diseased are not
diseased at all. For those who suffer from tertian and quartan periods, 16
when they experience a chill or fever, are in an affected state; but
when their unhealthy condition changes and they are not experiencing
any of these things but are in the intervals, as we call them, they are
outside the affection. A person might compare their sickly state, I 17
think, to persons who are mourning or are affected by love or envy
or something else of that kind. When these persons are drowsy or 18
are thinking of something else, they are outside their affection; when
presently they recall it, they enter a state similar to a recurring attack
of fever. Those who are not involved in mourning or some present
desire or anger are like persons in physical health. But since some of 19
these (healthy persons) are easy prey to disease and some are not,
so some of the healthy in soul will resemble the one set, some the
other; nevertheless they will not be said to be diseased in soul any
more than those others are called diseased in body.

But by heaven, some Stoic may say – as indeed they do say –, 20
there is not the same analogy between soul and body in respect of
affections and diseases and health. But why then, good people, we 21
would reply to them, do you compare the soul's affections to the
affections and diseases of the body? Why does Chrysippus write as
follows in his treatise on the Ethics of the Affections? "It is not true 22
that whereas there is an art, called medicine, concerned with the
diseased body, there is no art concerned with the diseased soul, or
that the latter (art) should be inferior to the former in the theory
and treatment of individual cases. Therefore just as the physician 23
of the body must be 'inside', as they say, the affections that befall
the body and the proper cure for each, so it is incumbent on the phy-
sician of the soul to be 'inside' both of these (things) in the best pos-
sible way. And a person might understand that this is so, since the 24
analogy with them was set up at the start. For the correlative af-
finity with them will also make evident to us, as I think, the simi-
larity of the cures and in addition, the analogy that the two kinds
of healing have with each other." It has become clear, I think, that 25
they intend an analogy between the (affairs) of the soul and those of
the body; (this is evident) not only from the passage just quoted but

γε διὰ τῆς προγεγραμμένης ῥήσεως ἀλλὰ καὶ δι' ὧν ἐφεξῆς γράφει τόνδε
26 τὸν τρόπον ἐχόντων· «καθάπερ γὰρ καὶ ἐπὶ τοῦ σώματος θεωρεῖται
ἰσχύς τε καὶ ἀσθένεια, εὐτονία καὶ ἀτονία [καὶ τόνος], πρὸς δὲ τούτοις
ὑγίειά τε καὶ νόσος, καὶ εὐεξία τε καὶ καχεξία», καὶ τἄλλα ὅσα τούτοις
ἑξῆς καταλέγει πάθη τε καὶ ἀρρωστήματα καὶ νοσήματα, «κατὰ τὸν
αὐτόν», φησί, «τρόπον ἀνάλογόν τινα πᾶσι τούτοις καὶ ἐν ψυχῇ λογικῇ
27 συνίσταταί τε καὶ ὀνομάζεται». εἶθ' ἑξῆς ἐπιφέρων φησίν, «ὡς οἴομαι,
ἀπὸ τῆς τοιαύτης ἀναλογίας τε καὶ ὁμοιότητος καὶ τῆς ἐν αὐτοῖς συνω-
415 νυμίας γεγενημένης· καὶ γὰρ καὶ κατὰ ψυχήν τινας λέγομεν ἰσχύειν / καὶ
ἀσθενεῖν καὶ εὐτόνους καὶ ἀτόνους εἶναι καὶ ἔτι νοσεῖν καὶ ὑγιαίνειν, οὕτω
πως καὶ τοῦ πάθους καὶ τοῦ κατ' αὐτὴν ἀρρωστήματος λεγομένου καὶ τῶν
28 τούτοις παραπλησίων.» ἐναργῶς γὰρ ἐν τούτοις ὁ Χρύσιππος ἀναλογίαν |
439 τινὰ βούλεται σῴζεσθαι τῶν ἐν τῇ ψυχῇ τοῖς κατὰ τὸ σῶμα καὶ παθῶν
πρὸς πάθη καὶ ἀρρωστημάτων πρὸς ἀρρωστήματα καὶ νοσημάτων πρὸς
νοσήματα καὶ ὑγιείας πρὸς ὑγίειαν καὶ εὐεξίας πρὸς εὐεξίαν καὶ ἰσχύος
πρὸς ἰσχὺν καὶ ἀσθενείας πρὸς ἀσθένειαν καὶ ἁπλῶς εἰπεῖν ἁπάντων τῶν
συνωνύμως λεγομένων πρὸς ἅπαντα· καὶ γὰρ τοὔνομα καὶ τὸν λόγον
29 αὐτῶν εἶναι τὸν αὐτὸν εἴ γε δὴ συνώνυμά φησιν ὑπάρχειν αὐτά. ὥστε
ὅπως ἄν τις ὁρίζηται καθόλου τὴν ἐν τῷ σώματι νόσον, ἀναγκαῖον εἶναι
τούτῳ καὶ τὴν ἐν ψυχῇ κατὰ τὸν αὐτὸν τρόπον ὁρίζεσθαι.

Ὅτι μὲν οὖν πρόκειται τῷ Χρυσίππῳ ⟨τὴν⟩ ἀναλογίαν ἅπασαν
30 ἐξηγεῖσθαί τε καὶ φυλάττειν, ἐκ τούτων δῆλον. εἰ δὲ ἐπιχειρήσας αὐτὸ
ποιεῖν οὐ τυγχάνει τοῦ προτεθέντος, οὐκ ἀποστατέον ἐστὶ τῆς ὁμοιότητος
416 ἀλλὰ / τῇ διδασκαλίᾳ μεμπτέον ὡς οὐκ ἀληθεῖ. τοῦτο δ' οὐδὲν ἧττον
αὐτῇ καὶ κατὰ τὸν ἐφεξῆς ὑπάρχει λόγον ἅπαντα τὸν ἐν τῷ Περὶ παθῶν
31 Ἠθικῷ. γράφει γοῦν ὧδε· «διὸ καὶ κατὰ τρόπον προῆκται Ζήνωνι
440 λόγος. ἡ δὲ τῆς ψυχῆς νόσος ὁμοιοτάτη ἐστὶ | τῇ τοῦ σώματος ἀκαταστα-
σίᾳ. λέγεται δὲ εἶναι σώματος νόσος ἡ ἀσυμμετρία τῶν ἐν αὐτῷ, θερμοῦ
32 καὶ ψυχροῦ, ξηροῦ καὶ ὑγροῦ.» καὶ μετ' ὀλίγα, «ἡ δ' ἐν τῷ σώματι
ὑγίεια εὐκρασία τις καὶ συμμετρία τῶν διειρημένων»· καὶ πάλιν ἐφεξῆς,
«οἶμαι γὰρ εἶναι εὐεξίαν σώματος τὴν ἀρίστην τῶν ῥηθέντων εὐκρασίαν»·
33 καὶ πάλιν ἐφεξῆς, «λέγεται δὲ καὶ ταῦτα οὐκ ἀπὸ τρόπου ἐπὶ τοῦ σώ-
ματος, διότι ἡ ἐν θερμοῖς καὶ ψυχροῖς καὶ ὑγροῖς καὶ ξηροῖς γενομένη
συμμετρία ἢ ἀσυμμετρία ἐστὶν ὑγίεια ἢ νόσος, ἡ δ' ἐν νεύροις συμμετρία
ἢ ἀσυμμετρία ἰσχὺς ἢ ἀσθένεια καὶ εὐτονία ἢ ἀτονία, ἡ δ' ἐν τοῖς μέλεσι
417 34 συμμετρία ἢ ἀσυμμετρία κάλλος / ἢ αἶσχος.» ἀλλὰ ταῦτα μέν, ὦ γεν-
ναιότατε Χρύσιππε, καλῶς ἅπαντα διῆλθες, ἀπόδος δ' ἡμῖν, ὡς

17–18] SVF III, p. 121 *cf.* Arist. Categ. 1: 1 a 6–7 21–36] SVF III, p. 121

3 καὶ τόνος *del. Müller* 4 καὶ[II] *del. Ald.* 6 φησί] φύσει H ἀνάλογά *Müller* 8 συνωνῦ' (μ supra) H: συνωνυμία M: *corr. Ald.* 11 πῶς H: *corr. Chart.* 18 *ante* εἶναι *add.* βούλεται *Müller* 21 τὴν *add. Petersen* 24 ἀληθῆ H: *corr. Ald.* 25 αὐτῷ *Müller* ὑπαρ' (χ supra) H: ὑπάρχειν R *Ald.*: *corr. Kühn* 30 διηρημένων H: *corr. Einarson*: δ' εἰρημένων *Müller* 33 γινομένη *Müller* 34 *post* ἀσυμμετρία *add. et del.* ἰσχὺς ἢ ἀσθένεια *(lin. 35)* H

also from what he writes immediately thereafter, which goes as follows: "Just as strength and weakness, firmness and softness, are ob- 26
served in the body, and also health and disease, robustness and sickliness", and all the other affections, infirmities, and diseases that he goes on to list, "in the same way", he says, "there are certain things in the rational soul that exist and are named analogously to all of
these". He then continues: "I fancy that this sort of analogy and sim- 27
ilarity has led to the sameness of their names. For we do in fact say that some persons are strong or weak also in soul, and firm or soft, diseased or healthy; and we speak in this way of affection, infirmity,
and the like in the soul." Clearly Chrysippus wishes to preserve 28
here a certain analogy between soul and body in their affections, infirmities, diseases, health, robustness, strength, weakness, and, in a word, everything that has the same name in both; for they have both the same name and the same definition, since he calls them 'same
in name'. Therefore whatever universal definition is given to disease 29
in the body, the soul's disease must be defined in the same way.

From this it is clear that Chrysippus' purpose is to
explain and preserve the entire analogy. If he tried and failed, we 30
must not give up the similarity but rather condemn his teaching as untrue. This applies no less to the teaching of all the subsequent
account in his Ethics of the Affections. He writes: "Therefore Zeno's 31
argument proceeds as it should. And disease of the soul is most similar to an unsettled state of the body. Disease of the body is said to be the lack of proportion in its components, hot and cold, dry and
wet." A little later he says, "Health in the body is a kind of blend 32
and proportion of the (things) expressly stated"; and then, "for in my opinion robustness of body is the best blend of the (things) men-
tioned"; and after that, "It is not out of place to say this of the body, 33
because proportion or lack of proportion in its components, hot, cold, wet, dry, is health or disease; proportion or lack of it in the sinews is strength or weakness, firmness or softness; and proportion
or the lack of it in the limbs is beauty or ugliness." All this, most 34
noble Chrysippus, you explained very well; but give us, as you

ἐπηγγεἰλω, τὴν ἀναλογίαν τῶν ἐν τῇ ψυχῇ συνωνύμως αὐτοῖς ὠνομα-
35 σμένων ἀρξάμενος ἀπὸ τῆς ὑγ⟨ι⟩είας τε καὶ τῆς νόσου. ὥσπερ γὰρ ὑγίεια
σώματός ἐστιν ἡ συμμετρία τῶν ἁπλουστάτων αὐτοῦ μορίων, ἃ δὴ καὶ
441 στοιχεῖα προσαγορεύομεν – τοῦ | θερμοῦ λέγω καὶ ψυχροῦ καὶ ξηροῦ
καὶ ὑγροῦ –, κατὰ τὸν αὐτὸν τρόπον εἴη ἂν οἶμαι καὶ ἡ τῆς ψυχῆς
ὑγίεια συμμετρία τις τῶν ἁπλῶν αὐτῆς μορίων· ἅτινά ποτ' ἐστὶ καὶ
ὁπόσα καὶ ὅπως ἔχοντα πρὸς ἄλληλα, διελθεῖν ἀναγκαῖον ἔσται σοι
36 μέλλοντί γε μηδὲν παραλείψειν ὧν ἐπηγγεἰλω. καὶ δὴ καὶ ἡ νόσος ἡ τῆς
ψυχῆς ὡσαύτως ἀσυμμετρία τις ἔσται καὶ στάσις πρὸς ἄλληλα τῶν
37 αὐτῶν τούτων μορίων, ὧν ἡ συμμετρία τῆς ψυχῆς ἦν ὑγίεια. τὰ δὲ
μόρια ταῦτα κατὰ τὸν Πλάτωνα τὸ θυμοειδές ἐστι καὶ τὸ λογιστικὸν
ἔτι τε πρὸς τούτοις τρίτον τὸ ἐπιθυμητικόν· ὥστε σῴζεσθαι τήν τε τῆς
ὑγιείας καὶ τὴν τῆς νόσου κατὰ πᾶν ὁμοιότητα τῆς ψυχῆς πρὸς τὸ
418 38 σῶμα. συμφωνοῦντα μὲν γὰρ ἀλλήλοις τὰ τρία καὶ / κατὰ μηδὲν στασιά-
ζοντα τὴν ὑγίειαν τῆς ψυχῆς ἀπεργάζεται, διαφωνήσαντα δὲ καὶ στασιά-
σαντα τὴν νόσον.
39 Ἔστι γὰρ ἡ νόσος ἀνωτέρω καὶ καθόλου μᾶλλον ἢ ὡς μικρὸν
ἔμπροσθεν εἴρηται. περιλάβωμεν οὖν αὐτῆς τὴν ἔννοιαν· ἡ τοῦ φύσει συγ-
γενοῦς ἔκ τινος ⟨διαφορᾶς⟩ διαφ⟨θ⟩ορά· οὕτως γὰρ ἐν Σοφιστῇ Πλάτων
442 40 ὡρίσατο. | ὅτι δ' ἀνωτάτω τ' ἐστὶν ἡ ἀπόδειξις ἥδε καὶ πάσας τὰς κατὰ
μέρος νόσους ἀκριβῶς ἐπιλαμβάνει, τάς τε τῆς ψυχῆς ἡμῶν καὶ τὰς τοῦ
σώματος καὶ τὰς ἐν τοῖς ἄλλοις ζῴοις τε καὶ φυτοῖς, ἤδη δὲ κἀν ταῖς
41 πόλεσιν ὅλαις, οὐ χαλεπὸν καταμαθεῖν. οὕτω γὰρ οἶμαι καὶ τὰς στασια-
ζούσας πόλεις ἐμφυλίῳ πολέμῳ νοσεῖν ἐν ἑαυταῖς λέγομεν, ὡς ἂν εἰς
42 μάχην ἀφιγμένων τῶν ἐν αὐταῖς φύσει συγγενῶν. αὕτη μὲν ἡ γενικωτάτη
νόσου πάσης ἔννοια. τῶν δ' ἁπλουστάτων μορίων ἡ πρὸς ἄλληλα
στάσις ἧττον ταύτης ἐστὶ γενική, καὶ ταύτης ἔθ' ἧττον ἐπειδὰν θερμῶν /
419 καὶ ψυχρῶν καὶ ξηρῶν καὶ ὑγρῶν ἀμετρία τις εἶναι λέγηται. σώματος γὰρ
αὕτη γε μόνου καὶ οὐδενὸς τῶν ἄλλων ἐστὶ νόσος, ὥσπερ γε καὶ ἡ τοῦ
λογιστικοῦ στάσις οὐδενὸς τῶν ἄλλων ἐστὶ πλὴν ψυχῆς νόσος.
43 Ὁ δὲ Χρύσιππος ἁμαρτάνει διττὰ κατὰ τὴν ἐν τούτοις διδασκα-
λίαν· πρῶτον μὲν ὅτι διαφέρεται πρὸς αὐτὸν ἐν μὲν τῷ Περὶ παθῶν Ἠθικῷ
συνωνύμως ὠνομάσθαι λέγων τὴν ἐν τῇ ψυχῇ νόσον τῇ κατὰ τὸ σῶμα,
443 διὰ δὲ τοῦ πρώτου τῶν | Λογικῶν εἰκάζων αὐτὴν εὐλύτῳ καὶ εὐδιαφθάρ-
τῳ ὑγιείᾳ· ἔπειθ' ὅτι μηδ' ὅπερ [ἀληθῶς] ὑπέσχετο κατὰ τὸ Θεραπευτι-

4–5] *cf. infra*, PHP 679.6–9 Müller 17–18] *cf. supra*, p. 300.18–20 18–20] Plat. Soph. 228 a 7–8 *cf. infra*, p. 310.26 26–27] *cf. supra*, lin. 3 32–33] *cf. supra*, p. 300.8–9, 17–18 34–35] *cf.* SVF III, p. 117 *supra*, p. 294. 33–36 *infra*, p. 308.5–6 35–304.1] *cf. infra*, p. 308.8–10

1 συνωνύμως] ω[I] *ex* ε *corr.* H 2 ὑγείας H: *corr. Ald.* ὑγεία H: *corr. Bas.* 6 ἅ τίνα *Kühn Kalbfleisch* 8 παραλείψειν] ει[I] *ex* η *corr.* H 17 *post* ἀνωτέρω *add.* τι *Corn.* καὶ] κ *ex* γ *corr.* H ἢ ὡς] ἐπὶ H: ὡς *Ald.*: ἢ *Kalbfleisch*: *corr. Einarson* 18 περιλάβομεν H: *corr. Chart.* *ante* ἡ *add.* ἔστι δ' *Schöne* 19 διαφορᾶς διαφθορά *ex Plat. Einarson*: διαφθορᾶς διαφορά *Ricci Corn. (cf. infra, p. 310.26)* 21 περιλαμβάνει *Kühn* 30 *post* λογιστικοῦ *inseruerit* καὶ τοῦ θυμοειδοῦς καὶ τοῦ ἐπιθυμητικοῦ *Müller* 35 ἀληθῶς *del. Einarson, ante* ὅπερ *trsp. Müller*

promised, the analogy of the things in the soul that have the same
names as these (bodily things), beginning with health and disease.
For as health of body is the proportion of its simplest parts, which 35
we also call its elements – I mean hot, cold, dry, wet –, in the same
way, I suppose, health of the soul would be a proportion of its sim-
plest parts. You must explain what these parts are, how many they are,
and how related to one another, if you are not to omit anything of
what you promised. Similarly, disease of the soul will be a dispro- 36
portion and mutual conflict in these very same parts whose proportion
was the soul's health. These parts, on Plato's view, are the spirited, 37
rational, and desiderative, so that the analogy of soul to body in health
and disease is preserved in every respect. For when the three parts are 38
in harmony with each other and are not in conflict at all, they produce
health of soul, but when in disharmony and conflict, (they produce)
disease.

Disease is a higher and more general term than was indicated by 39
the statement I made a moment ago. Let us therefore give a compre-
hensive definition of the concept: it is 'the destruction of what is by
nature congenial as a result of some dissension'. That was Plato's
definition in the Sophist. It is not difficult to ascertain that this 40
formulation is at a higher level and accurately covers all particular
diseases, those of our soul, those of our body, those found in other
animals and plants, and even those of whole cities. Thus we say, I 41
believe, that cities divided by civil war are internally diseased, as
though their components, congenial by nature, had come to blows.
This is the most generic concept of all disease. The mutual conflict of 42
the simplest parts is less generic than this, and still less generic is the
statement that disease is a lack of proportion of things hot, cold, dry
and wet. For this (last) is disease of the body only, and of nothing else,
just as the conflict of the rational is disease of nothing but the soul.

Chrysippus commits a double error in his teaching on these 43
matters: first, he contradicts himself when he says in his Ethics of the
Affections that disease of soul is the 'same in name' as disease of body,
but throughout the first (book) on the Theory (of the Affections)
compares it to unstable and precarious health; and second, he was not
able to demonstrate the very thing that he promised to demonstrate

44 κὸν καὶ 'Ηθικὸν ἐπιγραφόμενον βιβλίον ἠδυνήθη δεῖξαι. τί δ' ἐστὶ τοῦτο;
τῶν μερῶν τῆς ψυχῆς ἡ πρὸς ἄλληλα συμμετρία ⟨τε καὶ ἀσυμμετρία⟩
45 καθ' ἣν ὑγιαίνειν τε λέγεται καὶ νοσεῖν. πάντα γὰρ αὐτῆς τά τε πάθη
καὶ τὰ νοσήματα καθ' ἓν ὑποθέμενος γίγνεσθαι τὸ λογιστικὸν εἰκότως
ἀπορεῖ δεικνύναι τίνων μέν ἐστι μορίων ἡ τῆς ψυχῆς ὑγίεια συμμετρία. /
420 46 κατὰ δὲ τὸν αὐτὸν τρόπον ἐν συμμετρίᾳ μερῶν ὑποθέμενος γίγνεσθαι τὸ
κάλλος, ἐν ἀμετρίᾳ δέ τινι τὸ αἶσχος, εἰκότως ἀπορεῖ δεικνύναι ποίων μὲν
τῆς ψυχῆς μερῶν ἡ συμμετρία κάλλος ἐστί, ποίων δὲ ἀμετρία αἶσχος.
47 καίτοι γράφει γ' ἐφεξῆς ὧν ὀλίγον ἔμπροσθεν αὐτοῦ παρεθέμην ῥήσεων
ὡδί· «διὸ καὶ καλὴ ἢ αἰσχρὰ ψυχὴ ἀνάλογον ῥηθήσεται κατὰ συμμετρίαν
48 ἢ ἀμετρίαν τοιῶνδέ τινων μερῶν.» ὅτι μὲν οὖν κατὰ συμμετρίαν τέ τινα
καὶ ἀσυμμετρίαν τοιῶνδέ τινων μερῶν τῆς ψυχῆς ἢ καλὴν ἢ αἰσχρὰν |
444 αὐτὴν εἶναι λεκτέον ἐστὶ καὶ ὑγιαίνουσαν καὶ νοσοῦσαν, ὀρθῶς εἴρηται
τῷ Χρυσίππῳ· τίνα δ' ἐστὶ ταῦτα τὰ τῆς ψυχῆς μόρια μὴ δυνάμενος
εἰπεῖν, ὡς ἂν ἐν ἑνὶ μόνῳ τῷ λογιστικῷ καὶ τὴν ὑγίειαν αὐτῆς καὶ τὴν
νόσον καὶ τὸ κάλλος καὶ τὸ αἶσχος τιθέμενος, ἀναγκάζεται περιπλέκειν τε
49 τὸν λόγον καὶ τῶν ἐνεργειῶν αὐτῆς ὡς μερῶν μνημονεύειν. ἐφεξῆς γοῦν
421 οἷς παρεθέμην ὡδὶ γράφει· «ἔστι δὲ τῆς ψυχῆς μέρη δι'/ ὧν ὁ ἐν αὐτῇ
λόγος συνέστηκε καὶ ἡ ἐν αὐτῷ διάθεσις. καὶ ἔστι καλὴ ἢ αἰσχρὰ ψυχὴ
κατὰ τὸ ἡγεμονικὸν μόριον ἔχον ⟨οὕτως⟩ ἢ οὕτως κατὰ τοὺς οἰκείους
50 μερισμούς.» ποίους οἰκείους μερισμούς, ὦ Χρύσιππε, προσγράψας
51 ἐφεξῆς ἀπαλλάξεις ἡμᾶς πραγμάτων. ἀλλ' οὔτ' ἐνταῦθα προσέγραψας
οὔτ' ἐν ἄλλῳ τινὶ τῶν σεαυτοῦ βιβλίων, ἀλλ' ὥσπερ οὐκ ἐν τούτῳ τὸ
πᾶν κῦρος ὑπάρχον τῆς περὶ τῶν παθῶν πραγματείας, ἀποχωρεῖς τε
παραχρῆμα τῆς διδασκαλίας αὐτοῦ καὶ μηκύνεις τὸν λόγον ἐν τοῖς οὐ
προσήκουσι, δέον ἐπιμεῖναι καὶ δεῖξαι τίνα ποτέ ἐστι τὰ μόρια τοῦ
λογιστικοῦ τῆς ψυχῆς.

445 52 'Επειδὴ τοίνυν σὺ | παρέδραμες εἴθ' ἑκὼν εἴτ' ἄκων τὸν λόγον – οὐ
γὰρ ἔχω συμβαλεῖν –, ἐγὼ πειράσομαι τοῖς σοῖς δόγμασιν ἑπόμενος
ἐξευρεῖν τέ σου τὸ βούλημα καὶ διασκέψασθαι περὶ τῆς ἀληθείας αὐτοῦ
τὴν ἀρχὴν ἀπὸ τῆς προγεγραμμένης ῥήσεως ποιησάμενος ἐχούσης
ὧδε·

3. «Ἔστι δέ γε τῆς ψυχῆς μέρη δι' ὧν ὁ ἐν αὐτῇ λόγος συνέστηκεν»·
422 ἀναμιμνῄσκων ἴσως / ἡμᾶς τῶν ἐν τοῖς Περὶ τοῦ λόγου γεγραμμένων ὧν
2 σὺ διῆλθες, ὡς ἔστιν ἐννοιῶν τέ τινων καὶ προλήψεων ἄθροισμα. ἀλλ'
εἴπερ ἑκάστην τῶν ἐννοιῶν καὶ προλήψεων εἶναι μόριον νομίζεις τῆς

2–3] *cf. supra*, p. 302.6–7 9–11] SVF III, p. 121 14–27] SVF III, pp. 121–122 33–306.8] SVF II, p. 228 33] *cf. supra*, lin. 18–19 35] *cf. infra*, p. 314.20–21

2 τε καὶ ἀσυμμετρία *add. Müller* 5 *post* συμμετρία *add.* τίνων δὲ ἡ νόσος ἀσυμμετρία *Müller*, καὶ νόσος ἀσυμμετρία *v. Arnim* 8 ἡ *om. Müller* *post* κάλλος *add. et del.* μερῶν H 10 ἀνάλογον] λ *ex* γ *corr.* H 11 ἢ ἀμετρίαν] τέ τινα καὶ ἀσυμμετρίαν *Ald.* 16 ἀναγκάζει H: *corr. Kühn* 18 *post* δὲ *add.* γε *Müller* (*cf. infra, lin. 33*) 20 οὕτως[I] *add. Ricci Corn.* 24 ἀποχωρήσεις H: *corr. Müller*: ἀπεχώρησας *Einarson* 25 μηκυνεῖς *Kühn* 34 ἀναμιμνήσκεις *Müller* *ante* ὧν *add.* διὰ *Müller*

in his book called Therapy and Ethics. What was that thing? The 44
mutual proportion and disproportion of the soul's parts by reference
to which the soul is said to be healthy or diseased. As he supposes that 45
all its affections and diseases arise in a single part, reason, it is not
surprising that he is unable to explain what those parts are, the
proper proportion of which is the soul's health. Similarly, as he sup- 46
poses that beauty arises in a proportion of parts, and ugliness in a
disproportion, it is not surprising that he is unable to explain what is
the nature of those parts of the soul whose proportion is beauty and
whose disproportion is ugliness. And yet immediately after the 47
passages I quoted a moment ago he writes: "Therefore by analogy the
soul will also be called beautiful or ugly in terms of the proportion or
disproportion of certain parts of such and such a kind." Chrysippus 48
was correct in saying that the soul should be called beautiful or ugly,
healthy or diseased, in terms of a certain proportion or disproportion
of certain parts of such and such a kind. But as he was unable to say
what these parts of the soul are, since he placed its health and disease,
beauty and ugliness in one part only, the rational, he was compelled
to twist the argument and to count the soul's activities as its parts.
Thus he continues: "They are parts of the soul through which its 49
reason and the disposition of its reason are constituted. And a soul is
beautiful or ugly by virtue of its governing part being in this or that
state with respect to its own proper divisions." If you would go on to 50
state what its own proper divisions are, Chrysippus, you would
relieve us of our difficulty. But you did not go on to state them here 51
or in any other of your writings; instead, as though the entire validity
of your treatment of the affections did not depend on this, you sud-
denly withdraw from explaining it and prolong the discussion in
irrelevancies. You should rather have dwelt on this matter and
pointed out (to us) whatever are the parts of the rational part of the
soul.

Since, then, you passed over the account, whether deliberately 52
or not – I cannot conjecture which –, I shall try by inference from your
doctrines to discover your intention and inquire into its truth, taking
my start from the passage already quoted, which says:

3. "They are parts of the soul through which its reason is con-
stituted." Perhaps you are reminding us of what you said in your
treatise On Reason, that reason is a 'collection of notions and concepts'.
But if you think that each notion and concept is a part of the soul, you 2

ψυχῆς, ἁμαρτάνεις διττά. πρῶτον μὲν γὰρ οὐ ψυχῆς ἐχρῆν ἀλλὰ λόγου
ταῦτ' εἶναι μόρια φάσκειν, ὥσπερ οὖν καὶ γράφεις ἐν τῇ Περὶ λόγου πραγ-
3 ματείᾳ· οὐ γὰρ δήπου ταὐτόν ἐστι ψυχὴ καὶ λόγος. ἄλλως τε καὶ διὰ τῆς
προγεγραμμένης ῥήσεως ἐνεδείξω τῶν ἐν τῇ ψυχῇ συνισταμένων ὡς ἕν
τι καὶ ὁ λόγος ἐστίν· οὐ ταὐτὸν δὲ ψυχή ἐστι καὶ τὸ ἐν αὐτῇ συνιστάμε-
4 νον. ἔπειτα δ' εἰ καὶ τοῦτό τις ἐάσειεν ἀνέλεγκτον, ἀλλά τοι τάς γ'
446 ἐννοίας καὶ προλήψεις | οὐ μόρια τῆς ψυχῆς εἶναι λεκτέον ἀλλ' ἐνεργείας
5 τινάς. οὐδὲν δ' ἐκ τῶν οἰκείων ἐνεργειῶν σύγκειται, οὔτε οὖν ὁ ὀφθαλμὸς
οὔτε τὸ οὖς οὔτε χεὶρ οὔτε σκέλος οὔτ' ἄλλο τῶν πάντων οὐδέν· ἀλλ'
εἰσὶν ἐνέργειαι μὲν ὀφθαλμοῦ αἱ τῶν χρωμάτων ἑκάστου διαγνώσεις,
λευκοῦ καὶ μέλανος καὶ ξανθοῦ καὶ φαιοῦ καὶ τῶν ἄλλων ἁπάντων,
423 ὥσπερ γε καὶ ὠτὸς αὖ αἱ τῶν φωνῶν, / ὀξείας καὶ βαρείας καὶ μεγάλης
καὶ μικρᾶς καὶ λείας καὶ τραχείας, οὐ μὴν τά γε μόρια ταῦτ' ἐστὶν οὔτ'
6 ὠτὸς οὔτ' ὀφθαλμοῦ. ἀλλ' οἶσθα δήπου καὶ σὺ σαφῶς ὡς κερατοειδής τέ
τίς ἐστι χιτὼν καὶ ῥαγοειδὴς ἕτερος καὶ ἔτι κρυσταλ⟨λ⟩οειδές τε καὶ
ὑαλοειδὲς ὑγρὸν ἕτερά τε τοιαῦτα μόρια τῶν ὀφθαλμῶν, ὥσπερ γε καὶ
7 ὠτὸς ὀστᾶ καὶ χόνδροι καὶ νεῦρα καὶ ὑμένες ὅσα τε ἄλλα τοιαῦτα. μὴ
τοίνυν μηδὲ ἐπὶ τῆς ψυχῆς σύγχει τὰ μόρια ταῖς ἐνεργείαις. αἱ μὲν γὰρ
ἔννοιαι καὶ αἱ προ[σ]λήψεις ἐνέργειαι, ⟨μόρια δὲ⟩ τῆς ψυχῆς, ὡς αὐτὸς σὺ
δι' ἑτέρων ἐκδιδάσκεις, τό τε ἀκουστικὸν πνεῦμα καὶ τὸ ὀπτικὸν ἔτι τε
447 πρὸς τούτοις φωνητικόν τε καὶ γεννητικὸν καὶ πρὸ | πάντων αὐτῶν τὸ
ἡγεμονικόν, ἐν ᾧ καὶ τὸν λόγον ἔφης συνίστασθαι, καθ' ὃ δὴ καὶ μάλιστα
8 μόριον [δὴ] τῆς ψυχῆς αἶσχος καὶ κάλλος ἐγγίνεσθαι λέγεις αὐτῇ. τοῦτ'
οὖν τὸ πνεῦμα δύο μὲν κέκτηται μόριά τε καὶ στοιχεῖα καὶ καταστάσεις, /
424 δι' ὅλων ἀλλήλοις κεκραμ[μ]ένα, τὸ ψυχρὸν καὶ θερμόν, εἴπερ δ' ἑτέροις
ὀνόμασι καὶ ἀπὸ τῶν οὐσιῶν ἐθέλοι τις αὐτὰ προσαγορεύειν, ἀέρα τε καὶ
πῦρ· οὐ μὴν ἀλλὰ καὶ ἰκμάδα τινὰ προσείληφεν ἀπὸ τῶν σωμάτων ἐν οἷς
9 διαιτᾶται. ἀλλὰ θαυμάζοιμ' ἂν εἰ τὴν τούτων συμμετρίαν ὑγίειαν ἢ κάλλος
εἶναι βουλήσῃ τοῦ ἡγεμονικοῦ. τοῦ μὲν γὰρ σώματος αὐτοῦ τὴν ὑγίειαν
ἐν τούτοις τίθεσθαι προσῆκεν, ὡς ἡγεμονικοῦ δὲ ψυχῆς οὐκέτ' ἐν τούτοις
10 οὐδὲ κατ' αὐτὸν σέ. διέφθαρται τοίνυν ἡμῖν ὅλον τὸ παράδειγμα καὶ ἡ
τῆς συνωνυμίας ἐπαγγελία παντάπασιν οἴχεται μὴ δυνηθεῖσιν ἐπιδεῖξαι
τὸν αὐτὸν τρόπον ἐν τῷ τῆς ψυχῆς ἡγεμονικῷ νόσον ἢ ὑγίειαν ἢ κάλλος
11 ἢ αἶσχος συνιστάμενα καθάπερ ἐν ὅλῳ τῷ σώματι. καίτοι τοῦτό γ'
448 ὑπέσχου πρότερον ὀρθῶς γινώσκων καὶ φυλάττων | τὴν ἔννοιαν ἁπάν-
των τῶν εἰρημένων, οὐ μὴν ἀκολουθῆσαί γε μέχρι παντὸς ἠδυνήθης οὐδ'

3–5] *cf. supra*, p. 304.18–19, 33 18–22] SVF II, p. 228 *cf. supra*, p. 170. 10–16 23–28] SVF II, p. 228

5 ψυχή 'στιν *Petersen* 12 αὖ *del. Petersen (cf. infra, lin. 16–17)* 15 κρυσταλοειδές H: *corr.* R *Bas.* 19 αἱ *del. Müller* προσλήψεις H: π. . . .ήψεις L: *corr. Ald.* μόρια δὲ *add. v. Arnim*: *post* ψυχῆς *add.* μόρια δὲ αὐτῆς *Müller*, εἰσι· τὰ δὲ μόρια *Corn.* 22 καθὸ H L: *corr. Ald.* 23 δὴ *del. Ald.* 24 καὶ καταστάσεις *secl. Müller* 25 κεκραμμένα H L: *corr. Bas.* ἤπερ L δ' *om.* L 26 ἐθε' (λ supra) L 29 βουλήσει H τοῦ[II] *om.* L ὕγειαν L 30 ὡς] τοῦ *Müller* 31 ὑμῖν *Alexanderson* 33 νόσον ἢ] ὅσον L 36 γε *om.* L

are twice wrong. First, they should not be called parts of the soul but
of reason, as you yourself write in your treatise On Reason; for soul
and reason are surely not the same. And besides, you indicated in the 3
passage quoted above that reason is one of the things constituted in
the soul; but the soul is not the same as that which is constituted in it.
Secondly, even if we should let this pass unchallenged, nevertheless 4
notions and concepts must not be called parts, but activities, of the
soul. Nothing is composed of its own activities, not the eye, ear, arm, 5
leg, or any other thing at all. The activities of the eye are the discern-
ment of the several colors, white, black, yellow, grey, and all the rest;
of the ear, the discernment of sounds, high, low, loud, faint, soft,
harsh. But these are not the parts of eye or ear. Surely you too are 6
well aware that there is a hornlike tunic, another that is grape-like,
and there are also the moist crystalline and hyaloid bodies, and other
such parts of the eye, and that the parts of the ear, similarly, are bones,
cartilages, nerves, membranes, and a number of other things of that
description. Then in the soul too you must not confuse parts with 7
activities. Notions and concepts are activities, whereas the soul's parts,
as you yourself explain fully elsewhere, are the auditory pneuma, the
optic (pneuma), and in addition the vocal and generative (pneumas),
and over all of them the governing (pneuma) in which, you said, reason
is constituted; and you say that it is primarily with reference to this
part of the soul that ugliness and beauty are found in it. Now this 8
pneuma has two parts, elements, or states, that are intermingled
throughout, the cold and the hot, or, if you wish to use different
appellations and give them the names of their substances, air and fire;
and it also takes some moisture from the bodies in which it dwells.
But I would be surprised if you should wish to call the proportion of 9
these the health or beauty of the governing part. For the health of
its body is properly assigned to them, but as the governing part
of the soul, its health does not reside in them, even on your view.
Thus the whole pattern is destroyed and the claim to the same name 10
is completely gone if we cannot show that disease and health, beauty
and ugliness, are constituted in the soul's governing part in the same
way as in the whole body. And yet you promised earlier to show this, 11
rightly recognizing and preserving the meaning of all that had been
said; but you were not able to follow through to the end and you did

ἐξηγήσω τὴν ἀναλογίαν τε καὶ ὁμοιότητα τῶν κατὰ τὴν ψυχὴν ἐγγιγνο-
425 μένων / τοῖς κατὰ τὸ σῶμα.
12 Αὖθις οὖν ἀναλήψομαι τὸν λόγον ἵνα δή τι πέρας ἱκανὸν νῦν
ἀπολάβῃ. τῆς νόσου τὴν ἔννοιαν ἐν μὲν τῷ πρώτῳ Περὶ παθῶν συνέχεεν
ὁ Χρύσιππος ἀνάλογον ἔχειν φάμενος τὴν ἐν τῇ ψυχῇ νόσον τῇ τοῦ
σώματος καταστάσει, καθ' ἣν εὐεμπτώτως εἰς πυρετοὺς ἢ διαρροίας ἤ τι
13 τοιοῦτον ἔχει· κατὰ μέντοι τὸ Θεραπευτικὸν ἐφυλάξατο μὲν τὴν ἔννοιαν
τῆς νόσου τῆς πρὸς ἑαυτὸν οὐδὲν φροντίσας ἐναντιολογίας, ἐξηγήσασθαι
δ' ὡς ὑπέσχετο τὴν ἐν τῇ ψυχῇ νόσον ἅμα τοῖς ἄλλοις οἷς ἀνάλογον
ὑπάρχειν αὐτῇ φησι πρὸς τὸ σῶμα παντάπασιν ἠδυνάτησε, μετὰ τοῦ καὶ
14 συγχεῖν εἰς ταὐτὸν τήν θ' ὑγίειαν τῆς ψυχῆς καὶ τὸ κάλλος. ἐπὶ μὲν γὰρ
τοῦ σώματος ἀκριβῶς αὐτὰ διωρίσατο τὴν μὲν ὑγίειαν ἐν τῇ τῶν στοι-
15 χείων συμμετρίᾳ θέμενος, τὸ δὲ κάλλος ἐν τῇ τῶν μορίων. ἐδήλωσε γὰρ
σαφῶς τοῦτο διὰ τῆς προγεγραμμένης ὀλίγον ἔμπροσθεν ῥήσεως ἐν ᾗ τὴν
449 μὲν | ὑγίειαν τοῦ σώματος ἐν θερμοῖς καὶ ψυχροῖς καὶ ξηροῖς καὶ ὑγροῖς /
426 συμμετρίαν εἶναί φησιν, ἅπερ δὴ στοιχεῖα δηλονότι τῶν σωμάτων ἐστί,
τὸ δὲ κάλλος οὐκ ἐν τῇ τῶν στοιχείων ἀλλ' ἐν τῇ τῶν μορίων συμμετρίᾳ
συνίστασθαι νομίζει, δακτύλου πρὸς δάκτυλον δηλονότι καὶ συμπάντων
αὐτῶν πρός τε μετακάρπιον καὶ καρπὸν καὶ τούτων πρὸς πῆχυν καὶ
πήχεως πρὸς βραχίονα καὶ πάντων πρὸς πάντα, καθάπερ ἐν τῷ Πολυ-
16 κλείτου Κανόνι γέγραπται. πάσας γὰρ ἐκδιδάξας ἡμᾶς ἐν ἐκείνῳ τῷ
συγγράμματι τὰς συμμετρίας τοῦ σώματος ὁ Πολύκλειτος ἔργῳ τὸν
λόγον ἐβεβαίωσε δημιουργήσας ἀνδριάντα κατὰ τὰ τοῦ λόγου προστάγ-
ματα καὶ καλέσας δὴ καὶ αὐτὸν τὸν ἀνδριάντα, καθάπερ καὶ τὸ σύγγραμ-
17 μα, Κανόνα. τὸ μὲν δὴ κάλλος τοῦ σώματος ἐν τῇ τῶν μορίων συμμετρίᾳ
κατὰ πάντας ἰατροὺς καὶ φιλοσόφους ἐστίν, ἡ δ' ὑγίεια τῶν στοιχείων
18 αὖ πάλιν, ἅττα ποτ' ἂν ᾖ, πρὸς ἄλληλά ἐστι συμμετρία. εἴτε γὰρ ἐξ
ὄγκων καὶ πόρων ὡς Ἀσκληπιάδης ὑπέθετο τὰ τῶν ζῴων σύγκειται
450 σώματα, συμμετρία τούτων ἐστὶν ἡ ὑγίεια· | εἴτ' ἐξ ἀτόμων ὡς Ἐπί-
427 κουρος εἴτ' ἐξ / ὁμοιομερῶν ὡς Ἀναξαγόρας εἴτ' ἐκ θερμοῦ καὶ
ψυχροῦ καὶ ξηροῦ καὶ ὑγροῦ καθάπερ ὅ τε Χρύσιππος δοξάζει καὶ
πάντες οἱ Στωϊκοὶ καὶ πρὸ αὐτῶν Ἀριστοτέλης καὶ Θεόφραστος
καὶ πρὸ τούτων ἔτι Πλάτων καὶ Ἱπποκράτης, ἡ τῶν στοιχείων κατὰ
19 πάντα⟨ς⟩ συμμετρία τὴν ὑγίειαν ἐργάζεται. εἰ τοίνυν ἐθέλοι τις ἅπασαν
τὴν ἀναλογίαν [αὐ]τῶν κατὰ τὸ σῶμα τοῖς κατὰ τὴν ψυχὴν διασῴζειν,
ὡς ὑπέσχετο Χρύσιππος, ἐπιδεῖξαι χρὴ τοῦτον ἔκ τινων ἁπλῶν ὡσανεὶ

5–7] *cf. supra*, p. 294.33–36 7–10] *cf. supra*, pp. 302.32–304.1 10–18] SVF III, p. 122 13–26] Polyclit. fr. A 3 D.-K. 13–16] *cf. supra*, p. 300.28–34 26–34] *cf.* Gal. In Hipp. De nat. hom. comm. I 20: CMG V 9.1, p. 33.4–11 30] *cf.* Gal. De elem. sec. Hipp. I 9: I 484 K. 30–31] *cf. supra*, p. 300.28–29, 33–34

1 τὴν^{II} *om.* L 3 ἱκανὸν νῦν] ἱκνούμενον L 4 ἀπολαύῃ H 6 πυρεττοὺς L 7 [ἔχειν L μέντοι] μὲν L ἐφυλάξατο μὲν] ἐφυλάξαμεν L: ἐφύλαξε μὲν *Müller* 10 *ante* αὐτῇ *add.* ἐν *Müller* 11 ὑγείαν H L: *corr. Bas.* 23 κατὰ – 24 ἀνδριάντα *om.* L 26 *ante* καὶ *add.* τὲ L ὑγεία H 27 προσάλληλα L 30 ἀνομοιομερῶν L 34 πάντα H L: *corr. Einarson* 35 αὐτῶν H L: *corr. Müller* διασῴζειν] ἴδια σῴζειν L 36 τοῦτον] τοῦ τὴν L

not expound the analogy and similarity between the things that arise in the soul and those that arise in the body.

I shall once more review the argument, so that it may now be 12 brought to an adequate conclusion. Chrysippus in his first (book) On the Affections confused the notion of disease by saying that disease in the soul is analogous to the physical state in which the body is prone to fevers or diarrhoea or something of the kind. In his Therapy 13 (of the Affections), however, he preserved the notion of disease, taking no notice of the self-contradiction; but he was utterly unable to fulfil the promise he had made to account for disease in the soul or for the other things which he said were analogous in soul and body. And at the same time he confused the health of the soul with its beauty. For 14 he distinguished them accurately in the case of the body, placing health in the proportion of the elements, and beauty in the proportion of the members. He showed this clearly in the passage that I quoted 15 a short time ago, in which he says that health of body is proportion in things that are hot, cold, dry, and wet, which are obviously elements of bodies; but he believes that beauty does not lie in the proportion of the elements but of the members: of finger, obviously, to finger, of all the fingers to palm and wrist, of these to forearm, of forearm to upper arm, and of all to all, as is written in Polycleitus' Canon. Polycleitus first gave us full information in that book about all the 16 proportions of the body, then he confirmed his account in action by fashioning a statue in accordance with the demands of the theory; and he gave to the statue, as he did to the treatise, the name Canon. All physicians and philosophers place beauty of body in the proportion 17 of the members, and health in the proportion of the elements, whatever they may be, to each other. If living bodies are formed from solid 18 masses and the passages between them, as Asclepiades supposed, health is the proportion of these; or if from Epicurus' atoms, or Anaxagoras' homoeomeries, or from hot, cold, dry, and wet, as Chrysippus and all the Stoics teach, and Aristotle and Theophrastus before them, and Plato and Hippocrates even earlier, for all these men the proportion of the elements produces health. Now 19 if a person should wish to preserve, as Chrysippus promised, the entire analogy between the body's affairs and those of the soul, he

στοιχείων συγκειμένην τὴν ὅλην ψυχὴν ἵνα ἐν τῇ τούτων πρὸς ἄλληλα
συμμετρίᾳ τὴν ὑγίειαν καὶ τὴν νόσον αὐτῆς εὕρῃ γιγνομένην, ὅπερ ὁ
20 Πλάτων ἐποίησε. Χρύσιππος δ' οὔτε ταύτην ἠδυνήθη τὴν ὁμοιότητα
διδάξαι καίτοι ὑποσχόμενος οὔτε τὴν τοῦ κάλλους τῆς ψυχῆς, ἀλλὰ εἰς
21 ταὐτὸν συνέχεεν ὑγιείᾳ τὸ κάλλος. κατὰ γὰρ τοὺς οἰκείους τοῦ λόγου μερι-
σμοὺς καλὴν ἢ αἰσχρὰν ἔφησε γίγνεσθαι ψυχήν, ὑγιαίνουσα δ' ἢ νοσοῦσα
πῶς ἂν γένοιτο παρέλιπεν εἰς ταὐτόν, οἶμαι, συγχέων ἄμφω καὶ μὴ δυνά-
451 428 μενος | ἀκριβῶς τε καὶ ὡρισμένως ὑπὲρ αὐτῶν ἀποφή/νασθαι, καθάπερ ὁ
Πλάτων ἐποίησεν ἐν ἄλλοις τέ τισι καὶ τῷ Σοφιστῇ, τὴν μὲν τῶν μερῶν
τῆς ψυχῆς πρὸς ἄλληλα στάσιν ἀποφηνάμενος εἶναι νόσον ψυχῆς, τὰς
δὲ παραφόρους τε καὶ ἀμέτρους κινήσεις αὐτῆς, τουτέστι τὰς ἐνεργείας
τὰς καθ' ὁρμήν, αἶσχος, ὥσπερ γε τὴν μὲν συμφωνίαν τε καὶ συμμετρίαν
πρὸς ἄλληλα τῶν μορίων αὐτῆς ὑγίειαν, τὴν δὲ συμμετρίαν τῶν κινήσεων
22 [τὸ] κάλλος. ὥσπερ γὰρ τὸ σῶμα τὸ καλὸν ἐν τῇ συμμετρίᾳ τῶν μο-
ρίων τὴν γένεσιν ἴσχει, κατὰ τὸν αὐτὸν τρόπον ἐνέργεια καλὴ διὰ τὴν
23 τῶν κατὰ μέρος κινήσεων γίγνεται συμμετρίαν. οὕτω γοῦν καὶ ὀρχεῖσθαι
καὶ παγκρατιάζειν καὶ παλαίειν καὶ βαδίζειν εὐσχημόνως καὶ καλῶς
λέγονταί τινες, ἕτεροι δ' ἀσχημόνως τε καὶ αἰσχρῶς. ἐν μὲν ⟨γὰρ⟩ τῇ
συμμετρίᾳ τῶν κατὰ μέρος κινήσεων τὸ κάλλος τῶν ἐνεργειῶν ἐστι
γνώριμον, κατὰ δὲ τὰς ἀμετρίας τὸ αἶσχος.
429 24 Ἔχουσι δὲ καὶ αἱ τοῦ Πλάτωνος ῥήσεις ἐκ τοῦ / Σοφιστοῦ τόνδε
452 τὸν τρόπον· «δύο μὲν εἴδη κακίας περὶ ψυχῆς ῥητέον. | — ποῖα; — τὸ
μὲν οἷον νόσον ἐν σώματι, τὸ δ' οἷον αἶσχος ἐγγιγνόμενον. — οὐκ ἔμαθον.
— νόσον ἴσως καὶ στάσιν οὐ ταὐτὸν νενόμικας; — οὐδ' αὖ πρὸς τοῦτο
25 ἔχω τί χρή με ἀποκρίνασθαι. — πότερον ἄλλο τι στάσιν ἡγούμενος
ἢ τὴν τοῦ φύσει συγγενοῦς ἔκ τινος διαφορᾶς διαφ⟨θ⟩οράν; — οὐδέν.
— ἀλλ' αἶσχος ἄλλο τι πλὴν τὸ τῆς ἀμετρίας πανταχοῦ δυσειδὲς ὂν γέ-
26 νος; — οὐδαμῶς ἄλλο.» οὕτως μὲν ἐν τῷ καθόλου περὶ νόσου τε καὶ
αἴσχους ὁποῖόν τι τὴν φύσιν ἑκάτερον αὐτῶν ἐστιν ἐδίδαξεν ἡμᾶς ὁ
Πλάτων. καὶ ὅπως ἐγγίγνονται ταῖς ψυχαῖς ἐφεξῆς διδάσκων, περὶ
27 μὲν τῆς νόσου ταῦτα γράφει· «τί δέ; ἐν ψυχῇ δόξας ἐπιθυμίαις καὶ /
430 θυμὸν ἡδοναῖς καὶ λόγον λύπαις καὶ πάντα ἀλλήλοις ταῦτα τῶν φλαύ-

5–8] SVF III, p. 122 5–6] *cf. supra*, p. 304.19–21 22–28] Plat. Soph. 227 d 13–228 b 1 25–26] *cf. supra*, p. 302.18–19 31–312.3] Plat. Soph. 228 b 2–9

1 ἵνα] σύν, *ut vid.*, L 2 ὑγείαν L εὕρῃ *ex* ἄρα *(?) corr.* L 3 ἐποίησε] ε[II] *ex* εν *corr.* H 4 διδάξαι] δεῖξαι L *post* καίτοι *add.* γ' *Petersen* 5 *post* συνέχεεν *add.* τῇ *Ald.* 6 ἢ[II]] ἡ H 10 *ante* ψυχῆς[II] *add.* τῆς L 11 τὰς ἐνεργείας *om.* L 14 τὸ[I] *om.* F: *del. Müller* γὰρ] γε L 15 ἐνεργεία καλῇ H L: *corr.* F 16 γί(γ)νεσθαι H L: γίνεται F *Corn.* 18 γὰρ *add.* F *supra lin.* 19 τοῦ κάλλους ταῖς ἐνεργείαις L 20 γνώριμον] χρήσιμον L τὴν ἀμετρίαν F τοῦ αἴσχους L 21 σοφιστικοῦ L 22 εἴδη περὶ κακίας ῥητέον περὶ ψυχῆς L ψυχὴν *ex Plat.* F *Ald.* ποῖα] ὧν L 23 ἐν σώματι] σῶ' (μτ *supra*) L 25 χρή *om.* L ἀποκρίνεσθαι H πρότερον L 26 διαφορᾶς διαφοράν H: διαφορὰν L *(cf. supra, p. 302.19)* 27 ἄλλο τι πλὴν] ἀλλ' ὅτι δὴ L δυσειδὲς] υ *ex* ε *corr.* H 28 ἄλλως L[2?] 29 ἐστὶν ἑκάτερον αὐτῶν L 30 καὶ ὅπως *om.* L 31 νόσου *ex* ψυχῆς *corr.* L[2] ἐπιθυμίας L 32 ἡδονὰς L λύπας L τῶν] τε L

must show that the soul as a whole is composed of certain simple
elements, so to speak, so that he may discover its health and its disease
in their mutual proportion, as Plato did. But Chrysippus, in spite 20
of his promise, could give an account neither of this similarity nor of
the similarity in the soul's beauty, but he confused its beauty with its
health. He said that the soul becomes beautiful or ugly in terms of the 21
divisions proper to reason, but he neglected to say how it could
become well or ill; for it is my opinion that he confused the two and
was unable to make any precise or definite statement about them,
such as Plato made in a number of places, notably in the Sophist,
where he stated that the conflict of the soul's parts with each other is
disease of the soul, while its disordered and immoderate movements,
that is, conative acts, are ugliness, just as he held that the harmony
and mutual proportion of its parts is health, but proportion in its
movements is beauty. For as a beautiful body has its origin in the 22
proportion of the members, so a beautiful act arises through the pro-
portion of the particular movements. Thus some persons are said to 23
dance, perform the pancration, wrestle, and walk gracefully and
beautifully, others with awkwardness and ugliness. For beauty of
actions is recognized in the proportion of the particular movements,
and ugliness in their lack of proportion.

The passages from Plato's Sophist are as follows: "We must say 24
that there are two forms of evil in the soul. – What forms (are they)? –
One is like a disease infecting the body, the other like ugliness. – I do
not understand. – Perhaps you have not considered that disease and
internal conflict are the same thing? – I do not know what I should
answer to that, either. – Do you believe internal conflict to be any- 25
thing but the destruction of what is by nature congenial as a result of
some dissension? – It is nothing but that. – And is ugliness anything
other than the class of disproportion, which is everywhere unsightly?
– No; it is nothing else." Thus Plato instructs us in universal terms 26
about disease and ugliness, describing the nature of each. Next he tells
us how they enter the soul. He says of disease: "Answer me this: have 27
we not seen opinions at odds with desires, anger with pleasures, reason
with distress, and all of these with all the others, in the souls of worth-

ρως ἐχόντων οὐκ ᾐσθήμεθα διαφερόμενα; — καὶ σφόδρα γε. — ξυγγενῆ
γε μὴν ἐξ ἀνάγκης ξύμπαντα γέγονε. — πῶς γὰρ οὔ; — στάσιν ἄρα καὶ
453 28 νόσον τῆς ψυχῆς πονηρίαν λέγοντες ὀρθῶς ἐροῦ|μεν.» εἶτ' ἐφεξῆς ὅπως
αἶσχος ἐγγίνεται ψυχαῖς διεξιών φησι· «τί δ'; ὅσα κινήσεως μετέχοντα καὶ
σκοπόν τινα θέμενα πειρώμενα τούτου τυγχάνειν καθ' ἑκάστην ὁρμὴν πα-
ράφορα αὐτοῦ γίγνεται καὶ ἀποτυγχάνει, πότερον αὐτὰ φήσομεν ὑπὸ
συμμετρίας τῆς πρὸς ἄλληλα ἢ τοὐναντίον ὑπὸ ἀμετρίας αὐτὰ πά-
σχειν; — δῆλον ὡς ὑπὸ ἀμετρίας. — ἀλλὰ μὴν ψυχήν γε ἴσμεν ἄκουσαν
29 πᾶσαν πᾶν ἀγνοοῦσαν. — σφόδρα γε. — τό γε μὴν ἀγνοεῖν ἐστιν ἐπ'
431 ἀλήθειαν / ὁρμωμένης ψυχῆς παραφόρου συνέσεως γιγνομένης οὐδὲν
ἄλλο ἢ παραφροσύνη. — πάνυ μὲν οὖν. — ψυχὴν ἄρ' ἀνόητον αἰσχρὰν
30 καὶ ἄμετρον θετέον.» οὕτω μὲν ἐν τῷ Σοφιστῇ Πλάτων ἀπεφήνατο
καὶ καθόλου καὶ κατὰ μέρος ὑπὲρ ὑγιείας τε καὶ κάλλους, αἴσχους τε
καὶ νόσου, καθόλου μὲν ὑπογράψας τὴν ἔννοιαν αὐτῶν, κατὰ μέρος
δὲ ὅπως ἐγγίγνεται ταῖς ψυχαῖς διδάξας.

31 Τὰς δ' ἄλλας αὐτοῦ ῥήσεις οὐκ ὀλίγας οὔσας ἐν πολλοῖς τῶν συγ-
454 γραμμάτων ἐν | οἷς ὑπὲρ ὑγιείας τε καὶ κάλλους αἴσχους τε καὶ νόσου διῆλ-
θεν οὔ μοι δοκεῖ νῦν εἶναι παρατίθεσθαι καιρός· ἀλλ' ἐπειδὰν ὑπὲρ ὑγιείας
τε καὶ νόσων ὁ λόγος ἡμῖν περαίνηται δεικνύουσιν ὡσαύτως Ἱππο-
κράτει τὸν Πλάτωνα γιγνώσκειν ὑπὲρ αὐτῶν, ἐπὶ πλέον ἐν ἐκείνοις
τῶν τοιούτων μνημονεύσω ῥήσεων. /

432 4. Νυνὶ δέ, οὔτε γὰρ ἁπλῶς περὶ κάλλους ἢ ὑγιείας ἢ αἴσχους ἢ
νοσημάτων ὁ λόγος οὔτε περὶ μόνων τῶν τοῦ σώματος ἀλλὰ περὶ τῶν
παθῶν τῆς ψυχῆς ἐξ ἀρχῆς ἡμῖν προὔκειτο, παραλείψω μὲν τἄλλα, τὸ
2 προκείμενον δ' αὐτὸ μόνον ἀναλήψομαι. πρόκειται δὲ δεικνύειν ὡς
οὔτε καθ' ἓν μόριον τῆς ψυχῆς οὔτε κατὰ μίαν αὐτῆς δύναμιν αἵ τε
κρίσεις γίγνονται καὶ τὰ πάθη συνίσταται, καθάπερ ὁ Χρύσιππος
ἔφασκεν, ἀλλὰ καὶ δυνάμεις πλείους αὐτῆς εἰσιν ἑτερογενεῖς καὶ μόρια
3 πλείω. τὸ μὲν δὴ τὰς δυνάμεις τῆς ψυχῆς τρεῖς εἶναι τὸν ἀριθμόν, αἷς
ἐπιθυμοῦμέν τε καὶ θυμούμεθα καὶ λογιζόμεθα, καὶ Ποσειδώνιος
ὁμολογεῖ καὶ Ἀριστοτέλης· τὸ δὲ καὶ τοῖς τόποις αὐτὰς ἀλλήλων |
455 κεχωρίσθαι καὶ τὴν ψυχὴν ἡμῶν μὴ μόνον ἔχειν ἐν ἑαυτῇ δυνάμεις πολ-
λάς, ἀλλὰ καὶ σύνθετον ἐκ μορίων ὑπάρχειν ἑτερογενῶν τε καὶ δια-
φερόντων ταῖς οὐσίαις Ἱπποκράτους ἐστὶ καὶ Πλάτωνος δόγμα.
433 4 καί μοι πολλὰ μὲν ἤδη περὶ τῆς ἀληθείας αὐτοῦ διὰ τῶν / ἔμπροσθεν
εἴρηται, πολλὰ δ' ἐν τοῖς ἐφεξῆς εἰρήσεται.

4–12] Plat. Soph. 228 c 1 – d 4 29–34] Posid. fr. 142 Edelstein-Kidd

1 εἰθίσμεθα L 2 γε] τε H L: *ex Plat. corr. Ald.* 3 εἶθ' ἑξῆς L 4 γίγνεται L ὅσα] ὀστᾶ L 5 τιθέμενα L πειρόμενα L τυγχάνει L παραφορὰ H 6 αὐτοῦ] αὐτῶν L καὶ ἀποτυγχάνει *om.* L 7 τῆς *om.* L ἢ *om.* L 8 γε ἴσμεν] μὲν L 9 πασ. . . . οὐ νοοῦσαν L γε[II]] δὲ L *ante* ἀγνοεῖν *add. et del.* ἐπ' ἀλήθειαν ἀγνοεῖν ἐστὶν H 10 ὁρμουμένης L 13 ὑπὲρ] ὑπὸ H: περὶ F ὑγείας L 14 ἀπογράψας L 15 ἐνδιδάξω L 16 δ' *om.* L ἐν – συγγραμμάτων *post* κάλλους *(lin. 17) trsp.* L 17 αἷς L 18 δοκεῖ νῦν] δοκεῖν L 20 αὐτοῦ L ἐκείνῳ *Müller* 22 δ' H 24 ἐξ ἀρχῆς *om.* H παραλείψωμεν H: παραλείψομεν L: *corr. Chart.* 25 ἀναλήψομεν H *(in -ομαι corr.)* L 27 συνίστανται L 31 τοῖς τόποις αὐτὰς] τῶν τότε αὐτὰ L 32 κεχωρῆσθαι H τῇ ψυχῇ L 36 ταῖς H

less persons? – Yes, indeed. – But surely all these things are necessar-
ily akin? – Of course. – Then we shall be correct when we speak of
baseness as an internal conflict and disease of the soul." Then he goes 28
on to explain how ugliness arises in the soul: "But what of those parts
of the soul that have a share in motion and having set a goal for
themselves try to reach it but at every attempt swerve to the side and
miss it? Shall we say that they fail because they are in mutual propor-
tion, or, on the contrary, because of a lack of proportion? – Clearly
because of a lack of proportion. – But we know that all ignorance in
every soul is involuntary. – Quite so. – And when a soul aims at the 29
truth and misses the way that leads to understanding, its ignorance is
nothing other than misunderstanding. – That is very true. – Therefore
we must set it down that the unintelligent soul is ugly and lacks pro-
portion." Thus in the Sophist Plato spoke of health and beauty, 30
ugliness and disease in both universal and particular terms; he gave
a universal description of the concept of them, and a particular account
of the way in which they arise in the soul.

This is not the proper occasion, I think, to cite the other passages, 31
no few in number in many of his writings, in which he spoke of health
and beauty, ugliness and disease. But when our account has come to
health and diseases, when we show that Plato had the same views
about them as Hippocrates, I shall there discuss such passages at
length.

4. For the present, since our purpose from the start has been
neither to give simply an account of beauty or health or ugliness or
diseases, nor to discuss those of the body only, but to deal with the
affections of the soul, I shall omit the rest and consider only the matter
before us. My purpose is to show that it is not in a single part of the 2
soul nor by virtue of a single power of it that both judgments and
affections occur, as Chrysippus claimed, but that the soul has both
a plurality of powers of different kinds, and a plurality of parts.
Posidonius and Aristotle grant that the powers of the soul are 3
three in number, and that by them we desire, feel anger, and reason;
but that they are also spatially separate from each other, and that our
soul not only contains many powers but is composed of parts that
differ in kind and in substance, this is the doctrine of Hippocrates
and Plato. I have said much about the truth of it throughout the 4
preceding discussion, and I shall have much to say in what follows.

5 Νυνὶ δ' ἐπὶ τὸν Χρύσιππον αὖθις ἐπάνειμι μήτε τὰς εἰρημένας
δυνάμεις ὁμολογοῦντα κατὰ τὴν ψυχὴν ἡμῶν ὑπάρχειν, ἀλλὰ πᾶσαν
ἐνέργειάν τε καὶ πάθος ἐν τῷ λογιστικῷ μόνῳ συνίστασθαι φάσκοντα,
μήθ' ὅπως ἰᾶσθαι χρὴ τὰ πάθη γενόμενα μήθ' ὅπως κωλῦσαι γενέσθαι
6 διδάσκοντα. διηνέχθη μὲν οὖν καὶ περὶ τούτου πρὸς ἑαυτόν, ὥσπερ καὶ
περὶ παμπόλλων ἑτέρων, ἐν μὲν τῷ προτέρῳ Περὶ ψυχῆς τιθέμενος εἶναι
ταύτας δυνάμεις τῆς ψυχῆς ἃς ἐν τῷ πρὸ τούτου γράμματι παραθέ-
μενος αὐτοῦ τὰς ῥήσεις ἐπέδειξα, κατὰ δὲ τὰ Περὶ τῶν παθῶν βιβλία
κρίσεις τινὰς ὑπάρχειν τὰ πάθη τοῦ λογιστικοῦ τῆς ψυχῆς ἀποφηνά-
7 μενος. ἀλλ' ἡμεῖς ἃ μὲν ἀληθῶς εἶπε μαρτύρια τῶν Ἱπποκράτους
τε καὶ Πλάτωνος δογμάτων οὐ τὰ τυχόντα νομίζομεν ὑπάρχειν,
456 εἰρημένα γε | πρὸς ἀνδρὸς οὐ συνετοῦ μόνον ἀλλὰ καὶ σπεύδοντος ἅπαντι
τρόπῳ τὸ παλαιὸν δόγμα διαβαλεῖν. ἡ γὰρ παρὰ τῶν τοιούτων μαρτυ-/
434 ρία καταναγκαζομένων ὑπὸ τῆς ἀληθείας εἴωθε γίγνεσθαι.

8 Μεταβάντες δὲ πάλιν ἐφ' ἕτερα τῶν ὑπ' αὐτοῦ γεγραμμένων εἰς
τὸ προκείμενον ἐπιδείξομεν ὅπως καὶ τούτων ἔνια μὲν οἷς αὐτὸς εἶπεν
οὐ συμφωνεῖ, ἔνια δ' αὖ τοῖς ἐναργέσι μάχεται, τινὰ δὲ κατ' ἄμφω πε-
9 πλημμέληται. καὶ πρῶτόν γε πάλιν ἀναλαβὼν εἰς ὅπερ ἐτελεύτησεν ὁ
προγεγραμμένος μοι λόγος, ὡς ὑγίεια καὶ νόσος αἶσχός τε καὶ κάλλος
ψυχῆς ἐν τοῖς μέρεσι γίγνεται αὐτῆς καὶ ὡς τὰ μέρη ταῦτα ἔννοιαί τε
καὶ προλήψεις εἰσί, συγχωρήσω μὲν αὐτῷ τήν γε πρώτην· ὅτι μὲν γὰρ
ὅλως οὐ χρὴ κατὰ τὰς ἐνεργείας τίθεσθαι νόσον ἢ ὑγίειαν ἀλλ' αἶσχος
10 ἢ κάλλος μόνον, εἴρηταί μοι πρόσθεν. ὅτι δ' οὐδ' εἴ τις οὕτω συγχωρή-
σειε τὰ γοῦν ἑξῆς ὀρθῶς εἴρηται, νῦν ἐπιδεῖξαι πειράσομαι. εἴπερ γὰρ
ἐν τῷ μάχεσθαι δύο κρίσεις ἀλλήλαις ἡ τῶν παθῶν ἐστι γένεσις, ἀνάγκη
457 τῶν δύο τούτων κρίσεων | ἤτοι τὴν ἑτέραν μὲν ὑπάρχειν ἀληθῆ, τὴν
435 ἑτέραν δὲ ψευδῆ, ἢ ἀμφοτέρας ψευδεῖς, εἴ τις καὶ τοῦτο / συγχωρήσειεν,
11 ἔχει γάρ τινα ζήτησιν λογικήν. εἴτε δὲ ἀμφοτέρας ψευδεῖς εἴτε τὴν ἑτέραν
αὐτῶν ἀληθῆ φαίημεν ὑπάρχειν, οὐδαμῶς ἡ μάχη τῶν κρίσεων ἔσται
12 τὸ πάθος. ἀλλ' εἰ μὲν ἰσάζοιέν πως ἀλλήλαις αἱ κρίσεις ὡς πρὸς πίστιν,
ἐπέχειν ἀναγκαῖον ἡμᾶς ἔσται περὶ τῆς τοῦ πράγματος ὑπάρξεως, εἰ
δ' ἡ ἑτέρα φαίνοιτο μακρῷ πιστοτέρα, συγκατατίθεσθαι μὲν καὶ πράτ-
τειν γέ τι κατὰ τὴν συγκατάθεσιν, οὐκ ἀπερισκέπτως δέ, καθάπερ εἰ
καί τις τὴν ἡδονὴν ἀγαθὸν οἰόμενος ὑπάρχειν ἔχοι τι βραχὺ περιέλκον
εἰς τοὐναντίον ἢ εἰ μόνον τὸ καλὸν ἀγαθὸν ὑπολαμβάνων ὅμως ἔτι καὶ

6–8] *cf. supra*, pp. 234.26–238.4 8–10] *cf. supra*, pp. 238.4–23; 292.7–18 19–20] *cf. supra*, pp. 300.24–304.22 20–21] *cf. supra*, p. 304.28–35 21–23] *cf. supra*, p. 310.8–20

1 μήτε] μὴ δὲ L 3 ἐνέργειάν τε] ἀνερ^γ' τὲ L μόνῳ] λόγω L 3–4 φάσκοντα, μήθ' ὅπως] πάσχο^τυ μηδόλως L 6 παμπόλων H προτέρῳ *post* ψυχῆς *trsp.* L 7 ταύτας] ταῦτα L τῆς *om.* L ἃς] ὡς L 8 τῶν *om.* L 10 μαρτυρία H 12 γε] τὲ H L: *corr. Schöne* 13 διαβάλλειν *Chart.* 14 καταναγκαζομένη L 16 οἷς – 17 συμφωνεῖ *om.* L 17 ἔνια δ' αὖ τοῖς] οὐδ' αὐτοῖς L 18 ἀναλάβωμεν H: ἀναλάβομεν L: *correxi* 20 ἀ^τυ γίγνε^τ L 21 συγχωρήσωμεν H: συγχωρήσομεν L: *correxi* αὐτῷ τήν] αὐτήν L 30 ἰσάζοιέ H 32 μικρῷ *Diels* 34 περιέλκων H

I now return to Chrysippus, who refuses to grant that the 5
powers mentioned are in our soul and says that all activity and
affection arise in the rational part alone; and he fails to teach us how
to heal the affections when they occur or to prevent their occurrence.
He contradicted himself in this matter, as he did in many others: in 6
the first book of his work On the Soul he states that the soul has those
powers that I mentioned in the preceding book, where I quoted his
own words; but in his work On the Affections he asserts that the
affections are certain judgments of the reasoning part of the soul. Now 7
in our opinion his true statements give no ordinary support to the
teachings of Hippocrates and Plato, as they were spoken by a man
who was not only intelligent but also eager to discredit the older view
in every way. Testimony from such persons is ordinarily due to their
being compelled by the truth to give it.

When we turn to other things that Chrysippus wrote on the 8
subject now before us, we shall show how some of these too are in
disagreement with his own statements, some again are in conflict
with evident facts, and some are faulty on both counts. Returning 9
first to the view that was under discussion at the end of the preceding
section, that the soul's health and disease, ugliness and beauty, are in
its parts, and that its parts are notions and conceptions, I shall grant
him this for the moment; for I said earlier that one must never count
disease or health as activities, but only ugliness or beauty. But I shall 10
now try to show that even if we grant this, his next statement, at any
rate, is not correct. For if the origin of affections is in the conflict
between two judgments, it is necessary either that one of these two
judgments is true and the other false, or that both are false – if you
will grant this latter point, for it involves a question of logic. But 11
whether we assert that both are false or that one of them is true, in no
case will the conflict of judgments be the affection. If the judgments 12
should be of more or less equal credibility, we must withhold decision
about the truth of the matter, but if one of them should appear far
more convincing, we must assent to it and perform some act in accord-
ance with our assent, not, however, without circumspection: for
example, one who thinks that pleasure is good may nevertheless have
some minor thing that draws him toward the opposite view, or the
person who makes the supposition that only the honorable is good may

αὐτὸς ἀντισπῶσαν ἑτέραν ὑπόληψιν ἔχοι πρὸς τὸ μὴ διατεταμένως
πιστεύειν ἢ εἰ καθάπερ ὁ Πύρρων, ἀμφοτέρας ὁμοτίμως τιθέμενος
13 ἐπέχοι περὶ τῆς ἀποφάσεώς τε καὶ συγκαταθέσεως. ἐν οὐδενὶ γὰρ τῶν
τοιούτων συνίσταται τὸ πάθος, ὥσπερ καὶ αὐτὸς ὁ Χρύσιππος ἐναρ-
γῶς ἐδήλωσε δι' ὧν ἐν τῷ πρὸ τούτου γράμματι παρεθέμην ῥήσεων, ἐν
458 14 αἷς φησιν | «οὐχὶ ⟨εἰ⟩ διημαρτημένως φέρεται καὶ παριδών τι κατὰ τὸν /
436 λόγον», ὅσα τ' ἄλλα τοιαῦτα προσέγραψε, συνίστασθαι τὸ πάθος,
ἀλλ' ὅταν ἀπειθὴς ἡ ὁρμὴ γίγνηται τῷ λόγῳ, ὥστε κἀνταῦθα πάλιν
ἐναντιολογίαν τινὰ εὑρίσκεσθαι τοῦ Χρυσίππου πρὸς ἑαυτόν, εἴπερ
ἀποχωρίσας τὸ πάθος τῶν διημαρτημένων κρίσεων αὖθις ἐν τῇ τῶν
κρίσεων πρὸς ἀλλήλας ⟨ἀν⟩ομολογίᾳ τά τε νοσήματα τῆς ψυχῆς καὶ
15 τὰ πάθη συνίστασθαι λέγει. μὴ τοίνυν θαυμάζωμεν ἔτι μηδ' ὅτι
τὰς θεραπείας τῶν παθῶν ὀρθῶς μὲν ὁ Πλάτων ἔγραψεν, ὡς καὶ ὁ
16 Ποσειδώνιος αὐτῷ μαρτυρεῖ, μοχθηρῶς δ' ὁ Χρύσιππος. ὁ γὰρ μήτε
πάσας τὰς αἰτίας τῶν παθῶν ἀποφήνασθαι τολμήσας, ἀλλ' ἐν ταῖς
κυριωτάταις ἀπορεῖν ὁμολογήσας, ὡς ἐν τῷ πρὸ τούτου δέδεικται γράμ-
ματι, μήτ' ἐν αἷς ἐτόλμησεν εἰπεῖν τι καλῶς ἀποφηνάμενος, οὗτος οὐκ ἄν,
17 οἶμαι, δύναιτο τὴν θεραπείαν αὐτῶν ποιήσασθαι κατὰ τρόπον. ἀλλ'
ὅπερ εἶπον ἤδη καὶ πρόσθεν, εἴ τις ἐξελέγχοι τὰ τέσσαρα τοῦ Χρυσίπ-
που βιβλία, πολὺ πλεόνων αὐτῷ δεήσει συγγραμμάτων. /|
437 459 5. Ὅσα τοίνυν ἀναγκαιότατα πρὸς τὴν προκειμένην ἡμῖν πραγ-
ματείαν ἐστί, ταῦτα ἐπέλθωμεν μόνα καὶ πρῶτόν γε αὐτῶν προχει-
2 ρισώμεθα τὸ περὶ τῆς τῶν παιδίων διοικήσεως. οὔτε γὰρ ὑπὸ λόγου
τὰς ὁρμὰς αὐτῶν ἐπιτροπεύεσθαι δυνατὸν εἰπεῖν, οὐ γὰρ ἔχουσιν ἤδη
τὸν λόγον, οὔθ' ὡς οὐ θυμοῦταί τε καὶ λυπεῖται καὶ ἥδεται καὶ γελᾷ
καὶ κλαίει καὶ τοιαῦθ' ἕτερα πάθη πάσχει μυρία. πολὺ γὰρ δὴ καὶ πλείω
3 καὶ σφοδρότερα τὰ πάθη τοῖς παιδίοις ἐστὶν ἢ τοῖς τελείοις. οὐ μὴν
ἀκολουθεῖ γε ταῦτα τοῖς Χρυσίππου δόγμασιν, ὥσπερ οὐδὲ τῷ μηδε-
μίαν οἰκείωσιν εἶναι φύσει πρὸς ἡδονὴν ἢ ἀλλοτρίωσιν πρὸς πόνον.
ᾄττει μὲν γὰρ ἀδιδάκτως ἅπαντα τὰ παιδία πρὸς τὰς ἡδονάς, ἀποστρέ-
4 φεται δὲ καὶ φεύγει τοὺς πόνους. ὁρῶμεν δ' αὐτὰ καὶ θυμούμενα καὶ

6–8] *cf. supra*, pp. 240.26–27; 242.30–32; 256.1–2 8–9] *cf. supra*, p. 294.2 12–14] Posid. fr. 167 Edelstein-Kidd 12–14 μαρτυρεῖ] *cf. supra*, pp. 284.33–286.1 Pohlenz, 1898, p. 559 14–17] *cf. supra*, pp. 284.19–22, 25; 288.12–13 *infra*, pp. 318.21; 330.32–33; 332.5–8 Plut. Mor. 1015 B Pohlenz, 1921, pp. 173–174 18–20] *cf. supra*, pp. 234.7–9; 294.8–11 21–322.26] Posid. fr. 169 Edelstein-Kidd 22–29] SVF III, p. 54 24–25] *cf. supra*, p. 294.20 *infra*, pp. 340.18–19; 356.6–7

2 ἢ *om.* L πύρων H ἀμφοτρ' L ὁμοτίμους *Alexanderson* 6 εἰ *add.* *Corn.* (*cf. supra*, *p.* 242.30) *post* διημαρτημένως *add.* ὡς L *ante* κατὰ *add.* ὁ L 8 τοῦ λόγου L 9 ἐναντιολογίαν] ἢ ἀντιλογ' L 10 ἀποχωρήσας H 11 ὁμολογ' H L: "*fortasse* οὐχ ὁμολογίᾳ *vel* ἀνομολογίᾳ" *Müller*: ἐναντιολογίᾳ *Ricci Corn.* τά] ὅσά L 12 λέγοι H L: *corr. Kühn* 13 καὶ *om.* H 17 οὗτος *ex* οὕτως *corr.* H: *om.* L 19 εἴ τις] εἴτε L 20 πολὺ *om.* L αὐτῶν L 21 πραγματείαν ἡμῖν L 22 προχειρισώμεθα *ex* -όμεθα *corr.* L: προχειρησώμεθα H 23 τῶν παιδίων] ποδῶν L ὑπὸ] ἐπὶ L 24 ἐπιτρέπεσθαι L ἔχει *Müller* *post* ἤδη *add.* πω L 25 τε *om.* L 26 πάθη *om.* L 27 ἢ] οὐ H L: *corr.* R² *Corn.* 28 οὔτε τὸ H L: *corr. Müller*

himself have yet another supposition that pulls against his trusting it
earnestly; or someone may, like Pyrrho, assign equal value to both
and withhold his decision about assertion and assent. In none of these 13
situations does affection arise, as Chrysippus himself made quite
clear in the passages that I quoted in the preceding book, where he
says that affection does not arise "if he is carried away by error and 14
from a misapprehension of something that is in accord with reason",
and the other things of this kind that he added in his account; it arises
rather when conation becomes disobedient to reason. So here again
Chrysippus is discovered contradicting himself, since he first separa-
ted affection from mistaken judgments and then said that the diseases
and affections of the soul arise when judgments are in mutual disagree-
ment. Let us no longer marvel, then, that Plato described correctly 15
the cure of the affections, as Posidonius also testifies, and Chry-
sippus incorrectly. For a man who lacked the courage to state all the 16
causes of the affections, and who confessed to being perplexed about
the most important causes, as I pointed out in the preceding book,
and in those places where he had the courage to speak stated nothing
well, that man, I believe, would not be able to find the proper treat-
ment for them. But as I have already said, if one were to write an 17
answer to Chrysippus' four books, many more volumes would be
needed.

5. Let us therefore consider only those things that are most
essential to the present treatise, and of these let us first present the
matter of the governing power in little children. We cannot say that 2
their conations are supervised by reason, for they do not yet possess
reason, or that they do not feel anger, distress and pleasure, or do not
laugh and cry and experience countless other such affections. In fact,
the affections are much more numerous and more intense in children
than in adults. But these (facts) do not follow from the doctrines of 3
Chrysippus or from the view that there is no natural feeling of
kinship with pleasure or alienation from pain. For all children rush
untaught toward pleasures and turn and flee from pains. And we see 4

λακτίζοντα καὶ δάκνοντα καὶ νικᾶν ἐθέλοντα καὶ κρατεῖν τῶν τοιούτων,
438 ὥσπερ ἔνια τῶν ζῴων, οὐδενὸς ἄθλου προβαλ⟨λ⟩ομένου παρὰ / τὸ
5 νικᾶν αὐτό. φαίνεται δ' ἐναργῶς τὸ τοιοῦτον ἐπ' ὀρτύγων καὶ ἀλεκ-
460 τρυόνων καὶ περδίκων ἰχνεύμονός τε καὶ ἀσπίδος [τε] καὶ | κροκοδείλου
6 καὶ μυρίων ἑτέρων. οὕτως οὖν οἰκειοῦσθαι καὶ τὰ παιδία φαίνεται καὶ
πρὸς ἡδονὴν καὶ πρὸς νίκην, ὥσπερ ὕστερόν ποτε δείκνυσιν, ἐπειδὰν
προβαίνῃ κατὰ τὴν ἡλικίαν, ὅτι πρὸς τὸ καλὸν ἔχει τινὰ φυσικὴν οἰκείω-
7 σιν. αἰδεῖται γοῦν ἁμαρτάνοντα προϊούσης αὐτοῖς τῆς ἡλικίας καὶ
χαίρει τοῖς καλοῖς ἔργοις καὶ δικαιοσύνης καὶ τῶν ἄλλων ἀρετῶν ἀντι-
ποιεῖται καὶ πράττει πολλὰ κατὰ τὰς τῶν ἀρετῶν τούτων ἐννοίας,
ἔμπροσθεν, ἡνίκα ἦν ἔτι σμικρά, κατὰ πάθος ζῶντα καὶ τῶν ἐκ τοῦ λόγου
8 προσταγμάτων οὐδεμίαν φροντίδα ποιούμενα. τριῶν οὖν τούτων ἡμῖν
οἰκειώσεων ὑπαρχουσῶν φύσει καθ' ἕκαστον τῶν μορίων τῆς ψυχῆς
εἶδος, πρὸς μὲν τὴν ἡδονὴν διὰ τὸ ἐπιθυμητικόν, πρὸς δὲ τὴν νίκην διὰ
τὸ θυμοειδές, πρὸς δὲ τὸ καλὸν διὰ τὸ λογιστικόν, Ἐπίκουρος μὲν
439 τὴν τοῦ χειρίστου μορίου τῆς ψυχῆς / οἰκείωσιν ἐθεάσατο μόνην, ὁ δὲ
Χρύσιππος τὴν τοῦ βελτίστου, φάμενος ἡμᾶς οἰκειοῦσθαι πρὸς μόνον
τὸ καλόν, ὅπερ εἶναι δηλονότι καὶ ἀγαθόν. ἁπάσας δὲ τὰς τρεῖς οἰκειώ-
461 σεις θεάσασθαι μόνοις τοῖς παλαιοῖς ὑπῆρξε | φιλοσόφοις.
9 Ἐάσας οὖν τὰς δύο ὁ Χρύσιππος εἰκότως ἀπορεῖ περὶ τῆς κατὰ
τὴν κακίαν γενέσεως οὔτ' αἰτίαν ἔχων εἰπεῖν αὐτῆς οὔτε τρόπους τῆς
συστάσεως οὔθ' ὅπως ἁμαρτάνει τὰ παιδία δυνάμενος ἐξευρεῖν, ἅπερ εὐ-
λόγως οἶμαι πάντα καὶ ὁ Ποσειδώνιος αὐτοῦ καταμέμφεται καὶ ἐλέγχει.
10 εἰ γὰρ δὴ πρὸς τὸ καλὸν εὐθὺς ἐξ ἀρχῆς ᾠκείωται τὰ παιδία, τὴν κακίαν
οὐκ ἔνδοθεν οὐδ' ἐξ ἑαυτῶν ἀλλ' ἔξωθεν μόνον ἐχρῆν αὐτοῖς ἐγγίγνε-
11 σθαι. ἀλλὰ μὴν ὁρᾶταί γε, κἂν χρηστοῖς ἔθεσιν ἐντρέφηται καὶ προσηκόν-
τως παιδεύηται, πάντως ἐξαμαρτάνοντά τι, καὶ τοῦτ' αὐτὸ καὶ ὁ
12 Χρύσιππος ὁμολογεῖ. καίτοι γ' ἐνῆν αὐτῷ ὑπεριδόντι τῶν ἐναργῶς
φαινομένων αὐτὸ μόνον ὁμολογῆσαι τὸ ταῖς ἰδίαις ὑποθέσεσιν ἀκόλουθον,
440 εἰ καλῶς / ἀχθείη τὰ παιδία, πάντως αὐτὰ φάσκοντι σοφοὺς ἄνδρας
13 γενήσεσθαι τοῦ χρόνου προϊόντος. ἀλλ' οὐκ ἐτόλμησε τοῦτό γε κατα-
ψεύσασθαι τῶν φαινομένων, ἀλλὰ κἂν ὑπὸ φιλοσόφῳ τρέφηται μόνῳ
462 καὶ μηδὲν μήτε θεάσηται μήτ' ἀκούσῃ πώποτε παράδειγμα | κακίας,
14 ὅμως οὐκ ἐξ ἀνάγκης αὐτὰ φιλοσοφήσειν· διττὴν γὰρ εἶναι τῆς δια-

12–23] SVF III, p. 54 Posid. fr. 160 Edelstein-Kidd 12–15] *cf. infra*, p. 330.4–6 15–16] Usener, Epicurea, p. 275 21] *cf. supra*, p. 316.14–16 26–320.2] SVF III, pp. 54–55 34–320.2] *cf.* Diog. Laert. vii. 89 = SVF III, p. 53 Cic. De leg. i. 47

2 προβαλομένου H: *corr.* R *Ald.*: προκαλεῖ μὲν οὐ L 4 τε^II *del. Ald.* 5 ᾠκειῶσθαι *Müller* 6 δεικνύουσιν L 7 τὸ *om.* L 8 αὐτῆς L 12 προσταγμάτων] πραγματειῶν L 13 *ante* καθ' *add.* μιᾶς *Müller* 16 χωριστοῦ L 17 οἰκειῶσθαι H: ὠκειῶσθαι L: *corr. Bas.* 20 Ἐάσας] ἅτε L ἀπορεῖ περὶ] ἀπορεῖν ἐρεῖ H L: *corr. Diels apud Kalbfleisch* 23 καὶ ἐλέγχει] τε καὶ λέγει L 26 γε] τὲ L κἂν L ἐντρέφεται H προσήκον^τ L 27 καὶ^II *om.* L 28 γ' ἐνῆν] γέγονεν L 30 φάσκοντα L 32 φιλοσόφων L μόνῳ – 33 θεάσηται *om.* L 33 ἀκούσειε H: ἀκούσῃ μήτε L: *corr. Kühn* 34 ὅμως] ὅπως L αὐτῶ H: αὐ^τ L: *corr. Kühn* *post* φιλοσοφήσειν *add.* φησί *Sandbach apud Edelstein-Kidd*

them angry, kicking, biting, wanting to win and get the better of
their own kind, as some animals do, when no prize is offered beyond
victory itself. Such behavior as this is clearly observed in quail, cocks, 5
partridges, the ichneumon, the asp, the crocodile, and thousands of
others. In the same way children also appear to feel a kinship with 6
pleasure and victory, and at some later time, as they grow older, they
show that they have a certain natural kinship with what is right. Thus 7
they are ashamed of their errors as they grow older, they take pleasure
in noble acts, they lay claim to justice and the other virtues, and they
perform many acts in accordance with their notions of these virtues;
but earlier, when they were still small, they lived by their affections
and took no notice of the commands of reason. Thus there are these 8
three things with which we feel a natural kinship, corresponding to
each form of the soul's parts: pleasure, through the desiderative (form);
victory, through the spirited (form); and what is morally excellent,
through the rational (form). Epicurus saw only the kinship felt by
the worst part of the soul, Chrysippus only that felt by the best,
saying that we have a kinship only with what is morally excellent,
which, he holds, is obviously also good. The ancient philosophers were
the only ones who saw that we have a kinship with all three.

Since Chrysippus omitted two of them, it is not surprising that 9
he was perplexed about the origin of vice. He could not state its cause
or the ways in which it comes to exist; and he could not discover how
it is that children err. On all these points it was reasonable, I think, for
Posidonius to censure and refute him. For if from the start children 10
felt a kinship with moral excellence, their misconduct could not arise
internally or from themselves, but would necessarily come to them only
from the outside. But even though they are brought up in good habits 11
and are given the education that they ought to have, yet they are
invariably observed doing something wrong; and Chrysippus
acknowledges this fact. To be sure, he could have ignored the obvious 12
facts and have admitted only the conclusion that follows from his own
suppositions; he could have claimed that if children are well trained
they will surely become wise men in due time. But he did not venture 13
on this particular falsification of the facts; he granted that even if
children were raised under the exclusive care of a philosopher and
never saw or heard any example of vice, nevertheless they would not
necessarily become philosophers. There are two causes (he says) of 14

στροφῆς τὴν αἰτίαν, ἑτέραν μὲν ἐκ κατηχήσεως τῶν πολλῶν ἀνθρώπων
ἐγγιγνομένην, ἑτέραν δὲ ἐξ αὐτῆς τῶν πραγμάτων τῆς φύσεως. ἐγὼ δὲ
ὑπὲρ ἑκατέρας αὐτῶν ἀπορῶ καὶ πρώτης γε τῆς ἐκ τῶν πέλας γιγνο-
15 μένης. καὶ γὰρ διὰ τί θεασάμενα καὶ ἀκούσαντα παράδειγμα κακίας
οὐχὶ μισεῖ τοῦτο καὶ φεύγει τῷ μηδεμίαν οἰκείωσιν ἔχειν πρὸς αὐτό,
θαυμάζειν ἐπέρχεταί μοι, καὶ πολὺ δὴ μᾶλλον ἐπειδὰν μήτε θεασάμενα
16 μήτ' ἀκούσαντα πρὸς αὐτῶν τῶν πραγμάτων ἐξαπατηθῇ. τίς γὰρ ἀνάγκη
τοὺς παῖδας ὑπὸ μὲν τῆς ἡδονῆς ὡς ἀγαθοῦ δελεάζεσθαι μηδεμίαν οἰκείω-
441 σιν ἔχοντας πρὸς αὐτήν, ἀποστρέφεσθαι δὲ καὶ φεύγειν / τὸν πόνον
17 εἴπερ μὴ καὶ πρὸς τοῦτον ἠλλοτρίω⟨ν⟩ται φύσει; τίς δ' ἀνάγκη πρὸς
μὲν τοὺς ἐπαίνους καὶ τὰς τιμὰς ἵεσθαί τε καὶ χαίρειν αὐτοῖς, ἄχθεσθαι
δὲ καὶ φεύγειν τούς τε ψόγους καὶ τὰς ἀτιμίας, εἴπερ μὴ καὶ πρὸς ταῦτα
18 φύσει τινὰ ἔχουσιν οἰκείωσίν τε καὶ ἀλλοτρίωσιν; εἰ γὰρ μὴ ταῖς φωναῖς,
463 ἀλλὰ τῇ γε δυνάμει τῶν λεγομένων ὁμολογεῖν | ἔοικεν ὁ Χρύσιππος
ὡς ἔστιν οἰκείωσίς τέ τις ἡμῖν καὶ ἀλλοτρίωσις φύσει πρὸς ἕκαστον τῶν
19 εἰρημένων. ἐπειδὰν γὰρ λέγῃ τὰς περὶ ἀγαθῶν καὶ κακῶν ἐγγίνεσθαι
τοῖς φαύλοις διαστροφὰς διά τε τὴν πιθανότητα τῶν φαντασιῶν καὶ τὴν
κατήχησιν, ἐρωτητέον αὐτὸν τὴν αἰτίαν δι' ἣν ἡδονὴ μὲν ὡς ἀγαθὸν
20 ἀλγηδὼν δ' ὡς κακὸν πιθανὴν προβάλλουσι φαντασίαν. οὕτως δὲ καὶ
διὰ τί τὴν μὲν νίκην τὴν [ἐν] Ὀλυμπίασιν καὶ τὴν τῶν ἀνδριάντων
ἀνάθεσιν ἐπαινούμενά τε καὶ μακαριζόμενα πρὸς τῶν πολλῶν ἀκούοντες
ὡς ἀγαθά, περὶ δὲ τῆς ἥττης τε καὶ τῆς ἀτιμίας ὡς κακῶν, ἑτοίμως πει-
442 21 θόμεθα; καὶ / γὰρ καὶ ταῦθ' ὁ Ποσειδώνιος μέμφεται καὶ δεικνύναι
πειρᾶται πασῶν τῶν ψευδῶν ὑπολήψεων τὰς αἰτίας ἐν μὲν τῷ θεωρητικῷ
⟨γίγνεσθαι δι' ἀμαθίας, ἐν δὲ τῷ πρακτικῷ⟩ διὰ τῆς παθητικῆς ὁλκῆς,
προηγεῖσθαι δ' αὐτῆς τὰς ψευδεῖς δόξας ἀσθενήσαντος περὶ τὴν κρίσιν
τοῦ λογιστικοῦ· γεννᾶσθαι γὰρ τῷ ζῴῳ τὴν ὁρμὴν ἐνίοτε μὲν ἐπὶ τῇ τοῦ
λογιστικοῦ κρίσει, πολλάκις δ' ἐπὶ τῇ κινήσει τοῦ παθητικοῦ.
22 Συνάπτει δ' εἰκότως τοῖς λόγοις τούτοις ὁ Ποσειδώνιος τὰ κατὰ
464 τὸν | φυσιογνώμονα φαινόμενα· καὶ γὰρ τῶν ζῴων καὶ τῶν ἀνθρώπων
ὅσα μὲν εὐρύστερνά τε καὶ θερμότερα θυμικώτερα πάνθ' ὑπάρχει⟨ν⟩

13–23] SVF III, p. 55 23–28] *cf.* Pohlenz, 1898, pp. 560; 564–565; 621 n. 1 Pohlenz, Die Stoa II. p. 113 29–322.8] Posid. fr. 102 Jacoby (Fr. Gr. Hist. II A, p. 282) *cf.* Pohlenz, 1898, pp. 565–566; 621 Edelstein, 1936, p. 307 nn. 83; 86 Foerster, Scriptores Physiognomonici II, p. 273

2 αὐτῶν L 4 διὰ] ἰδία L 5 τὸ H: *om.* L: *corr. Corn.* αὐτὰ L 7 ἐξηπατῆ' (θ supra) L 8 ἀγαθοῦ] εἰῶ' (θ supra) L 10 ἠλλοτρίωται H L: *corr. Müller* 11 ἵεσθαί H L: *correxi*: ἥδεσθαί *Ald.* 13 μὴ] μὴ καὶ L: καὶ μὴ *Müller* 14 τῶν λεγομένων *om.* L 16 τὰς] τίς L ἀγαθοῦ καὶ κακοῦ L καὶ κακῶν *del. Müller* 18 ἡδονὴν L 19 ὡς] ὢ H προβαλούση φαντασία L 20 ἐν ὀλυμπιάσι(ν) H L: *corr. Charitonides* 22 κακὰ H L: *corr. Müller* 24 θεωρηματικῶ L 25 γίγνεσθαι – πρακτικῷ *addidi*: σκέμματι γινομένων διὰ τῆς τῶν ὄντων οὐχ ἱκανῆς ἐμπειρίας, ἐν δὲ τῷ πρακτικῷ *add. Pohlenz*, σκέμματι γινομένων διὰ τῆς ἀμαθίας, ἐν δὲ τῷ πρακτικῷ *Edelstein*, γίνεσθαι *post* ὁλκῆς *Müller* 26 αὐταῖς L ἀσθενήσαντας H: ἀσθενήσαν (τ supra) L: *corr. Chart.* *post* κρίσιν *add.* τὴν H 27 τῶν ζώων L 29–30 τὰ κατὰ τὸν φυσιογνώμονα] κατὰ τὴν φυσιογνωμονίαν τὰ L 31 μὲν *om.* L ὑπάρχει H L: *corr. Kühn*

their corruption; one arises in them from the conversation of the
majority of men, the other from the very nature of the things (around
them). I have objections to both of these causes, beginning with that
which arises from associations (with men). It occurs to me to wonder 15
why it is that when they have seen and heard an example of vice, they
do not hate it and flee from it, since they feel no kinship with it; and
I wonder all the more that they should be corrupted when they have
neither seen nor heard such examples and are deceived by the very
things themselves. What necessity is there that children be enticed by 16
pleasure as a good thing, when they feel no kinship with it, or that
they avoid and flee from pain if they are not by nature also alienated
from it? And what necessity is there that they be eager for praise and 17
honor and take delight in them, but are distressed by dispraise and
disgrace and try to avoid them, if they do not feel some natural
kinship and alienation relative to these things also? If Chrysippus 18
does not actually say so, yet his words seem to imply acceptance of
the view that we feel a natural kinship and alienation relative to each
of the things mentioned. For when he says that corruption arises in 19
inferior men in regard to good and evil because of the persuasiveness
of appearances and the talk of men, we must ask him why it is that
pleasure projects the persuasive appearance that it is good, and pain
that it is evil. Similarly, when we hear the majority of men praise and 20
glorify victory at Olympia and the erection of one's statue as good
things, and when we hear them speak of defeat and disgrace as evil,
why is it that we are readily persuaded? Indeed, Posidonius censures 21
(Chrysippus) on these points also, and he tries to show that the
causes of all false suppositions arise in the theoretical sphere through
ignorance, and in the practical through the pull of the affections, but
that false opinions precede this pull, because the reasoning part has
become weak in judgment. For conation (he says) is sometimes generated in the animal as a result of the judgment of the reasoning part,
but often as a result of the movement of the affective part.

Posidonius plausibly attaches to this discussion the obser- 22
vations of the physiognomist: men and animals that are broad-chested
and warmer are all by nature more given to anger, but those that have

23 φύσει, ὅσα δὲ πλατυΐσχιά τε καὶ ψυχρότερα δειλότερα. καὶ κατὰ τὰς
χώρας δὲ οὐ σμικρῷ τινι διενηνοχέναι τοῖς ἤθεσι τοὺς ἀνθρώπους εἰς
δειλίαν καὶ τόλμαν ἢ τὸ φιλήδονόν τε καὶ φιλόπονον, ὡς τῶν παθητικῶν
κινήσεων τῆς ψυχῆς ἑπομένων ἀεὶ τῇ διαθέσει τοῦ σώματος, ἣν ἐκ τῆς
443 24 κατὰ τὸ περιέχον κράσεως / οὐ κατ' ὀλίγον ἀλλοιοῦσθαι. καὶ γὰρ δὴ
καὶ τὸ αἷμα διαφέρειν ἐν τοῖς ζῴοις φησὶ θερμότητι καὶ ψυχρότητι καὶ
πάχει καὶ λεπτότητι καὶ ἄλλαις [φησὶ] διαφοραῖς οὐκ ὀλίγαις, ὑπὲρ ὧν
25 Ἀριστοτέλης ἐπὶ πλεῖστον διῆλθεν. ἡμεῖς δὲ κατὰ τὸν οἰκεῖον καιρὸν
ἐπὶ προήκοντι τῷ λόγῳ μνημονεύσομεν αὐτῶν, ἡνίκα ἂν καὶ αὐτὰς τὰς
Ἱπποκράτους τε καὶ Πλάτωνος ῥήσεις περὶ τούτων παραγράφωμεν.
26 ἐν δὲ τῷ παρόντι πρὸς τοὺς περὶ τὸν Χρύσιππον ὁ λόγος ἐνέστηκέ
μοι μήτ' ἄλλο τι γιγνώσκοντας τῶν κατὰ τὰ πάθη μήθ' ὡς αἱ τοῦ
σώματος κράσεις οἰκείας ἑαυταῖς ἐργάζονται τὰς παθητικὰς κινήσεις· |
465 27 οὕτως γὰρ ὁ Ποσειδώνιος ὀνομάζειν εἴωθεν. Ἀριστοτέλης δ' ἄντι-
κρυς ἤθη καλεῖ τῶν ζῴων ἁπάσας τὰς τοιαύτας τῆς ψυχῆς καταστά-
σεις ἐξηγεῖταί τε καθ' ὅντινα τρόπον ἐπὶ ταῖς διαφερούσαις κράσεσι
28 συνίσταται. διόπερ, οἶμαι, καὶ ἡ τῶν παθῶν τῆς ψυχῆς ἴασις ἐπ' ἐνίων
444 μὲν εὔκολός τε καὶ ῥᾳδία / διὰ τὸ μήτε τὰς παθητικὰς κινήσεις αὐτοῖς
ἰσχυρὰς ὑπάρχειν μήτε τὸ λογιστικὸν ἀσθενὲς φύσει καὶ ἀσύνετον ἀλλὰ
δι' ἀμαθίαν καὶ μοχθηροὺς ἐθισμοὺς ἐμπαθῶς ἀναγκάζεσθαι ζῆν τοὺς
τοιούτους ἀνθρώπους, ἐνίοις δὲ χαλεπὴ καὶ δύσκολος ὅταν κινήσεις αἱ
κατὰ πάθος αἱ διὰ τὴν τοῦ σώματος κατασκευὴν ἀναγκαίως γιγνόμεναι
μεγάλαι δή τινες οὖσαι τύχωσι καὶ σφοδραὶ τό τε λογιστικὸν ἀσθενὲς
29 καὶ ἀσύνετον φύσει. χρὴ γὰρ καὶ τοῦτο μὲν ἐπιστήμην λαβεῖν τῶν ἀληθῶν
καὶ τὰς κατὰ πάθος δὲ κινήσεις ἀμβλυνθῆναι χρηστοῖς ἐπιτηδεύμασιν
ἐθισθείσας εἴ τις μέλλοι βελτίονα τὸ ἦθος ἀποδείξειν τὸν ἄνθρωπον.
30 Οὕτω δὲ καὶ πλάττειν ἐξ ἀρχῆς ἄνθρωπον χρὴ πρὸς τὸ βέλτιστον
ἁπάντων μὲν πρῶτον αὐτῶν τῶν σπερμάτων προνοουμένους, οἷς |
466 ἐφεξῆς τῆς διαίτης ἣν ἡ κυοῦσα διαιτήσεται κατά τε τὰς τροφὰς καὶ τὰ
πόματα καὶ τὰ γυμνάσια καὶ τὰς ἡσυχίας καὶ τοὺς ὕπνους καὶ τὰς ἐγρη-
445 γόρσεις ἐπιθυμίας τε καὶ θυμοὺς ὅσα τ' ἄλλα τοιαῦτα, περὶ ὧν / ἁπάντων
31 ὁ μὲν Πλάτων ἀκριβέστατα διῆλθεν. ὁ δὲ Χρύσιππος οὐ μόνον αὐτὸς

11–13] SVF III, p. 55 12–14] *cf. supra*, lin. 3–4; pp. 286.24; 288.28; 290.6 Posid. fr. 153 Edelstein-Kidd 27–326.8] Posid. fr. 31 Edelstein-Kidd 32–324.2] SVF III, p. 55

1 πλατυΐσχυά L 2 δὲ *om.* H οὐ σμικρῷ τινι] ὡς μικρο$^{\tau\rho}$' L 3 δει$^{\lambda}$' καὶ τόλμας L ἢ τὸ] ἤτοι L 4 ἣν] ἵν' L 7 φησὶ *del. Müller*: φυσικαῖς *coni. Einarson* 9 αὐτὰς] ταύτας H L: *corr. Kühn* *post* τὰς *add.* περὶ τοῦ L 10 τοῦτον L περιγράφωμεν H L: *corr. Ald.* 12 τι *om.* H *ante* τῶν *add.* περὶ *Müller* τὰ *om.* L 13 κράσεις] κρ^{ι}' L 15 ἤδη H: ἤδει L: *correxi* καλεῖν L ζωΐων L ἁπάσας *post* καταστάσεις *(lin. 16) trsp.* L 17 συνίστανται *Corn.* 18 αὐτῆς L 20 ζῆν τοὺς] ζητοῦσι L 21 χαλεπῶς καὶ δυσκο$^{\lambda}$' L ὅταν κινήσεις αἱ] ὅτε αἱ κινήσεις L 22 πα$^{\vartheta}$' H: τὰ πάθη L: *corr. Ald.* 23 τό τε] τότε τὸ L ἀσθενὲς *om.* L 24 τού^{T} L: τοῦτον *Ald.* 25 αὐληθῆναι L 26 ἐθισθεῖσαν H: ἐθισθεῖσαι L: *corr. Müller* εἰ μέλλοιμεν L ἀποδεῖξαι L 29 ἐφεξῆς] ἔθ' ἑξῆς L ἡ κυοῦσα] οἰκείως ἂν L διαιτήσηται L

wide hips and are colder are more cowardly. And he says that in 23
different localities men's characters exhibit no small differences in
cowardice and daring, in love of pleasure and of toil, the supposition
being that the affective movements of the soul in every case follow the
physical state, which is altered in no small degree by the mixture (of
elements) in the environment. For even the blood in animals differs, 24
he says, in warmth and coldness, thickness and thinness, and in many
other properties, which Aristotle discussed at great length. We shall 25
mention these properties at the appropriate time as the discussion
proceeds, when we quote the actual passages from Hippocrates and
Plato that deal with them. For the present my argument is with 26
Chrysippus and his followers, who know nothing else that pertains
to the affections, nor yet that each mixture in the body produces its
own set of 'affective motions' – that is the name that Posidonius
habitually gave them. But Aristotle comes straight out and calls all 27
settled states of this kind in the souls of animals their 'characters', and
he explains how they arise from different mixtures. For that reason, 28
I suppose, the cure of the soul's affections is in some persons agreeable
and easy, since their affective motions are not strong and their reason-
ing part is not by nature weak and uncomprehending; instead it is
ignorance and bad habits that compel such men to live under the sway
of the affections. But in others the cure is difficult and disagreeable,
when the affective motions, occurring of necessity because of the
construction of the body, are great and violent, and the reasoning part
is by nature weak and uncomprehending. For two things must be 29
done: this latter part must acquire knowledge of the truth, and the
affective movements must be blunted by habituation to good practices,
if one is to point to an improvement in the man's character.

Thus from the start one should mold a human being with an eye 30
to what is best, with forethought first of all for the very seed, then for
the regimen that the pregnant mother will follow in food and drink,
exercise and rest, sleep and waking, desire and anger, and the like, all
of which Plato discussed with the greatest exactness. But Chry- 31

οὐδὲν ἱκνούμενον εἶπεν, ἀλλ' οὐδὲ τῶν ἀπ' αὐτοῦ τινι κατέλιπεν ἀφορμὴν
32 εὑρέσεως μοχθηρὰν ὑποβαλλόμενος τῷ λόγῳ τὴν κρηπῖδα. ταῦτά τοι
καὶ ὁ Ποσειδώνιος αὐτῷ μέμφεται μετὰ τοῦ καὶ θαυμάζειν ὅσα Πλά-
των εἶπεν ὑπὲρ τῆς τῶν παίδων ἔτι τε κυουμένων ἐν τῇ μήτρᾳ διαπλά-
σεως ἀποκυηθέντων τε τροφῆς καὶ παιδείας, καὶ γέγραφεν οἷον ἐπιτομήν
τινα κατὰ τὸ πρῶτον αὐτοῦ Περὶ παθῶν σύγγραμμα τῶν ὑπὸ Πλά-
τωνος εἰρημένων, ὡς χρὴ τρέφεσθαι καὶ παιδεύεσθαι τοὺς παῖδας ὑπὲρ
τοῦ τὸ παθητικόν τε καὶ ἄλογον τῆς ψυχῆς σύμμετρον ἀποφαίνεσθαι
33 ταῖς κινήσεσι καὶ τοῖς τοῦ λόγου προστάγμασιν εὐπειθές. «αὕτη γὰρ
ἀρίστη παίδων παιδεία[ς], παρασκευὴ τοῦ παθητικοῦ τῆς ψυχῆς, ὡς
34 ἂν ἐπιτηδειοτάτη ᾖ πρὸς τὴν ἀρχὴν τοῦ λογιστικοῦ.» μικρὸν μὲν γὰρ
467 *446* τὰ πρῶτα καὶ | ἀσθενὲς ὑπάρ/χειν τοῦτο, μέγα δὲ καὶ ἰσχυρὸν ἀποτε-
λεῖσθαι περὶ τὴν τεσσαρεσκαιδεκαέτην ἡλικίαν, ἡνίκα ἤδη κρατεῖν τε
καὶ ἄρχειν αὐτῷ προσήκει καθάπερ ἡνιόχῳ τινὶ τοῦ ζεύγους τῶν συμ-
φύτων ἵππων ἐπιθυμίας τε καὶ θυμοῦ μήτ' ἰσχυρῶν ὑπαρχόντων ἄγαν
μήτε ἀσθενῶν μήτ' ὀκνηρῶν μήτ' ἐκφόρων μήτε δυσπειθῶν ὅλως ἢ ἀκόσμων
ἢ ὑβριστῶν, ἀλλ' εἰς ἅπαν ἑτοίμων ἕπεσθαί τε καὶ πείθεσθαι τῷ λογι-
35 σμῷ. τούτου δ' αὐτοῦ τὴν παιδείαν γε καὶ τὴν ἀρετὴν ἐπιστήμην εἶναι
τῆς τῶν ὄντων φύσεως, ὥσπερ τοῦ ἡνιόχου τῶν ἡνιοχικῶν θεωρη-
μάτων· ἐν γὰρ ταῖς ἀλόγοις τῆς ψυχῆς δυνάμεσιν ἐπιστήμας οὐκ ἐγγί-
γνεσθαι, καθάπερ οὐδὲ ἐν τοῖς ἵπποις, ἀλλὰ τούτοις μὲν τὴν οἰκείαν
ἀρετὴν ἐξ ἐθισμοῦ τινος ἀλόγου παραγίγνεσθαι, τοῖς δ' ἡνιόχοις ἐκ
διδασκαλίας λογικῆς.

36 Ἕπεται δ' εὐθὺς τοῖσδε καὶ ὁ περὶ τῶν ἀρετῶν λόγος, καὶ αὐτὸς
447 ἔχων τὸ σφάλμα διττόν, εἴτε ἐπιστήμας τις ἁπάσας αὐτὰς εἴτε / δυνάμεις
37 ὑπολάβοι. τῶν μὲν γὰρ ἀλόγων τῆς ψυχῆς μερῶν ἀλόγους ἀνάγκη
468 καὶ τὰς ἀρετὰς | εἶναι, τοῦ λογιστικοῦ δὲ μόνου λογικήν. ὥστ' εὐλόγως
ἐκείνων μὲν αἱ ἀρεταὶ δυνάμεις εἰσίν, ἐπιστήμη δὲ μόνου τοῦ λογιστικοῦ.
38 Χρύσιππος δὲ μεγάλα σφάλλεται οὐχ ὅτι μηδεμίαν ἀρετὴν ἐποίησε
δύναμιν – οὐ γὰρ μέγα τὸ τοιοῦτον σφάλμα ἐστὶν οὐδὲ διαφερόμεθα

2–9] *cf.* Pohlenz, 1921, p. 170 Edelstein, 1936, p. 307 n. 85 Reinhardt, 1953, col. 753 3–23] Pohlenz, 1898, pp. 622–624 9–11] Posid. fr. 148 Edelstein-Kidd 20–23] Reinhardt, 1953, col. 753 20–21] Posid. fr. 148 Edelstein-Kidd 24–326.8] SVF III, pp. 61–62 24–28] *cf.* Edelstein, 1936, p. 312 n. 104 24–25] *cf.* Pohlenz, 1898, p. 566 Reinhardt, 1953, col. 742–743 26–27] *cf.* Pohlenz, 1898, p. 624 29–326.2] *cf.* Reinhardt, 1953, col. 743

1 ἱκνούμενον H L: *corr.* p *Bas.* 2 μοχθηρὰν – κρηπῖδα *om.* L ὑποβαλό-μενος *e corr.* p 3 αὐτὰ L 4 μητρὶ L 6 σύγκρα (μ supra lin.) L 7 ὡς] "*f.* πῶς" *Bake* 9 ταῖς *om.* L *post* γὰρ *inseruerit* φησί *Müller* 10 παιδείας H L: *corr. Müller* 12 καὶ[II] *om.* L 13 τεσσαρεσκαιδεκαετὴν L: τεσσαρεσκαιδεκαετῆ H: *corr. Petersen* ἤδει L 14 αὐτὸ H: αὐτῶν L: *corr. Kühn* προσήκειν L συμφύτων] συντρόφων L, *sed cf. Plat. Phaedr. 246 a 6* 17 ἢ *om.* L 18 γε] τε F *Ald.* 19 *post* ἡνιόχου *add.* τὴν F 20 τοῖς L 21 οἰκείαν] εἰκό (ν supra lin.)' L 22 παραγίνεσθαι M *Ald.*: περιγίγνεσθαι H L: *correxi* 24 εὐθὺς] αὖθις *Ald.* ὁ *om.* L *aut* καὶ αὐτὸς *aut* αὐτοῖς *Reinhardt*: αὐτὸς *Corn.*: αὐτὰς H: ἐπιστήμας τίς ἀπάσας αὐτὰς (αὐτὰς *ex* -ῶν *corr.*) καὶ αὐτ' L: αὐτοῦ *Müller* 25 ἔχων *om.* L: ἐλέγχων *Müller*, *sed cf. Kalbfleisch, 1892, p. 34* 27 λογικήν] λογιστικὴν L 29 οὐχ (ου *e corr.*) H L 30 διαφερόμενον L

sippus not only said nothing himself that was adequate; he did not
even leave to any of his followers a starting point for the investigation,
as he rested his argument on a faulty foundation. Posidonius cen- 32
sures him for this, while he admires what Plato said about the shaping
of unborn children in the womb and about their rearing and training
after birth; and in his first book On the Affections he wrote a kind of
epitome of Plato's remarks about children, how they must be reared
and trained in order that the affective and irrational part of their soul
may exhibit due measure in its motions and obedience to the commands
of reason. "For this is the best training of children: preparation of the 33
affective part of the soul in such a way that it may be most amenable
to the rule of the rational part." At first (he says) this (rational part) is 34
small and weak, but it acquires size and strength at about the four-
teenth year, which is the proper time for it to take control and to rule,
as a kind of charioteer, the team of horses conjoined with it, namely,
desire and anger, so long as they are not excessively strong or weak,
sluggish or restive, or in general disobedient or disorderly or lawless,
but ready to follow and obey reason in everything. The education and 35
the virtue of the rational part itself (he says) is the knowledge of the
nature of things, just as the education and virtue of the charioteer is
the knowledge of the rules of chariot-driving, for knowledge does not
arise in the irrational powers of the soul any more than it does in hor-
ses: the horses get their proper virtue from a kind of irrational habitua-
tion, the charioteers from rational instruction.

The account of the virtues follows directly on this, and it too 36
contains a double error, whether the supposition be that all the virtues
are kinds of knowledge, or that all are powers. Of necessity the virtues 37
of the irrational parts of the soul are irrational; that of the rational
alone is rational. Therefore it is reasonable that the virtues of the
other parts are powers, and knowledge is the virtue only of the rational
part. Chrysippus, however, committed a major blunder, not in 38
failing to make any virtue a power – that kind of error is of little
consequence, and we are not attacking it – but in saying that there are

πρὸς αὐτό —, ἀλλ' ὅτι πολλὰς ἐπιστήμας τε καὶ ἀρετὰς εἶναι φήσας μίαν
39 ἔφησεν εἶναι δύναμιν τῆς ψυχῆς. οὐ γὰρ ἐνδέχεται μιᾶς δυνάμεως ἀρετὰς εἶναι πολλάς, εἴ γε μηδὲ τελειότητας πολλὰς ἑνὸς πράγματος. μία γὰρ ἑκάστου τῶν ὄντων ἡ τελειότης, ἡ δ' ἀρετὴ τελειότης ἐστὶ τῆς ἑκάστου
40 φύσεως, ὡς αὐτὸς ὁμολογεῖ. κάλλιον οὖν Ἀρίστων ὁ Χῖος οὔτε πολλὰς εἶναι τὰς ἀρετὰς τῆς ψυχῆς ἀποφηνάμενος, ἀλλὰ μίαν ἣν ἐπιστήμην
448 ἀγαθῶν τε καὶ κακῶν εἶναί φησιν, οὔτε / περὶ τῶν παθῶν ἐναντία ταῖς ἰδίαις ὑποθέσεσι γράψας, ὥσπερ ὁ Χρύσιππος.

6. Ἀλλὰ περὶ μὲν τῶν ἀρετῶν ἐν τοῖς ἑξῆς ἐροῦμεν, ἐπειδὴ καὶ περὶ τούτων ὁ Χρύσιππος ἐπηρεάζει τὸν Πλάτωνα. νυνὶ γὰρ ἐξ ἀκολου-
469 θίας τινὸς αὐτῶν ἐμνημόνευσα, τῷ περὶ | τῶν παθῶν δόγματι καὶ τοῦ περὶ τῶν ἀρετῶν ἐξ ἀνάγκης ἑπομένου, ὥσπερ καὶ ὁ Ποσειδώνιός φησιν ὧδέ πως γράφων αὐτοῖς ὀνόμασι κατὰ τὸ πρῶτον Περὶ παθῶν
2 οὐ μετὰ πολλὰ τῆς ἀρχῆς τοῦ βιβλίου· «νομίζω γὰρ καὶ τὴν περὶ ἀγαθῶν καὶ κακῶν καὶ τὴν περὶ τελῶν καὶ τὴν περὶ ἀρετῶν ἐκ τῆς περὶ παθῶν ὀρθῶς διασκέψεως ἠρτῆσθαι.»

3 Ὅτι μὲν οὖν τὴν περὶ τῶν ἀρετῶν ὀρθῶς δόξαν ἐζεῦχθαι συμβέβηκε τῇ περὶ τῶν παθῶν, αὐτάρκως ἐνδεδεῖχθαί μοι δοκῶ· ὅτι δὲ καὶ τὴν περὶ ἀγαθῶν τε καὶ τοῦ τέλους, ἀρκεῖ μοι τὰ Ποσειδωνίου παραγράψαι
4 τόνδε τὸν τρόπον ἔχοντα· «τὸ δὴ τῶν παθῶν αἴτιον, τουτέστι τῆς τε
449 ἀνομολογίας καὶ τοῦ κακοδαίμονος / βίου, τὸ μὴ κατὰ πᾶν ἕπεσθαι τῷ ἐν αὐτῷ δαίμονι συγγενεῖ τε ὄντι καὶ τὴν ὁμοίαν φύσιν ἔχοντι τῷ τὸν ὅλον κόσμον διοικοῦντι, τῷ δὲ χείρονι καὶ ζῳώδει ποτὲ συνεκκλίνοντας
5 φέρεσθαι. οἱ δὲ τοῦτο παριδόντες οὔτε ἐν τούτοις βελτιοῦσι τὴν αἰτίαν τῶν παθῶν οὔτ' ἐν τοῖς περὶ τῆς εὐδαιμονίας καὶ ὁμολογίας ὀρθοδο-
470 ξοῦσιν· οὐ γὰρ βλέπουσιν ὅτι πρῶτόν ἐστιν ἐν αὐτῇ τὸ | κατὰ μηδὲν ἄγεσθαι ὑπὸ τοῦ ἀλόγου τε καὶ κακοδαίμονος καὶ ἀθέου τῆς ψυχῆς.»
6 ἐν τούτοις φανερῶς ὁ Ποσειδώνιος ἐδίδαξε πηλίκον ἁμαρτάνουσιν οἱ περὶ τὸν Χρύσιππον οὐ μόνον ἐν τοῖς περὶ τῶν παθῶν λογισμοῖς,

3–5] *cf. infra*, PHP 588.14–589.1 Müller 5–7] *cf. infra*, PHP 591.4–7 Müller In Theaet. comm. anon. col. xi. 33–40 10–13] Reinhardt, 1953, col. 742 12–16] Posid. fr. 30 Edelstein-Kidd *cf.* Pohlenz, 1898, p. 610 Reinhardt, 1921, p. 294 Reinhardt, 1953, col. 733 Edelstein, 1936, p. 308 Nock, 1959, p. 11 n. 54 17–332.31] Posid. fr. 187 Edelstein-Kidd 18–27] *cf.* Pohlenz, 1898, p. 625 Reinhardt, 1921, p. 329 Reinhardt, 1953, col. 747–748 Edelstein, 1936, pp. 314–315 Nock, 1959, p. 10 20–328.2] SVF III, pp. 111–112 21–23] *cf.* SVF III, p. 4.4–7 = Diog. Laert. vii. 88

1 αὐτὸν L: αὐτὸν διὰ τοῦτο *Reinhardt* μίαν – 2 ψυχῆς *om.* L 3 τελειο^{ττ}' (τ^{I} *ex* λ *corr.*) H L: *corr. Corn.* μία] μὴ L 4 τελειότης^{II} *om.* L 5 αὐτὸς *ex* αὐτοῦ, *ut vid.*, *corr.* L καλλίων H χίος H L: *corr. Chart.* 6 μίαν] μόνην L 7 ἐναντία *om.* L 11 ἑαυτῶν H *ante* τῷ *add.* ἐν L 12 ἑπομένων L 13 φησιν *om.* L 15 *ante* ἀγαθῶν *add.* τῶν L 17 ἔδοξαν L 18 τῇ] τῆς H L: *corr. Ald.* περὶ τῶν] τῶν περὶ L 19 ἀρκεῖ] ἀρ *e corr.* L παραγράψαν, *ut vid.*, L^{2} 21 ὁμολο^{γ}' L ἕπεσθαι] εσθ *in ras.* H τῷ] τῶν L 22 αὐτῷ H L: *corr. Bake*: αὐτοῖς F δαίμονι] δὲ μο^{λ}' L 23 συγκλίνοντας L 24 οἱ δὲ] οὐδὲ L παριδόντας L βελτιοῦσι] βλέπουσι *Reinhardt* 26 πρῶτόν ἐστιν] περιττὸν L τὸ *supra lin. add.* H 27 ἀλόγου] λο^{γ}' L 28 φανερῶς] φασί, *ut vid.*, L

many kinds of knowledge and many virtues, yet that the power of the
soul is single. For it is impossible that a single power have many 39
virtues, since it is impossible that a single thing have many perfect
states. The perfect state of each thing that exists is single, and virtue
is the perfect state of the nature of each, as he himself agrees. Ariston 40
of Chios did better: he said that the soul does not have a plurality of
virtues, but only one, which he called knowledge of things good and
evil; and in his account of the affections he did not contradict his own
presuppositions, as Chrysippus did.

6. We shall speak of the virtues at a later time, since on that sub-
ject too Chrysippus scoffs at Plato. I have mentioned them here
because of a kind of logical necessity, inasmuch as the doctrine of the
virtues necessarily follows from the doctrine of the passions. Posi-
donius also says this; in the first (book) of his work On the Affections,
not far from the beginning, he writes these very words: "For I believe 2
that the examination of things good and evil, of ends and of virtues,
depends on a genuine examination of the affections."

I think that I have given sufficient indication that correct opinion 3
about the virtues has been joined to correct opinion about the affec-
tions. To establish that this is true also of correct opinion about what
is good and about the end, it is enough for me to quote the following
words of Posidonius: "The cause of the affections, that is, of 4
discord and the unhappy life, is that men do not follow in everything
the divinity in themselves which is akin and by nature similar to the
divinity that rules the whole universe, but sometimes they turn aside
in the company of that part of them which is inferior and beastlike and
let it carry them along. Those who have failed to see this give no better 5
cause for the affections in those matters, nor do they have correct
views in the matter of happiness and concord. For they do not see that
what is of first importance in happiness is that one should not be led in
anything by the irrational, unhappy and godless part of the soul." In 6
this passage Posidonius clearly taught us the extent to which
Chrysippus and his followers err, not only in their reasoning about

7 ἀλλὰ καὶ περὶ τοῦ τέλους. οὐ γὰρ ὡς ἐκεῖνοι λέγουσιν ἀλλ' ὡς ὁ Πλάτων
8 ἐδίδαξε, τὸ τῇ φύσει ζῆν ὁμολογουμένως ἐστίν. ὄντος γὰρ ἐν ἡμῖν τοῦ
μὲν βελτίονος τῆς ψυχῆς μέρους τοῦ δὲ χείρονος, ὁ μὲν τῷ βελτίονι
450 συνεπόμενος ὁμολογουμένως ἂν λέγοιτο τῇ φύσει ζῆν, ὁ δὲ τῷ / χείρονι
μᾶλλον ἑπόμενος ἀνομολογουμένως· ἔστι δ' οὗτος μὲν ὁ κατὰ πάθος
9 ζῶν, ἐκεῖνος δὲ ὁ κατὰ λόγον. οὐκ ἀρκεσθεὶς δὲ τούτοις ὁ Ποσειδώνιος
ἐναργέστερόν τε καὶ σφοδρότερον καθάπτεται τῶν περὶ τὸν Χρύσιππον
10 ὡς οὐκ ὀρθῶς ἐξηγουμένων τὸ τέλος. ἔχει δὲ ἡ ῥῆσις ὧδε· «ἃ δὴ παρέντες
ἔνιοι τὸ ὁμολογουμένως ζῆν συστέλλουσιν εἰς τὸ πᾶν τὸ ἐνδεχόμενον
ποιεῖν ἕνεκα τῶν πρώτων κατὰ φύσιν, ὅμοιον αὐτῷ ποιοῦντες τῷ
σκοπὸν ἐκτίθεσθαι τὴν ἡδονὴν ἢ τὴν ἀοχλησίαν ἢ ἄλλο τι τοιοῦτον.
471 11 ἔστι δὲ μάχην ἐμφαῖνον | κατ' αὐτὴν τὴν ἐκφοράν, καλὸν δὲ καὶ εὐδαι-
μονικὸν οὐδέν· παρέπεται γὰρ κατὰ τὸ ἀναγκαῖον τῷ τέλει, τέλος δὲ
12 οὐκ ἔστιν. ἀλλὰ καὶ τούτου διαληφθέντος ὀρθῶς, ἔξεστι μὲν αὐτῷ χρῆσθαι
πρὸς τὸ διακόπτειν τὰς ἀπορίας ἃς οἱ σοφισταὶ προτείνουσι, μὴ μέντοι
γε τῷ κατ' ἐμπειρίαν τῶν κατὰ τὴν ὅλην φύσιν συμβαινόντων ζῆν, ὅπερ
451 ἰσοδυνα/μεῖ τῷ ὁμολογουμένως εἰπεῖν ζῆν ἡνίκα μὴ τοῦτο μικροπρεπῶς
συντείνει[ν] εἰς τὸ τῶν διαφορῶν τυγχάνειν.»
13 Ἤρκει μὲν οὖν ἴσως καὶ τοῦτο πρὸς ἔνδειξιν τῆς ἀτοπίας ὧν ὁ
Χρύσιππος εἴρηκε περὶ τοῦ τέλους ἐξηγούμενος ὅπως ἄν τις τυγχάνοι
τοῦ ὁμολογουμένως τῇ φύσει ζῆν· ἄμεινον μὴν ἡγοῦμαι καὶ τὰ τούτοις
ἑξῆς ὑπὸ τοῦ Ποσειδωνίου γεγραμμένα παραθέσθαι τόνδε τὸν τρόπον
14 ἔχοντα· «ταύτην τε δὴ τὴν ἀτοπίαν διέλυσεν ἡ αἰτία τῶν παθῶν ὁρα-
θεῖσα καὶ τὰς ἀρχὰς ἔδειξε τῆς ἐν τοῖς ὀρεκτοῖς καὶ φευκτοῖς διαστροφῆς
καὶ τοὺς τρόπους τῆς ἀσκήσεως διεῖλε καὶ τὰ διαπορούμενα περὶ τῆς
15 ἐκ πάθους ὁρμῆς ἐξέφηνεν.» οὐ σμικρά γε οὐδὲ τὰ τυχόντα φησὶν ἡμᾶς
472 ἀπολαύσειν ἀγαθὰ τῆς αἰτίας | τῶν παθῶν εὑρεθείσης. εἰς γὰρ τὸ μαθεῖν
ἀκριβῶς οἷόν τι τὸ ὁμολογουμένως τῇ φύσει ζῆν ἐστιν, ἐκ τῆς τῶν
16 παθῶν αἰτίας εὑρεθείσης ὠφελήθημεν. ὁ μὲν γὰρ κατὰ πάθος οὐχ /
452 ὁμολογουμένως ζῇ τῇ φύσει, ὁ δὲ μὴ κατὰ πάθος ὁμολογουμένως ζῇ
τῇ φύσει. ἕπεται γὰρ ὁ μὲν τῷ ἀλόγῳ καὶ ἐμπλήκτῳ τῆς ψυχῆς, ὁ δὲ

6–18] SVF III, p. 5 8–18] *cf.* Pohlenz, 1898, p. 626 Reinhardt, 1921, pp. 330–331 Reinhardt, 1953, col. 749–750 O. Rieth, Hermes 69 (1934), pp. 34–44 Edelstein, 1936, pp. 313–314 21–27] Posid. fr. 150b Edelstein-Kidd 23–26] Pohlenz, 1898, pp. 568; 626–627 O. Rieth, Hermes 69 (1934), p. 36

1 *ante* περὶ *add.* τοῖς L 2 ἐστίν] ὀρθῶς ἂν λέγοιτο *aut* ὀρθῶς λέγοιτ' ἂν *Castiglioni* 3 ὃ L 4 συνεπόμενον L λέγοι τὸ H: *corr. Ald.*: λέγοιτο τὸ L ὃ L 5 μᾶλλον ἑπόμενος] μαχουμένως τὲ καὶ L οὕτως L 6 ἐκείνως L 7 ἐγκαθάπτεται L 10 αὐτὸ M 12 ἐμφαίνων *Edelstein* καλὸν *ex* μᾶλλον *corr.* H 15 ἃς *om.* L μὴ *om.* L 16 τῷ] τὸ H L: *corr. Bake*: πρὸς τὸ *Wyttenbach apud Bake*: τὰς κατὰ τὸ *Reinhardt* τῶν] τὸ L ἀμβαινόντων, *ut vid.*, L 17 ἰσοδυναμεῖν *Hirzel* εἶπε *Hirzel* ζῆν ἡνίκα] ζήνωνι· καὶ L 18 συντείνειν H L: *corr. Corn.*: συστέλλειν *Bake*: συντείνειν φαμὲν *Reinhardt* εἰς τὸ] εἴς τι *Wyttenbach apud Bake* ἀδιαφόρων *Wyttenbach apud Bake*: διαφόρων *Bake* τυγχάνει *Ald.* 20 τυγχάνει L 21 ὁμολογημένως H 23 τε] δὲ L αἰτία] ἀτοπία L εὑρεθεῖσα *Müller* 24 τῆς *ex* τοῖς *corr.* H ὀρεκτοῖς] ὁρατοῖς H L: *corr. Ald.* (ὀρεκτ.): αἱρετοῖς *Müller* 27 *ante* γὰρ *add.* τε L 30 ὁ – 31 φύσει *om.* L

the affections, but also about the end. For the end is to 'live in concord 7
with nature', not as they explain the phrase, but as Plato taught (us).
For as one part of the soul in us is better, another worse, the person 8
who follows the better (part) would be said to live in concord with nature, but the person who rather follows the worse (part), in discord. The latter person is one who lives by the affections; the former, one
who lives by reason. But Posidonius, not content with this, makes a 9
more obvious and more forceful attack on Chrysippus and his school,
charging that their explanation of the end is not correct. The passage 10
is as follows: "Some persons, neglecting these matters, reduce 'living in concord' to doing everything possible for the sake of the things that are 'first by nature', thereby taking an action that is similar to actually setting up pleasure or freedom from troubles or something else of that
kind as the goal. But the very statement of their position contains an 11
inconsistency, and it presents nothing that is noble or conducive to happiness. For those things necessarily follow on the end, but they
are not the end. When this distinction has been properly made, it can 12
be used for resolving the questions that the sophists pose; but one cannot so use the view that the end is 'living in accord with one's experience of the things that happen in accord with the whole nature' – which is equivalent to saying, 'live in concord when this does not tend unworthily toward hitting on differences'."

Perhaps this quotation would be sufficient to indicate the absurd- 13
ity of the things Chrysippus said about the end, as he explained how a person might succeed in living in concord with nature; but it is better, I think, to quote the passage that comes next in Posido-
nius' work: "When the cause of the affections was seen, it removed 14
this absurdity; it showed the sources of distortion in what is to be sought and avoided; it distinguished the methods of training; and it cleared up the difficulties about the conation that arises from affection."
These are no small or chance benefits that he says we shall derive from 15
the discovery of the cause of the affections. Indeed, the discovery of the cause of the affections helped us to understand precisely what
sort of thing it is to 'live in concord with nature'. For the person who 16
lives by the affections does not live in concord with nature, and the person who does not live by the affections lives in concord with nature. The one follows the irrational and unstable part of the soul, the other

17 τῷ λογικῷ τε καὶ τῷ θείῳ. «καὶ τὰς ἀρχὰς δὲ τῆς ἐν τοῖς αἱρετοῖς τε καὶ
18 φευκτοῖς διαστροφῆς ἐδίδαξεν ἡ αἰτία τῶν παθῶν εὑρεθεῖσα.» τὰ γὰρ
οἰκεῖα ταῖς ἀλόγοις δυνάμεσι τῆς ψυχῆς ἐξαπατώμενοί τινες ὡς ἁπλῶς
οἰκεῖα δοξάζουσιν οὐκ εἰδότες ὡς τὸ μὲν ἥδεσθαί τε καὶ τὸ κρατεῖν τῶν
πέλας τοῦ ζῳώδους τῆς ψυχῆς ἐστιν ὀρεκτά, σοφία δὲ καὶ πᾶν ὅσον
19 ἀγαθόν τε καὶ καλὸν ἅμα τοῦ λογικοῦ τε καὶ θείου. «καὶ τοὺς τρόπους
δέ», φησί, «τῆς ἀσκήσεως ἡ τῶν παθῶν αἰτία γνωρισθεῖσα διωρίσατο.»
20 τοὺς μὲν γὰρ ἐν τοιοῖσδε ῥυθμοῖς ἅμα καὶ ἁρμονίαις καὶ ἐπιτηδεύμασι,
τοὺς δὲ ἐν τοιοῖσδε διαιτᾶσθαι κελεύσομεν, ὥσπερ ὁ Πλάτων ἡμᾶς
ἐδίδαξε, τοὺς μὲν ἀμβλεῖς καὶ νωθροὺς καὶ ἀθύμους ἔν τε τοῖς ὀρθίοις |
478 ῥυθμοῖς καὶ ταῖς κινούσαις ἰσχυρῶς τὴν ψυχὴν ἁρμονίαις καὶ τοῖς τοιού-
453 τοις ἐπιτηδεύμασι / τρέφοντες, τοὺς δὲ θυμικωτέρους καὶ μανικώτερον
21 ᾄττοντας ἐν ταῖς ἐναντίαις. ἐπεὶ διὰ τί πρὸς θεῶν — ἐρωτήσω γὰρ ἔτι
τοῦτο τοὺς ἀπὸ τοῦ Χρυσίππου —, Δάμων ὁ μουσικὸς αὐλητρίδι
παραγενόμενος αὐλούσῃ τὸ Φρύγιον νεανίσκοις τισὶν οἰνωμένοις καὶ
μανικὰ ἄττα διαπραττομένοις ἐκέλευσεν αὐλῆσαι τὸ Δώριον, οἱ δ'
22 εὐθὺς ἐπαύσαντο τῆς ἐμπλήκτου φορᾶς; οὐ γὰρ δήπου τὰς δόξας τοῦ
λογιστικοῦ μεταδιδάσκονται πρὸς τῶν αὐλημάτων, ἀλλὰ τὸ παθητικὸν
τῆς ψυχῆς ἄλογον ὑπάρχον ἐπεγείρονταί τε καὶ πραΰνονται διὰ κινήσεων
ἀλόγων. τῷ μὲν γὰρ ἀλόγῳ διὰ τῶν ἀλόγων ἥ τε ὠφέλεια καὶ ἡ βλάβη,
τῷ λογικῷ δὲ δι' ἐπιστήμης τε καὶ ἀμαθίας.
23 Καὶ ταῦτ' οὖν ἐκ τῆς τῶν παθῶν αἰτίας γνωσθείσης ὠφελεῖσθαί φησιν
ἡμᾶς ὁ Ποσειδώνιος καὶ προσέτι «τὰ διαπορούμενα», φησί, «περὶ τῆς
24 ἐκ πάθους ὁρμῆς ἐξέφηνεν.» εἶτ' αὐτὸς ἄττα ποτ' αὐτά ἐστιν ἐπιφέρων
ἐξηγεῖται τόνδε τὸν τρόπον· «οἶμαι γὰρ ὅτι πάλαι βλέπετε πῶς διὰ
454 474 λόγου μὲν πεισθέντες κακὸν /| ἑαυτοῖς παρεῖναι ἢ ἐπιφέρεσθαι οὔτε φο-
βοῦνται οὔτε λυποῦνται, φαντασίας δ' ἐκείνων αὐτῶν λαμβάνοντες.
25 πῶς γὰρ ἄν τις λόγῳ κινήσειε τὸ ἄλογον, ἐὰν μή τινα ἀναζωγράφησιν
26 προσβάληται αἰσθητῇ παραπλησίαν; οὕτως γοῦν ἐκ διηγήσεώς τινες
εἰς ἐπιθυμίαν ἐκπίπτουσιν καὶ ἐναργῶς ἐγκελευσαμένου φεύγειν τὸν
27 ἐπιφερόμενον λέοντα οὐκ ἰδόντες φοβοῦνται.» ταῦτά τε οὖν εἴρηται
καλῶς τῷ Ποσειδωνίῳ καὶ τὰ τούτων ἐφεξῆς ἔτι συμπάσας τὰς αἰτίας
ἐξηγουμένῳ τῶν ἀπορηθέντων ὑπὸ τοῦ Χρυσίππου, περὶ ὧν κατὰ
τὸ πρὸ τούτου γράμμα διῆλθον ἐπὶ τῆς τελευτῆς· ὅθεν μοι δοκῶ καὶ

1–6] Posid. fr. 161 Edelstein-Kidd 1–2] *cf. supra*, p. 328.23–25 2–6] *cf.* O. Rieth, Hermes 69 (1934), p. 41 n. 2 Reinhardt, 1953, col. 753 4–6] *cf. supra*, p. 318.12–15 6–21] Posid. fr. 168 Edelstein-Kidd 6–7] *cf. supra*, p. 328.25 14–17] Damon. fr. A 8 D.-K. 22–31] Posid. fr. 162 Edelstein-Kidd 23–24] *cf. supra*, p. 328.25–26 25–332.7] Pohlenz, 1898, pp. 627–628 Reinhardt, 1921, p. 296 31–332.4] Posid. fr. 174 Edelstein-Kidd

1 τῷ[II] *om.* L τῆς *ex* τοῖς *corr.* H 5 ζοώδους L 8 τοιοῖσδε] τοῖς τε L 10 ἀμελεῖς L 13 ᾄττοντας] -τας *ex* -τες *(?) corr.* H 14 ὑπὸ L 15 νεανί| H: νεανίαις R² 16 ἄττα H L: *corr. Kühn* δόριον H οἶδ' H L: *corr.* R 21 λογικῷ] κ *ex* στ *corr.* H εὐμαθίας H 24 ἐκ πάθους] ἐμφανοῦς L αὐτά *om.* L 27 λαμβάνονται H 28 πῶς γὰρ *in ras.* L λόγῳ] λόγος L 29 προσβάλληται L οὖν H 30 *post* ἐγκελευσαμένου *inseruerit* του *Bake* 32 σὺν πάσας H 33 ἐξηγουμένων L

the rational and divine. "And the discovery of the cause of the affec- 17
tions taught (us) the sources of distortion in what is to be sought and
avoided." Some persons mistakenly suppose that what is suitable to 18
the irrational powers of the soul is suitable without qualification; they
do not know that to experience pleasure and to rule over one's neigh-
bors are objects sought by the animal-like part of the soul, but wisdom
and all that is good and noble are objects sought by that (part) which
is rational and divine. "And", he says, "when the cause of the affec- 19
tions was recognized it distinguished the methods of training." We 20
shall prescribe for some persons a regimen of rhythms and scales and
exercises of such and such a sort, and for others another sort, as Plato
taught us. We shall rear the dull and heavy and spiritless in high-
pitched rhythms and in scales that move the soul forcibly and in
exercises of the same kind; and we shall rear those who are too high-
spirited and who rush about too madly in the opposite kind. Why was 21
it, in heaven's name – I shall address this question also to Chrysippus'
followers – that when Damon the musician came upon a flute girl
playing in the Phrygian mode to some young men who were over-
come with wine and acting madly, he told her to play in the Dorian
mode, and the youths immediately dropped their wild behavior?
Obviously they are not taught anything by the music of the flute that 22
changes the opinions of their rational faculty; but since the affective
part of the soul is irrational, they are aroused or calmed by means of
irrational motions. For the irrational is helped and harmed by irration-
al things, the rational by knowledge and ignorance.

These too, then, are benefits that Posidonius says we derive 23
from the knowledge of the cause of the affections; and in addition, he
says, "it cleared up the difficulties about the conation that arises from
affection." Then he himself goes on to explain what these difficulties 24
are, in the following way: "For I fancy that you have long observed
how men do not experience fear or distress when they have been
rationally persuaded that evil is present or is approaching, but they
do so when they get an image of those same things. For how could you 25
stir the irrational by means of reason, unless you place before it a
picture, as it were, that resembles a picture perceived by the eye?
Thus some persons fall victim to desire as a result of a verbal account, 26
and when realistically ordered to flee the charging lion, even though
they have not seen it they are afraid." Posidonius' statements here 27
are correct, and also those that follow, as he explains all the causes of
the difficulties encountered by Chrysippus, which I discussed at
the end of the preceding book. I have decided therefore to conclude

νῦν ἐνταῦθα καταπαῦσαι τὸν λόγον μίαν ἔτι τὴν ἐφεξῆς αὐτοῦ παρα-
28 γράψας ῥῆσιν ἔχουσαν ὧδε· «καὶ μὴν οἱ προκόπτοντες μεγάλα κακὰ
δοκοῦντες ἑαυτοῖς ⟨παρεῖναι⟩ οὐ λυποῦνται· φέρονται γὰρ οὐ κατὰ τὸ
ἄλογον τῆς ψυχῆς οὕτως, ἀλλὰ κατὰ τὸ λογικόν.»
455 29 Εἶτ' ἐφεξῆς οὗτος / διὰ τί τὰ χρονίζοντα [τε] τῶν παθῶν ἡσυχέστερά
τε καὶ ἀσθενέστερα γίγνεται, τὴν αἰτίαν ἀποδίδωσιν ὑπὲρ ἧς ὁ Χρύ-
475 30 σιππος ἐν | τῷ δευτέρῳ Περὶ παθῶν ἀπορεῖν ὡμολόγησεν. εἴρηται δὲ
περὶ αὐτῆς ὑφ' ἡμῶν ἐπὶ τῇ τελευτῇ τοῦ τετάρτου καὶ νῦν δ' εἰρήσεται
διὰ βραχέων οἷον ἐπιτομή τις τῆς Ποσειδωνίου ῥήσεως μακρᾶς ὑπαρ-
31 χούσης. τὸ τοίνυν παθητικὸν τῆς ψυχῆς ἐν τῷ χρόνῳ τοῦτο μὲν ἐμπίπλα-
ται τῶν οἰκείων ἐπιθυμιῶν, τοῦτο δὲ κάμνει ταῖς πολυχρονίοις κινήσεσιν,
ὥστε δι' ἄμφω καθησυχάσαντος αὐτοῦ καὶ μέτρια κινουμένου κρατεῖν
ὁ λογισμὸς ἤδη δύναται, ὥσπερ εἰ καὶ ἵππου τινὸς ἐκφόρου τὸν ἐπιβάτην
ἐξενεγκόντος βιαίως, εἶτα κάμνοντός τε ἅμα τῷ δρόμῳ καὶ προσέτι
καὶ ἐμπλησθέντος ὧν ἐπεθύμησεν αὖθις ὁ ἡνίοχος ἐγκρατὴς κατασταίη.
32 φαίνεται γὰρ τοῦτο πολλάκις γιγνόμενον καὶ οἵ γε παιδεύοντες τὰ νέα
τῶν ζῴων ἐπιτρέψαντες αὐτοῖς κάμνειν τε ἅμα καὶ ἐμπλησθῆναι κατὰ
33 τὰς ἐκφόρους κινήσεις, ὕστερον ἐπιτίθενται. περί τε οὖν τῶν τοιούτων
456 ἠπόρησεν ὁ Χρύσιππος ὡς ἂν οὐ δυνάμενος εἰς / τὸ παθητικὸν τῆς
ψυχῆς ἀναφέρειν αὐτῶν τὰς αἰτίας, καὶ προσέτι – καὶ γὰρ καὶ τοῦτο
δείκνυσιν ἐν τοῖς ἑξῆς ὁ Ποσειδώνιος –, οὐ τοῖς φαινομένοις μόνοις |
476 34 ἀλλὰ καὶ Ζήνωνι καὶ Κλεάνθει διαφέρεται. τὴν μὲν οὖν τοῦ Κλεάνθους
γνώμην ὑπὲρ τοῦ παθητικοῦ τῆς ψυχῆς ἐκ τῶνδε φαίνεσθαί φησι τῶν
ἐπῶν·

35 «Τί ποτ' ἔσθ' ὃ βούλει, θυμέ; τοῦτό μοι φράσον.
'Εγώ, λογισμέ; πᾶν ὃ βούλομαι ποιεῖν.
⩡ βασιλικόν γε· πλὴν ὅμως εἶπον πάλιν.
'Ως ἂν ἐπιθυμῶ, ταῦθ' ὅπως γενήσεται.»

36 ταυτὶ τὰ ἀμοιβαῖα Κλεάνθους φησὶν εἶναι Ποσειδώνιος ἐναργῶς
ἐνδεικνύμενα τὴν περὶ τοῦ παθητικοῦ τῆς ψυχῆς γνώμην αὐτοῦ, εἴ γε
37 δὴ πεποίηκε τὸν λογισμὸν τῷ θυμῷ διαλεγόμενον ὡς ἕτερον ἑτέρῳ. ὁ δὲ

5–31] Posid. fr. 166 Edelstein-Kidd 6–8] *cf. supra*, p. 316.14–17 10–18] Pohlenz, 1898, p. 628 *cf.* Reinhardt, 1921, p. 308 Reinhardt, 1953, col. 738 10–11] *cf. supra*, p. 288.9–10 13–14] *cf. supra*, p. 238.16–17 *infra*, PHP 495.14 Müller 18–22] Posid. test. 93 Edelstein-Kidd 22–31] SVF I, pp. 129–130 *cf.* Pohlenz, 1898, p. 629 Wilamowitz, Hermes 54 (1919), p. 68 Powell, Collectanea Alexandrina, Oxonii, 1925, p. 230 Verbeke, Kleanthes van Assos, Bruxellae, 1949, pp. 167–168 31–334.10] Posid. fr. 33 Edelstein-Kidd

3 παρεῖναι *add. Pohlenz*, παρεῖναι ἢ ἐπιφέρεσθαι *Müller* 5 οὗτος] οὕτως L τε *del. Kühn* 8 δ' *om.* H 11 πολυχρονίαις H 13 λόγος L εἰ *om.* H ἐπιβάτην] τ *ex* ν *corr.* H 19 ἠπόρει L 20 ἀναφέρεσθαι H L: *corr. Müller* καὶ[III] *om.* L 22 οὖν *om.* H τοῦ *om.* L 25 ποτε H ὃ *ex* ὅτε *corr.* H: ὅτι *Ald.* 26 'Εγώ] λέγω *Powell*: σέ γ' ὦ *v. Arnim* 27 βασιλικόν γε] ἢ βασιλικόν γε *Powell*: ναὶ βασιλικόν γε *Meineke*: βασιλικὸν εὖ γε *Scaliger*: βασιλικὸν εἶπες *v. Arnim*: βασιλικὰ μέν γε *Wilamowitz*: τυραννικόν γε *Cobet* 28 'Ως] ὧν *Corn.*: ὅσ' *Wyttenbach apud Bake* ἐπὶ θυμῶ H "*ich glaube* ..., *daß* ταῦτα ... *aus* πάντα *verdorben ist*" *Wilamowitz* 30 ἐνδεικνύμενος H L: *corr. Bake* εἴ] ἢ L

the present account now at this point, after quoting one more passage which comes next in his book and is as follows: "Indeed, persons who 28 are progressing are not distressed at the thought that they are in the presence of great evils; for they are carried to this belief not by the irrational part of the soul, but by the rational."

He next explains why it is that affections after a time become 29 quieter and weaker, a question that Chrysippus raised in the second book On the Affections and confessed he could not answer. I spoke of 30 this at the end of the fourth book; I shall now review it briefly, giving a kind of summary of the Posidonian passage, which is long. For 31 one thing, the affective part of the soul gets its fill of its own desires in the lapse of time; and for another, the affective part is wearied by motions that continue over a long period. Therefore, when for both of these reasons it has become quiet and its movements are moderate, reason is now able to take control. It is as if some runaway horse carried off the rider by force, but then as it grows weary with running and has in addition fulfilled its desire, the man who holds the reins once more establishes control. This is often observed to happen; and 32 trainers of young animals first permit them to weary themselves and take their fill of uncontrolled movement, and afterwards they take them in hand. About these matters, then, Chrysippus was per- 33 plexed, being unable to refer their causes to the affective part of the soul; and besides – Posidonius makes this point also in what follows –, he disagrees not only with observed facts but also with Zeno and Cleanthes. Cleanthes' opinion about the affective part 34 of the soul is disclosed, he says, in these lines of verse:

"What, Anger, do you wish? Pray tell me that. 35
I, Reason? To do everything I wish.
Why that is royal; yet say it once again.
That all that I desire may come to pass."

Posidonius says that this dialogue clearly reveals Cleanthes' 36 opinion about the affective part of the soul, since Cleanthes portrayed reason talking to anger as two different things. Chrysippus, however, 37

457 Χρύσιππος οὐθ' ἕτερον / εἶναι νομίζει τὸ παθητικὸν τῆς ψυχῆς τοῦ
λογιστικοῦ καὶ τῶν ἀλόγων ζῴων ἀφαιρεῖται τὰ πάθη φανερῶς ἐπιθυμίᾳ
τε καὶ θυμῷ διοικουμένων, ὡς καὶ ὁ Ποσειδώνιος ὑπὲρ αὐτῶν ἐπὶ
38 πλέον διεξέρχεται. ὅσα μὲν οὖν τῶν ζῴων δυσκίνητά τ' ἐστὶ καὶ προσ-
πεφυκότα δίκην φυτῶν πέτραις ἤ τισιν ἑτέροις τοιούτοις, ἐπιθυμίᾳ μόνῃ
διοικεῖσθαι λέγει [αὐτά], τὰ δ' ἄλλα τὰ ἄλογα σύμπαντα ταῖς δυνάμεσιν
ἀμφοτέραις χρῆσθαι, τῇ τ' ἐπιθυμητικῇ καὶ τῇ θυμοειδεῖ, τὸν ἄνθρω-
477 πον | δὲ μόνον ταῖς τρισί, προσειληφέναι γὰρ καὶ τὴν λογιστικὴν ἀρχήν.
39 ταῦτά τε οὖν ὀρθῶς εἴρηται τῷ Ποσειδωνίῳ καὶ ἄλλα πάμπολλα καθ'
ὅλην τὴν Περὶ τῶν παθῶν πραγματείαν. ὥσπερ οὖν ὁ Χρύσιππος ἐσφαλ-
μένος ἐν αὐτοῖς, ὡς ἄν τις εἴποι, τοῖς στοιχείοις τῆς περὶ τῶν παθῶν θεω-
ρίας ἐξ ἀνάγκης πάμπολλα κακῶς εἶπεν, οὕτως ἀνάγκη τὸν ἀληθέσι
ταῖς ἀρχαῖς χρησάμενον εἰ μὲν ἀκριβῶς φυλάξειε τὸ πρὸς αὐτὰς ἀκόλου-
458 θον, ἅπαν εἰπεῖν ὀρθῶς, εἰ δ' οὐκ ἀκριβῶς ἀλλὰ τά / γε πλεῖστα κατορ-
θῶσαι.

40 Δοκῶ μοι καταπαύσειν ἤδη τὸν ἐνεστῶτα λόγον ἐν τῷδε. τὸ γὰρ
ἐπισκέπτεσθαι νῦν ὁποίας τινὸς ἔχεται γνώμης ὁ Ζήνων οὐ κατὰ τὸν
41 ἐξ ἀρχῆς ἄν μοι προτεθέντα γίγνοιτο σκοπόν. ἕνεκα γὰρ τοῦ μὴ μακρο-
λογεῖν ἀποχωρήσειν μὲν ἔφην τῶν ἄλλων Στωϊκῶν, ἐξετάσειν δὲ μόνα
τὰ Χρυσίππου. καὶ γὰρ οὐδὲ τί ποτε ἕκαστος ἐγίγνωσκε τῶν
φιλοσόφων ὑπὲρ ψυχῆς ὑπεσχόμην ἐν τῇδε τῇ πραγματείᾳ διελθεῖν ἀλλ'
ὅπως ἀληθείας ἔχει τὰ Πλάτωνός τε καὶ Ἱπποκράτους δόγματα
478 42 διασκέψασθαι. ὥστε καὶ τὰ πρὸς τὸν Χρύσιππον ἀντειρημένα | μοι διὰ
τὸ προκείμενον ἐγένετο, καὶ Ζήνων, εἰ μὲν τὰ αὐτὰ βούλοιτο Χρυσίπ-
πῳ, τοῖς αὐτοῖς ἐγκλήμασιν ὑπεύθυνος καθεστήξεται, εἰ δὲ ταῖς τοῦ
Πλάτωνος ἀρχαῖς ἕποιτο Κλεάνθει τε καὶ Ποσειδωνίῳ παραπλησί-
ως, τῆς ἡμετέρας ἂν οὕτω μετέχοι φιλοσοφίας, εἰ δ', ὅπερ ἐγὼ πείθομαι,
κρίσεσιν ἐπιγίνεσθαι τὰ πάθη νομίζοι, μέσος ἂν εἴη τῆς τε χειρίστης
459 ὑπὲρ αὐτῶν αἱρέσεως τῆς Χρυσίππου / καὶ τῆς ἀρίστης ἣν Ἱππο-
43 κράτης τε καὶ Πλάτων ἁπάντων πρῶτοι μετεχειρίσαντο. Ποσειδώνιος
δὲ καὶ Πυθαγόραν φησίν, αὐτοῦ μὲν τοῦ Πυθαγόρου συγγράμματος
οὐδενὸς εἰς ἡμᾶς διασῳζομένου τεκμαιρόμενος δ' ἐξ ὧν ἔνιοι τῶν μαθητῶν
αὐτοῦ γεγράφασιν. ἀλλ' ὅπερ εἶπον ὀλίγον ἔμπροσθεν, οὐχ ἱστορίαν
δογμάτων παλαιῶν ὁ λόγος διδάξειν ἐπηγγείλατο μόνα δὲ τὰ πρὸς

4–8] *cf.* Pohlenz, 1898, pp. 568–569; 619 n. 7 Pohlenz, Die Stoa I, p. 227; II p. 114 Reinhardt, 1921, p. 309 Reinhardt, 1953, col. 777 Nemes. De nat. hom. 1: pp. 41.3–43.6 Matth. Jaeger, Nemesios, p. 116 23–33] Posid. test. 91 Edelstein-Kidd fr. 151 Edelstein-Kidd 28] *cf. supra*, pp. 238.21; 240.7–8; 292.19–20 30–33] *cf. supra*, p. 290.2–4 Pohlenz, 1898, p. 629 Reinhardt, 1953, col. 768 Pythag. fr. 18 D.-K.

1 οὐθ' ἕτερον] οὐδέτερον L 3 ὁ *om.* H 4 δυσκίνητά τ'] δυσκίνητ' H 6 λέγων H L: *corr. Ald.* αὐτά *del. Petersen* τὰ^{II} *del. Müller* 8 γὰρ] μὲν L 9 τε *om.* L πάμπολα H 10 ἐσφαλμένως L 12 πάμπολα H 13 αὐτὸ L 17 νῦν] με L 18 προστεθέντα H γίγνοιτο *in ras.* H ἕνεκα] ἐνταῦθα L 19 ἔφη L ἐξετάζειν H 20–21 τῶν φιλοσόφων ἐγίγνωσκεν L 23 διὰ] παρὰ *Ricci* 24 βούλοι τῷ H 27 ὑμετέρας L 28 νομίζει H 29 τῆς^{I} *ex* τοῦ *corr.* L

does not believe that the affective part of the soul is other than the rational, and he denies affections to the irrational animals, although they are obviously ruled by desire and anger, as Posidonius also explains more fully in his discussion of them. All animals, he says, that 38
are not easily moved and are attached like plants to rocks or the like are ruled by desire alone; all other irrational animals make use of both powers, the desiderative and the spirited; and only man employs three, for he has acquired a rational principle also. Posidonius was correct 39
in what he said about this and about much else in the whole of his treatise On the Affections. Just as Chrysippus, then, who erred in the very elements, one might say, of the theory about the affections, was necessarily mistaken on many points, so a person who has employed true principles, if he observes carefully what follows from them, would necessarily give an entirely correct account; and if he does not observe carefully, he would at least be correct in most things.

I have decided to end the present discussion at this point. An 40
investigation at this time into Zeno's position would not be in accord with the goal I set for myself at the start. For in order to avoid ex- 41
cessive length I said I would pass over the other Stoics and examine only Chrysippus' doctrines. I did not promise to review in this work the opinion of every philosopher on the soul, but only to inquire whether the teachings of Plato and Hippocrates are true. Therefore 42
I gave a refutation of Chrysippus, because my plan demanded it. As for Zeno, if the position he took was the same as that of Chrysippus, he will be liable to the same criticisms; if he followed Platonic principles, as Cleanthes and Posidonius did, he would accordingly be a partner in our philosophy; but if, as I believe, he thought that affections supervene on judgments, he would be intermediate between the worst view of the matter – that of Chrysippus – and the best view, which Hippocrates and Plato were the very first to expound. Posidonius says that Pythagoras also held this view; he 43
infers this from the writings of some of Pythagoras' pupils, as no work of Pythagoras himself has been preserved up to our time. But as I said just now, my account did not claim that it would record the history of ancient doctrines, but only that it would investigate what

44 Ἱπποκράτους καὶ Πλάτωνος εἰρημένα διασκέψεσθαι. καί μοι τοῦτο
καθ' ὅσον οἷός τ' ἦν περαίνεται διὰ βραχυτάτων. οὐ γὰρ ὅτι πολύβιβλος
ἡ πραγματεία χρὴ σκοπεῖν ἀλλὰ τοῦτο μὲν εἰς τὸ πλῆθός τε καὶ τὸ
479 μέγεθος ὧν ἂν ἐπισκεπτώμεθα δογμάτων ἀναφέρειν, ἐξετά|ζειν δὲ καὶ
σκοπεῖν εἰ περὶ τῶν αὐτῶν ἐνεχώρει βραχύτερον εἰπεῖν ἄνευ τοῦ παρα-
λιπεῖν τι τῶν ἀναγκαίων, ὡς τοῦτό γε καὶ ἐξ αὐτῶν ὧν ἔγραψε Χρύ-
45 σιππος Περὶ παθῶν ἔνεστι καταμαθεῖν. τεττάρων γὰρ βιβλίων οὕτω
μεγάλων αὐτῷ γεγραμμένων ὥσθ' ἕκαστον εἶναι διπλάσιον τῶν ἡμετέ-
460 ρων, ὅμως ἡμεῖς / οὐδ' ἐν ὅλοις δύο τὴν περὶ τῶν παθῶν αὐτοῦ γνώμην
ἐξητάκαμεν εὐθὺς καὶ τῶν τῷ Ποσειδωνίῳ γραφέντων εἰς τὴν αὐτὴν
46 πραγματείαν ἐπιμνησθέντες. ἡ μὲν δὴ πρὸς Χρύσιππον ἀντιλογία
τέλος ἐχέτω. νομίζω γὰρ εἰ μέν τις προσέσχε τὸν νοῦν τοῖς εἰρημένοις οὐκ
ἂν χαλεπῶς αὐτὸν ἐξευρεῖν ὅσα κατὰ μέρος ἐν ὅλῃ τῇ πραγματείᾳ
διημάρτηται, εἰ δέ τις οὐ προσέσχε τούτοις, οὐδ' ἂν ἔτι πλείω γράφηται,
προσέξει.

7. Μεταβήσομαι δ' ἤδη πρὸς τὴν ὑπὸ Πλάτωνος εἰρημένην
ἐπίδειξιν ἐν τῷ τετάρτῳ τῆς Πολιτείας ὑπὲρ τοῦ τρία τῆς ψυχῆς εἶναι
2 μόρια τὰ καθ' ὁρμὴν ἡμᾶς κινοῦντα. γινώσκειν δὲ χρὴ κἀνταῦθα τὸ μὲν
ὅτι μόρια διαφέροντ' ἀλλήλων ἐστίν, οὐκ ἀναγκαστικῶς ἀποδεικνύμε-
480 νον· | οὐδὲ γὰρ μᾶλλον τρεῖς εἶναι δυνάμεις ἢ τρία μόρια δείκνυσιν ὁ
λόγος· ὅτι μέν⟨τοι⟩ γε τρία τὰ σύμπαντ' ἐστὶν εἴτε μόρια ψυχῆς εἴτε /
461 δυνάμεις ὑφ' ὧν ὁ βίος ἡμῶν διοικεῖται, βιαστικῶς τε καὶ ἀναντιρρήτως
3 ἀποδείκνυται. ὥστε καὶ ἐκ τῶν νῦν λεχθησομένων ἡ μὲν τοῦ Χρυσίππου
διαβληθήσεται δόξα κατασκευασθήσεται δὲ τὸ κοινὸν Ἀριστοτέλει
καὶ Πλάτωνι καὶ Ποσειδωνίῳ δόγμα, τὸ καθ' ἑτέραν μὲν ἡμᾶς δύνα-
4 μιν λογίζεσθαι, καθ' ἑτέραν δὲ θυμοῦσθαι, κατ' ἄλλην δ' ἐπιθυμεῖν. ὅτι
μέντοι καὶ ταῖς οὐσίαις ἀλλήλων ταῦτα διαφέρει καὶ πολὺ μᾶλλον ὅτι κατὰ
διαφέροντας ἵδρυται τόπους ἐκ μὲν τῶν νῦν λεχθησομένων ἐπιστημο-
νικὴν ἀπόδειξιν οὐκ ἔνεστι λαβεῖν· ἐν δὲ τῷ μετὰ ταῦθ' ὑπομνήματι
γραφησομένῳ μοι, τῆς ὅλης πραγματείας ἕκτῳ γενήσεσθαι μέλλοντι,
δι' ἐναργῶν λημμάτων ἀποδειχθήσεται κατὰ τὰς Ἱπποκράτους τε
καὶ Πλάτωνος μεθόδους.

5 Ἰστέον δ' ὅτι καὶ ὁ Πλάτων αὐτὸς ἐπίσταται τὴν δύναμιν τῶν λε-
χθησομένων ἀποδείξεων. ἄρχεσθαι γοῦν αὐτῶν μέλλων τάδε προὔγραψε·

6–10] SVF III, p. 111 6–8] *cf. supra*, p. 238.4–6 7–11] Posid. test. 63 Edelstein-Kidd 24–26] Posid. fr. 143 Edelstein-Kidd

1 διασκέψασθαι H L: *corr. Kühn* 2 οἷον τ' ἦν *Ald.*: οἷόν τέ ἐστι *Müller* 3 τὸ^II *om.* L 4 ἂν *om.* L ἐπισκεπτόμεθα H L: *corr. Chart.* δὲ] τὲ H L: *corr. Müller* 6 τούτω L ἔγ(ραψε) L: ἔγραφε *v. Arnim* 9 ἡμεῖς] ει *ex* ι *(?)* *corr.* H γνῶσιν L 10 ἐξητάκημεν H τῶν *om.* L 13 χαλεπὸν L 17 ἀπόδειξιν *(e corr.)* F 20 οὐδὲ] οὐδὲν *Ald.* τρεῖς – μόρια] τρία μόρια ἢ τρεῖς εἶναι δυνάμεις F 21 μέντοι] μέν H L: *suppl.* F τρία τὰ] τρία μόρια H: τρία μόνα *Al. Just.* 22 ἀναντιρρητικῶς *ex* ἀντιρρητικῶς *mut.* L 23 μὲν *e corr.* H 26 ὅτι] ἔτι L 33 ὁ *om.* L 34 προὔγραψεν L

was said by Hippocrates and Plato. And this is being accomplished 44
to the best of my ability in the briefest possible form. One ought not
look at the fact that the treatise fills many books, but credit this to the
number and magnitude of the doctrines I am examining, and look
into the matter and consider whether it would have been possible to
speak more briefly of these same things without omitting some essen-
tial point. The answer may be got even from the very treatise of
Chrysippus On the Affections: he wrote four books, so long that 45
each of them is double the length of mine; yet we took not quite two
full (books) to examine directly his view of the affections, and we have
also mentioned the comments that Posidonius made on that same
treatise. So let there be an end to our refutation of Chrysippus. I 46
believe that anyone who has listened attentively to my remarks would
have no difficulty in discovering by himself the particular errors in the
whole treatise; and if he has not listened attentively, he will not do so
even if I should write still more.

7. I shall now pass to Plato's proof in the fourth (book) of the
Republic that the parts of the soul that move us by conation are three
in number. Here again one must acknowledge that he does not give a 2
necessary proof that they are parts, each differing from the others, for
the argument is no more a proof that the three are powers than that
they are parts. But that they are three in all, whether parts of the soul
or powers, by which our life is controlled, this he proves cogently and
irrefutably. Therefore the things we are about to say will overthrow 3
the Chrysippean view and will establish the doctrine common to
Aristotle, Plato, and Posidonius, that by one power we reason,
by another we are angry, and by a third we desire. That they differ 4
also in their substances, and even more that they are stationed in
different places, cannot be scientifically demonstrated from the
statements now to be made; but in the next book, which will be the
sixth of the entire treatise, these things will be demonstrated from
evident premises, in accord with the methods of Hippocrates and
Plato.

It must be recognized that Plato himself understood the force of 5
the proofs here to be presented. Thus as he was about to enter upon

481 6 «καὶ εὖ γ' ἴσθι, ὦ Γλαύκων, | ὡς ἡ ἐμὴ δόξα ἀκριβῶς μὲν τοῦτο
462 ἐκ τοιούτων / μεθόδων οἵαις δὴ νῦν ἐν τοῖς λόγοις χρώμεθα, οὐ μή ποτε
7 λάβωμεν· ἄλλη γὰρ μακροτέρα καὶ πλείων ὁδός» ἐστι, δι' ἧς ἀποδείκνυται
τρία τῆς ψυχῆς ἡμῶν εἶναι τὰ μέρη οὐ μόνον τοῖς τόποις τοῦ σώματος,
ἀλλὰ καὶ ταῖς οὐσίαις καὶ ταῖς δυνάμεσι καὶ ταῖς ἐνεργείαις διαφέροντα,
ὡς κατὰ τὸν ἑξῆς λόγον ἐπιδείξω, καθ' ὃν καὶ τὴν μέθοδον αὐτὴν ἣν
8 ἐνταῦθ' αἰνίττεται μέλλω διεξέρχεσθαι. διὰ τί δὲ καίτοι μὴ θαρρῶν ᾗ
μέλλει λέγειν ἀποδείξει, ὅμως χρῆται, πρόδηλον ὑπάρχειν οἶμαι τῷ γε
προσεσχηκότι τὸν νοῦν οἷς [δὲ] ἀρτίως ἐλέγομεν, ὡς ὅτι μὲν τρεῖς εἰσιν αἱ
διοικοῦσαι τὸν βίον ἡμῶν δυνάμεις ἐναργῶς ἀποδείκνυται, μὴ μέντοι τὸ
9 ὅτι διαφέρουσαι ταῖς οὐσίαις. πρὸς δὲ τὴν προκειμένην αὐτῷ πραγματείαν
ἐν τῇ Πολιτείᾳ, τὴν περὶ δικαιοσύνης τε καὶ τῶν ἄλλων ἀρετῶν, ὑπὲρ
463 ἁπασῶν γὰρ ἐν τοῖς ἑξῆς ποιεῖται τὸν λόγον, ἤρκει τὸ / δειχθῆναι τρεῖς
10 εἶναι δυνάμεις ἑτερογενεῖς. οὕτω γοῦν καὶ ὁ Ποσειδώνιος ὑπολαβὼν
482 ἀπεχώρησέ τε τοῦ Χρυσίππου καὶ μᾶλλον ἠκολούθησεν | Ἀριστοτέ-
λει καὶ Πλάτωνι. προσέθηκα δὲ τῷ λόγῳ τὸ μᾶλλον ἐπειδὴ κατὰ μέρος
εὑρίσκονταί τινα διαφωνοῦντες οἱ τρεῖς ἄνδρες ὑπὲρ τῆς τῶν ἀρετῶν
11 διαφορᾶς, κατὰ δὲ τὸ σύμπαν ὁμολογοῦσιν ἀλλήλοις. ἐπιδείξω δὲ καὶ
αὐτὸ τοῦτο σαφῶς ἡνίκ' ἂν ἐν τοῖς ἔπειτα τὸν ὑπὲρ τῶν ἀρετῶν διεξέρχω-
μαι λόγον· ἐν δὲ τῷ παρόντι τῶν ἐν τῷ τετάρτῳ τῆς Πολιτείας ὑπὸ
τοῦ Πλάτωνος εἰρημένων ἀποδείξεων ἤδη μνημονεύσω προγράψας
12 τὴν ῥῆσιν ἀφ' ἧς ἄρχεται τοῦ λόγου· ἔχει δὲ ὧδε· «ταὐτὸν δηλονότι
τἀναντία ποιεῖν ἢ πάσχειν [ἢ] κατὰ ταὐτόν τε καὶ πρὸς ταὐτὸν οὐκ
13 ἐθελήσει ἅμα.» εἶθ' ἑξῆς πιστωσάμενός τε τοῦτο καὶ περὶ τῶν δοκούντων
464 μάχεσθαι διελθὼν ἐπιφέρει «ἆρ' οὖν, ἦν δ' ἐγώ, / τὸ ἐπινεύειν τῷ ἀνα-
νεύειν καὶ τὸ ἐφίεσθαί τινος λαβεῖν τῷ ἀπαρνεῖσθαι καὶ τὸ προσάγεσθαι
τῷ ἀπωθεῖσθαι, πάντα τὰ τοιαῦτα τῶν ἐναντίων ἀλλήλοις θείης εἴτε
ποιημάτων εἴτε παθημάτων; οὐδὲν γὰρ ταύτῃ διοίσει. – ἀλλ', ἦ δ' ὅς,
14 τῶν ἐναντίων. – τί οὖν, ἦν δ' ἐγώ, διψῆν καὶ πεινῆν καὶ ὅλως τὰς ἐπιθυ-
μίας καὶ αὖ τὸ ἐθέλειν καὶ τὸ βούλεσθαι, οὐ ταῦτα πάντα εἰς ἐκεῖνά ποι ἂν
483 θείης τὰ | εἴδη τὰ νῦν λεχθέντα; οἷον ἀεὶ τὴν τοῦ ἐπιθυμοῦντος ψυχὴν

1–3] Plat. Resp. iv: 435 c 9 – d 3 11–18] Posid. test. 96 Edelstein-Kidd 11–16] Posid. fr. 144 Edelstein-Kidd 14–18] Posid. fr. 183 Edelstein-Kidd 14–16] *cf.* Pohlenz, 1898, pp. 569; 572 22–24] Plat. Resp. iv: 436 b 8–9 *cf. infra*, PHP 818.13–14 Müller 25–340.6] Plat. Resp. iv: 437 b 1 – d 1 25–28] *cf. infra*, PHP 498.4–8 Müller 29–340.6] *cf. infra*, PHP 498.9–499.4 Müller

1 γ' *cum Plat.* L: *om.* H ··μὲν *supra lin. add.* L² τοῦτο *om.* L 2 οἵαις] αἷς H: οἷα L: *ex Plat. corr. Chart.* 3 πλείω H 4 τρία (ω supra lin.) L 6 ὡς *om.* L καθὸ L 7 ᾗ *om.* L 8 μέλλοι L 9 οἷς] ὡς L δὲ *del. Müller*: δὴ *Corn.* ἔλε-γον L εἰσιν αἱ] εἰσὶ H 11 ὅτι] τί L *(cf. Pohlenz, 1898, p. 569 n. 4)* αὐτῶν H L: *corr.* F 12 τὴν περὶ] τῇ περὶ τῆς L τε *om.* L 13 ἤρκει τὸ] ἠρκεῖτο δὴ L 15 τοῦ τε L 16 τὸ *om.* L 18 κατὰ δὲ] καὶ L 19 ὑπὲρ] περὶ L διεξέρ(χται supra lin.) L 21 προσγράψας L 22 *post* ὧδε *add.* ἠδί L 23 ἢ[II] *sec. Plat. del. Corn.* τε] γε *ex Plat. Corn.* 25 ἦν δ'] οἶδ' L 28 οὐδὲ L ταῦ-τα L ἦ δ' ὅς] ἡ ὁδὸς L 29 ἦν] ἢ L πεινῆν] ει *ex* ι *corr.* H 30 *post* πάντα *add.* τὰ L 31 εἴδη] ἤδη L τὰ[II] *om.* L

them, he first wrote the following words: "Be assured, dear Glaucon, 6
that in my opinion we shall never get a precise understanding of the
matter from the kind of methods we are now using in our discussion.
Another longer and fuller way" exists which leads to the demonstration 7
that there are three parts of the soul, differing not only in their
location in the body, but also in their substances, powers, and activi-
ties, as I shall show in the next book, where I shall also recount the
actual way at which he is here hinting. Why he uses this proof, even 8
though he does not have full confidence in it, is clear, I believe, to
anyone who has been attentive to what we said just now: the argument
clearly proves that the powers controlling our life are three, but not
that they differ in their substances. For Plato's purpose in the 9
Republic, where the concern is with justice and the other virtues, all
of which he subsequently discusses, it was sufficient to prove that
there are three powers different in kind. Thus Posidonius, who also 10
saw the matter in this light, parted company with Chrysippus and
followed Aristotle and Plato to a greater extent. I have added the
qualification 'to a greater extent', since on particular points the three
men are found to have some disagreements about the difference in the
virtues, but on the whole they agree. I shall also clarify this point 11
later on, when I give my detailed account of the virtues. In the present
(book) I shall now proceed with my account of the proofs that Plato
gives in the fourth book of the Republic; I shall first quote the passage
with which he begins the argument. It is as follows: "Obviously the 12
same thing will not consent to do or undergo opposite things at the
same time in the same respect and in relation to the same object."
Then, after having confirmed this and examined things apparently 13
inconsistent with it, he continues, "Well then, I said, what about
assent as against dissent, seeking to obtain a thing as against refusing
it, and drawing it to oneself as against pushing it away? Would you
not put all such things in the class of opposites to each other, whether
they are things we do or things done to us? For that will make no
difference. – Yes, he said, in the class of opposites. – Then, said I, 14
what about thirst and hunger and the desires generally, and also con-
senting and wishing? Would you not assign them all to one or another
of those classes just now mentioned? For example, would you not say
that in every case the soul of the person who desires a thing either

οὐχὶ ἤτοι ἐφίεσθαι φήσεις ἐκείνου οὗ ἂν ἐπιθυμῇ, ἢ προσάγεσθαι τοῦτο
ὃ ἂν βούληταί οἱ γενέσθαι, ἢ αὖ οὐ καθ' ὅσον ἐθέλει τί οἱ πορισθῆναι,
ἐπινεύειν τοῦτο πρὸς αὑτὴν ὥσπερ τινὸς ἐρωτῶντος ἐπορεγομένην
15 αὐτοῦ τῆς γενέσεως; — ἔγωγε. — τί δέ; τὸ ἀβουλεῖν καὶ μὴ ἐθέλειν μηδ'
465 ἐπιθυμεῖν οὐκ εἰς τὸ ἀπωθεῖν καὶ / ἀπελαύνειν ἀπ' αὐτῆς καὶ εἰς ἅπαντα
τἀναντία ἐκείνοις θήσομεν; — πῶς γὰρ οὔ;»

16 Ἐν ταύτῃ τῇ ῥήσει καὶ ταῖς ἑξῆς ἁπάσαις δείκνυσιν ἕτερον εἶναι
μέρος τῆς ψυχῆς τὸ ἐπιθυμοῦν τοῦ λογιζομένου πῶς καὶ τίνα τρόπον ἐν
μὲν τῷ πεινῆν ἐφιέμεθα πληρωθῆναι σιτίων, ἐν δὲ τῷ διψῆν πόματος.
17 ἀλλὰ παῖδες μὲν ὄντες ὁμοίως τοῖς ἀλόγοις ζῴοις ἑτοίμως ἐπὶ τὸ πληρω-
θῆναι ἐρχόμεθα μήτ' εἰ συνοίσει τοῦτο μήτ' εἰ βλάψει σκοπούμενοι· κατὰ
δὲ τὴν ἡλικίαν καὶ τὸν λογισμὸν γενόμενοι πολλάκις μὲν οὐδ' ὅλως
πίνομεν ἐπειδὰν πεισθῶμεν ὑπὸ τοῦ πόματος βλάβην ἔσεσθαι, πολλάκις
δὲ ὀλιγώτερον ἢ ὅσον ἐπιθυμοῦμεν εἰ κἀνταῦθα μέλλοι βλάψειν τὸ πλέον, |
484 ἐνίοτε δ' ὕδωρ πίνομεν οἶνον ἐπιθυμοῦντες πιεῖν ἢ σφοδρῶς ὀρεγόμενοι
18 ψυχροῦ θερμὸν προσφερόμεθα. οἱ δέ γε ἀλόγιστοι τῶν ἀνθρώπων
ὡσαύτως τοῖς βρέφεσι καὶ θηρίοις οὔτε τὸν καιρὸν ἀναμένουσιν οὔτε
19 ποσότητα καὶ ποιότητα τοῦ πόματος ἐπισκέπτονται. τὸ μὲν δὴ μὴ
466 χρῆσθαι λογισμῷ μήτε τὰ / θηρία μήτε τὰ βρέφη καὶ πρὸς τῶν περὶ τὸν
Χρύσιππον ὡμολόγηται· τὸ δὲ ὑπὸ δυνάμεώς τινος ἑτέρας παρὰ τὸν
λογισμὸν ἐπὶ τὴν ἀπόλαυσιν ὧν ἐπιθυμοῦσιν ἔρχεσθαι ποτὲ μὲν ὁμολο-
γοῦσιν, ἔστιν ὅτε δ' ἀρνοῦνται περιπλέκοντες ἄνω καὶ κάτω τοὺς
λόγους, ἐνὸν ὡς ἄνδρας ἐραστὰς ἀληθείας ἐκ προχείρου συλλογίζεσθαι
δύναμίν τινα ὑπάρχειν ἄλογον ἐπὶ τὴν τοῦ πόματος ἀπόλαυσιν ἄγουσαν
οὐ τὰ βοσκήματα μόνα καὶ τοὺς παῖδας, ἀλλὰ καὶ τοὺς βοσκήμασιν
20 ὁμοίους ἀνθρώπους. εἰς μὲν οὖν τὴν τοιαύτην ἀπόδειξιν ὁ λόγος ἡμᾶς
ἤγαγε προτέραν ἐξ ἀκολουθίας τινὸς οὐ σμικρὰ συντελοῦσαν οὐδ' αὐτὴν
ταῖς ὑπὸ τοῦ Πλάτωνος λεγομέναις.

21 Ἐπὶ δὲ τοὺς ἤδη τελείους ἄνδρας οὐ κατὰ τὴν ἡλικίαν μόνον, ἀλλὰ
485 καὶ κατὰ | τὸν λογισμὸν ἀφικόμενοι τῷ λόγῳ θεασώμεθα ἤδη τὴν ἐν
αὐτοῖς μάχην τῆς λογιστικῆς δυνάμεως πρὸς τὴν ἐπιθυμητικὴν ἔν τε νόσοις
καὶ ἄλλαις πολλαῖς περιστάσεσιν ἐν αἷς οὔπω δοκεῖ καιρὸς εἶναι προσφέ-
467 ρεσθαι πόμα τὸν διψῶντα / καὶ σιτία τὸν πεινῶντα καὶ θάλπεσθαι τὸν
ῥιγοῦντα καὶ ψύχεσθαι τὸν θαλπόμενον ἀφροδισίοις τε χρῆσθαι τὸν ἐπὶ

22–23] *cf. supra*, p. 214.25

1 φήσεις] φύσει H L: *ex Plat. corr. Corn.* ἐπιθυμεῖ H ἢ *om.* L 2 οἱ γενέσθαι] γενέσθαι μοι H: γενέσθαι L: *ex Plat. corr. Corn.* αὖ οὐ] οὐ L: αὖ *ex Plat. Corn.* ἐθέλοι L οἱ[II]] οἳ H 3 πρὸς αὑτήν H: *ex Plat. corr. Müller*: πορισθῆναι L ἐπορεγομένην] -ην *ex* -ου *corr.* H: ἐπωρεγμένην L 4 τοῦ ἀβουλεῖν H: *corr. Kühn*: τὸ ἀποβουκολεῖν L 5 ἀπ' αὐτῆς *e corr.* L 8 ἐπιθυμεῖν H *ante* πῶς *add.* καὶ *Müller* 11 ἐχόμεθα H 14 ὅσων *Müller* 18 πόματος] σώματος H L: *corr. Al. Just.* ἐπισκέπτεσθαι H L: *corr. Corn.* 19 χρήσασθαι L 21 ποτὲ μὲν ὁμολογοῦσιν *bis scr.* L 23 ἀλῆ (θ' *supra*) H: *corr.* M: ἀληθοῦς L 24 πόματος] σώματος H L: *corr. Müller* 25 μόνον L 26 εἰς] εἰ L 30 θεασόμεθα L ἐν *om.* H 31 ἐπιθυμητικὴν] αἰσθητικὴν L 32 καιρὸς εἶναι *supra lin. add.* L[2] 33 σῖτον L 34 ῥιγῶντα L

seeks the thing it desires or draws to itself the thing it wishes to possess,
or again, to the extent that it is willing that something be brought to
it, does it not assent with a nod to itself as though (in answer) to a
question, and yearn for the occurrence of the thing? – I would say so. –
And what of not wishing and not consenting or desiring? Shall we not 15
put them in the class of repelling and rejecting from oneself, and all
that is opposite to the former class? – Of course."

In this passage and in all that follows Plato shows that the part of 16
the soul which desires is other than the part which rationally deter-
mines how and in what manner we seek to be filled with food when we
are hungry, and with drink when we are thirsty. When we are children 17
we readily proceed to get filled, like irrational animals, without con-
sidering whether it will benefit or harm (us); but when we have arrived
at maturity and rationality it often happens that we do not drink at
all when we are persuaded that harm would result from the drink;
and often we drink less than we desire if here too the greater amount
would be harmful; and sometimes we drink water when our desire is
to drink wine, or we take a warm drink when we strongly crave a
cold one. Unreasoning persons, however, are like children and beasts: 18
they do not wait for the opportune time and do not consider the amount
or kind of drink. Now Chrysippus and his followers have admitted 19
that beasts and children do not employ reason; and sometimes they
admit that beasts and children proceed to the satisfaction of their
desires through the agency of some power contrary to reason, but at
other times they deny it, twisting the arguments up and down. And
yet as truth-loving men they could have readily concluded that there
is an irrational power which leads not only cattle and children but also
cattle-like men to the enjoyment of drink. Thus our account has led us 20
first to a proof such as this, a proof which by virtue of a certain logical
necessity also gives no small support to the words of Plato.

As we have now come to the consideration of men who are already 21
mature not only in years but in rationality, let us proceed to examine
in them the struggle of the rational power against the desiderative in
times of illness and in many other circumstances where the time is
not yet thought to be right for the thirsty man to take drink or the
hungry man food, for the cold man to be warmed or the warm man

22 ταῦτ' ὀργῶντα. ἡ μὲν γὰρ ἄλογος ἐν ἡμῖν δύναμις ἐφ' ἕκαστον τῶν
ἐπιθυμουμένων ἕλκει τὸν δεόμενον, ὁ δὲ λογισμὸς ἀντισπᾷ καὶ κατέχει τὴν
οὐκ ἐν καιρῷ φοράν. καὶ μάχη γε πολλάκις ἑκατέρων ἰσχυρὰ γίγνεται
πρὸς ἄλληλα φανερῶς ἐνδεικνυμένη διττὴν εἶναι φύσιν ἐν ἡμῖν τῶν στα-
23 σιαζουσῶν ἀλλήλαις δυνάμεων. εἴπερ γὰρ ἦν μία μόνη καθάπερ ἐν τοῖς
παισίν, οὐδὲν ⟨ἂν⟩ ἐκώλυεν ἀκαίρως ἡμᾶς ἀπολαύειν τῶν ἐπιθυμου-
μένων ὥσπερ γε καὶ εἰ μόνος ὁ λογισμὸς ἦν πρὸς οὐδὲν ἀνθέλκειν τε καὶ
στασιάζειν εἰθισμένος οὐδὲν ἂν ἦν πρᾶγμα διψῶντα μὴ πίνειν ἢ πεινῶντα
μὴ ἐσθίειν οὐδ' ἐγκρατὴς οὐδὲ σώφρων ἂν ὁ μὴ πίνων ὠνομάζετο καθ-
24 άπερ οὐδ' ὁ μὴ βαδίζων εἰ μὴ βούλοιτο. νυνὶ δ' ἐπεὶ διτταί τινές εἰσιν αἱ
486 τὸν ἄνθρωπον | ἐπισπώμεναι δυνάμεις, ἔστι δὲ ἄλογος ἡ τοῦ πόματος
468 ἐπιθυμοῦσα, / ἡ δὲ κατέχουσα ταύτην λογική, σωφροσύνης ἐν τῷ
25 τοιούτῳ καὶ ἐγκρατείας ἡ γένεσις. ἀλλὰ τοῦτο μὲν ἡμῖν οὐ σμικρὸν ἐν
παρέργῳ δειχθὲν εἰς τὸν περὶ τῶν ἀρετῶν λόγον μνημονευέσθω μήτ'
ἐγκράτειαν εἶναί τι μήτε σωφροσύνην ἀναιρεθείσης τῷ λόγῳ τῆς ἐπιθυ-
μητικῆς δυνάμεως.
26 Ἐπὶ δὲ τὸ προκείμενον αὖθις ἐπάνειμι, ὡς ἡ τοῦ διψῶντος μὲν μὴ
βουλομένου δὲ πίνειν ψυχὴ κατὰ μέν τινα τῶν ἑαυτῆς δυνάμεων ἢ μερῶν
ἐφίεται ποτοῦ, καθ' ἕτερον δέ τι φεύγει καὶ ἀποτρέπεται· ἑνὶ γὰρ καὶ
ταὐτῷ προσίεσθαί τι καὶ ἀπαρνεῖσθαι καὶ διώκειν καὶ φεύγειν οὐκ
27 ἐνδέχεται. εἴτε δὲ προσίεσθαι καὶ φεύγειν λέγεις εἴτε διώκειν εἴτ' ἐφίεσθαι
διαφέρει οὐδέν, ὥσπερ οὐδὲ εἰ βούλεσθαι ἢ ὀρέγεσθαι ἢ ἀντιποιεῖσθαι ἢ
28 ἀσπάζεσθαι ἢ ἐπιθυμεῖν. ἡ γὰρ τῶν τοιούτων ὀνομάτων διαίρεσις
οὐδὲν εἰς τὴν παροῦσαν σκέψιν ὀνίνησιν, ἀλλ' αὐτὸ τοὐναντίον ἄκαιρός τ'
ἐστὶ καὶ τὴν περὶ τῶν πραγμάτων ζήτησιν εἰς τὴν περὶ τῶν ὀνομάτων
469 487 29 ἀμφισβήτησιν ἀπάγει. / διὸ καὶ τεχνάζονταί τινες ἐξεπίτηδες ὑπὲρ | τοῦ
μηδὲν περανθῆναι πρὸς ἕκαστον τῶν ὀνομάτων ἐνίστασθαι· εἰ μὲν ὀρέ-
γεσθαι πόματος εἴποις τὸν διψῶντα, μὴ συγχωροῦντες ὀρέγεσθαι λέγειν·
ἀστεῖον γάρ τι τὴν ὄρεξιν εἶναι καὶ μόνου τοῦ σοφοῦ, ὑπάρχειν γοῦν
αὐτὴν ὁρμὴν λογι[στι]κὴν ἐπί τι⟨νος⟩ ὅσον χρὴ ἥδοντος· ἂν δὲ ἐπιθυμεῖν,
οὐδὲ οὕτως ὀνομάζειν συγχωροῦντες, τὸ μὲν γὰρ διψῆν οὐκ ἐν τοῖς
φαύλοις μόνον ἀλλὰ καὶ τοῖς ἀστείοις γίγνεσθαι, τὴν δ' ἐπιθυμίαν αὐτήν
τε φαύλην εἶναι καὶ μόνοις τοῖς φαύλοις ἐγγίγνεσθαι, εἶναι γὰρ ὄρεξιν

21–344.6] SVF III, pp. 107–108   29–30] *cf. supra*, pp. 238.36–37; 250.8–9, 11–12

4 *post* φανερῶς *add.* δ' L   στασιαζουσῶν] ζ *ex* σ *corr.* H   5 ἦν] ἡ (η *ex* ει *corr.*) L   6 ἂν *add. Kühn*   7 ἀνθέλκειν *et* ἀνθέλκων H: ἀνθέλκων L   8 στασιάζειν *et* στασιάζων H: στασιάζων L   9 πεινῶν L   11 τῶν ἀνθρώπων L   ἔστι δὲ] εἴη δ' L   12 ἡ δὲ] ἣ L   ταύτην λογική] ταῦτ' ἣ λογικῆς L   13 ἡ *om.* H   14 μνημονεύσω L   19 τι *om.* L   20 τι] τε *Müller*   ἀπαρνεῖσθαι – καὶ[III] *om.* H   20–21 οὐκ ἐνδέχεται] ἀδύνατον L   21 καὶ φεύγειν *om.* L   λέγοις H   22 οὐδὲν διαφέρει *Petersen*   25 πραγματειῶν L   ὀνομάτων] πραγμάτων H   26 τεχνάζοντές L   ἐξεπίτηδες *om.* L   27 ἐνίστανται L   28 συγχωροῦντα L   29 ἀστεῖον] αἴτιον H L: *corr. Hirzel (cf. infra, lin. 32)*   30 λογιστικὴν H L: *corr. Petersen*   τι H L: *correxi (cf. infra, comm. ad p. 238.36–37)*   ἥδοντος] ἤδη ὄντος L: ἦδον *Müller*   ἂν] αὐτῶν L: αὐτῷ εἰ *Müller*.   33 γίγνεσθαι L

cooled, or for sexual appetite to be indulged. The irrational power in 22
us draws the person who feels the need to each of the desired objects,
while reason pulls in the opposite direction and checks the untimely
motion. And often the conflict between the two becomes violent, thus
indicating clearly that the nature of the contending powers in us is
two-fold. If there were only one (power), as in children, nothing would 23
prevent our enjoying inopportunely the things we desire; and similarly,
if there were only the rational power, not accustomed to resist and
contend with anything, then it would be nothing for the thirsty man
not to drink, or the hungry man not to eat; and you would not call the
person who does not drink self-controlled or temperate, any more than
you would the person who does not walk if he does not wish to. But as 24
it is, since there are two powers that pull the human being, since there
is an irrational (power) that desires the drink and a rational (power)
that holds the irrational in check, in that sort of situation temperance
and self-control have their origin. But let this matter of no small 25
importance, which we have proved in passing, be remembered for our
discussion of the virtues, that there is no such thing as self-control or
temperance if the desiderative power is eliminated in our theory.

I return to the matter before us, that the soul of the person who 26
is thirsty but does not wish to drink seeks drink through one of its
powers or parts but through another flees from it and turns away;
for it is not possible that through one and the same part it should
accept and reject a thing, or pursue and avoid it. It makes no difference 27
whether you say that it accepts and avoids, or pursues, or seeks, or whether
you say it wishes, or has an appetition, or lays claim to, or welcomes
or desires. The differentiation of these terms contributes nothing to 28
the present inquiry; quite the contrary, it is untimely and it diverts
the investigation of things to a dispute about names. Some persons 29
therefore deliberately contrive to raise objections to every term, in
order that no conclusion may be reached. If you say that the thirsty
man 'has an appetition' for drink, they will not agree to the term
appetition; for appetition is something commendable and pertains
only to the sage: it is in fact a rational conation for something that
gives pleasure to the extent that it should. But if you say that he
'desires' (drink), they will not admit this word either; for thirst is
found not only among inferior men but also among the better sort,
whereas desire is itself inferior and arises only in inferior persons, for

30 ἀθρόως ῥεπτικὴν πρὸς τὸ τυγχάνειν. εἰ δέ ⟨τις⟩ μὴ μακρὸν οὕτως αὐτῆς
ὁρισμὸν ποιήσειεν ἀλλ' ὄρεξίν γε ἄλογον ὑπάρχειν εἰπών, ἐπιτιμήσει
μάλα σεμνῶς ἀνδρὶ πολλάκις οὐκ ἐν τῇ τῶν πραγμάτων ἐπιστήμῃ
31 μόνον, ἀλλὰ κἀν τῇ τῶν ὀνομάτων χρήσει μυρίον διαφέροντι. τοιοῦτοι δ'
470 ἀμέλει καὶ τῶν παλαιῶν ἦσαν οὐκ ὀλίγοι καθάπερ καὶ / αὐτὸς ὁ Πλάτων
φησίν, ὀνόμασι χρώμενοι καινῶς μετωνομασμένοις· δι' οὓς μοι δοκεῖ καὶ
488 νῦν οὐχ ἓν ἁπλῶς γράψαι κατὰ τὸν προκείμενον | λόγον ὄνομα, χρήσασθαι
32 δὲ ἐξεπίτηδες ἅπασιν οἷς ἐγχωρεῖ ταὐτὸν δηλῶσαι πρᾶγμα. τῷ τε γὰρ
ὀρέγεσθαι καὶ τῷ ἐπιθυμεῖν καὶ τῷ ἐφίεσθαι καὶ τῷ ἐπινεύειν ἐπορέγεσθαί
τε καὶ θέλειν καὶ βούλεσθαι καὶ προσάγεσθαι καὶ μέντοι καὶ τοῖς ἐναντίοις
αὐτῶν ἐπὶ τοῦ ἑνὸς πράγματος φαίνεται χρώμενος, τῷ ἀβουλεῖν καὶ μὴ
33 ἐθέλειν. ἐνδείξασθαι γὰρ αὐτῷ πρόκειται καὶ δηλῶσαι σαφῶς ὃ βούλεται,
περὶ τὴν ἀπόδειξιν ἐσπουδακότι καὶ δουλεύοντι διὰ τῆς λέξεως τῇ
μηνύσει τοῦ πράγματος, οὐ τερθρευομένῳ περὶ τὰς συλλαβάς.
34 Ἐκ μὲν δὴ τῶν προειρημένων ἕτερον ἐπέδειξε τὸ ἐπιθυμοῦν τοῦ
λογιζομένου. παραγράφειν γὰρ ἁπάσας αὐτοῦ τὰς ῥήσεις μακρὸν ἔδοξέ
μοι δυναμένου γε παντὸς τοῦ βουλομένου τὸ ἐφεξῆς ἅπαν ἀναγνῶναι τοῦ
35 βιβλίου χωρίον. εἰ δὲ καὶ τὴν ἐπὶ τῆς τελευτῆς ὅλου τοῦ λόγου δέοι
471 παραγράψαι ῥῆσιν, ὡς / ἔμοιγε δοκεῖ, χάριν τοῦ σαφεστέραν γενέσθαι
36 τὴν ἐπὶ τὸ δεύτερον κεφάλαιον μετάβασιν, οὐδὲ ταύτην παρήσω· ἔχει δ'
ὧδε· «ἆρα τοῦ διψῶντος ἡ ψυχὴ καθ' ὅσον δὴ διψῇ οὐκ ἄλλο τι βούλεται
37 ἢ πιεῖν καὶ τούτου ὀρέγεται καὶ ἐπὶ τοῦτο ὁρμᾷ; — δῆλον δή. — οὐκοῦν |
489 εἴ ποτέ τι αὐτὴν ἀνθέλκει διψῶσαν, ἕτερον ἄν τι ἐν αὐτῇ εἴη αὐτοῦ τοῦ
διψῶντος καὶ ἄγοντος ὥσπερ θηρίου ἐπὶ τὸ πιεῖν; οὐ γὰρ δή φαμεν τό
γε αὐτὸ τῷ αὐτῷ ἑαυτοῦ περὶ τὸ αὐτὸ ἅμα τἀναντία πράττειν. — οὐ γὰρ
38 οὖν. — ὥσπερ γε, οἶμαι, τοῦ τοξότου οὐ καλῶς ἔχει λέγειν ὅτι αὐτοῦ ἅμα
αἱ χεῖρες τὸ τόξον ἀπωθοῦνταί τε καὶ προσέλκονται, ἀλλ' ὅτι ἄλλη μὲν ἡ
ἀπωθοῦσα χείρ, ἑτέρα δ' ἡ προσαγομένη. — παντάπασι μὲν οὖν, ἔφη. —
πότερον δὴ φῶμέν τινας ἔστιν ὅτε διψῶντας οὐκ ἐθέλειν πιεῖν; — καὶ
472 39 μάλα / γ' ἔφη πολλοὺς καὶ πολλάκις. — τί οὖν, ἔφην ἐγώ, φαίη τις ἂν
τούτων πέρι; οὐκ ἐνεῖναι μὲν ἐν τῇ ψυχῇ αὐτῶν τὸ κελεῦον, εἶναι δὲ τὸ
κωλῦον πιεῖν ἄλλο ὄν, τὸ κρατοῦν τοῦ κελεύοντος; — ἔμοιγ' ἔφη δοκεῖ. —

5–6] Plat. Theaet. 180 a 3–6 *cf.* Brenner, Primit. Czern., p. 77 21–346.7] Plat. Resp. iv: 439 a 9 – d 8

1 εἰ δὲ H: *suppl. Müller*: εἴπερ L αὐτὴν L 2 ἀλλ' *delendum censet Einarson* γε] τε H L: *corr. Müller*: *del. v. Arnim* εἴποι *v. Arnim* ἐπιτιμῶσι *v. Arnim*: ἐπιτιμηθήσεται *Müller* 4 μυρίων H L: *corr. Einarson (cf. Plat. Theaet. 166 d 3)* 6 κενῶς L 7 χρῆσθαι L 8 ἐξεπίτηδες] καὶ ἐπίτηδες L 12 βούλεται] κοίλεται L 17 δυναμένω γε παντὶ τῶ βουλομένω H L: *corr. Petersen*: δυνάμενόν γε παντὶ τῷ βουλομένῳ *Müller* 18 ὅλου] ὁμοῦ H L: *corr. Corn.* 19 προσγράψαι L 21 ἆρα *ex* ἄρα *corr.* H δὴ *cum Plat. codd. om.* L διψεῖ H 23 τι[I]] ἐπ' L ἀνθέλκειν H 23–24 αὐτοῦ τοῦ διψῶντος] α. . . . . . .ω.τος H 24 ἄγοντος ὥσπερ] ἄ. . . . . . .σπερ H θηρίον *Ald.* ποιεῖν L δὴ φαίημεν H: *ex Plat. corr. Chart.*: διψᾷ μὲν L 25 αὐτὸ[I]] αὐτ᾽ H: αὐτ̊᾽ L: *corr. Müller* τῷ αὐτῷ] . . αὐτῶ H: *corr.* M: *om.* L πράττοι L 26 γε *om.* H 27 μὲν ἄλλη H 28 παντάπασι μὲν] παντάπασιν L 31 εἶναι] ἐνεῖναι *ex Plat. Kühn*: ἐν εἶναι *Chart.* 32 ὂν *om.* L τὸ] καὶ *ex Plat. Corn.*

desire is an appetition that moves in a rush to the attainment of its
object. If one does not define it at such length but says that it is at 30
any rate an irrational appetition, then our opponent will very solemnly
censure a man who is on many occasions vastly superior not only in
the knowledge of things but also in the use of words. Even among the 31
ancients there were no few men of that kind, as Plato himself tells
(us), who used words in strange new meanings. It was because of them,
I think, that here again he did not simply write down a single term in
the passage before us but intentionally used all the terms with which
it is possible to refer to the same thing. Thus we see that Plato uses 32
the terms 'have an appetition for', 'desire', 'seek', 'nod assent to',
'yearn for', 'be willing', 'wish', 'draw to oneself', and indeed he uses
their opposites also, 'not wish', 'be unwilling', with reference to just
one thing. For it is his aim to indicate and express clearly what he 33
wishes to say. He is intent on the proof; he uses language in the service
of conveying meaning; and he does not quibble about syllables.

Now in the passage quoted above Plato pointed out that that 34
which desires is other than that which reasons. It seemed to me tedious
to copy out all that he says, as anyone who wishes may read in its
entirety the part that comes next in his book. If it should be necessary, 35
as I think it is, to transcribe also the passage at the end of the whole
discussion in order to make a clearer transition to the second main
head, I shall not fail to do so. It is as follows: "Then the soul of the 36
thirsty man, insofar as it is thirsty, has no other wish than to drink;
it has a craving for drink, and is impelled toward it? – That is clear. –
Then if ever anything exerts a contrary pull on the thirsty soul, that 37
would be something in it other than the part which is thirsting and,
like a brute, is leading it to drink? For we would not say that the
same thing acts in opposite ways at the same time on the same object
with the same part of itself. – No indeed. – For example, it would not 38
be right, I think, to say of the archer that his hands simultaneously
push and pull the bow, but rather that one hand pushes and the
other pulls. – Quite so, he said. – Now shall we say that some thirsty
persons are sometimes unwilling to drink? – Yes, he said; many persons, and many times. – What then, I said, would one say about 39
these men? Would it not be that there is in their soul something that
commands them to drink, but that there is some other thing that
forbids it, the master of the former? – That is my opinion, he said. –

ἆρ' οὖν οὐ τὸ μὲν κωλῦον τὰ τοιαῦτα ἐγγίγνεται, ὅταν ἐγγένηται, ἐκ
τοῦ λογισμοῦ, τὰ δὲ ἄγοντα καὶ ἕλκοντα διὰ παθημάτων τε καὶ νοσημά-
40 των παραγίγνεται; — φαίνεται. — οὐ δὴ ἀλόγως, ἦν δ' ἐγώ, ἀξιώσομεν
490 αὐτὰ διττά τε καὶ ἕτερα ἀλλήλων εἶναι, τὸ | μὲν ᾧ λογίζεται λογιστικὸν
προσαγορεύοντες τῆς ψυχῆς, τὸ δ' ᾧ ἐρᾷ τε καὶ πεινῇ καὶ διψῇ καὶ περὶ
τὰς ἄλλας ἐπιθυμίας ἐπτόηται ἀλόγιστόν τε καὶ ἐπιθυμητικόν, πληρώ-
41 σεών τινων καὶ ἡδονῶν ἑταῖρον.» διὰ τούτων ἔδειξεν ἕτερον εἶδος εἶναι
42 ψυχῆς τὸ λογιστικὸν τοῦ ἐπιθυμητικοῦ. ἀλλ' ὡς εἶπον καὶ πρόσθεν,
οὔπω μοι πρόκειται δεικνύειν ὡς ἕτερα τῷ εἴδει ταυτὶ τὰ δύο μέρη τῆς
473 ψυχῆς ἐστιν, ἀλλ' εἷς / γε τὸ προκείμενον ἀπόχρη τὸ περαινόμενον ἀναμ-
φισβητήτως, ὅτι μὴ τῆς αὐτῆς ἐστι δυνάμεως τό τε λογίζεσθαι καὶ τὸ
σιτίων ἢ ποτῶν ἢ ἀφροδισίων ἐπιθυμεῖν, ὅπερ οὐκ οἶδ' ὅπως ὁ Χρύσιπ-
43 πος ἅμα πολλοῖς Στωϊκοῖς ἠγνόησεν. ἀλλὰ τὸ μὲν ἀγνοῆσαί τι
συγγνωστόν, ὡς καὶ πρόσθεν ἔλεγον, οὐ συγγνωστὸν δὲ τὸ πλημμελῶς
οὕτως μεταχειρίσασθαι τὸν λόγον ὥστε τῶν μὲν τοῖς κωμικοῖς ἢ τραγι-
κοῖς ποιηταῖς εἰρημένων μνημονεύειν εἰς τηλικούτου δόγματος ἀπόδειξιν —
ἀνθρώποις οὐδ' ἐπιχειροῦσιν ἀποδεικνύειν οὐδὲν ἀλλὰ μόνον οἷα ἂν αὐτοῖς
δόξῃ πρέπειν τῷ λέγοντι προσώπῳ κατὰ τὸ δρᾶμα, κοσμοῦσι διὰ τῆς
491 ἑρμηνείας —, | τῶν δ' ὑπὸ Πλάτωνος εἰρημένων εἰς τὴν ἀπόδειξιν αὐτοῦ
μήτε μνημονεῦσαι μήτ' ἀντειπεῖν ἐπιχειρῆσαι, ἀλλ' ἐξ ἑτοίμου τε καὶ
προχείρου λαμβάνειν ὡς ἔνθ' ἂν ᾖ τὰ πάθη τῆς ψυχῆς, ἐνταῦθ' ἐστὶ καὶ
τὸ λογιζόμενον.

44 Χρύσιππος μὲν οὖν ἀεὶ τοιοῦτος. ὁ δὲ Πλάτων ἐπειδὴ διώρισται
474 ἐν τῇ προγεγραμμένῃ ῥήσει τὸ / ἐπιθυμητικὸν τοῦ λογιστικοῦ, μετὰ
45 ταῦτα πειρᾶται καὶ τὸ θυμοειδὲς αὐτῶν διορίζειν· ἔχει δ' ἡ ἀρχὴ τῆς
ῥήσεως ὧδε· «ταῦτα μὲν τοίνυν, ἦν δ' ἐγώ, δύ' ἡμῖν ὡρίσθω εἴδη ἐν
ψυχῇ ἐνόντα· τὸ δὲ δὴ τοῦ θυμοῦ καὶ ᾧ θυμούμεθα πότερον τρίτον ἢ
τούτων ποτέρῳ εἴη ἂν ὁμοφυές; — ἴσως, ἔφη, τῷ ἑτέρῳ, τῷ ἐπιθυμητικῷ.
46 — ἀλλ', ἦν δ' ἐγώ, ποτὲ ἀκούσας τι πιστεύω τούτῳ, ὡς ἄρα Λεόντιος ὁ
Ἀγλαΐωνος ἀνιὼν ἐκ Πειραιέως ὑπὸ τὸ βόρειον τεῖχος ἐκτὸς αἰσθόμε-
νος νεκροὺς παρὰ τῷ δημίῳ κειμένους ἅμα μὲν ἰδεῖν ἐπιθυμοῖ, ἅμα δὲ
δυσχεραίνοι καὶ ἀποτρέποι ἑαυτὸν καὶ τέως μὲν μάχοιτό τε καὶ παρα-

8] *cf. supra*, p. 336.16–26 14] *v. supra*, p. 248.15 *cf. supra*, pp. 84.18; 252.7–8 19–20] *cf. supra*, p. 172.4–7 *infra*, p. 348.22–26; PHP 652.11–14 Müller 21–22] *cf. supra*, p. 292.9–10 26–348.5] Plat. Resp. iv: 439 e 2 – 440 a 7

1 οὖν οὐ τὸ] οὐκ εἰ τοῦτο L *post* κωλῦον *add.* ἐστὶ L ἐγγίγνεσθαι H 2 τοῦ *om.* L ἕλκοντα] θέλοντα L νοσημάτων τε καὶ παθημάτων L 7 ἑταῖ-ρον — ἔδειξεν *om.* L 8 λογιστικὸν] λο *ex* λι *corr.* H 9 ἑτέρα H 10 γε] τε L ἀναμφισβητήτως] ἀν *e corr.* H: ἀναμφισβήτως L 13 *post* πολλοῖς *ras. unius litt.* (τ *ut vid.*) L 15 οὕτω L τῶν] τῶ *(ex* τὸ *mut.)* H 16 μνημο-νεύειν *ex* μνημονεύων *corr.* L[2] εἰς] ἢ L 17 ἀνθρώπων . . . ἐπιχειρούντων H L: *corr. Müller* μόνον οἷα] μόνων ὧν L 18 πρέπει H κοσμούντων H L: *corr. Müller* 19 τῶν δ' *om.* L 23 διώρισεν *coni. Müller* 26 τοίνυν *inser.* H ἦν L δύ' ἡμῖν] ἡμῖν *ex* ὑμῖν *corr.* H: δὴ μὲν L εἰ δὴ L 27 δὴ *om.* L πρό-τερον L 28 τοῦτο L πρότερον L 29 τοῦτο H L: *ex Plat. corr. Corn.* 30 ἀγλαώνιος L πειρέως H: πειραιῆς, *ut vid.*, L: *corr. Chart.* 31 ἐπιθυμεῖ L

Then does not that which forbids such actions arise, when it arises,
from reasoning, while the things that draw and pull (the soul) enter
through affections and diseases? – It appears so. – Then, I said, it 40
will not be unreasonable for us to judge them to be two, each differ-
ent from the other, and to call the one by which the soul reasons
its rational part, and the one by which it loves, hungers, thirsts,
and flutters over the other desires, its irrational and desiderative part,
the companion of certain repletions and pleasures." By these (words) he 41
showed that the rational part of the soul is different in kind from the
desiderative. But as I said earlier, my aim is not yet to show that these 42
two parts of the soul are different in kind; for my present purpose
it is sufficient to conclude indisputably that it is not within the pro-
vince of the same power both to reason and to desire food or drink
or sexual pleasure, a fact that somehow escaped Chrysippus and
many Stoics. Ignorance of a thing is pardonable, as I said before; 43
but it is not pardonable to handle the argument so ineptly as to cite
as proof of so important a doctrine the words of comic and tragic
poets – men who do not try to prove anything but only adorn with
beauty of language the speeches they think appropriate to the char-
acter speaking in the play – and to fail to mention what Plato
said in proof of it, and to make no attempt to answer him, but to
assume readily and without question that where the soul's affections
are, there its rational part is also.

Now Chrysippus always behaves in this way. But Plato, 44
after distinguishing the desiderative from the rational in the passage
quoted above, next tries to distinguish also between them and the
spirited part. The passage begins as follows: "Well then, said I, let 45
us accept these as two distinct forms present in the soul. But is the
form of anger, and that by which we experience anger, a third, or
would it be of the same nature as one of the other two? – Perhaps,
he said, the same as one of the others, the desiderative. – But, I said, 46
I accept as trustworthy a story I once heard, that when Leontius,
son of Aglaion, was coming up from the Peiraeus outside the north
wall and became aware of corpses lying by the place of public execu-
tion, he desired to look at them, yet at the same time was repelled
and turned away; for a time he resisted and covered his head, but

καλύπτοιτο, κρατούμενος δ' οὖν ὑπὸ τῆς ἐπιθυμίας διελκύσας τοὺς
492 ὀφθαλμοὺς προσδραμὼν πρὸς τοὺς | νεκρούς, 'Ἰδοὺ ὑμῖν' ἔφη 'ὦ κακοδαί-
μονες, ἐμπλήσθητε τοῦ καλοῦ θεάματος'. — ἤκουσα, ἔφη, καὶ αὐτός. —
475 47 οὗτος μέντοι, ἔφην, ὁ / λόγος σημαίνει τὴν ὀργὴν πολεμεῖν ἐνίοτε ταῖς
48 ἐπιθυμίαις ὡς ἄλλο ὂν ἄλλῳ. — σημαίνει γε, ἔφη.» πάλιν κἀν τούτοις ὁ
Πλάτων ἐπιδείκνυσιν ὡς ἕτερόν ἐστι τὸ ἐπιθυμητικὸν τοῦ ὀργιζομένου,
προσχρώμενος δηλονότι τῷ κατ' ἀρχὰς ὑποκειμένῳ ἀξιώματι ὡς οὐκ
ἐνδέχεται τὸ ἀκριβῶς ἓν καὶ ἁπλοῦν καὶ ἀσύνθετον ὀρέγεσθαί τινος καὶ
ἀποτρέπεσθαι καὶ χαίρειν τῷ αὐτῷ καὶ δυσχεραίνειν ἀλλ' ἀναγκαῖον ἕτερον
μὲν τὸ ἐπιθυμοῦν θεάσασθαι τοὺς νεκρούς, ἕτερον δὲ τὸ κωλῦον θεάσασθαι,
καὶ ὡς τῷ μὲν ἐπιθυμοῦντι πάντως πού τις ἡδονὴ κατὰ τὴν θέαν ἤμελλεν
49 ἔσεσθαι, τῷ δὲ κωλύοντι δυσχέρειά τε καὶ ἀνία. τὸ γὰρ ὀργίζεσθαι τῷ
ἐπιθυμοῦντι καὶ δυσχεραίνειν αὐτοῦ ταῖς ὁρμαῖς καὶ κωλύειν ἐθέλειν τε
ταῖς ἐπιθυμίαις ἐπιτιμᾶν τε καὶ μέμφεσθαι καὶ πάνθ' ὅσα τοιαῦτα μέρους
476 ἑτέρου τῆς ψυχῆς ἔργον ἐστίν, οὐκ αὐτοῦ τοῦ ἐπιθυ/μοῦντος· εἰ δὲ καὶ
50 μὴ μέρους ἀλλὰ δυνάμεώς γε πάντως ἑτέρας. εἴρηται γὰρ ἤδη γε τοῦτο
493 πολλάκις, | ὡς οὐδέπω κατὰ τόδε τὸ βιβλίον ἀγωνιζόμεθα πρὸς Ἀρι-
στοτέλην καὶ Ποσειδώνιον ὁμολογοῦντας μὲν ἑτέροις ἀλλήλων
λογίζεσθαί τε καὶ θυμοῦσθαι καὶ ἐπιθυμεῖν ἡμᾶς, οὐ μὴν εἴδεσί γε ἢ
μορίοις ψυχῆς ἀλλὰ δυνάμεσιν· ἐν γὰρ τοῖς ἐφεξῆς λόγοις ἐπιδείξομεν
ὅτι μὴ δυνάμεσι μόνον, ἀλλὰ καὶ μέρεσι τῆς ψυχῆς ἑτέροις ἀλλήλων κατ'
51 εἶδος. ἐν δὲ τῷδε τῷ νῦν ἐνεστῶτι τοῦτ' ἀρκεῖ μόνον ἀποδεῖξαι πρὸς
ἔνδειξιν τῆς Χρυσίππου περὶ τὰ τοιαῦτα ῥᾳθυμίας, ὡς αὐτὸς ἰσχυρῶν
λόγων ὑπὸ Πλάτωνος ἠρωτημένων εἰς ἀπόδειξιν τοῦ νῦν ἡμῖν ζητου-
μένου δόγματος οὔτ' ἐμνήσθη τινὸς αὐτῶν οὔτ' ἀντειπεῖν ἐπεχείρησε,
καίτοι πληρώσας λόγων μακρῶν, μᾶλλον δὲ ποιητικῶν ἐπῶν, ὅλον τὸ
52 πρῶτον βιβλίον Περὶ ψυχῆς, ἐν ᾧ περὶ ἡγεμονικοῦ διεξῆλθεν. οὐ μόνον
477 δὲ κατὰ τοῦτο / τελέως ἐσιώπησε τοὺς τοῦ Πλάτωνος λόγους ἀλλὰ καὶ
κατὰ τὰ Περὶ παθῶν συγγράμματα, τά τε τρία τὰ λογικὰ καὶ τὸ χωρὶς
αὐτῶν ἰδίᾳ γεγραμμένον ὑπ' αὐτοῦ, τὸ Θεραπευτικόν τε καὶ Ἠθικὸν
ἐπιγραφόμενον.

7–10] *cf. supra*, pp. 338.22–24; 342.14–21 16–20] Posid. fr. 145 Edelstein-Kidd *cf. supra*, pp. 312.29–34; 346.8–13 *infra*, PHP 501.10–11 Müller 23–26] *cf. supra*, pp. 172.4–7; 346.19–20 26–27] *cf. supra*, pp. 174.27–28; 178.3–4; 194.31–34 28–31] SVF III, p. 113 *cf. supra*, p. 238.4–7

1 οὖν] αὖ M *Ald.* 4 οὕτως L σημαίνει] χαλεπαίνειν H ἐνίοτε πολεμεῖν L 5 ἄλλο ὂν ἄλλῳ] ἄλλον ἄλλως L σημαίνει τὲ H: σημαίνηται L: *corr. Einarson*: σημαίνει γὰρ *ex Plat. Corn.* 7 προσχρώμενον L δηλονότι] δηλῶν οὐ L_{μ}, οὐκ] οὖν L 13 καὶ[II] *ex* κω *(?) corr.* H κωλύειν] κελεύειν L 14 τὰς ἐπιθυ L 15 οὐκ] οὐ κατ' L 16 γε[I]] τε L τοῦτο γε L 17 οὐδέποτε H 19 ἢ *om.* L 22 τῷδε *om.* L τοῦτο L 23 ὡς αὐτὸς] ὡσαύτως L 25 αὐτὸς L 26 πληρῶσαι L 29 κατὰ *om.* L *ante* παθῶν *add.* τῶν L τὸ] τὰ H L: *corr. Müller* 30 αὐτῶν] αἰτιῶν H καὶ ἰδία L γεγραμμένα H L: *corr. Müller*

being overcome none the less by the desire, he opened his eyes wide
and ran over to the corpses and said, 'Look, you wretches; take your
fill of the beautiful sight'. – I too have heard it, he said. – This story, 47
I said, indicates that anger sometimes fights against the desires, as
one thing against another. – Yes, it does, he said." Again in this 48
passage Plato shows that that which desires is other than that which
is angered, obviously using as a premise the initial postulate, that a
thing that is strictly one, single, and uncompounded cannot have an
appetition for something and also reject it, or be pleased and displeased
by the same object; there must be one thing that desires to see the
corpses, another that tries to prevent it. And he shows that the sight
would surely give a certain pleasure to the part that desires it, but
displeasure and distress to the part that opposes. For to be angry 49
with the part that desires, displeased at its conations and opposed
to them, to be willing to reprove and censure the desires, and all
things of this kind, are the act of another part of the soul, not that
which has the desire – or if not of another part, at any rate of another
power. I have already stated repeatedly that in this book I am not yet 50
challenging Aristotle and Posidonius, who agree that reasoning,
being angry, and desiring are effected in us by agencies that differ
from one another, yet who say that these agencies are powers, not
forms or parts, of the soul. In subsequent books I shall show that they
are not powers only, but also parts of the soul that differ from each
other in form. In the present book, in order to indicate Chrysippus' 51
carelessness in such matters, it is enough merely to demonstrate that
he did not mention any of the strong arguments formulated by Plato
for the proof of the doctrine we are now investigating, nor did he try
to answer them, although he filled the whole of his first book On the
Soul, in which he discussed the ruling part, with lengthy discourses,
or rather, with verses from the poets. Not only in this (book) was he 52
completely silent about Plato's arguments, but also in his writings
On the Affections, both the three (books) of theory and the separate
(book) that he wrote entitled Therapy and Ethics.

53 Ἐπὶ τὰς ὑπολοίπους οὖν τοῦ Πλάτωνος ῥήσεις ἴωμεν ἐχούσας
494 ὧδε· | «οὐκοῦν καὶ ἄλλοθι, ἔφη⟨ν⟩, πολλαχοῦ αἰσθανόμεθα ὅταν βιά-
ζωνταί τινα παρὰ τὸν λογισμὸν ἐπιθυμίαι, λοιδοροῦντά τε αὑτὸν καὶ
θυμούμενον τῷ βιαζομένῳ ἐν αὑτῷ καὶ ὥσπερ δυοῖν στασιαζόντοιν
54 σύμμαχον τῷ λόγῳ γιγνόμενον τὸν θυμὸν τοῦ τοιούτου; ταῖς δ' ἐπιθυ-
μίαις αὐτὸν κοινωνήσαντα αἱροῦντος λόγου μὴ δεῖν τι πράττειν οἶμαί σε
οὐκ ἂν φάναι γενομένου ποτ' ἐν ἑαυτῷ τοιούτου αἰσθέσθαι, οἶμαι δ' οὐδ'
478 55 ἐν ἄλλῳ. – οὐ μὰ τὸν Δία, ἔφη.» κατὰ μὲν οὖν τὴν προτέραν ῥῆσιν / ὁ
Πλάτων ἐν ᾗ τοῦ ποθοῦντος θεάσασθαι τοὺς νεκροὺς ἐμνημόνευσεν,
ἐναργῶς μὲν ἀπέδειξεν ἕτερον ὑπάρχειν τὸ θυμούμενον τοῦ ἐπιθυμοῦντος,
οὐ μὴν ὅτι τὸ λογιζόμενον ἕτερον ἀμφοῖν ἐστιν ἐναργῶς εἶπεν, ἀλλ'
ἐνεδείξατο καὶ κατ' ἐκεῖνον μέν πως τὸν λόγον, ἐνταυθοῖ δ' ἱκανῶς ἐπ-
56 εξέρχεται. ὅταν γάρ τινα βιάζηταί τις ἐπιθυμία παρὰ τὸν λογισμόν,
ὥσπερ τὸν ἔμπροσθεν εἰρημένον Λεόντιον, ὁ θυμὸς ἐνταῦθα κινεῖται
συμμαχῶν τῷ λογισμῷ καὶ πολλάκις μὲν ἐκράτησεν ἅμα τῷ λογισμῷ τῆς
495 ἀμέτρου κινήσεως τοῦ ἀκολάστου τῆς ψυχῆς εἴδους καὶ | κατέσχε τε καὶ
διεκώλυσεν αὐτὸ καὶ τῆς ὁρμῆς ἐπέσχεν, ὥσπερ οὖν καὶ ὁ Λεόντιος
ἐδυνήθη λοιδορηθεὶς ἑαυτῷ τῆς περὶ τὸ θεάσασθαι τοὺς νεκροὺς ἀκρασίας
παρελθεῖν μὴ θεασάμενος αὐτούς, ἐνίοτε δ' ἀμφοτέρων τῶν μερῶν τῆς
ψυχῆς ἀγχόντων τε καὶ λοιδορουμένων ἀντιπραττόντων τε καὶ ἀνθελ-
κόντων ἐκράτησε τὸ ἐπιθυμητικόν, ὥσπερ ἐπ' αὐτοῦ τοῦδε τοῦ θεασα-
479 μένου τοὺς νεκροὺς ὁ Πλάτων / διηγεῖται γενέσθαι συνενδεικνύμενος ἐν
57 τῷ λόγῳ πολλά. καὶ γὰρ ὅτι τὸ θυμαινόμενον ἕτερόν ἐστι τοῦ ἐπιθυ-
μοῦντος καὶ ὅτι τὸ λογιζόμενον ἀμφοῖν ἄλλο καὶ ὡς τὸ θυμαινόμενον
οὐδέποτε συμμαχεῖ τῷ ἐπιθυμητικῷ, δι' ἑνὸς ἐνεδείξατο τοῦδε τοῦ προ-
58 ειρημένου παραδείγματος. οὐδεὶς γοῦν ἐπετίμησεν ἑαυτῷ ποτε καὶ
59 ὠργίσθη, διότι τῶν ἀκαίρων ἐπιθυμιῶν ἀφίστασθαι προαιρεῖται. τίς
γὰρ ἐν νόσῳ τῶν ἀμέτρως διακαιομένων ἐπιθυμούντων τε πόματος
ψυχροῦ λογισάμενος ὄλεθρον οἴσειν αὐτῷ τὸ πόμα καὶ βλάβην ἐσχάτην,
εἶτ' ἐπισχὼν τὴν ὁρμὴν καὶ καθησυχάσας ἐπετίμησεν αὑτῷ καὶ ὠργίσθη,
496 60 διότι καλῶς ἐλογίσατο; οὐδεὶς ὡς οἶμαι τῶν πάντων. ἀλλ' | ἔνθα μὲν ἂν

2–8] Plat. Resp. iv: 440 a 8 – b 8

2 ἄλλοθι] ἀλλό τι L ἔφη H L: *ex Plat. corr. Chart.* πολλαχ῀ H: τινὸς ἀλλαχοῦ L: *corr. Müller* ἠσθανόμεθα L 3 παρὰ *et* περὶ H αὐτὸν H L: *ex Plat. corr. Müller* 4 ἑαυτῷ H: αὐτῷ L: *corr. Müller* στασιαζόντων L 5 τῷ *ex* τὸν *corr.* H τὸν θυμὸν *et* τῷ θυμῷ H δ' *om.* L 6 αὐτῶν L κοινωνήσαντος H L: *ex Plat. corr. Corn.* αἱροῦντος *om.* L τί πράττειν H L: *corr. Ald.*: ἀντιπράττειν *ex Plat. Corn. (cf. infra, lin. 20)* 7 οὐκ ἂν φάναι γενομένου] οὐ κακουμένου L σεαυτῷ *ex Plat. Chart.* 7–8 δ' οὐδ' ἐν *om.* L 8 ἄλλου L οὔ H L: *corr.* R οὖν *om.* L 9 ἐν ᾗ] εἰ L 12 καὶ *del. Müller* ἐνταυ῀ H ὑπεξέρχεται H 14 ὥσπερ] ὡς ἐπὶ H 15 ἐκράτησεν] ἐκράτησε συμμαχῶν L 17 διεκώλυεν, *ut vid.*, L ἐπέσχε τὴν ὁρμὴν *Petersen coll. lin. 30* 18 ἠδυνήθη L τοὺς *om.* L 19 προελθεῖν H: πρόελθεῖν L: *corr. Müller* δ' *om.* L 20 ἀκόντων L 26 ἐπεθύμησεν L 27 ἀκαίρως H 28 διακαιομένων ἐπιθυμούντων] διακαιομ.......... H 29 οἴσειν H αὐτῷ H *(ex* αὐτὸ *mut.)* L: *corr. Müller* πόμα καὶ βλάβην] πόμ. κ...... H 30 καὶ καθησυχάσας *scripsi*: καὶ κατὰ τὰς ψυχὰς ἃς H L: *del. Corn.*: κατὰ τὴν ψυχὴν *Müller* αὐτῷ L ὠργίσθη H 31 ἁπάντων L

Let us now pass to the remainder of the Platonic passage, which 53
is as follows: "And on many other occasions also, I said, when desires
are driving a man to go against reason, do we not observe him scolding himself and angry at that part of himself which would force him; and as in a struggle between two hostile factions, do we not observe
the anger of such a man taking the side of reason? But that anger 54
should ally itself with the desires and perform some act when reason decides it ought not, I imagine you would say that you have never perceived this sort of thing happening in yourself or in anyone else. –
No indeed, he said." In the former passage, where Plato mentioned 55
the man who had a craving to see the corpses, he clearly demonstrated that the part that feels anger is other than the part that desires, but he did not clearly state that the reasoning part is other than both; yet even in that argument he gave some indication of this latter point,
and now he presents an adequate account of it. For when a desire 56
exerts a force on someone against his reason, as it did on the abovementioned Leontius, in that situation anger is aroused as an ally of reason, and often in company with reason it overpowers the immoderate movement of the intemperate form of the soul; it restrains and impedes it, and checks the impulse. So Leontius too could have scolded himself for incontinence about viewing the corpses and then passed by without looking at them. But sometimes when both parts of the soul are pressing and scolding, the desiderative part overcomes their opposition and contrary pull, just as Plato describes its happening to this very man who viewed the corpses. With this story
Plato indicates many things at once. By this one aforementioned 57
example he indicated that the part which feels anger is other than the part which desires, that the rational part is different from both,
and that the angry part never allies itself with the desiderative. No one 58
ever censured himself and got angry at himself for choosing to abstain
from untimely desires. What sick person, who has a high fever and de- 59
sires a cold drink but reasons that the drink will destroy him and do him the utmost harm and so checks the urge and stills it, has censured himself or been angered at himself for reasoning correctly? None at
all, I think. Where the rational part (of the soul) voluntarily follows 60

480 ἑκὼν ὁ λογισμὸς ἕπηται τῷ ἐπιθυμητικῷ, / συνέπεται καὶ τὸ θυμοειδὲς τῷ
λογισμῷ — τούτῳ γὰρ ὑπηρετεῖν καὶ συμπράττειν ὥσπερ τις κύων
κυνηγέτῃ κατὰ τοῦ τρίτου τῆς ψυχῆς εἴδους ὑπὸ τῆς φύσεως ἐδόθη —·
ἔνθα δὲ ἐναντιοῦται καὶ στασιάζει καὶ μάχεται, μετὰ τοῦ λογισμοῦ
61 γίγνεται καὶ τούτῳ συμμαχεῖ. ὅτι δὲ τῷ λογιστικῷ τὸ θυμοειδὲς ἀεὶ κατὰ
τοῦ ἐπιθυμητικοῦ συμμαχεῖ καὶ διὰ τῆς ἐπιφερομένης ῥήσεως δῆλον
62 ποιεῖται γράφων ὧδε· «τί δέ; ἦν δ' ἐγώ· ὅταν τις οἴηται ἀδικεῖν, οὐχ
ὅσῳ ἂν γενναιότερος ᾖ τοσούτῳ ἧττον δύναται ὀργίζεσθαι καὶ πεινῶν
καὶ ῥιγῶν καὶ ἄλλο ὁτιοῦν τῶν τοιούτων πάσχων ὑπ' ἐκείνου ὃν ἂν
οἴηται δικαίως ταῦτα δρᾶν, καὶ ὃ λέγω οὐκ ἐθέλει πρὸς τοῦτον αὐτοῦ
63 ἐγείρεσθαι ὁ θυμός; — ἀληθῆ, ἔφη. — τί δέ; ὅταν ἀδικεῖσθαί τις ἡγῆται,
481 οὐκ ἐν τούτῳ ζητεῖ τε καὶ χαλεπαίνει[ν] / καὶ συμμαχεῖ[ν] τῷ δοκοῦντι
δικαίῳ καὶ διὰ τὸ πεινῆν καὶ διὰ τὸ ῥιγοῦν καὶ πάντα τὰ τοιαῦτα πάσχειν
ὑπομένων καὶ νικᾷ καὶ οὐ λήγει[ν] τῶν γενναίων πρὶν ἂν ἢ διαπράξηται
497 ἢ τελευτήσῃ ἢ ὥσπερ κύων ὑπὸ | νομέως ὑπὸ τοῦ λόγου τοῦ παρ' αὐτῷ
ἀνακληθεὶς πραϋνθῇ;»
64 Ἐν ταύτῃ τῇ ῥήσει πάλιν ὁ Πλάτων ἐμνημόνευσεν δυοῖν ἀνθρώ-
πων, ἀμφοῖν μὲν ταὐτὰ πασχόντων ὑπό τινος ἄρχοντός τε καὶ κρατοῦντος
ὡς καὶ πεινῆν καὶ διψῆν καὶ ῥιγοῦν, ἀλλὰ τοῦ μὲν ἑτέρου δικαίως
πεπεισμένου πάσχειν αὐτά, τοῦ δὲ ἑτέρου ἀδίκως· εἶτά φησιν ὡς ὁ μὲν
ἕτερος ὅστις ἂν οἴηται δικαίως πάσχειν ταῦτα διὰ τὸ πρότερον αὐτὸς
ἀδικεῖν τι, φέρει πράως αὐτὰ καὶ οὐκ ὀργίζεται τῷ δικαίως κολάζοντι,
65 καὶ τοσούτῳ γε μᾶλλόν φησιν ὅσῳπερ ἂν καὶ γενναιότερος. εἴρηκε δὲ
τοῦτο περὶ αὐτοῦ τοῦ κολαζομένου· οὗτος γὰρ ὅσῳπερ ἂν εὐγενέστερος /
482 ὑπάρχῃ φύσει, τοσούτῳ μᾶλλον ὑπομένει γενναίως τὰς κολάσεις. ὁ δ'
ἕτερος, ὅστις ἂν ἀδικεῖσθαι νομίζῃ, θυμοῦται καὶ χαλεπαίνει καὶ συμμαχεῖ
66 τῷ δοκοῦντι δικαίῳ. ταῦθ' ὁσημέραι τὰ γιγνόμενα κἀπὶ τῶν οἰκετῶν
ἔστι θεάσασθαι· ὅσοι μὲν γὰρ ἂν αὐτῶν ἢ κλέπτοντες ἤ τι τοιοῦτον
ἕτερον δρῶντες ἁλῶσι, καὶ μαστιγούμενοι καὶ λιμαγχονούμενοι καὶ
498 ἀτιμαζόμενοι πρὸς τῶν δεσποτῶν οὐκ ὀργίζονται· ὅσοι δ' ἂν | οἰηθῶσιν

2–3] *cf. supra*, p. 184.26 *infra*, lin. 15; p. 356.15–16; PHP 505.5–7; 738. 12–13 Müller 7–16] Plat. Resp. iv: 440 c 1 – d 3 20–22] *cf.* Arist. Rhet. ii. 3: 1380 b 16–18 [Xenoph.] Ath. Pol. 3.13 26] *cf.* Arist. Eth. Nic. v. 8: 1135 b 28–29 ἐπὶ φαινομένῃ γὰρ ἀδικίᾳ ἡ ὀργή ἐστιν

1 ἕπηται] ἐπί τε L 2 ὑπηρετεῖ L συμπράττει L 3 κατὰ – εἴδους *uncis incl. Müller* 4 δὲ] γὰρ L: δὲ ἂν *Müller* ἐναντιῶται H (ἐναντιῶται ... στασιάζῃ ... μάχηται *Müller*): *corr. Bas.*: ἠναντίωται L 5 καὶ τούτῳ] τοῦτο L συμμαχεῖν L ὅτι δὲ *om.* L 6 συμμαχεῖ *om.* L δῆλον *om.* L 7 ποιεῖ *Müller* ἀδικεῖν – 8 ᾖ *om.* L 8 τοσώτω H 10 ἐθέλει] ἐγείρεσθαι θέλει L τούτων αὐτῶν L 11 ἐγείρεσθαι ὁ *om.* L ἀδικεῖσθαί] ἀδικῆ γέ L ἡγεῖται H L: *corr. Kühn* 12 ζητεῖ τε] ζητεῖται H: ζητεῖν τὲ L: *ex Plat. corr. Einarson*: ζεῖ τε *Corn. (cf. infra, p. 354.12)* χαλεπαίνειν H L: *corr. Corn.* συμμαχεῖν H L: *corr. Corn.* 13 δικαίως H (ς *eras.*) L 14 καὶ ὑπομένων *Corn.* νικᾶν H L: *corr. Corn.* λήγειν H L: *corr. Corn.* 15 τελευτή H αὐτῶ, *ut vid.*, L 16 ἀνακλιθεὶς H 17 ἐμνημόνευσε L 18 ταῦτα L 20 τοῦ δὲ] καθ' L 21 ὅστις ἂν *om.* L 22 φέρειν L ὀργίζεσθαι L 23 καὶ^{II} *om.* H: ᾖ *Kühn*: ᾖ *post* γενναιότερος *add. Müller* 24 τοῦ *om.* L 25 ὑπαρ^χ' H L: *corr. Chart.* 26 θυμοῦται καὶ] θυμῶ τὲ L 27 ταῦτα L τὰ *om. Ald.* 28 θεᾶσθαι L

the desiderative, there the spirited part follows along with the rational
– for the spirited was given by nature to the rational as a hound to a
hunter to serve and help it against the third form of the soul –; but
where the rational part opposes, dissents and fights, the spirited
accompanies it and fights beside it. That the spirited part always sides 61
with the rational against the desiderative Plato makes clear also in
the next passage, where he writes: "Tell me, I said; when a person 62
believes himself the author of an unjust act, is he not the less able,
the nobler he is, to be angry when he suffers hunger or cold or any-
thing of that kind at the hands of the man who, he believes, is treating
him justly, and, as I say, is not his anger unwilling to be aroused
against that person? – That is true, he said. – But what happens when 63
a person thinks that he is the victim of injustice? Does not his anger
seek about in this situation and become indignant and ally itself with
what it thinks just? And because it is suffering hunger, cold, and
everything of that kind, does it not persevere and triumph and refuse
to leave off its noble acts until it has accomplished its purpose or
died or, like a dog called back by the shepherd, it is called back by
reason, which stands beside it, and is calmed?"

Again in this passage Plato mentions two men, both of whom 64
receive the same treatment at the hands of some powerful ruler, so
that they are hungry, thirsty, and cold; but one of them is persuaded
that he is justly treated, the other that he is not. Then Plato says
that the one who considers the treatment just, because earlier he had
himself acted unjustly, submits calmly and is not angry at the man
who justly punishes him; and the nobler he is (Plato says), the more
calmly he submits. He was referring here to the man who is actually 65
being punished: the nobler this man is by nature, the more nobly he
endures the punishment. But the other man, who believes himself
a victim of injustice, is angry and indignant and allies himself with
what he thinks is just. Behavior of this kind can also be seen every 66
day in slaves. Those who are caught stealing or doing something
else of that kind, even when whipped, starved and disgraced by their
masters, are not angry; but those who believe they are suffering or

ἀδίκως τι τούτων ἢ πάσχειν ἢ πεπονθέναι, ἀεὶ τούτων ἔνδον ὁ θυμὸς
ἀγριούμενός ἐστι καὶ ποθῶν ἀντιτιμωρήσασθαι τὸν ἀδικοῦντα.
67 Δηλοῦται δ' ἐξ ἀμφοτέρων τῶν παραδειγμάτων ὡς τὸ θυμοειδὲς
ὑπὸ τῆς φύσεως ἡμῖν ἐδόθη σύμμαχον τῷ λογιστικῷ. τούτῳ γοῦν δὴ
φαίνεται συμμαχοῦν, ὅταν ὑπό τινος ἢ ἔνδοθεν ἢ ἔξωθεν ἀδικεῖσθαί τε καὶ
68 βιάζεσθαι δοξάζῃ. τὸ μὲν οὖν δοξάζειν ἀδικεῖσθαι τοῦ λογιστικοῦ, τὸ
69 δ' ἐπαμύνειν αὐτῷ κατὰ τοῦ βιαζομένου τοῦ θυμοειδοῦς ἴδιον. ἐπειδὰν
483 μὲν οὖν ἀμέτρως ἐπί τι φερό/μενον τὸ τῆς ψυχῆς ἐπιθυμητικὸν ἄκοντα τὸν
λογισμὸν ἕλκῃ βιαίως, κατ' ἐκείνου σύμμαχον τῷ λογιστικῷ τὸ θυμοειδὲς
γίγνεται· ὅταν δὲ ἔξωθεν ᾖ τις ἀδικῶν, ἐκεῖνον ἀντιτιμωρεῖσθαι σπεύδει.
70 ἐπειδὰν δ' ὑπὸ μηδενὸς ἀδικεῖσθαι δοξάζῃ τὸ λογιστικόν, οὐδ' ὁ θυμὸς
ἀναζεῖ τηνικαῦτα, κἂν ὅτι μάλιστα κολάζηται τὸ σῶμα δικαίως ὑπό
71 τινος ἢ ῥιγοῦν ἢ πεινῆν ἢ διψῆν ἀναγκαζόμενον. ᾧ δῆλον ὡς ταῖς δόξαις
ἕπεται τοῦ λογιστικοῦ κατὰ φύσιν ἔχον τὸ θυμοειδές. ἐνδέχεται γάρ ποτε |
499 72 καὶ τοῦτο μοχθηρῶς διακείμενον ἀπειθῶς κινεῖσθαι τῷ λογισμῷ. μετ'
ὀλίγα γοῦν καὶ αὐτὸς ὁ Πλάτων ἐνδεικνύμενος τοῦτό φησιν «ἢ καθάπερ
ἐν τῇ πόλει συνεῖχεν αὐτὴν τρία ὄντα γένη, χρηματιστικόν, ἐπικουρητικόν,
βουλευτικόν, οὕτω καὶ ἐν ψυχῇ τοῦτο τρίτον ἐστὶ τὸ θυμοειδές, ἐπί-
κουρον ὂν τῷ λογιστικῷ φύσει, ἐὰν μὴ ὑπὸ κακῆς τροφῆς διαφθείρηται;»
73 τίνες μὲν οὖν εἰσιν αἱ διαφθοραὶ τοῦ θυμοειδοῦς, οὐκ ἐν καιρῷ νῦν λέ-
484 γειν· ἐν γὰρ τῷ μετὰ τοῦτον / λόγῳ περί τε τῶν παθῶν τῆς ψυχῆς,
ὡς ἐδόκει Πλάτωνι, καὶ περὶ νοσημάτων καὶ ἁμαρτημάτων τῶν κατ'
αὐτὴν ἁπάσης ⟨τε⟩ τῆς κακίας, ὅπως γίγνεταί τε καὶ θεραπεύεται
μετὰ τὸ γενέσθαι, διελθεῖν ἔγνωκα καὶ δὴ καὶ περὶ κάλλους τε καὶ ὑγι-
είας αὐτῆς ἁπασῶν τε τῶν ἀρετῶν· οὐ σμικρὰ γὰρ οὐδ' ἐν τούτοις ὁ
Χρύσιππος σφάλλεται.
74 Νυνὶ δὲ ἔτι μίαν ῥῆσιν ὑπογράψαι βούλομαι τοῦ Πλάτωνος
ἐν ᾗ δείκνυσιν ἕτερον ὑπάρχειν τὸ θυμοειδὲς τοῦ λογιστικοῦ. γέγραπται
500 δ' ἐφεξῆς τῶν προειρημένων ἐν τῷ τετάρτῳ τῆς | Πολιτείας τόνδε τὸν
75 τρόπον· «καὶ γὰρ ἐν τοῖς παιδίοις τοῦτό γ' ἄν τις ἴδοι, ὅτι θυμοῦ μὲν
εὐθὺς γενόμενα μεστά ἐστι, λογισμοῦ δ' ἔνιοι μὲν ἔμοιγε δοκοῦσιν οὐ-
δέποτε μεταλαμβάνειν, οἱ δὲ πολλοὶ ὀψέ ποτε. — ναὶ μὰ Δία, ἦν δ' ἐγώ,
καλῶς εἶπες. ἔτι γ' ἐν τοῖς θηρίοις ἄν τις ἴδοι ὃ λέγεις, ὅτι οὕτως ἔχει.
485 76 πρὸς δὲ τούτοις καὶ ὃ ἄνω που ἐκεῖ εἴπομεν, τὸ τοῦ Ὁμήρου / μαρ-

11–12] *cf. infra*, PHP 576.14–577.3 Müller *comm. ad* p. 352.12 16–19] Plat. Resp. iv: 440 e 10 – 441 a 3 30–356.5] Plat. Resp. iv: 441 a 7 – c 2 34 ἄνω που] Plat. Resp. iii: 390 d 4

2 ἐστι] τε L τὸν] τὰ L 3 δηλοῦνται L 4 ἡμῶν L 6 τὸ[II]] τοῦ H 10 ἐκείνων L 13 πινῆν H 16 ᾖ] εἰ L 18 θυμοειδές] ει *ex* ϊ *corr.* H 20 διαφοραὶ L 21 τούτω H 22 *post* καὶ[II] *add.* περὶ L τῶν *om.* H 23 ἁπάσης τε *Diels*: ἁπασῶν H *(post* ἁπασῶν *add. et del. ex lin. 25sq.* τε – Χρύσιππος H*)* L: ἁπασῶν καὶ *Müller* 24 μετὰ τὸ *om.* L καὶ[II] *om.* L ὑγείας L 25 ὁ *om.* L 30 τοῦτον L ἴδη H: *ex Plat. corr. Chart.*: εἴδοι *Corn.*: εἶναι L 31 γενόμενα, *ut vid.*, H: γεννώμενα L μὲν] ἢ L 32 μεταλαμβάνειν – ποτε *om.* H Δία] δί' L 33 *post* καλῶς *inser.* δ', *ut vid.*, L ἔτι γ'] οὐδ' L λέγω H 34 ὁ ἄνω πούς L ἐκεῖ *ex Plat. scr. Chart.*: *om.* H: καὶ L εἴπωμεν L μαρτυϑ/ H: *corr. Corn.*: μάρτυσι L

have suffered any of these things unjustly have inside them an anger
that is always savage and craves vengeance on the wrong-doer.

Both examples make it clear that the spirited part was given us 67
by nature as an ally of the rational. Thus it is observed to be on the
side of reason when it believes that it is being wronged and coerced
by something either internal or external. Now the belief that one is 68
being wronged pertains to the rational part, but help in combatting
the coercive force is the special function of the spirited part. When 69
the desiderative part of the soul is carried immoderately toward some-
thing and forcibly pulls reason against its will, the spirited part be-
comes an ally of reason against the desiderative; and when the in-
justice is the work of someone outside, the spirited part is eager to
avenge itself on him. But when the rational part believes it is not 70
wronged by anyone, then anger does not boil up either, even if the
body is severely punished by being justly compelled by someone to
undergo cold or hunger or thirst. Hence it is clear that the spirited 71
part in its natural state follows the opinions of the rational part.
For it is possible that this (part) too, if in a corrupted condition, may
sometimes move in disobedience to reason. Plato himself indicates 72
this a little further on, when he says: "Or as in the city the classes
that held it together were three, the money-makers, the defenders and
the deliberators, so in the soul this spirited part is the third class,
by nature a defender of the rational, if it is not corrupted by evil nur-
ture." This is not the place for a discussion of the corruptions of the 73
spirited part; for in the next book I have decided to treat in detail
Plato's view of the affections of the soul, its diseases and errors
and all its vices, how they arise and how after arising they are cured,
and again its beauty and health and all its virtues; for in these mat-
ters too Chrysippus makes no small mistakes.

For the present I wish to append one more passage from Plato 74
in which he shows that the spirited part is other than the rational. It
follows immediately after the passages already quoted from the fourth
book of the Republic: "This much, at least, can be seen in children: 75
right from birth they are full of anger; and some, as I believe, never
get a share of reason, while the majority get it late. – Yes indeed,
I said; you put it very well. And one can see in the brutes too that
what you say is true. And besides, the line of Homer that we quoted 76
earlier in that other discussion will testify to it, the line (that says),

τυρήσει, τὸ

‘στῆθος δὲ πλήξας κραδίην ἠν[ε]ίπαπε μύθῳ·’

ἐνταῦθα γὰρ δὴ σαφῶς ὡς ἕτερον ἑτέρῳ ἐπιπλῆττον πεποίηκεν Ὅμηρος
τὸ ἀναλογισάμενον περὶ βελτίονός τε καὶ χείρονος τῷ ἀλογίστω⟨ς⟩ θυμου-
77 μένῳ.» ἐν τούτοις ἐναργῶς ὁ Πλάτων ἐπιδείκνυσιν ἕτερον ὑπάρχον τὸ
θυμούμενον τοῦ λογιζομένου. οἱ γοῦν παῖδες ὥσπερ καὶ τὰ θηρία θυμοῦ
78 μὲν πλήρεις εἰσί, λογισμοῦ δὲ ἥκιστα μετέχουσιν. ἐπὶ μὲν οὖν τῶν θηρίων
ἐτόλμησαν ἔνιοι λέγειν οὔτε θυμὸν οὔτ' ἐπιθυμίαν ἐνυπάρχειν αὐτῶν ταῖς
79 ψυχαῖς, ἐπὶ δὲ τῶν παίδων οὐκ οἶδ' ὅ τι φήσουσιν. οὐ γὰρ δή γε καὶ τὰ |
501 τούτων πάθη διὰ συλλογισμοῦ χρὴ μαθεῖν, ἀλλ' ἀναμνησθῆναι μόνον
αὔταρκες ὡς οὐκ ἄλλως μὲν νῦν ἄλλως δὲ παῖδες ὄντες θυμούμεθα· καὶ
486 80 γὰρ δύναμις ἡ αὐτὴ καὶ ὁ τρόπος τῆς τοῦ / πάθους γενέσεως ὅμοιος. ἓν
δὲ μόνον ἐξαίρετον ὑπάρχει τοῖς τελείοις ἀνδράσιν, ὅταν γε μὴ κατὰ πάθος
ζῶσιν ἀλλὰ λογισμὸς αὐτῶν ἐξηγῆται τοῦ βίου· κατέχουσιν ἐν πολλαῖς
πράξεσι τὸν θυμόν, ὥσπερ τις νομεὺς κύνα γενναῖον ἀγριώτερον ἐκφερό-
81 μενον ἐπὶ τοὺς πέλας. ἐν δὲ τοῖς παισὶν οὐδὲν γίγνεται τοιοῦτον, ὥσπερ
οὐδὲ ἐν τοῖς θηρίοις, ὅτι τοῖς μὲν οὐδέπω τοῖς δὲ οὐδέποτε λογισμὸς ἄρχει
82 τῶν ὁρμῶν. ταῦτα μὲν οὖν ὀρθῶς εἴρηται τῷ Πλάτωνι καὶ προσέτι τὸ
κατὰ τὴν τελευτὴν τῆς ῥήσεως γεγραμμένον, ἔνθα τὸν Ὅμηρον ἐπάγεται
μάρτυρα ταυτὶ λέγοντα·

«στῆθος δὲ πλήξας κραδίην ἠν[ε]ίπαπε μύθῳ·»

«ἐνταῦθα γάρ», φησίν, «ὡς ἕτερον ἑτέρῳ πεποίηκεν ἐπιπλῆττον τὸ ἀνα-
502 λογισάμενον περὶ τοῦ βελτίονός τε καὶ χείρονος | τῷ ἀλογίστως θυμου-
μένῳ.»

83 Ἠβουλόμην δ' ἂν καὶ τὸν Χρύσιππον ἀνεγνωκέναι τε τὴν ῥῆσιν
487 αὐτοῦ προσεσχηκέναι τε τὸν νοῦν / αὐτῇ. πάντως γὰρ ἄν τι καὶ αὐτὸς
ὤνητο μαθὼν ὁπηνίκα τε προσήκει καλεῖν Ὅμηρον μάρτυρα καὶ περὶ
84 τίνων πραγμάτων. οὔτε γὰρ ἐν ἀρχῇ τῶν λόγων, ἀλλ' ἐπειδὰν ἱκανῶς
ἀποδείξῃ τις τὸ προκείμενον ἀνεπίφθονον ἤδη καὶ τοὺς πρεσβυτέρους
ἐπικαλεῖσθαι μαρτυρήσοντας οὔτε περὶ πραγμάτων ἀδήλων παντάπασιν
ἀλλ' ἤτοι περὶ φαινομένων ἐναργῶς ἢ παρακειμένην αἰσθήσει τὴν ἔν-

2] Hom. Od. xx. 17 *cf. supra*, pp. 178.10; 184.18; 186.23 *infra*, lin. 21 6–7] *cf. supra*, pp. 316.31–318.5 21–24] *cf. supra*, lin. 2–5 25–358.3] Posid. fr. 156 Edelstein-Kidd 28–358.3] Posid. test. 87 Edelstein-Kidd

2 ἠνείπαπε H L: *corr. Kühn* 3 ἐπιπλήττων H L: *corr. Chart.* (ἐπιπλήττον *Ald.)* 4 τὸ ἀναλογισόμενον H: *ex Plat. corr. Corn.*: τῶ ἀναλογισαμένω L *post* περὶ *add.* τοῦ *Müller (cf. infra, lin. 23)* ἀλογίστω H L: *ex Plat. corr. Corn.* θυμούμενος L 5 ὑπάρχειν L 7 λογισμὸν ... ἔχουσιν L οὖν *om.* L 12 αὐτὴ] *lac. 6 litt. in* H τῆς *om.* H γενέσεως τοῦ πάθους L 13 ὑπάρχειν L ὅταν] οἱ δ' ἂν L: ὅτι, ὅταν *Müller* 14 ζῶσιν *ex* ὦσιν *corr.* H ἐξηγεῖται H L: *corr. Kühn* 16 ἐν] ἔνια L οὐδὲν γίγνεται] οὐκ ἐγίγνετο L τοιοῦτον *ex* τοιαῦτα *corr.* H 17 ἀρχὴ L 18 μὲν] τε *Müller* 18–19 τὰ ... γεγραμμένα L 20 μαρτυρία H 21 ἠνείπαπε H *(ex* εἴπατε *mut.)* L: *corr. Kühn* 22 ἐπιπλήττων L 23 ἀλογίστω H: ἀναλογίστως L: *ex Plat. corr. Corn.* 25 ῥῆσιν] γνῶσιν L 26 πάντως] π *ex* κ *corr.* H 27–28 περί τινων L 29 ἴδη L 30 οὗτοι L 31 περιφαινομένων H

'Striking his breast he rebuked his heart with words.'

Here Homer has clearly presented the two parts as distinct: the part
that has reflected on what is better or worse rebukes the part that
is irrationally angry." In this passage Plato clearly shows that the 77
angry part is other than the rational. Thus children, and brutes too,
are full of anger and have no share at all in reason. Some persons 78
have dared to say of animals that there is neither anger nor desire
in their souls, and I don't know what they will say of children. But 79
surely no reasoning is needed to teach us about children's affections;
it is sufficient merely to recall that there is no difference between the
way we are angry now and the way we were angry as children. The
power is the same and the manner in which the affection occurs is
similar. Only one thing is peculiar to mature persons, whenever they 80
do not live by affections but make reason their guide in life: they
check their anger in many actions, as a shepherd checks his noble
dog when it rushes too fiercely at persons close by. But nothing of 81
the sort happens in children or in brutes because the conations of the
former are not yet ruled by reason, and those of the latter are never
so ruled. Plato stated this correctly, and what he wrote at the end 82
of the passage is also correct, where he introduces the testimony of
Homer:

"Striking his breast he rebuked his heart with words."

"Here", Plato says, "Homer has presented the two parts as distinct: the part that has reflected on what is better or worse rebukes the part that is irrationally angry."

I could have wished that Chrysippus had read this passage 83
and given it his attention. He would surely have derived some profit
from it himself, by learning on what occasions one may properly call
Homer as a witness, and about what subjects. For one thing, witnesses 84
should not be called at the beginning of the argument, but when you
have proved adequately what you set out to prove, then there is no objection to calling on men of earlier times to testify; and also, they should not be called to testify about matters that are utterly obscure but either about evident facts or about things the indication of which

δειξιν ἐχόντων, οἷά πέρ ἐστι τὰ πάθη τῆς ψυχῆς, οὐ μακρῶν λόγων οὐδ'
ἀποδείξεων ἀκριβεστέρων δεόμενα, μόνης δὲ ἀναμνήσεως ὧν ἑκάστοτε
85 πάσχομεν, ὡς καὶ Ποσειδώνιος εἶπεν. ὅτι μὲν γὰρ ἐν ἐγκεφάλῳ τὸ
λογιζόμενόν ἐστιν ἢ ἐν καρδίᾳ τὸ θυμούμενον οὐ μεγάλην μοῖραν πρὸς
πίστιν ἐκ τῶν μαρτύρων, ἀλλ' ἀποδείξει χρὴ τὸ πᾶν ἐπιτρέπειν ἐνταῦθα·
86 τὸ δὲ ἕτερον εἶναι τοῦ θυμουμένου τὸ λογιζόμενον οὔτ' ἀποδείξεως δεῖται
508 μακρᾶς οὔτε | σοφῶν τῶν μαρτυρησόντων ἀλλ' ἀρκεῖ μὲν καὶ Ὅμηρος
488 ἐπὶ τοῖς ἀρτίως ῥηθεῖσι μαρτυρῶν, ἀρκεῖ δὲ καὶ / Θουκυδίδης λέγων
«καὶ οἱ λογισμῷ ἐλάχιστα χρώμενοι θυμῷ πλεῖστα εἰς ἔργον καθίστανται»,
ἀρκεῖ δὲ καὶ Δημοσθένης εἰπὼν «ἀλλὰ μὴν ἄν τις ἄφνω τὸν λογισμὸν
φθάσας ἐξαχθῇ, πράξεις ὑβριστικῶς ποιήσει, δι' ὀργήν γ' ἔνι [Πλάτων]
φῆσαι πεποιηκέναι»· πρὸς τούτοις οἱ λοιποὶ πάντες καὶ ῥήτορες καὶ
ποιηταὶ καὶ μυθολόγοι· διὰ γὰρ τὴν ἐνάργειαν τοῦ πράγματος οὐδεὶς
87 ἔστιν ὃς οὐχ οὕτω γιγνώσκει. προσεκτέον οὖν ἐστι τῇ προγεγραμμένῃ
τοῦ Πλάτωνος ῥήσει τῶν τε ἄλλων ἕνεκα καὶ ὅπως ἀσφαλῶς οὐ περὶ
τοῦ κατὰ μὲν τὸν ἐγκέφαλον εἶναι τὸ λογιζόμενον, ἐν καρδίᾳ δὲ τὸ
θυμούμενον, ἐπεκαλέσατο μαρτυρήσοντα τὸν Ὅμηρον, ἀλλὰ περὶ
μόνου τοῦ διαφέρειν τὸ θυμούμενον τῆς ψυχῆς τοῦ λογιζομένου. τοῦτο
μὲν γὰρ ἅπαντες ἄνθρωποι γιγνώσκουσι δι' ἐνάργειαν, ἐκεῖνο δ' οὐκέθ'
88 ὁμοίως ἅπαντες, ἀλλ' ἀποδείξεως αὐτὸ δεῖ. διό μοι δοκῶ κἀγὼ καταπαύειν
504 489 μὲν ἤδη τὸν | ἐνεστῶτα λόγον, / ἐν δὲ τῷ μετ' αὐτὸν ἐπὶ τὴν ἀπόδειξιν
τρέπεσθαι τοῦ καὶ τοῖς τόποις διωρίσθαι τὰ τρία μόρια τῆς ψυχῆς. /|

1–3] *cf. supra*, p. 356.9–11 *infra*, PHP 732.3–4 Müller Posid. Rel., p. 230 Bake Zeller, Philos. der Gr. III 1^5, p. 601 n. 2 9] Thuc. ii. 11.7 10–12] Demosth. Or. 21.41

4 θυμούμενον] μου *ex* μο *corr.* H *post* μεγάλην *add.* ἔχει *Müller* 6 ἕτερον] πρότερον H L: *corr. Ricci Corn.* 8 ἐπὶ] ἐν L 11 πράξις H ὑβριστικὰς H 11–12 γ' ἔνι φῆσαι *ex Demosth. scr. Müller*: δ' ὁ πλάτων ἔφησε H: τὲ πλάτων ἔφησε L 12 καὶ ῥήτορες *om.* L 13 ἐνέργειαν L 13–14 οὐδεὶς ἔστιν *om.* L 16 μὲν τοῦ κατὰ H 19 ἐνερ (γ' *suprascr.*) L 20 αὐτῶ L 22 τόποις] τό H: τρόποις L: *corr. Ricci Corn.* τρία *om.* L γαληνοῦ περὶ τῶν ἱπποκράτους καὶ πλάτωνος δογμάτων, τὸ *(om. H)* ε̄ *subscr.* H L

lies close to sense-perception – as is the case with the affections of the soul –, which do not require extended arguments or more precise proofs, but only reminders of what we experience on each occasion, as Posidonius also said. Witnesses contribute little to the proof 85
that the reasoning part is in the brain or the angry part in the heart; there the entire matter must be turned over to scientific demonstration. But no lengthy proof or testimony of sages is required to establish 86
that the rational part (of the soul) is other than the angry part. It is enough to quote the evidence of Homer in the passages just cited, or again of Thucydides when he says, "And those who least use reason most often turn to action in anger"; or even of Demosthenes, who says, "Indeed if a person is carried away suddenly, outstripping his reason, he will perform acts lawlessly; it can be said that he did them in anger"; and in addition, of all the other orators, poets, and storytellers. For because the fact is so clear there is no one who does not understand it in this way. The passage from Plato quoted above 87
must therefore be read attentively for a number of reasons, and especially in order to observe how unerringly he called upon Homer, not for testimony that reason is in the brain and anger in the heart, but only that the angry part of the soul is not the same as the rational. All men know the latter, because it is obvious; but they do not all know the former in the same way, and the point itself requires demonstration. I have decided, therefore, to terminate the present book 88
at this point and to turn in the next (book) to the proof that the three parts of the soul are spatially separate.

FSC
www.fsc.org
MIX
Papier | Fördert
gute Waldnutzung
FSC® C083411

Kolibri 360 GmbH
Ferdinand-Jühlke-Straße 7
99095 Erfurt, Deutschland
produktsicherheit@kolibri360.de